CRITICAL SURVEY OF
Poetry
Fourth Edition

European Poets

CRITICAL SURVEY OF
Poetry
Fourth Edition

European Poets

Volume 2
Paul Haavikko—Vasko Popa

Editor, Fourth Edition
Rosemary M. Canfield Reisman
Charleston Southern University

SALEM PRESS
Pasadena, California
Hackensack, New Jersey

Editor in Chief: Dawn P. Dawson

Editorial Director: Christina J. Moose   *Research Supervisor:* Jeffry Jensen
Development Editor: Tracy Irons-Georges   *Research Assistant:* Keli Trousdale
Project Editor: Rowena Wildin   *Production Editor:* Andrea E. Miller
Manuscript Editor: Desiree Dreeuws   *Page Design:* James Hutson
Acquisitions Editor: Mark Rehn   *Layout:* Mary Overell
Editorial Assistant: Brett S. Weisberg   *Photo Editor:* Cynthia Breslin Beres

Cover photo: Rainer Maria Rilke (The Granger Collection, New York)

Some of the essays in this work, which have been updated, originally appeared in the following Salem Press publications, *Critical Survey of Poetry, English Language Series* (1983), *Critical Survey of Poetry: Foreign Language Series* (1984), *Critical Survey of Poetry, Supplement* (1987), *Critical Survey of Poetry, English Language Series, Revised Edition*, (1992; preceding volumes edited by Frank N. Magill), *Critical Survey of Poetry, Second Revised Edition* (2003; edited by Philip K. Jason).

∞ The paper used in these volumes conforms to the American National Standard for Permanence of Paper for Printed Library Materials, X39.48-1992 (R1997).

Library of Congress Cataloging-in-Publication Data

Critical survey of poetry. — 4th ed. / editor, Rosemary M. Canfield Reisman.
    v. cm.
Includes bibliographical references and index.
    ISBN 978-1-58765-582-1 (set : alk. paper) — ISBN 978-1-58765-756-6 (set : European poets : alk. paper) — ISBN 978-1-58765-757-3 (v. 1 : European poets : alk. paper) — ISBN 978-1-58765-758-0 (v. 2 : European poets : alk. paper) — ISBN 978-1-58765-759-7 (v. 3 : European poets : alk. paper)
1. Poetry—History and criticism—Dictionaries. 2. Poetry—Bio-bibliography. 3. Poets—Biography—Dictionaries. I. Reisman, Rosemary M. Canfield.
    PN1021.C7 2011
    809.1'003--dc22

                             2010045095

First Printing

CONTENTS

COMPLETE LIST OF CONTENTS

VOLUME 1

VOLUME 2

Contents

VOLUME 3

RESOURCES

INDEXES

PRONUNCIATION KEY

To help users of the *Critical Survey of Poetry* pronounce unfamiliar names of profiled poets correctly, phonetic spellings using the character symbols listed below appear in parentheses immediately after the first mention of the poet's name in the narrative text. Stressed syllables are indicated in capital letters, and syllables are separated by hyphens.

VOWEL SOUNDS

Symbol	Spelled (Pronounced)
a	answer (AN-suhr), laugh (laf), sample (SAM-puhl), that (that)
ah	father (FAH-thur), hospital (HAHS-pih-tuhl)
aw	awful (AW-fuhl), caught (kawt)
ay	blaze (blayz), fade (fayd), waiter (WAYT-ur), weigh (way)
eh	bed (behd), head (hehd), said (sehd)
ee	believe (bee-LEEV), cedar (SEE-dur), leader (LEED ur), liter (LEE tur)
ew	boot (bewt), lose (lewz)
i	buy (bi), height (hit), lie (li), surprise (sur-PRIZ)
ih	bitter (BIH-tur), pill (pihl)
o	cotton (KO-tuhn), hot (hot)
oh	below (bee-LOH), coat (koht), note (noht), wholesome (HOHL-suhm)
oo	good (good), look (look)
ow	couch (kowch), how (how)
oy	boy (boy), coin (koyn)
uh	about (uh-BOWT), butter (BUH-tuhr), enough (ee-NUHF), other (UH-thur)

CONSONANT SOUNDS

Symbol	Spelled (Pronounced)
ch	beach (beech), chimp (chihmp)
g	beg (behg), disguise (dihs-GIZ), get (geht)
j	digit (DIH-juht), edge (ehj), jet (jeht)
k	cat (kat), kitten (KIH-tuhn), hex (hehks)
s	cellar (SEHL-ur), save (sayv), scent (sehnt)
sh	champagne (sham-PAYN), issue (IH-shew), shop (shop)
ur	birth (burth), disturb (dihs-TURB), earth (urth), letter (LEH-tur)
y	useful (YEWS-fuhl), young (yuhng)
z	business (BIHZ-nehs), zest (zehst)
zh	vision (VIH-zhuhn)

CRITICAL SURVEY OF
Poetry
Fourth Edition

European Poets

H

PAAVO HAAVIKKO

Born: Helsinki, Finland; January 25, 1931
Died: Helsinki, Finland; October 6, 2008

PRINCIPAL POETRY

Tiet etäisyyksiin, 1951
Tuuliöinä, 1953
Synnyinmaa, 1955
Lehdet lehtiä, 1958
Talvipalatsi, 1959 (*The Winter Palace*, 1968)
Puut, kaikki heidän vihreytensä, 1966
Selected Poems, 1968
Neljätoista hallitsijaa, 1970
Runoja matkalta salmen ylitse, 1973
Kaksikymmentä ja yksi, 1974 (*One and Twenty*, 2007)
Runoelmat, 1975
Runot, 1949-1974, 1975
Viiniä, kirjoitusta, 1976
Rauta-aika, 1982 (*The Age of Iron*, 1982)
Kullervon tarina, 1983
Sillat: Valitut Runot, 1984
Toukokuu, ikuinen, 1988
Talvirunoja, 1990
Runot! Runot, 1984-1992, 1992
Kahden vuoden päiväkirja: Muistiinmerkittyä vuosilta, 1995-1998, 2001
Prosperon runot: 45 runoa, 2001
Talvipalatsi: Varhaisversion rekonstruktio vuodelta 1959, 2001
Valitut runot, 1949-2001, 2006

OTHER LITERARY FORMS

Paavo Haavikko (HAW-vihk-koh) was one of the most prolific Finnish writers; he published more than fifty books in his native language and wrote equally masterfully in every literary genre. He made his debut in the 1950's with collections of lyrical poems, and

in the following decades, he published novels, short stories, epic poems, and plays, in addition to which he wrote two opera librettos, based on his plays: *Ratsumies* (1974; *The Horseman*, 1974) and *Kuningas lähtee Ranskaan* (1984; *The King Goes Forth to France*, 1984). The music for both operas was composed by Aulis Sallinen, and they were first performed at the Savonlinna Opera Festival in Finland. They have since been staged in West Germany, New Mexico, and London's Covent Garden.

History has provided some of the major themes for Haavikko's poetry and plays, and he also published nonfiction in that field. His literary work includes collections of aphorisms, scripts for films, and radio and television plays. Some of Haavikko's work has been translated into English, French, German, and Swedish. Haavikko also published three volumes of memoirs and continued to write opera libretti. In 2000, he collaborated with the composer Tuomas Kantelinen on an opera about the early twentieth century Olympic long-distance runner Paavo Nurmi. This work, titled *Paavo Suuri, Suuri juoksu, Suuri uni*, was directed by Kalle Holmberg and received widespread exposure throughout Europe.

ACHIEVEMENTS

From the very start of his literary career, Paavo Haavikko never sought favor with the reading public; in fact, he rebelled against the thought that art and literature should be "pretty" or popular; for him, a poet's greatest achievement is the writing itself. His unique contributions in the forefront of post-World War II literature were early recognized, and consequently he was awarded the Finnish Government Literature Prizes for his work in the years 1958, 1960, 1962, 1964, 1966, 1969, 1970, and 1974. In 1966, Haavikko received the Aleksis Kivi Prize (which is named after the writer of the first Finnish-language novel, published in 1870), and in 1969, he was awarded the Finnish Government Drama Prize and an honorary doctorate from the University of Helsinki. A symposium was held in 1976 in Joensuu, Finland, at which the participants, who represented the academic disciplines of literature, history, political science, and economics, analyzed and examined Haavikko's work. In 1978, he received the Order of the White Rose of Finland for his literary achievements. Haavikko's four-part television drama, *Rauta-aika* (based on his poem), which has also been published in book form, won for him the Prix d'Italia as best European television series of the year 1982.

Only a sampling of Haavikko's poetry, plays, and other literary work has been translated into other languages. As Philip Binham, one of the English-language translators of Haavikko's work, has pointed out, Finnish is particularly difficult to render in translation the subtlety and rhythm of Haavikko's language; indeed, Haavikko's poetic expression has often posed problems even to native Finnish readers. In the 1960's, however, some of Haavikko's work began to appear in translations, and in 1984, Haavikko won the Neustadt Prize, administered by the University of Oklahoma, which is given to non-American writers for a particularly substantive and challenging body of work. He also won the Nordic Prize of the Swedish Academy in 1993. He received the Nossack Prize in 2002 and the America Award from the Contemporary Arts Educational Project for lifetime contribution to international writing in 2007. Haavikko has, over the entire course of his career, been one of the world's leading poets.

BIOGRAPHY

Paavo Juhani Haavikko was born on January 25, 1931, in Helsinki, the capital city of Finland, a city in which the poet lived all his life and about which he wrote a book. Haavikko's father was a businessman, and after his high school graduation in 1951 and customary service in the Finnish army, Haavikko also entered the business world, working as a real estate agent. Like many Finnish modern poets, Haavikko consistently maintained a second profession alongside his literary career; in fact, he believed that an author who is solely occupied by writing loses touch with the realities of life. Indeed, in his poetry Haavikko never seems to be an observer on the sidelines; he appears to be in the middle of the events and freely uses concepts and imagery from commerce and the business world in his creative writing, most of which he did on weekends. Haavikko was the literary editor for Otava, a major Finnish publishing company, from 1967-1983. In 1989, he formed his own publishing company, the Art House,

and served as managing director until the age of seventy, when he retired, although he continued as a board member. In 1955, Haavikko married poet and writer Marja-Liisa Vartio; she died in 1966. Haavikko and literary historian Ritva Rainio Hanhineva were married in 1971.

In his work, Haavikko always showed a great skepticism toward any political or philosophical ideology: "If the philosophy is wrong, all deeds become crimes." Varying political ideologies are much the same in Haavikko's eyes: "Socialism! so that capitalism could begin to materialize./ Capitalism! the Big Money!/ They spend their evenings in a small circle,/ hand in hand, fingers linked in fingers, and like to remember their youth." Haavikko's stand was that of an antiutopian realist, to whom an individual's uniqueness and freedom are the highest values; in his view, man had "perhaps a two percent margin" in the maze of corporations, institutions, and governments and their bureaucracies, or simply in the complexity of life and in facing fate. To Haavikko, the most positive aspects of life were nature, the biological world, and the human mind.

In his own country, Haavikko was generally seen as a conservative and patriotic poet, who paradoxically has often through his work questioned some of his society's most cherished myths and values. Beginning in the 1980's, Haavikko was a regular columnist for the magazine *Suomen Kuvalehti*. By this point in his career, Haavikko had become a well-known figure in Finnish cultural life, even to people who did not particularly follow poetry. Gray-haired, distinguished-looking, and wearing thick eyeglasses, Haavikko became a national sage without suffering the decrease in literary quality often associated with such a status. He died October 6, 2008, after a long illness.

ANALYSIS

Paavo Haavikko belongs to the generation of Finns who experienced World War II as children, growing into maturity in the immediate postwar years, a period that in many ways constituted a watershed for the Finnish society, in that a major, still ongoing culture change began in the 1950's. The largely rural society (70 percent of the population lived in the countryside until the postwar years) had been a major source of literary themes for the prewar writers and poets. Finnish as a creative literary language was still relatively new, Finland having been part of the Swedish kingdom for six hundred years and of the Russian empire for one hundred years, during which time Swedish was the language of culture and education. In the nineteenth century, a smoldering nationalistic movement gained impetus, under the influence of the ideas of the German philosopher Johann Gottfried von Herder, and in 1863, the Finnish language was granted equal status with Swedish. The following decades produced an abundance of writers of Finnish-language literature, which reflected continental European trends and the "national neo-Romanticism." The latter was partly a product and a culmination of the struggle for the country's independence, which was gained in 1917.

World War II broke the continuity of Finnish literature. The war experience and the resulting circumstances and conditions caused a reevaluation of prewar ideas and ideology. It was a time of careful assessments of history and of the present possibilities for the country's political, economic, and cultural survival. New influences from the Anglo-Saxon world, especially in the form of translated literature, reached Finland, and in the late 1940's, a new generation of poets entered the literary scene.

Many of the representatives of the new poetry experimented with a number of styles, not immediately finding one distinctly their own. Not so with Haavikko. His first poetry collection, *Tiet etäisyyksiin* (the roads to far away), published in 1951, when the writer was twenty years old, showed him following his own instincts and philosophy about the nature of poetry and of language, humankind, and the world. The poets of the new era of modernism strove for fresh forms of expression, rejecting the preexisting poetic structures and in their themes avoiding any sort of ideology or sentimental self-analysis. Haavikko took these aims further than anybody else. He constructed his poems in nonrhyming, rhythmical language, attempting to get as close as possible to the spoken idiom.

He set out to examine the "eternal issues" of love, death, the identities of man and woman and their relationship to each other, and the possibilities for the indi-

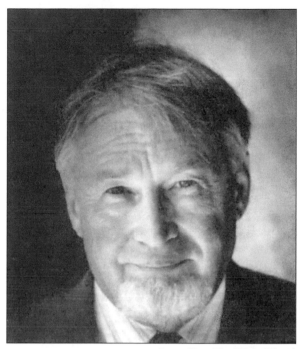

Paavo Haavikko (©Irmeli Jung)

vidual human being in an ever-changing world, in which the human character, man's psyche and behavior, and his actions and passions stay the same. Haavikko also set out to find linguistic expressions that would most clearly and honestly define and depict all these phenomena. Haavikko saw language as restricting humanity's perception of human processes and thoughts, even causing an estrangement from the realities of life. In an early poem, he spoke of the limitations of his native language: "Finnish isn't a language, it's a local custom/ of sitting on a bench with hair over your ears,/ it's continual talking about the rain and the wind." In another poem, he spoke of his own role as a poet in improving the existing modes of expression: "I'm on a journey into the language/ of this people." On the other hand, Haavikko also realized the advantages of his mother tongue, whose structure allows a compactness and a poetic construction in which "the relations between one thing and another, the world picture, are the most important elements."

This last observation pertains to Finnish folk poetry, a rich warehouse of themes and frames for his work. Haavikko set out to clear from literary expression all empty rhetoric and pathos, taking words, which he perceived as "treacherous symbols," and using them to find the truth. In this never-ending search for truth—for ultimately there are no answers—Haavikko created poetry in fluid combinations of images and concepts, taken from nature, everyday urban surroundings, mythology and tales, and classical antiquity as well as more recent history.

The structures of Haavikko's poems are complex, multifaceted, and multilayered. His lyrics have been compared to rich tapestries, to top rough-edged crystals, and to modern Finnish objets d'art. All these descriptions are fitting, and perhaps one more could be added, a concept taken from nature: Haavikko's poems could be seen as many items frozen in a block of ice; the block may melt, the ice become water and part of the continuous life cycle, and the pieces encased may become recognizable and identifiable, or the ice block may remain an enigmatic, opaque object, beautiful to contemplate but giving no answers to the viewer. Haavikko's poetry has also been likened to music, its sound obviously being most resonant in the original language. In the end, the responsibility for an interpretation and an understanding of the poet's ideas is left to each individual reader.

As Kai Laitinen and others have pointed out, Haavikko's writing is deeply rooted in a cultural and geographic area and its social and historical processes; the poet's perspectives were those of a European and of a citizen of a small European nation. The small size of the Finnish reading public (and, for writers in the Finnish language, an international public without much innate potential) has led Finland's writers to be unusually versatile, working in several forms and often having different identities in different genres or milieus. At times, the author's work reflects not only an individual's loneliness and feeling of being different but also an entire nation's sense of isolation and separateness.

Besides that, Haavikko had much to say about the most central and universal issues of human existence—the identity of an individual, the relativity of values, and the difficulty of living—and about the concepts of society, history, and literature. He said it through complex anachronisms, analogies, and "precise ambiguities," all the while refining and defining language, which in his work, especially in the opera librettos and the aphorisms, became increasingly sparse and intense. He moved freely between literary genres, letting the subject matter determine the form of his writing.

In an interview, Haavikko stated that, when composing poems, he always let the entire poem take shape in his mind, before writing it down, for fear that the words would take over and begin to lead a life of their own. He might use concrete images or paradoxes to weave the thread of human experience through several time periods, illuminating the present through the past and speaking about the future at the same time:

> The Greeks populated Mycenae,
> the poets of Rome in their turn
> filled Greece with shadowless beings,
>
> there is no night when no one wrote
> someone's writing into these rooms too,
> poem-dressed lovers, when we are not saying
>
> The room is not free but full of breathing
> and embraces, light sleeping, hush,
> be still, so we don't wake, someone's writing
> into the night.

For Haavikko, there was no separation of time and space; human existence, behavior, interactions, and in the end human fate, remained the same.

From the early metaphysical lyrical poetry through the plays, opera librettos, epic poetry, aphorisms, and historical analyses, Haavikko's work continued to create lively debate, providing new perspectives and new insights through its oracle-like visions and presentation of world structures. In the meantime, Haavikko continued to search for "himself, woman, god, tribe, old age and the grave" and the uniqueness of things, "not wanting generalizations, either, but trying to make things concrete." For Haavikko, one who generalizes is a fool, and in his work, the poet never pontificated. He merely invited the reader onto new paths, to which he had opened the way.

THE WINTER PALACE

The collections of poems published by Haavikko in the 1950's firmly established him as the most original and brilliant representative of the modernist group. The nine-poem collection *The Winter Palace* is a synthesis of all the themes that had preoccupied Haavikko in his previous work. The collection derived its name from the imperial Russian palace in St. Petersburg, and within this frame of a center for historical events, the poet examines the nature of art, poetry, love and death, and political power. The first poem begins: "Chased into silver,/ side by side:/ The images./ To have them tell you." The poet warns the reader to be alert, to enter this experience with an open mind, and through personal perception to organize the kaleidoscope, which will follow, into a comprehensible whole.

As an eighteen-year-old high school student, Haavikko had read T. S. Eliot, who without doubt pointed him the way "into the unknown." At about that time, Haavikko wrote a poem that served as a declaration of his intentions: "Bridges are taken by crossing them/ Each return is a defeat." From then on Haavikko continued crossing bridges, and *The Winter Palace* has been described as the Finnish *Waste Land*:

> This poem wants to be a description,
> And I want poems to have
> only the faintest of tastes.
> Myself I see as a creature, hopeful
> As the grass.
> These lines are almost improbable
> This is a journey through familiar speech
> Towards the region that is no place.

HISTORY, POLITICS, AND COMMUNICATION

After *The Winter Palace*, Haavikko turned to writing prose. He had already in his earlier collections of lyrical poetry, particularly in *Synnyinmaa* (native land) and *Lehdet lehtiä* (leaves, pages), dealt with the issues of the politics of the day, especially examining the events during the war and its aftermath, illuminating and assessing, through similar historical events, the actions and reasoning of the principal Finnish statesmen, as well as probing the Finnish national identity and attitudes. Historical themes in general increased in Haavikko's work considerably in the next two decades; seventeen of his plays are within a historical framework.

Haavikko continued questioning the essence of power, the motives and aims of those wielding it, and

how they influence the world, in particular the fate of the individual, who is tied to a historical situation. Most of Haavikko's novels and plays deal with social problems and issues involving the state, the church, the judiciary and taxation systems, diplomacy, commerce, and the family unit. In these contexts, the writer examined the problem of communication, how different social roles are manifested in the speech act, and the ways in which language is used and manipulated by various interest groups and individuals.

For Haavikko, nonverbal communication was much less dangerous than verbal communication; generally, everything bad derives from words: "And so out of words grow war/ and war becomes real/ it eats men, horses, corn,/ fire devours houses, years gnaw on man." An individual's odds for survival, however, are increased if he is aware of and can master the largest possible body of the various ways of communicating and knows the requirements that certain social roles impose on speech. Women's language is different from that of men: "It is pleasant to listen to, difficult to speak,/ impossible to understand." One of Haavikko's themes was that of a woman's greater strength, compared with that of a man; men desire power, they plan and develop; women have more common sense and keep everything together, and they steer life along healthier lines. Haavikko's writing implies that the cruelties and injustices of the world usually derive from men's actions. There is a deep, underlying pessimism in his prose, but it is lightened by a special brand of humor, the Finnish "gallows humor," which is a mixture of absurdity and irony and which, alongside more classical satire, is embedded in all the poet's work.

AN ILLOGICAL WORLD

In 1966, Haavikko published his only collection of lyrical poems of that decade, *Puut, kaikki heidän vihreytensä* (trees in all their verdure), which in its direct and clear simplicity remains one of his major works, alongside the collections of 1973 and 1976, when he returned briefly to lyrical poetry, dealing with new and different subject matter. Haavikko's interest was turning increasingly toward economics and history, particularly Finnish history and toward Byzantium, both of which provided him with a background against which to examine the fate of rulers, political factions and their intrigues, and man's quest for power and riches. In short, Haavikko could study the entire world in microcosm. The world as expressed in Haavikko's poetry is illogical, it is a paradox, and it is merciless; once an individual comes to terms with this understanding of the world, however, "looking it into the eyes every moment," it is possible for him to live without fear and, characteristic of Haavikko, without hope.

NELJÄTOISTA HALLITSIJAA

Haavikko's epic poem *Neljätoista hallitsijaa* (fourteen rulers) consists of fifteen cantos, based on the events described in the chronicle of Michael Psellus, an eleventh century Byzantine court historian and philosopher. The first four songs are the poet's first-person prologue, after which he merges with Psellus, through whose eyes he draws the Byzantine worldview. The main themes are, as in much of Haavikko's work, the position of the individual, who cannot escape his fate though he himself also shapes that fate, and the frame of historical understanding, the historical process devouring the individual, who searches for permanence but finds it an illusion. In this cyclical world, however, in which everything is in flux, an individual must, in some way, influence the outcome of the events, and he must try to combat evil, which Haavikko includes in his term "fascism." The word represents to the poet, among some other aspects, all accumulated stupidity, in which an initially small, annoying amount may become dangerous. In Haavikko's terminology, the opposite of fascism is pragmatic caution in all human endeavor, perceiving realities, being prepared for the worst, all the while maintaining the ability to function and staying alive. Haavikko's interest in Byzantium links him to modernists such as the Irish poet William Butler Yeats and the Greek poet Constantine Cavafy. Like those two poets, Haavikko felt a concrete, historical sense of connection to the Byzantine Empire, as raiders from Finland had encountered Byzantine culture while on expeditions southward at the turn of the first millennium. The concrete historicism of *Neljätoista hallitsijaa*, combined with Haavikko's rigorously ironic view of history (his lack of credence in history's substantiality) endows it with both spectacle and skepticism.

ONE AND TWENTY

Haavikko's stylistic and thematic concerns and his preoccupation with human cognitive processes are expressed in the following lines: "Every house is built by many people/ and is never through,/ history and myth are told and told again/ contradicting halls lead to understanding." These concerns led the poet to begin telling old Finnish myths anew, by rewriting one of the central cycles of the *Kalevala* (1835, enlarged 1849 as *Uusi Kalevala*; English translation, 1888), an epic compiled and rewritten from folk poetry by Elias Lönnrot. This work became the national epic and had a great impact on the national culture, inspiring writers, painters, and composers, such as Jean Sibelius. *One and Twenty*, Haavikko's version of the Sampo cycle (which in folk tradition centers on a mythical talisman that brings good fortune) takes place in Byzantium, where, according to the poet, Finnish Vikings went in search of a coin-minting machine, which they hoped to plunder.

Haavikko continued following a partially economic point of view in his subsequent re-creations of the world of the folk poetry, which he inhabited with antiheroes, people modeled after those of modern times, while at the same time depicting the archetypal man. The poet acknowledged his indebtedness to his native oral traditions, which provided him with an inheritance of the world of the epic, and he interpreted that world in the language and with the techniques of the twentieth century.

OTHER MAJOR WORKS

LONG FICTION: *Yksityisia asioita*, 1960; *Toinen taivas ja maa*, 1961; *Vuodet*, 1962.

PLAYS: *Münchhausen*, pr. 1958; *Nuket*, pr., pb. 1960; *Agricola ja kettu*, pr., pb. 1968; *Ylilääkäri*, pb. 1968 (*The Superintendent*, 1978); *Sulka*, pr., pb. 1973; *Harald Pitkäikäinen*, pb. 1974; *Ratsumies*, pb. 1974 (libretto; music by Aulis Sallinen; *The Horseman*, 1974); *Näytelmät*, pb. 1978; *Viisi pientä draamallista tekstiä*, pb. 1981; *Kuningas lähtee Ranskaan*, pr. 1984 (libretto; music by Sallinen; *The King Goes Forth to France*, 1984); *Lastenkutsut*, pr. 2000; *Paavo Suuri, Suuri juoksu, Suuri uni*, pr. 2000 (libretto; music by Tuomas Kantelinen).

TELEPLAYS: *Rauta-aika*, 1982 (adaptation of his poem); *Kirkas ilta*, 1995; *Korkein oikeus*, 1999.

RADIO PLAYS: *Audun ja jääkarhu*, 1966; *Lyhytaikaiset lainat*, 1966; *Freijan pelto*, 1967.

NONFICTION: *Puhua, vastata, opettaa*, 1972; *Ihmisen ääni*, 1977; *Kan-sakunnan linja*, 1977; *Ikuisen rauhan aika*, 1981; *Pimeys*, 1984; *Yritys omakskuvaksi*, 1987; *Vuosien aurinkoiset varjot*, 1994; *Prospero*, 1995.

MISCELLANEOUS: *Romaanit ja novellit*, 1981 (novels and short fiction).

BIBLIOGRAPHY

Binham, Philip. "Dream Each Within Each: The Finnish Poet Paavo Haavikko." *Books Abroad* 50, no. 2 (1976): 337-341. A brief look at the first half of Haavikko's career, emphasizing its experimental aspect. Does not provide sufficient coverage of the poet's Byzantine and historical concerns but is otherwise reliable and insightful.

Haavikko, Paavo. *One and Twenty*. Translated by Anselm Hollo. Beaverton, Ont: Aspasia, 2007. In addition to the translation, this work contains several essays on Haavikko's work.

_____. "What Has the *Kalevala* Given Me?" *Books from Finland* 1 (1985): 65. The poet discusses his relationship to Finland's fundamental body of mythological legend and inferentially his stance toward story and history.

Laitinen, Kai. *Literature of Finland: In Brief*. 3d ed. Helsinki: Otava, 2001. Provides a good overall placement of Haavikko within the literary tradition of Finland.

Lyytikäinen, Pirjo. *Changing Scenes: Encounters Between European and Finnish Fin de Siècle*. Helsinki: Finnish Literature Society, 2003. Contains analysis of the poetry of Haavikko and several other poets, touching on national identity, naturalism, and modernism.

Paddon, Seija. "John Ashbery and Paavo Haavikko: Architects of Postmodern Space in Mind and Language." *Canadian Review of Comparative Literature/Revue Canadienne de Littérature Comparée* 20, nos. 3/4 (1993): 409-416. Compares Haavikko to Ashbery based on observed similarities and on Ashbery's lavish admiration for Haavikko's *The Winter Palace*. Paddon is a leading scholar of Finnish poetry in North America, and his article is one of few in English to provide sustained analysis of Haavikko's poetic techniques.

Schoolfield, George. *A History of Finland's Literature*. Lincoln: University of Nebraska Press, 1998. Provides a substantial overview of Haavikko's entire poetic career; also gives a sense of his comparative importance in the national literature and the cross-fertilizations between his work and that of his Finnish and Finnish-Swedish contemporaries.

World Literature Today 58, no. 4 (1984). A special issue devoted to Haavikko's work on the occasion of his winning the Neustadt Prize in 1984. Includes not only reprints of some of Haavikko's work but rigorous and laudatory analyses as well.

Tuula Stark
Updated by Nicholas Birns

HARTMANN VON AUE

Born: Swabia (now in Germany), c. 1160-1165
Died: Swabia (now in Germany); c. 1210-1220
Also known as: Hartmann von Ouwe

PRINCIPAL POETRY

Die Klage, c. 1180 (*The Lament*, 2001)

Erek, c. 1190 (*Erec*, 1982)

Gregorius, c. 1190-1197 (English translation, 1955, 1966)

Iwein, c. 1190-1205 (*Iwein: The Knight with the Lion*, 1979)

Der arme Heinrich, c. 1195 (English translation, 1931)

Arthurian Romances, Tales, and Lyric Poetry: The Complete Works of Hartmann von Aue, 2001

OTHER LITERARY FORMS

Although all extant works by Hartmann von Aue (HORT-mon vawn OW-uh) are in verse form, scholars have been tempted to consider the courtly epics *Erec*,

Iwein, *Gregorius*, and *Der arme Heinrich* as prototypes of modern prose forms such as the novella and the novel. Nevertheless, Hartmann is first and foremost an epic poet. Because he and his contemporaries drew no such generic distinctions, neither shall this survey.

ACHIEVEMENTS

In *The Emergence of German as a Literary Language* (2d ed., 1978), Eric Blackall describes the development of "an uncouth language into one of the most subtle literary media of modern Europe," attaining respectability, however, only after 1700. Blackall implies here that until the eighteenth century, German literature was essentially derivative, struggling to define itself in the presence of other, highly developed European languages and literatures. Seen in this light, the modest oeuvre of Hartmann von Aue—often topically repetitive and linguistically naïve by modern standards—can be appreciated for its true worth: as a giant stride toward vernacular poetry of the highest stature.

Hartmann's language is a model of consistency and moderation. His sentences are clearly constructed, his rhymes are natural and unaffected, and his mastery of various verse forms is assured. His was a poetry of reflection and reason, and he frequently employed devices that clarified the theme for his audience, particularly parallelism and contrasting imagery. In his verse, he presented problematic situations that would be of interest and application to a broad audience, avoiding bizarre plots that would defeat his didactic purposes. The same concerns are reflected in his language: Hartmann pruned outdated expressions, dialect words, and foreign phrases in favor of a language accessible to a broader geographical audience. In this respect, Hartmann anticipated Martin Luther's efforts to promote a standard German language. Finally, Hartmann is credited with introducing the Arthurian romance in Germany.

For his innovations in style, form, and language, Hartmann was respected by his contemporaries, honored by patron and audience alike, and frequently imitated by his colleagues. With Wolfram von Eschenbach and Gottfried von Strassburg, Hartmann is regarded as one of the three literary trendsetters of his age—at once exemplary and inimitable.

Perhaps of greater significance than his stylistic innovations, however, was the attitude that Hartmann brought to his works. His personal experiences and reflections are presented in a serious, contemplative mood, ennobling both the man and his writing. Furthermore, an earnest involvement with the social and moral issues of his society are hallmarks of his poetry. Hartmann's thoughtful treatment of the tensions existing between society and religious devotion illuminated one of the most enduring concerns for German culture, a concern mirrored in works of later authors as diverse as Hans Jakob Christoffel von Grimmelshausen, the Brothers Grimm, and Thomas Mann.

Hartmann's popularity and literary success resulted in part from his attempts to unify form and content. He constantly strove to make his language appropriate to the experiences and emotions described in the text. The tales themselves, of Erec and Iwein, of Gregorius and Heinrich, were certainly not extraordinary for his time; many of his contemporaries created more adventurous, more bizarre stories to captivate their audiences. Hartmann, however, was able to engage his listeners in a more intellectual fashion, by stating problems inherent in his society and by examining them thoughtfully and intelligently, so that the listener understood their import for his or her own life.

BIOGRAPHY

As is the case with many medieval poets, documentary evidence attesting the life and deeds of Hartmann von Aue is sparse. The few tantalizing clues that have survived have become the topic of continuing scholarly debate and controversy. From brief statements within the works of Hartmann and his fellow courtly poets, from contemporary events, and from astute speculation, a plausible biography has been established. Hartmann's birth date, for example, can be surmised only by backdating—that is, by assuming that his earliest work was composed at approximately the age of twenty. Thus, since the first work attributable to Hartmann appeared around 1180, he was probably born between 1160 and 1165. His noble appellation "von Aue" indicates that he lived in the German territory known as Swabia, located in present-day Germany. From the introduction to *Der arme Heinrich*, in which Hartmann describes himself as "learned"—that is, able to read Latin (and presumably French)—one can assume that he enjoyed an education, most likely in a monastery school. As an adult, Hartmann became an unpropertied knight in the administrative service of a noble lord.

Hartmann's earliest works convey his involvement in courtly society and its chivalric conventions, but his failure at *Minne* (courtly love), the death of his beloved lord and patron, and his eventual participation in a Crusade reflect a gradual but fundamental change in his life. Hartmann forsook the conventions of *Minne* and his role as *Minnesinger*, placing himself in the service of Christ and composing instead songs of the Crusades and of renunciation. Although *Iwein* appears to have been the last secular work that Hartmann wrote, scholars now believe that this work was merely the completion of an earlier commission and thus does not accurately reflect Hartmann's mature stance. There is no evidence that Hartmann wrote anything during the last ten or more years of his life. The date and circumstances of his death remain a mystery to this day. Poets of the time implied that Hartmann was still living in 1210, but by 1220 he was mentioned as being among the deceased.

ANALYSIS

The period of courtly love poetry presents several insoluble problems for the modern reader. Little is known of the poets as individuals, of the circumstances in which their songs were created and performed, or of the melodies that accompanied the songs. Few manuscripts survive, and these were often copied down generations after the fact; by the time individual songs were committed to parchment, deviations from the original text were inevitable. These factors impose limits on any analysis of Hartmann von Aue's poetry. Although his surviving works are few in number—sixteen songs and five works of substantial length—they are rich in variety, reflecting his changing concerns and the gradual refinement of his style.

THE LAMENT

The earliest work attributable to Hartmann is *The Lament*, a relatively youthful attempt at conventional courtly poetry. The title is somewhat misleading, for the content clearly represents disputation or rational debate. Here a young knight, unsuccessful in courtly love, engages the service of his "body" and "heart" to clarify their roles in this delicate struggle. This didactic piece, clearly a product of reflection and not of immediate personal suffering, recommends traditional chivalric qualities such as discipline, loyalty, and dependability; moderation and modesty; striving and denial. In spite of its relative superficiality and clumsy logic, *The Lament* represents the first rational clarification of the redemptive and civilizing qualities required by courtly society. Hartmann's goal here was no less than to determine those qualities that allow the individual to find favor in the eyes of God and of other people. This question and the contemplative search for an appropriate answer characterize Hartmann's entire oeuvre.

In the same period in which he wrote *The Lament*, Hartmann composed the first of his courtly love songs. These earliest poems also uncritically propagated the chivalric qualities necessary for attaining the favor of a noble lady, though Hartmann soon demonstrated his unwillingness to feign joy over the pains of unrequited love. Later poems reflected a greater sorrow that had befallen Hartmann—the death of his lord and patron. The poet had mentioned his failure to win the favor of a particular lady, but that was only a temporary disappointment when compared to the loss of his lord. (Although more recent scholarship questions the sincerity of the singer-patron relationship, suggesting that the poet's expression of gratitude was purely conventional, Hartmann was doubtless loyal and grateful to his patron. Obviously, the death of his lord had a lasting effect on Hartmann's life and thus on his poetry.)

In any case, Hartmann's failure in love prompted him to assess his position. While not questioning the conventions of courtly society in general or of courtly love in particular, Hartmann did come to the realization that he himself was not suited to such *Minne* service. As he wrote at the time: "True joy is never having loved." He was too honorable to place blame on the lady in question, reserving all culpability for himself. In truth, Hartmann was not made for such a contest. The protest against his personal suffering eventually grew into a denial of courtly love, couched in a typically objective critique. Hartmann no longer praised this idealized, unrequited love, celebrating instead a mutually harmonious relationship with a woman of less than noble stature beyond the stifling bounds of the court. At the same time, this shift in Hartmann's attitude toward courtly love was motivated by an intense spiritual reorientation: For the salvation of his and his patron's souls, Hartmann joined a Crusade, creating songs of dignified devotion as a religious stimulus to others of his class. These changes in Hartmann's outlook took place only gradually, and their development can be traced in his works.

EREC

Hartmann's *Erec* is German literature's first Arthurian romance, a genre that has retained its popularity to this day. Though Hartmann relied on an earlier work by Chrétien de Troyes for his source, he should not be accused of plagiarism: In the Middle Ages, it was assumed that authors would choose their themes from an established collection of plots; true *inventio*, or originality, appeared in the manner of presentation. One noticeable innovation in Hartmann's version is the role of the narrator; actual dialogue is subordinated to the third-person narrative, in which an objective distance from event and character is achieved.

While Chrétien had described the successes of a mature hero, Hartmann's story begins with an impetuous youth. Overwhelmed by his passion for the beautiful Enite, Erec ignores his obligations as knight and ruler, thus bringing dishonor on himself, his court, and his land. He can regain his honor only by renewed, mature striving within the dictates of courtly society; by doing precisely that, he, too, gains personally through a more mature and balanced relationship with his wife. Their love nurtures the well-being that now permeates their entire sphere of influence.

Hartmann's young Erec has failed abysmally and must undergo a lengthy and painful process of maturation, until he can prove himself worthy of being the leader of a court and the ruler of a kingdom. The major tension in this work is provided by the concepts of personal and social love. Personal, possessive love (that is, passion) must not prove destructive to the greater good represented by a harmonious, integrated society. The prevailing motif of beauty is subtly compared and contrasted to substantiate this point: Sensual beauty is destructive, for it lures the knight to thoughts and deeds of sexual excess, but beauty can also be the outward manifestation of inner harmony, as exemplified by Enite and the lovely ladies at King Arthur's court. Hartmann explores these conflicts to demonstrate how the individual can enjoy his personal life while remaining a constructive member of society.

Symmetrically placed episodes reinforce this theme: Erec's immature adventures at the outset of the work are paralleled by his mature successes at the conclusion. In tracing the development of the titular hero from a self-centered youth to a responsible ruler, Hartmann reminded his contemporaries of the responsibilities of the individual knight to others and to society as a whole; Hartmann saw the courtly social code calcifying into a set of rules for membership in an exclusive club.

IWEIN

Hartmann's *Iwein*, based on yet another tale by Chrétien, examines the responsibilities of the knight from a different point of view. Unlike Erec, Iwein is overly concerned with acquiring honor and, from a sense of rampant egoism, neglects equally important chivalric imperatives. Iwein is persuaded to leave his wife for a year (lest he end like Erec) to participate in jousting tournaments and adventures and thereby accumulate more honor. Iwein becomes so self-centered that he fails to return home at the end of the year's time and is consequently condemned before Arthur's court as unfaithful, having betrayed his wife's and society's trust. The accusation strikes Iwein so forcefully that he goes mad and lives in the wilderness as a wild man. Only through a number of painful learning experiences does he gradually regain his senses, his honor, his wife, and his position in society. The lion mentioned in the subtitle serves to accent the importance of loyalty; Iwein rescues a lion, which then becomes his faithful companion, truly a "noble" beast. The errant Iwein is also treated with kindness by others until he can learn to reciprocate their goodness unselfishly. In stages, Iwein learns loyalty, kindness, and consideration for others, and his selfless service is rewarded with honor and salvation.

From the large number of surviving manuscripts, it is evident that *Iwein* was Hartmann's most popular work. In recognition of its important theme and stylistic excellence, modern scholars have frequently referred to it as the classical work of the high courtly period. Nevertheless, *Iwein* is a problematic work, for it appears to have been written at widely separated intervals. The first one thousand lines exhibit characteristics of Hartmann's middle period, around 1190, while the remainder of the work is composed in a mature yet detached style. Scholars speculate that the work was commissioned while Hartmann was still involved in courtly service and attempting to accommodate himself to its demands; after a lengthy interruption, during which time Hartmann had disengaged himself from *Minne* conventions, he returned to the manuscript to fulfill, albeit mechanically, the commission. Since *Iwein* still accepts the precepts of courtly society unquestioningly, one can scarcely consider it as Hartmann's definitive statement on the subject, especially in the light of his mature personal convictions and the discrepancy in style. It is a tribute to Hartmann's artistry that he could complete such a work "mechanically" yet produce one of the most popular epics of the High Middle Ages.

GREGORIUS

Gregorius, Hartmann's courtly legend of the life of a fictive pope, was based on a contemporary French source, *Vie du Pape Gregoire*. Despite its explicit references to Sophocles' *Oidipous Tyrannos* (c. 429 B.C.E., *Oedipus Tyrannus*, 1715), *Gregorius* is an ingenious mixture of Asian and Occidental mythology and folklore, although Hartmann's version features a distinctly Christian accent with its traditional progression of innocence, sin and downfall, contrition, penance, and salvation. The plot itself is at once fascinating and convoluted. The devil succeeds in blinding two noble children, so that the brother seduces his own sister. The brother then dies on a pilgrimage, while the sister secretly nurses the child of the incestuous relationship. The child is set adrift at sea, accompanied only by a tablet on which is inscribed a message that explains his origin and begs that he pray for his parents' salvation. The foundling is raised by foster parents, educated at a monastery school, and named after the local abbot, Gregorius. All goes well until an argument reveals to the young man his parents' shame. Despite the Abbot's insistence that his namesake is predestined for the priesthood, young Gregorius flees to take up an adventuresome life as a knight. In his first encounter with the outside world, Gregorius frees a beleaguered city and claims the widowed queen as his bride. In all innocence, Gregorius has married his own mother, thus heaping incest upon incest. He now flees again, in complete despair. Taken to a remote island, he is chained to a rock, and the key to his bonds is thrown into the sea; thus, Gregorius spends the next seventeen years in bondage and isolation. In the meantime, a successor to the deceased pope is sought. The name of Gregorius appears in a dream to the electors, and two papal legates are dispatched to locate this holy man; they are led to the island, where, miraculously, the key to Gregorius's chains is found in the belly of a fish. Soon, the fame of the new pope draws the incestuous queen to Rome, in the hope of gaining absolution from her sins. Gregorius and his mother immediately recognize each other and are reunited and absolved of their mutual burden. The tale closes with an epilogue reminding the audience that all sins can be expiated through contrition and penance.

Aside from the titillating motif of incest, this work offers its audience several moral considerations to ponder: Is Gregorius somehow responsible for the sins of his parents? Should he be punished for unwittingly and unwillingly becoming a participant in incest himself? Despite the folklore surrounding such "sins," the Church of Hartmann's day would have considered neither of these sins to be culpable. As several scholars have indicated, Gregorius's actual transgression is against himself and his God. In agreement with the mother's original request, the Abbot had insisted that the youth devote his life to prayer for his parents' salvation; Gregorius's defection was thus a betrayal of his sacred duty. In choosing to sally forth as a knight in search of adventure, courtly love, and honor—duties required of the chivalric class—he was placing personal gratification and *superbia* (ego or self) before his obligation to others and to his God.

In criticizing Gregorius for his blind devotion to *Minne* and honor, Hartmann was in fact questioning the entire structure of courtly society. He showed that the arch virtues mentioned above could lead to sin and downfall, and could be expiated only through a long and horrible penance such as that which Gregorius suffered, chained to his island rock. To be sure, Hartmann did not completely undermine the values inherent in the courtly system, but he did expose them as less than absolutes. Even supposedly courtly virtues can be tools of the devil to tempt innocents from their divinely chosen paths. It is significant that a story that begins badly in worldly society can end happily in the religious seclusion of Rome. This qualified renunciation of the profane in favor of the sacred was the most pronounced development in Hartmann's life and found its poetic culmination in the songs he composed for the Crusades.

DER ARME HEINRICH

Der arme Heinrich, in its own time perhaps the least appreciated of Hartmann's works (if the small number of surviving manuscripts is any indication), has ironically become the most popular. Scarcely fifteen hundred lines in length, it has been considered the prototype of the modern German novella. It was the poem's treatment of its theme, however, and not its formal aspect, that made it revolutionary in Hartmann's day. Heinrich is the epitome of a medieval nobleman. He possesses all the knightly virtues; he enjoys riches and honor, power and fame. Suddenly and inexplicably, he is struck down by leprosy, the most odious illness imaginable. The man who was once the ideal of social virtue is now cast out by that very society, for his beauty has turned to ugliness, his honor to dishonor, his fame to infamy. In search of a medical cure for his affliction, Heinrich travels first to Montpellier and then to Salerno, but he learns that he can be saved only by the blood from the heart of a pure maiden. In despair, Heinrich retires to the country, where he is welcomed and nursed by a family of loyal tenants. The daughter is especially drawn to Heinrich and asks why he has been so cursed. His answer is that he had been a worldly fool, accepting happiness and success as his just reward and not as a sign of God's grace.

Just as Heinrich had been obsessed with his worldly possessions, the daughter becomes equally fanatic in her desire to die for his salvation. In extended discussions with her parents, the girl proclaims her desire to depart this life. Eventually, Heinrich accedes to her wishes, and they leave for Salerno, but at the moment the doctor is about to make the initial incision, Heinrich glimpses the beautiful girl and experiences a change of heart. He releases the girl unharmed, knowing that he cannot accept such a sacrifice and must reconcile himself to living the remainder of his life as a leper. The girl, however, is in despair and curses Heinrich for depriving her of escape from this world. At this point, both are miraculously "cured" through God's mercy: Heinrich is restored to a youthful state of good health and beauty, while the girl regains a healthy desire to live out her life on Earth, as Heinrich's wife. Together, they live a full and happy life before entering Heaven.

In this didactic tale, Hartmann again warned of the dangers of *superbia*, of selfishly living only for worldly goals or of selfishly desiring a premature death. Both Heinrich and the girl must learn to live in this world while still recognizing the divine scheme of things. This moral was directly aimed at the courtly society of which Heinrich is representative. With his unrestrained and unquestioning appreciation for worldly values, Heinrich fails to realize that all things come from God: Heinrich's successes, his suffering, and his ultimate salvation are all the result of God's grace. That Heinrich must overcome the courtly values as limitations, that he marries a girl beneath his social standing, that he lives out the remainder of his life far from court—these developments would have seemed foreign to a courtly audience and as such were obviously viewed as unwelcome provocations. This would account for the contemporary reception of Hartmann's text.

BIBLIOGRAPHY

Fiddy, Andrea. *The Presentation of the Female Characters in Hartmann's "Gregorius" and "Der arme Heinrich."* Göppingen, Germany: Kümmerle, 2004. Fiddy's work provides a feminist analysis through its examination of women characters in *Gregorius* and *Der arme Heinrich*.

Gentry, Francis G., ed. *A Companion to the Works of Hartmann von Aue.* Rochester, N.Y.: Camden House, 2005. A scholarly collection of essays covering a wide range of topics on Hartmann von Aue's works. Includes bibliography and index.

Hasty, Will. *Adventures in Interpretation: The Works of Hartmann von Aue and Their Critical Reception.* Columbia, S.C.: Camden House, 1996. A survey of criticism of Hartmann von Aue's work from the Enlightenment to postmodernism, which concludes that the interpretations by modern readers have been shaped mainly by critical trends.

Jackson, W. H. *Chivalry in Twelfth-Century Germany: The Works of Hartmann von Aue.* Rochester, N.Y.: D. S. Brewer, 1994. A study of Hartmann von Aue's poetic representation of knighthood and chivalric values with consideration of historical, literary, and linguistic influences.

Jackson, W. H., and S. A. Ranawake, eds. *The Arthur of the Germans: The Arthurian Legend in Medieval German and Dutch Literature.* Cardiff: University of Wales Press, 2000. A group of essays includes chapters on the emergence of the German Arthurian romance.

Pincikowski, Scott E. *Bodies of Pain: Suffering in the Works of Hartmann von Aue.* New York: Routledge, 2002. Pincikowski argues that the ideological system that informs courtly life causes suffering in both the physical body and the social body of the court.

Resler, Michael. Introduction to *Hartmann von Aue: "Erec."* Philadelphia: University of Pennsylvania Press, 1987. An extensive introduction including general historical and cultural background, specific information on the life of Hartmann, a discussion of Arthurian romance, and a full consideration of the sources, structure, and thematic issues of this work. This volume also contains a translation of *Erec* plus explanatory endnotes. Includes helpful selected bibliography, although the majority of the references are to sources in German.

Sullivan, Robert G. *Justice and the Social Context of Early Middle High German Literature.* New York: Routledge, 2001. A history of the Holy Roman Empire hinging on an examination of High German literature and its authors' focus on social, political, and spiritual issues during a time of transformation. Bibliographical references, index.

Thomas, J. W. Introduction to *Hartmann von Aue: "Erec."* Lincoln: University of Nebraska Press, 1982. Includes information on Hartmann's life and works, as well as the theme, plot structure, motifs, and style of the translated work. Explanatory notes

at the end provide bibliographical information on each of these topics. A readable translation of the text follows.

_____. Introduction to *Hartmann von Aue: "Iwein."* Lincoln: University of Nebraska Press, 1979. An informative introduction with an overview of Hartmann's works and discussions of the theme of *Iwein*, structure and motifs, and the narrative style. Notes include important bibliographical references as well as helpful information. The translation included in this volume is very readable.

Todd C. Hanlin

PIET HEIN

Born: Copenhagen, Denmark; December 16, 1905
Died: Fyn, Denmark; April 17, 1996
Also known as: Kumbel Kumbell

PRINCIPAL POETRY

Gruk, 1-20, 1940-1963 (as Kumbel Kumbell; *Grooks*, 1-6, 1966-1978)
Den tiende Muse, 1941
Vers i verdensrummet, 1941
Kumbels almanak, 1942
Vers af denne verden, 1948
Kumbels fødselsdagskalender, 1949
Du skal plante et træ, 1960
Husk at elske, 1962
Husk at leve, 1965
Lad os blive mennesker, 1967
I folkemunde, 1968
Runaway Runes, 1968
Det kraftens ord, 1969

OTHER LITERARY FORMS

While Piet Hein (hin) is known internationally for his aphoristic "grooks" (Danish *gruk*, his own coinage) and in Denmark is highly regarded for his more traditional strophic poetry as well, he also published collections of epigrams and prose aphorisms, expressing the same outlook that informs his poetry: *Man skal gaa paa*

Jorden—(1944; one has to walk on the Earth); its sequel, —*Selvom den er gloende* (1950; even if it is glowing); and the volume *Ord* (1949; words). *Vis Electrica* (1962), a Festschrift treating the nature and manifold uses of electricity, includes grooks and conventional poems as well; the harmony between scientific and humanistic perspectives was characteristic of Hein's entire career.

ACHIEVEMENTS

Between 1940 and 1963, Piet Hein published twenty collections of grooks. Altogether, he wrote about ten thousand grooks, and by 1971, his publishing house would announce that the grooks had been printed in 1,250,000 copies. They are also available on two long-playing records, read by Hein himself. They have been set to music, have formed the basis for twenty short features on television (by Ivo Caprino), and have been made available in numerous translations, including Indonesian, Iranian, Japanese, and Chinese. One entire volume was published in Esperanto, and Hein himself personally re-created his grooks in German, French, Spanish, and, in particular, English. Several grooks have been written directly in these languages and are not available in Danish.

Writing, however, was only one of Hein's means of expression. Quotations from the grooks in newspapers, books, and lectures have spread to ashtrays, salt and pepper shakers, and ceramic plaques. Most of these objects have the distinctive shape of a rectangular oval or "superellipse": Hein, a mathematician, inventor, and designer as well as a poet, created this unique geometrical form. The superellipse merges the circle and the rectangle into a newly perfected form: It has solved the traffic problem in central Stockholm, joining two freeways in a roundabout system only 210 yards long in an aesthetically appealing design. Hein's innovative design has gained world recognition; he applied his superellipse to the structure of furniture and lamps, to the planning of Mexico City's Olympic Stadium and of the city center in Canada's Peterborough, and to architectural projects in France. Its three-dimensional version, the "superegg," can be found both as a sculpture and—in smaller sizes—as a drink cooler and a stress-relief ball.

Hein's inventiveness and creativity were also evident in numerous other inventions and designs—especially in the design of board games and puzzles such as the Polygon Game and the three-dimensional SOMA Cube, which became favorite pastimes for thousands of people in Europe and the United States. The origin of these games was in Hein's fondness for "creative playing," which he shared with his friend Albert Einstein. In his essay "Et Menneske" ("A Man"), Hein quoted Einstein:

> There is a striking similarity, he said, between the usual games and the prime one: to discover the structure of nature. I cannot understand complicated things: therefore, I have tried to reduce the laws of nature to a simple formula. The great coherences in nature are simple. And when you see the perspective in things, nothing is small.

This holistic effort to find harmony in microcosm as well as in macrocosm was central not only to Hein's scientific achievements but also to his poetry.

For his literary and scientific achievements, Hein won a number of international honors, including the Alexander Graham Bell Silver Bell in 1968, the award Huitième Salon International du Lumière in 1973, and the International Aphia Prize in 1980. In 1970, he became a member of the British Society of Authors and won the Danish Design Council's Annual Award in 1989 and the Tietgen Medal in 1990. In 1972, he received an honorary doctorate in humane letters from Yale University. His speech of thanks attested to Hein's international outlook and humanist worldview:

> Science has a vital task in manifesting its own true nature: synthesis and openness, both in its own sphere and in the larger one of humankind. It must help both spheres to raise themselves above their present state of local habits in global worlds.

BIOGRAPHY

Piet Hein's creative versatility reflected his eclectic education. His father, civil engineer Hjalmar Hein, descended from a German-Dutch family; his mother, Estrid Hein, was a well-known Copenhagen ophthalmologist, a member of and prolific writer for the Danish women's movement, and a cousin to the writer Isak Dinesen. Hein's childhood home was located in Rungsted, north of Copenhagen, to which he returned to live for many years with his wife, Gerd Hein, an actress at The Royal Theater in Stockholm. Following her death in 1968, Hein moved to Poke Stoges in England; in 1976, he returned to Denmark and made his home at the Damsbo estate on the island of Funen.

Having received his high school and college education in Copenhagen, Hein passed his university entrance exams as a mathematics major in 1924. In 1925, however, after the obligatory examination in philosophy, he left Copenhagen for Stockholm to begin training as a painter at the Royal Academy of the Arts. In 1927, he returned to Copenhagen, where, until 1931, he studied philosophy and theoretical physics, both at the university and at the Niels Bohr Institute, without taking a degree. At the institute, Hein constructed a model that illustrated the principle of complementarity (formulated by Bohr in 1927), and his so-called atomarium, which, together with his participation in advanced colloquia concerning recent discoveries in atomic theory, earned him the greatest respect from his fellow scientists.

In the following years, Hein worked on various industrial designs and technical inventions, including an ingenious rotor engine. In 1947, he published *Helicopteren*, which was the result of an exhaustive study, and created a "coloroscope," a device to create light effects in which the spectrum could be moved from a spatial to a temporal state. During the 1930's, Hein began his creative authorship, concurrently joining a number of new liberal political movements. From 1935 to 1955, he was a member of the board of the Danish section of Open Door International and, from 1948 to 1949, president of the Danish section of the World Movement for World Federal Government. He also was active in organizations such as the International PEN Club and numerous Danish groups promoting world peace and tolerance. His membership in the Adventurers Club testified to his many travels and extensive stays in Europe and in North and South America. Likewise telling was Hein's membership in the Frensham Group—which he called "Ten-Wise-Men-and-Me"—an international organization furthering interdisciplinary research and contact between scientific and nonscientific groups. Hein died in 1996 in Denmark.

ANALYSIS

Throughout his entire career, Piet Hein strove for the harmony between scientific and humanistic perspectives. His dual perspective is apparent in *Kilden og krukken* (1963; the spring and the urn), a volume that intersperses brief philosophical prose texts, related to the classical fable, with some of Hein's numerous public lectures. The common theme is that while technology must serve humanity, the humanities must serve reason via the individual. Contemporary humans, however, must first have their original synthesis restored—ther balance of reason and emotion, of the objective and the subjective. Hein analyzes the disastrous split between the exclusively scientific, technological worldview on one hand and the exclusively humanistic worldview on the other. Hein's life's work was given to a reconciliation of these opposing outlooks.

Hein's vast literary canon—in particular, the grooks—is too multifaceted to be gathered under a single heading. A common denominator, however, was his precise, epigrammatic language. His speeches, aphorisms, grooks, and more conventional poetry were all informed by certain recurring themes that constituted his philosophy as well as his poetics. Thus, an aphorism from 1944, "Art is the solution to those problems which cannot be formulated clearly before they are solved," clearly expressed Hein's conviction that such scientific activities as the raising of new questions and the proving of new theories are fundamentally similar to the concerns of the artist. The natural sciences and the humanities have a common point of origin: human imagination. This insistence on the potential union of art and science was the subject of Hein's speech on having become an honorary member of the Danish Students' Association in 1970:

> In all areas it is a matter of seeing how the objects could be different from what we are used to, of generalizing the problem in a hitherto unnoticed dimension, and within the new, larger, more general multiplicity of choosing a specific case, a new and better solution. This process has been typical for all great innovations within science. This is the true form of imagination. Imagination is just a higher form of the sense of reality.

GROOKS

Hein insisted on viewing life's questions from new perspectives: "He on whom God's light does fall, sees the great things in the small." This point of view was precisely reflected, both in form and content, by the grooks (defined as a "small lyrical or intellectual aphorism in poetic form and with a point"):

> Infinity's taken
> by everyone
> as a figure-of-eight
> written sideways on.
> But all of a sudden
> I now apprehend
> that eight is infinity
> standing on end.

Hein began publishing short poems in Danish magazines and newspapers during the 1930's, in particular in one of the leading Copenhagen dailies, *Politiken*. Here the grooks were printed regularly after the German occupation of Denmark on April 9, 1940, often containing veiled allusions to the German forces. Originally, the grooks were published under the pseudonym Kumbel Kumbell. Gradually, however, as their popularity grew, Hein used only the signature "Kumbel" on all his collections of grooks; his other poetry is published under his own name. An important feature of the grooks is that almost all are accompanied by a drawing. Even in his first collection, Hein worked as his own illustrator, placing himself in the center of the universe of the drawings as a little poet, usually with hat, bow tie, and lyre. His line is slim and elegant, and the illustrations are indispensable supplements to the text, which is set either in Hein's characteristic handwriting or in the corresponding typeface, Helvetica, in order to emphasize the graphic effect.

"Grook" found its way into Danish dictionaries. Hein's grooks have their roots in the Old Norse Hávámál poems and share with them a wisdom about life expressed in concentrated form. With occasional sarcasm—yet free of any moralizing—they convey their message in a cathartic burst of humor, often based on paradoxical statements, puns, and other forms of wordplay, couched in sophisticated rhymes and rhythms. Underlying the grooks is always a cosmic and existen-

tial appeal—"As eternity is reckoned, there's a lifetime in a second"—as well as words to the wise on the art of living: "Love while you've got/ love to give./ Live while you've got/ life to live." Such injunctions to enjoy life here and now are frequently balanced, however, by warnings against intolerance and persecution: "Men, said the Devil,/ are good to their brothers:/ they don't want to mend/ their own ways, but each other's." Hein saw regimentation, ideology, and national and economic boundaries as barriers to human development. After World War II, there was no direct political sting in the grooks, but one would be hard-pressed to find a pithier warning to *Homo politicus* than Hein's rephrasing of Hamlet's "To be or not to be": "Coexistence/ or no existence."

DEN TIENDE MUSE

To his own generation, Hein was a traditionalist. His formal achievement lies in the turning of the common idiom toward the uncommon insight. Hein's intellectual and linguistic agility was most apparent in the grooks, but even in his more conventional poetry, the emotional and potentially sentimental elements were subordinated to the speculative. Thus, when Hein rapturously described Danish landscapes, his impressions of nature became points of departure for philosophical reflections. He employed the same method in poetically sketching various writers and scientists, congenial spirits to whom he felt closely related, while actually presenting his own worldview. In his first volume, *Den tiende Muse* (the tenth Muse), Hein addressed poems to three of the most prominent humanistic spirits of modern civilization: Niels Bohr, who since his youth had been a friend; Albert Einstein, whom he frequently visited at Princeton; and Norbert Wiener, the founder of cybernetics, who wrote his last book while staying at Hein's home in Rungsted. In this volume, as well as in the collections *Vers af denne verden* (verses from this world) and *Du skal plante et træ* (you shall plant a tree), Hein presented the quintessence of his worldview: a cosmic perspective, a strong contempt for pretense and artificiality, and an adjuration to fight prejudice and to rescue the planet from the threat of annihilation.

It is this appeal to humane reason, this urgent request for universal solidarity, which gives Hein's work its timeless authority. Poet and designer, scientist and philosopher, Hein was an exemplary humanist who urged people to look to the future and the well-being of humankind.

OTHER MAJOR WORKS

NONFICTION: *Helicopteren*, 1947.

MISCELLANEOUS: *Man skal gaa paa Jorden—*, 1944; *Ord*, 1949; *—Selvom den er gloende*, 1950; *Vis Electrica*, 1962; *Kilden og krukken*, 1963.

BIBLIOGRAPHY

Andersen, Hans Christian. "From Grook to Superellipsoid." *The Guardian*, May 4, 1996, p. 228. A lengthy obituary of Hein that looks at his numerous achievements.

Berdichevsky, Norman. "Piet Hein: A Dane to Remember." *Scandinavian Review* 92, no. 1 (Summer, 2004): 16-24. Contains a discussion of the life and works of the poet and scientist.

Claudi, J. *Contemporary Danish Authors*. Copenhagen: Danske Selskab, 1952. Contains a brief profile of Hein and his work up to 1950. Includes a historical outline of Danish literature.

Rossel, Sven H., ed. *A History of Danish Literature*. Vol. 1 in *A History of Scandinavian Literatures*. Lincoln: University of Nebraska Press, 1992. A historical and critical study of Danish Literature. Mentions Hein only briefly but provides background for understanding him. Includes bibliographic references and index.

Sven H. Rossel

HEINRICH HEINE

Born: Düsseldorf, Prussia (now in Germany); December 13, 1797
Died: Paris, France; February 17, 1856
Also known as: Christian Johann Heinrich Heine

PRINCIPAL POETRY

Gedichte, 1822 (*Poems*, 1937)
Tragödien, nebst einem lyrischen Intermezzo, 1823 (*Tragedies, Together with Lyric Intermezzo*, 1905)
Buch der Lieder, 1827 (*Book of Songs*, 1856)
Deutschland: Ein Wintermärchen, 1844 (*Germany: A Winter's Tale*, 1892)
Neue Gedichte, 1844 (8 volumes; *New Poems*, 1858)
Atta Troll, 1847 (English translation, 1876)
Ein Sommernachtstraum, 1847 (*A Midsummer Night's Dream*, 1876)
Romanzero, 1851 (English translation, 1859)
Gedichte, 1851-1857 (4 volumes; *Poems*, 1937)
Letzte Gedichte und Gedanken, 1869 (*Last Poems and Thoughts*, 1937)
Atta Troll, and Other Poems, 1876 (includes *Atta Troll* and *A Midsummer Night's Dream*)
Heinrich Heine: The Poems, 1937
The Complete Poems of Heinrich Heine, 1982

OTHER LITERARY FORMS

Although Heinrich Heine (HI-nuh) is best remembered for his verse, he also made significant contributions to the development of the feuilleton and the political essay in Germany. Experiments with prose accelerated his rise to fame as a writer. Among the most important of his nonfiction works are *Reisebilder* (1826-1831; *Pictures of Travel*, 1855), a series of witty essays that are spiced with poetic imagination and penetrating social commentary; *Zur Geschichte der neueren schönen Litteratur in Deutschland* (1833; *Letters Auxiliary to the History of Modern Polite Literature in Germany*, 1836), which was later republished and expanded as *Die romantische Schule* (1836; *The Romantic School*, 1876) and constitutes Heine's personal settlement with German Romanticism; *Französische Zustände* (1833; *French Affairs*, 1889), a collection of sensitive newspaper articles about the contemporary political situation in France; and *Vermischte Schriften* (1854), a group of primarily political essays.

Heine's attempts to create in other genres were unsuccessful. During his student years in Berlin, he began a novel, *Der Rabbi von Bacherach* (1887; *The Rabbi of Bacherach*, 1891), but it remained a fragment. Two dramas, *Almansor* and *William Ratliff*, published in *Tragedies, Together with Lyric Intermezzo*, failed on the stage, although *William Ratliff* was later employed by Pietro Mascagni as the basis of an opera.

ACHIEVEMENTS

Second only to Johann Wolfgang von Goethe in impact on the history of German lyric poetry in the nineteenth century, Heinrich Heine was unquestionably the most controversial poet of his time. He was a major representative of the post-Romantic literary crisis and became the most renowned love poet in Europe after Petrarch, yet for decades he was more celebrated abroad than in Germany. Anti-Semitism and negative reactions to his biting satire, to his radical inclinations, and to his seemingly unpatriotic love of France combined to prevent any consistent approbation in Heine's homeland. Nevertheless, he became the first Jewish author to break into the mainstream of German literature in modern times.

Heine's poetic reputation is based primarily on *Book of Songs*, which went through twelve editions during his lifetime. The collection achieved immediate popularity with the public and was well received by critics; since 1827, it has been translated into more than fifty languages. Lyrics that became part of the *Book of Songs* were set to music as early as 1822, and within a year after the book appeared, Franz Schubert used six poems from the "Heimkehr" ("Homecoming") section in his famous cycle *Schwanengesang* (1828; "Swan Song"). Robert Schumann's *Dichterliebe* (1840; love poems) features musical settings for sixteen poems from *Tragedies, Together with Lyric Intermezzo*. By 1840, Heine's works had become prime texts for German songs. In all, more than three thousand pieces of music have been written for the creations of Heine's early period.

In 1835, four years after he went into self-imposed exile in France, Heine's works were banned in Germany, along with the writings of the social reform and literary movement Junges Deutschland (Young Germany). The critics rejected him as a bad influence on Germany's youth. His immediate popularity waned as conflicts with government censors increased. In the late nineteenth century, attempts to reclaim his works for German literature touched off riots, yet by then his enchanting lyrics had become so ingrained in German

culture that it was impossible to expel them. The measure of Heine's undying significance for German poetry is perhaps the fact that even the Nazis, who formally prohibited his works once again, could not exclude his poems completely from their anthologies of songs.

BIOGRAPHY

Heinrich Heine was born Chaim Harry Heine, the son of a Jewish merchant. He spent his early years working toward goals set for him by his family. His secondary education ended in 1814 when he left the Düsseldorf Lyceum without being graduated. After failing in two apprenticeships in Frankfurt, he was sent to Hamburg to prepare for a career in commerce under the direction of a wealthy uncle. While there, he fell in love with his cousin Amalie. This unfulfilled relationship was a stimulus for verse that the young poet published in a local periodical. In 1818, his uncle set him up in a retailing enterprise, but within a year Harry Heine and Co. was bankrupt. Acknowledging that his nephew was unsuited for business, Uncle Salomon at last agreed to underwrite his further education.

Between 1819 and 1825, Heine studied in Bonn, Berlin, and Göttingen. His university years were very important for his development as a poet. While in Bonn, he attended lectures given by August Wilhelm von Schlegel, whose interest in his work stimulated Heine's creativity. In the fall of 1820, he moved to Göttingen. Besides law, he studied German history and philology until January, 1821, when he challenged another student to a duel and was expelled from the university. He continued his studies in Berlin and was rapidly accepted into prominent literary circles. Included among the writers with whom he associated were Adelbert von Chamisso, Friedrich Schleiermacher, and Christian Dietrich Grabbe. Rahel von Varnhagen helped in the publication of Heine's first collection of poems in 1822, and he quickly became known as a promising talent. During a visit to Hamburg in 1823, he met Julius Campe, who afterward published all Heine's works except a few commissioned essays that he wrote in Paris. Literary success persuaded him away from the study of law, but at his uncle's request Heine returned to Göttingen to complete work toward his degree. In the summer of 1825, he passed his examinations, though not with distinction. To facilitate a public career, he was baptized a Protestant, at which time he changed his name to Heinrich.

Travel was a significantly formative experience for Heine. Vacations in Cuxhaven and Norderney provided initial powerful impressions of the sea that informed the two North Sea cycles of the *Book of Songs*. Journeys through the Harz Mountains in 1824, to England in 1827, and to Italy the following year provided material for the *Pictures of Travel* series that elevated him to the literary mainstream of his time. Exposure to foreign points of view also aroused his interest in current political questions and led to a brief involvement as coeditor of Johann Friedrich von Cotta's *Politische Annalen* in Munich in 1827 and 1828.

When continued efforts to obtain permission to practice law in Hamburg failed, Heine moved to Paris in 1831, where he began to write articles for French and German newspapers and journals. Heine loved Paris, and during the next few years friendships with Honoré de Balzac, Victor Hugo, George Sand, Giacomo Meyerbeer, and other writers, artists, and composers contributed to his sense of well-being. When the German Federal Diet banned his writings, making it impossible for him to continue contributing to German periodicals, the French government granted him a modest pension.

The 1840's were a stormy period in Heine's life. In 1841, he married Cresence Eugénie Mirat (whom he called Mathilde), his mistress of seven years. Her lack of education and understanding of his writings placed a strain on their relationship and later contributed to the poet's increasing isolation from his friends. After returning from Hamburg in 1843, Heine met Karl Marx. Their association sharpened Heine's political attitudes and increased his aggressive activism. Salomon Heine's death in 1844 unleashed between the writer and his cousins a struggle for the inheritance. Eventually they reached an accommodation that guaranteed an annuity in exchange for Heine's promise not to criticize family members in his writings.

After a collapse in 1848, Heine spent his remaining years in unceasing pain. An apparent venereal disease attacked his nervous system, leaving him paralyzed.

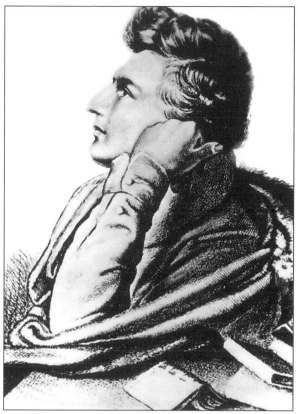

Heinrich Heine (Library of Congress)

Physical infirmities, however, did not stifle his creative spirit, and from the torment and loneliness of his "mattress grave," he wrote some of the best poetry of his career.

ANALYSIS

Unlike many poets, Heinrich Heine never stated a formal theory of poetry that could serve as a basis for interpreting his works and measuring his creative development. For that reason, confusion and critical controversy have clouded the picture of his oeuvre, resulting in misunderstandings of his literary orientation and intentions. The general concept that he was a poet of experience is, at the very least, an oversimplification. To be sure, immediate personal observations of life were a consistent stimulus for Heine's writing, yet his product is not simply a stylized reproduction of individual encounters with reality. Each poem reveals a reflective processing of unique perceptions of people, milieus, and events that transforms seemingly specific descriptions into generally valid representations of humankind's confrontation with the times. The poet's ability to convey, with penetrating exactitude, feelings, existential problems, and elements of the human condition that correspond to the concerns and apperceptions of a broad readership enabled him to generate lyrics that belong more to the poetry of ideas than to the poetry of experience.

A characteristic of Heine's thought and verse is a purposeful poetic tension between the individual and the world. The dissonance between the artistic sensibility and reality is presented in unified constructs that represent qualities that were missing from the poet's era: unity, form, constancy, and continuity. By emphasizing condition rather than event, Heine was able to offer meaningful illustrations in the juxtaposition of antithetical concepts: sunny milieu and melancholy mood, pain and witticism, affirmation and negation, enchantment of feeling and practical wisdom of experience, enthusiasm and pessimism, love and hate, spirit and reality, tradition and anticipation of the future. The magic and power of his verse arise from his ability to clothe these dynamic conflicts in deceptively simple, compact forms, pure melodic sounds and rhythms, and playfully witty treatments of theme, substance, motif, and detail.

More than anything else, Heine was a poet of mood. His greatest strengths were his sensitivity and his capacity to analyze, create, and manipulate feeling. A colorful interchange of disillusionment, scorn, cynicism, rebellion, blasphemy, playful mockery, longing, and melancholy is the essence of his appeal to the reader's spirit. The goal, however, is not the arousal of emotion but rather the intensification of awareness, achieved by drawing the audience into a desired frame of feeling, then shattering the illusion in a breach of mood that typifies Heine's poetry.

Although he was not a true representative of any single German literary movement, Heine wrote poems that reflect clear relationships to definite intellectual and artistic traditions. Both the German Enlightenment and German Romanticism provided him with important models. In matters of form, attitude, and style, he was a child of the Enlightenment. Especially visible are his epigrammatic technique and the tendency toward didactic exemplification and pointed representation. Gotthold Ephraim Lessing was his favorite among Enlightenment authors. Heine combined the technical aspects of Enlightenment literary approach with a pronounced Romantic subjectivity in the handling of substance, theme, and motif, particularly in the examination of self, pain, experience, and condition. The absolute status of the self is a prominent characteristic of his works. In the emancipation of self, however, he carried the thoughtful exploration of personal individuality a step beyond that of the early Romantics and in so doing separated himself from them. Other Romantic traits in his lyrics include a dreamy fantasy of feeling and a pronounced element of irony. Where Friedrich Schlegel employed irony to transcend the restrictive material world and unite humankind with a spiritual cosmos, Heine used it to expand the self to encompass the cosmos. The feature of Romanticism with which Heine most consciously identified was the inclination of Joseph von Eichendorff and others toward simple musical poems modeled on the German folk song. Heine specifically acknowledged the influence of Wilhelm Müller, whose cultivation of pure sound and clear simplicity most closely approximated his own poetic ideal.

In many respects, the polish of language and form that marked Heine's *Book of Songs* was never surpassed in later collections. At most a strengthening of intonation, an increase in wit, a maturing of the intellect subtly and gradually enhanced his writings with the passing years. Nevertheless, his literary career can be divided into four distinct phases with regard to material focus and poetic concern.

EARLY YEARS

Heine's initial creative period encompassed his university years and reached its peak in the mid-1820's. In *Poems*, the cycle of verse in *Tragedies, Together with Lyric Intermezzo*, and, finally, *Book of Songs*, the young poet opened a world of personal subjectivity at the center of which is a self that undergoes unceasing examination. Consciousness of the self, its suffering and loneliness, is the essence of melodic compositions that include poems of unrequited love, lyrical mood pictures, satires, romances, confessions, and parodies. Lines and stanzas deftly reflect Heine's ability to feel his way into nature, the magic of legend, and the spiritual substance of humankind, while the poetic world remains a fragmentary manifestation of the subjective truthfulness of the moment.

THE SELF AS A MIRROR OF THE TIMES

A major change in orientation coincided with Heine's move to Paris. The political upheaval in France and the death of Goethe signaled the end of an artistic era, and Heine looked forward to the possibility of a different literature that would replace the subjectivity of Romanticism with a new stress on life, time, and reality. He was especially attracted to the Saint-Simonian religion, which inspired within him a hope for a modern doctrine that would offer a new balance between Judeo-Christian ideals and those of classical antiquity. The lyrics in *New Poems*, the major document of this period, reveal a shift in emphasis from the self per se to the self as a mirror of the times. Heine's poetry of the 1830's is shallower than his earlier creations, yet it effectively presents the inner turmoil, confusion, and splintering of the era as Heine experienced it. Accompanying a slightly faded reprise of earlier themes is a new view of the poet as a heathen cosmopolitan who affirms material reality and champions the moment as having eternal value.

POLITICAL RADICALIZATION

The third stage in Heine's career is best described as a period of political radicalization. It most visibly affected his poetry during the mid-1840's, the time of his friendship with Marx. In the aggressively satirical epics *Atta Troll* and *Germany: A Winter's Tale*, he paired sharp criticism of contemporary conditions with revelations of his love for Germany, specifically attacking his own critics, radical literature, militant nationalism, student organizations, the German hatred of the French, the fragmented condition of the German nation, and almost everything else that was valued by the establishment.

LAST OF THE ROMANTICS

Profound isolation and intense physical pain provided the catalyst for a final poetic reorientation after Heine's physical collapse in 1848. Some of the poems that he wrote in his "mattress grave" are among his greatest masterpieces; they reflect a new religiosity in spiritual penetration of the self. In *Romanzero* and

other late poems, the poet becomes a kind of martyr, experiencing the world's illness in his own heart. The act of suffering generates a poetry of bleak glosses of the human condition, heartrending laments, and songs about death unequaled in German literature.

Although Heine styled himself the last of the Romantics, a significant difference in approach to substance distinguishes his early poems from those of the Romantic movement. Where Clemens Maria Brentano and Eichendorff celebrated existence as it opened itself to them, Heine sang of a life that had closed its doors, shutting him out. The dominant themes of his *Book of Songs* are longing and suffering as aspects of the experience of disappointed love. Combining the sentimental pessimism of Lord Byron with the objective portrayal of tangible reality, he succeeded in exploring love's frustrations and pain more effectively, more impressively, and more imaginatively than any of his forerunners and contemporaries had done. In dream images, songs, romances, and sonnets that employ Romantic materials yet remain suspicious of the feelings that they symbolize, the poet transformed the barrier that he felt existed between himself and the world into deceptively simple, profoundly valid treatments of universal problems.

BOOK OF SONGS

The poems of *Book of Songs* are extraordinarily flexible, self-contained productions that derive their charm from the combination of supple form and seemingly directly experienced and personally felt content. Colorful sketches of lime trees, an ancient bastion, a city pond, a whistling boy, gardens, people, fields, forests, a mill wheel, and an old tower contribute to a world of great fascination and sensual seduction. The verse is often bittersweet, however, focusing not on the sunny summer landscape but on the sadness of the poet who does not participate in a beauty that mocks him. The forceful presentation of the individual's isolation and conflict with the times represented a fresh direction in poetry that contributed greatly to Heine's early popularity. At the same time, the carefully constructed tension between the poet and his surroundings established a pattern that became characteristic of all his works.

An extremely important feature of these early lyrics is the break in mood that typically occurs at several levels, including tone, setting, and the lyricist's subjective interpretation of his situation. The tone frequently shifts from emotional to conversational, from delicate to blunt, while the settings of the imagination are shattered by the banal reality of modern society. As the poet analyzes his position vis-à-vis his milieu, his positive feeling is broken by frustration and defeat, his hope collapses beneath the awareness of his delusion, and his attraction to his beloved is marred by her unthinking cruelty. There is never any resolution of these conflicts, and the poem itself provides the only mediation between the writer and a hostile world.

Among the most exquisite compositions in *Book of Songs* are the rustically simple lyric paintings from "Die Harzreise" ("The Journey to the Harz") and the rhythmically powerful, almost mystical studies from the two cycles of "Die Nordsee" ("The North Sea"). Filled with the fairy-tale atmosphere of the Rhine and the Harz Mountains, "The Journey to the Harz" poems exemplify Heine's ability to capture the compelling musicality and inner tone of the folk song and to combine these elements with an overwhelming power of feeling in the formation of an intense poetry of mood. In "The North Sea," he cultivated a new kind of language, anticipating twentieth century verse in free rhythms that sounded the depths of elemental human experience. Constant motion, changing patterns of light, play of wind, and movement of ships and fish combine as parts of a unified basic form. Heine pinpointed the individuality of the ocean in a given moment, reproducing atmosphere with precision and intensifying impact through mythological or human ornamentation. The rolling flow of impression is a consistent product of Heine's poetic art in its finest form.

NEW POEMS

Two years after moving to Paris, Heine published *Letters Auxiliary to the History of Modern Polite Literature in Germany*, his most significant theoretical treatise on literature and a work that marked his formal break with Romanticism. The major poetic document of this transition to a more realistic brand of expression is *New Poems*, a less integrated collection than *Book of Songs*, containing both echoes of early themes and the first fruits of his increased political commitment of the 1840's. *New Poems* attests strongly a shift in approach

and creative concern from poetry as an absolute to the demand for contemporary relevance.

The first cycle of *New Poems*, "Neuer Frühling" ("New Spring"), returns to the motifs that dominate the "Lyric Intermezzo" and "Homecoming" segments of *Book of Songs* yet presents them with greater polish and distance. New variations portray love as a distraction, a nuisance that causes emotional turmoil in the inherent knowledge of its transitoriness. The tone and direction of the entire volume are established in the prologue to "New Spring," in which the poet contrasts his own subjection to the hindering influence of love with the strivings of others in "the great struggle of the times."

Among the other sections of the book, "Verschiedene" ("Variae"), with its short cycles of rather acidic poems about the girls of Paris, its legendary ballad "Der Tannhäuser" ("Tannhäuser"), and its "Schöpfungslieder" ("Songs of Creation"), is the least coherent, most disturbing group of poems that Heine ever wrote. Campe, his publisher, decried the lyricist's creation of what he called "whore and chamber-pot stories" and was extremely reluctant to publish them. Nothing that Heine wrote, however, is without artistic value, and there are nuggets of brilliance even here. Despite its artificiality and seeming inconsistency with Heine's true poetic nature, "Tannhäuser," for example, must be regarded as one of his greatest masterpieces. The deeply psychological rejuvenation of the old folk epic, which served as the stimulus for Richard Wagner's opera, reflects the poet's all-encompassing and penetrating knowledge of the human heart.

"Zeitgedichte" ("Poems of the Times"), the concluding cycle in *New Poems*, sets the pattern for Heine's harsh political satire of the 1840's. Some of the lyrics were written expressly for Karl Marx's newspaper *Vorwärts*. Most of them are informed by homesickness, longing, and the bitter disappointment that Heine felt as the expected dawn of spiritual freedom in Germany failed to materialize in the evolution of a more cosmopolitan relationship with the rest of Europe. Powerful poems directed against cultural, social, and political dilettantes anticipate the incisively masterful tones of his most successful epics of the period, *Atta Troll* and *Germany: A Winter's Tale*; irreverent assaults on cherished institutions, superficial political activism, and his own critics accent his peculiar love-hate relationship with his homeland.

ROMANZERO

Regarded by many critics as Heine's finest collection of poems, *Romanzero* presents his final attempts to come to grips with his own mortality. Rich in their sophistication, more coherent in tone than the lyrics of *New Poems* or even the *Book of Songs*, the romances, laments, and melodies of *Romanzero* reveal the wit, irony, and epigrammatic style for which Heine is famous in the service of a new, peculiarly transparent penetration of the self. Dominant in the poems is the theme of death, which confronts the individual in many forms. A new religiosity is present in the acknowledgment of a personal God with whom the poet quarrels about a divine justice that is out of phase with humankind's needs. Individual creations pass through the spectrum of human and religious history and into the future in the expectation of a new social order. Bitter pessimism unmasks the dreams of life, pointing to the defeat of that which is noble and beautiful and the triumph of the worse human being over the better as the derisive law of the world. Voicing the mourning and bitter resistance of the tormented soul, Heine transforms personal confrontation with suffering and death into a timeless statement of universal experience.

Romanzero is divided into three main parts, each of which projects a substantial array of feeling: seriousness, despair, goodness, compassion, a longing for faith, bitterness, and mature composure. The first section, "Historien" ("Stories"), is composed of discursive, sometimes rambling narrative ballads and romances dealing with the tragedies of kings, heroes, and poets. Some of them process through a temporal distance such typical Heine themes as the yearning for love, clothing them in historical trappings. Others, such as the cruel poem "Vitzliputzli" that ends the cycle, are profound discourses on humans' inhumanity toward their own kind. The poems of "Lamentationen" ("Lamentations"), the second major section, are directly confessional in form: deeply moving cries of anguish, sublime expressions of horror, statements of longing for home. The "Lazarus" poems that conclude this portion of *Romanzero* are especially vivid documents of the

poet's individual suffering in a world where God seems to be indifferent. In "Hebräische Melodien" ("Hebrew Melodies"), the last segment of the collection, Heine presented the essence of his reidentification with Judaism. Three long poems explore the broad dimensions of Jewish culture, history, and tradition, ending with an almost sinister medieval disputation between Christian and Jew that evolves into a tragicomic anticlerical satire. Thumbing his nose at irrational action, intolerance, and superstition, the poet offers a dying plea for humanism.

No other volume presents Heine so thoroughly in all his heights and depths, perfection and error, wit and seriousness. Captivating for the directness of despairing and contrite confession, repelling for its boastful, sometimes vicious cynicism, *Romanzero*, as perhaps no other work in the history of German lyric poetry, reveals the hubris of the problematic individual and penetrates the facade of the bright fool's drama that is life.

OTHER MAJOR WORKS

LONG FICTION: *Der Rabbi von Bacherach*, 1887 (*The Rabbi of Bacherach*, 1891).

SHORT FICTION: *Aus den Memoiren des Herrn von Schnabelewopsky*, 1910 (*The Memoirs of Herr von Schnabelewopski*, 1876).

PLAYS: *Almansor*, pb. 1821 (English translation, 1905); *Der Doktor Faust*, pb. 1851 (libretto; *Doktor Faust*, 1952).

NONFICTION: *Briefe aus Berlin*, 1822; *Reisebilder*, 1826-1831 (4 volumes; *Pictures of Travel*, 1855); *Die Bäder von Lucca*, 1829 (*The Baths of Lucca*, 1855); *Französische Zustände*, 1833 (*French Affairs*, 1889); *Zur Geschichte der neueren schönen Literatur in Deutschland*, 1833 (*Letters Auxiliary to the History of Modern Polite Literature in Germany*, 1836); *Der Salon*, 1834-1840 (4 volumes; *The Salon*, 1893); *Zur Geschichte der Religion und Philosophie in Deutschland*, 1835 (*On the History of Religion and Philosophy in Germany*, 1876); *Die romantische Schule*, 1836 (expansion of *Zur Geschichte der Religion und Philosophie in Deutschland*; *The Romantic School*, 1876); *Über die französische Bühne*, 1837 (*Concerning the French Stage*, 1891-1905); *Shakespeares Mädchen und Frauen*, 1838 (*Shakespeare's Maidens and Ladies*, 1891); *Ludwig Börne: Eine Denkschrift von H. Heine*, 1840 (*Ludwig Börne: Recollections of a Revolutionist*, 1881); *Les Dieux en exil*, 1853 (*Gods in Exile*, 1962); *Lutetia: Berichte über Politik, Kunst, und Volksleben*, 1854 (*Lutetia: Reports on Politics, Art, and Popular Life*, 1891-1905); *Vermischte Schriften*, 1854 (3 volumes); *De l'Allemagne*, 1855 (2 volumes).

MISCELLANEOUS: *The Works of Heinrich Heine*, 1891-1905 (12 volumes).

BIBLIOGRAPHY

Cook, Roger F., ed. *A Companion to the Works of Heinrich Heine*. Rochester, N.Y.: Camden House, 2002. A collection of essays that examine Heine's work; topics include the eroticism, Jewish culture, mythology, and modernity in his poems.

Heady, Katy. *Literature and Censorship in Restoration Germany: Repression and Rhetoric*. Rochester, N.Y.: Camden House, 2009. This work on the censorship of literature that occurred in Restoration Germany examines how the intellectual and political climate affected Heine.

Hermand, Jost, and Robert C. Holub, eds. *Heinrich Heine's Contested Identities: Politics, Religion, and Nationalism in Nineteenth-Century Germany*. New York: Peter Lang, 1999. A collection of essays concerning Heine's identity, which was formed and reformed, revised and modified, in relationship to the politics, religion, and nationalism of his era. The essays offer an understanding of Heine's predicaments and choices as well as the parameters placed on him by the exigencies of the time.

Justis, Diana Lynn. *The Feminine in Heine's Life and Oeuvre: Self and Other*. New York: Peter Lang, 1997. Heine's literary representations of women and interactions with women vividly demonstrate his position as a marginal German-Jewish writer of the nineteenth century. Heine, like many Jews of that era, internalized the European cultural stereotype of the Jew as "woman," that is, as essentially inferior and marginal.

Pawel, Ernst. *The Poet Dying: Heinrich Heine's Last Years in Paris*. New York: Farrar, Straus and Giroux, 1995. In this biography of Heine, Pawel portrays a poet at the height of his creativity in the last eight years of his life, when he was confined to his bed with a mysterious ailment.

Phelan, Anthony. *Reading Heinrich Heine*. New York: Cambridge University Press, 2007. Examines Heine's poetry from the earliest to his last, and argues that Heine is a major contributor to the articulation of modernity.

Lowell A. Bangerter

ZBIGNIEW HERBERT

Born: Lvov, Poland (now Lvov, Ukraine); October 29, 1924
Died: Warsaw, Poland; July 28, 1998

PRINCIPAL POETRY

Struna światła, 1956
Hermes, pies i gwiazda, 1957
Studium przedmiotu, 1961
Selected Poems, 1968
Napis, 1969
Poezje wybrane, 1970
Wiersze zebrane, 1971
Pan Cogito, 1974 (*Mr. Cogito*, 1993)
Selected Poems, 1977
Raport z oblężonego miasta i inne wiersze, 1983 (*Report from the Besieged City, and Other Poems*, 1985)
Elegia na odejście, 1990 (translation in *Elegy for the Departure, and Other Poems*, 1999)
Elegy for the Departure, and Other Poems, 1999
The Collected Poems, 1956-1998, 2007 (Robert Hass, editor)

OTHER LITERARY FORMS

Zbigniew Herbert (KEHR-behrt) was primarily a poet, but he was also a prose writer of considerable originality and distinction. A collection of essays titled *Barbarzyńca w ogrodzie* (*Barbarian in the Garden*, 1985) appeared in Poland in 1962; these essays are a unique combination of personal, richly poetic, firsthand description with analytical, scholarly research.

Herbert also wrote several plays, including radio plays as well as works for the stage; a collection of his dramatic works was published in 1970 under the title *Dramaty* (plays).

In addition, Herbert published works in a genre of his own invention, his "apocryphas." These prose pieces are a synthesis of the short story and the essay; they contest traditional accounts or interpretations of major historical events and present the very different ("apocryphal") interpretations of the author. Although most of Herbert's apocryphas take their subjects from Western European history, some go farther afield—to Chinese history, for example.

ACHIEVEMENTS

Zbigniew Herbert exerted great influence as a poet and as a moral force both in Poland and Western Europe. He was above all the spokesperson of the individual conscience. He excited interest as a political poet, but although his poems addressed major political issues, they went far beyond immediate issues and encompassed a broad range of problems that are both philosophical and personal. Herbert resisted categorization and never represented a group or school of any kind. He gave the impression of being entirely alone, answerable only to his conscience—yet he managed at the same time to pitch his voice in such a way that he was one of the most authentically public poets of the age. This was the paradox of Herbert that gives his poetry its particular stamp.

Although Herbert was an antirhetorical poet, it is difficult to separate the content of his writing from his style. His poetic forms and rhythms exerted a powerful influence on other poets. One of the two greatest living Polish poets (the other, Czesław Miłosz, has translated a number of Herbert's poems into English), his influence has been acknowledged not only by younger Polish poets such as Ryszard Krynicki, Stanisław Barańczak, and Jacek Bierezin but also by a wide range of poets in the United States and throughout the West.

Herbert's influence was recognized with several awards throughout his career. In 1958, he won the Polish Radio Competition Prize, and in 1964, he received the Millennium Prize from the Polish Institute of Arts and Sciences (United States). For his contribution to European literature, he was awarded the Nickolas Lenau Prize (Austria) in 1965. In 1973, he received both the Alfred Jurzykowski Prize and the Herder Prize. He also won the Petrarch Prize in 1979, the Bruno Schulz Prize in 1988, the Jerusalem Literature Prize in 1991, and a Jurzykowski Foundation Award.

BIOGRAPHY

Zbigniew Herbert grew up in the Polish city of Lvov; in 1939, when he was fifteen years old, this part of Poland was invaded by the Soviet Union. Herbert began to write poetry during World War II, and the war permanently shaped his outlook. The face of postwar Poland was permanently changed, socially, physically, and politically: Herbert's native city became part of the Soviet Union.

In 1944, Herbert studied at the Academy of Fine Arts in Kraków—he was always interested in painting, sculpture, and architecture—and a year later, he entered the Academy of Commerce, also in Kraków. In

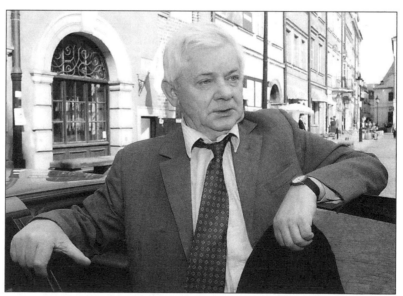

Zbigniew Herbert (AP/Wide World Photos)

1947, he received a master's degree in economics and moved to Toruń, where he studied law at the Nicolas Copernicus University. He received the degree of master of laws in 1950. Herbert stayed on in Toruń to study philosophy and was influenced by the philosopher Henryk Eizenberg. In 1950, he lived briefly in Gdańsk and worked there for the *Merchant's Review* before moving to Warsaw, where for the next six years, he held a variety of jobs: in the management office of the peat industry, in the department for retired pensioners of the Teachers' Cooperative, in a bank, in a store, and in the legal department of the Composers' Association.

Herbert's poems began to appear in periodicals in 1950, but no collection was published in book form; during the increasing social and cultural repression of the Stalinist years, several of the magazines publishing Herbert's work were closed by the government. It was only after the "thaw" of 1956 that his first two collections of poems were published, almost simultaneously. The event of publication after enforced silence is poignantly described in Herbert's poem "Drawer."

In the late 1950's, Herbert made his first trip to Western Europe. His collection of essays, *Barbarian in the Garden*, reveals the impact of this experience. Herbert spent 1965 to 1971 abroad, based in West Berlin but traveling to many countries, among them Greece, Italy, France, and the United States. He spent the 1970-1971 academic year teaching at California State University, Los Angeles. After returning to Poland to live in 1971, Herbert moved to West Berlin again in 1974, staying there intermittently until 1980, when he returned to Warsaw. He again left Poland in 1986 in protest of Communist policies but returned to Warsaw once communism was ended around 1990. Around this time, his health began to deteriorate and when, in 1996, the Nobel Prize was awarded to Wisława Szymborska (only seventeen years after another Pole and adopted Californian, Czesław Miłosz), the joy of this deserved distinction was mixed with a touch of regret for Herbert. For many, Herbert's achievements equaled those of his two honored compatriots, and there were those who considered him superior to both. He died in Warsaw on July 28, 1998.

ANALYSIS

Zbigniew Herbert was a member of the generation of poets who came to maturity during World War II. They are known as the War Generation, but they are also referred to in Polish literary criticism as *Kolumbowie* (Columbuses), because it was they who first "explored" the new postwar reality. This generation proved to be one of the most talented in twentieth century Polish literature, including, in addition to Herbert, such varied figures as Tadeusz Różewicz, Miron Bialoszewski, Tymoteusz Karpowicz, Szymborska, and Anna Swir. The war left an indelible imprint on all of them; as late as 1969, in the poem "Prologue," which introduced Herbert's fourth collection of poems, he wrote about those who took part in the war: "I must carry them to a dry place/ and make a large mound of sand/ before spring strews flowers for them/ and a great green dream stupefies them."

LESSONS FROM THE WAR

Few assumptions about the world and about civilization—what it is and what it is not—survived the war unscathed. The sense of continuity was broken, and many shared the vantage point of what might be called the "rubbish heap" of the present. Herbert's poem "Przebudzenie" ("Awakening"), from *Wiersze zebrane*, is a fine description of this attitude. It begins:

> When the horror subsided the floodlights went out
> we discovered that we were on a rubbish-heap in very
>   strange poses
> . . . .
> We had nowhere to go we stayed on the rubbish-heap
> we tidied things up
> the bones and sheet iron we deposited in an archive
> We listened to the chirping of streetcars to a
>   swallow-like voice of factories
> and a new life was unrolling at our feet.

The common experience of wartime destruction and of starting a "new life" united Herbert and the other members of his generation and gave them their unique temporal perspective. They drew very different conclusions from their experiences, however, and there is no consensus of attitude or ideology among them. Herbert is sometimes linked to Różewicz, another poet who lived through the war, because they were close in age and were both moralists. Their values, however, were in fundamental conflict. Różewicz's poetry after the war denied all previous values and emphasized purely personal experience, whereas Herbert arrived at entirely different conclusions. He wrote:

> Something makes me different from the "War Generation." It seems to me that I came away from the war without accepting the failure of the earlier morality. It is still attractive to me most of all because I painfully feel the lack of tablets of values in the contemporary world.

Herbert was a more positive poet than many other members of the War Generation, although rarely have positive values been won against greater opposition and with greater struggle.

USE OF THE PAST

One of the most striking features of Herbert's poetry was the manner in which he used the past. It was remarkably alive for him; historical figures frequently appeared in his poems with the vividness of contemporaries. In Western Europe and the United States, poetry that invokes the great traditions of Western culture is often associated with reactionary values. In Poland during the decade after World War II, however, a paradoxical situation arose in which some of the writers who had most completely rejected the prewar culture found that they had little basis for rebelling against the Stalinist present; on the other hand, a poet such as Herbert, who strived to repossess the culture of the past, was able to express revolt in one of its most intense and radical forms.

It is a mistake, however, to call Herbert a classicist, as he was sometimes labeled. For him, the past was not a static source of value; he is not an antiquarian, as his poem "Classic" made clear. For Herbert, the past represented living experience rather than lifeless forms. He did not adhere to the past at the expense of the present; instead, the past is the ally of the present. The distinction is a useful one and even crucial, for Herbert's use of the past was the opposite of that of a genuine classicist such as the contemporary Polish poet Jaroslaw Rymkiewicz. Herbert felt the dead are alive, made of flesh and blood. If there was a division between the past and the present, it was often spatial rather than temporal. In Herbert's famous poem "Elegy of Fortinbras,"

he assumed the persona of Fortinbras, who addresses Hamlet as his immediate contemporary; the poem ends by translating death into terms of spatial distance: "It is not for us to greet each other or bid farewell we live on archipelagos/ and that water these words what can they do what can they do prince." The ever-present tension and dialogue between past and present did not restrict Herbert's poetry; in fact, the reverse is true: He confronted the world in all its breadth, and his experience is placed in a seamless historical continuum.

AVANT-GARDE INFLUENCE

Herbert was influenced both by the Catastrophists, such as Miłosz, who stressed philosophical and historical themes in their poetry, and by the avant-garde poets of the 1920's and the 1930's, such as Jozéf Czechowicz, who eschewed punctuation. Several other poets of Herbert's generation who lived through the war also turned to the avant-garde in their search for poetic forms that were capable of rendering their experience. Many of Herbert's early poems shared the phenomenological preoccupations of the avant-garde; at the most fundamental level, poets were asking: How can one describe the world? How can one describe one's experience? Herbert's poems "I Would Like to Describe," "Attempt at a Description," "Voice," "Episode in a Library," "Wooden Bird," "Nothing Special," and the later "Mr. Cogito Thinks About the Voice of Nature and the Human Voice" all approached this concern from different angles.

Herbert's phenomenological preoccupations are particularly apparent in his handling of punctuation. Conventional punctuation was not automatically accepted by serious poets in Poland after the war, and Herbert was by no means alone in questioning its use. Prewar avant-garde poetry still enjoyed a high esteem among poets, and punctuation also had a political coloring: Lack of conventional punctuation became associated with revolt and with individualism. Herbert's first collection of poems, *Struna światła* (chord of light), which represented work done during the first postwar decade, eschewed conventional punctuation, particularly the use of periods. In a prose poem written somewhat later, "Period," he placed punctuation in a very broad historical and social context; the poem ends: "In fact the period, which we attempt to tame at any price, is a bone protruding from the sand, a snapping shut, a sign of a catastrophe. It is a punctuation of the elements. People should employ it modestly and with proper consideration, as is customary when one replaces fate." In other words, for Herbert, the "period" marked a hiatus in the texture of the world and of reality. Its thoughtless use is presumptuous and even destructive, violating the living tissue and the continuities of the real world.

In England and America, the traditional use of punctuation was—with notable exceptions—maintained after the war; accepted practice had not been put into doubt by new experience. In Central and Eastern Europe, however, especially in those countries that had experienced the worst destruction during the war and that had suffered under Nazi occupation, conventional punctuation was sharply questioned, along with other inherited poetic practices. Indeed, punctuation became one of the major topoi, or themes, of postwar Eastern European literature.

THE PROSE POEM

Parallel to Herbert's radical reduction of punctuation (he frequently employed dashes, as well as occasional parentheses and question marks) was his development of the prose poem; much of the prose poetry written in Poland since 1957 was influenced by Herbert's explorations in the genre. While his first collection of poems was restricted to largely punctuation-free verse, his second, *Hermes, pies i gwiazda* (Hermes, dog and star), had a separate section of prose poems, comprising sixty of the book's ninety-five poems. Originally, Herbert intended these prose poems to constitute a separate volume, and he called them *bajeczki* (little fairy tales). His project was thwarted by an editor, however, and they were included in his second volume of poems. In subsequent volumes, Herbert intentionally interspersed prose poems among his punctuation-free verse poems, and this became his regular practice.

In his third collection, *Studium przedmiotu* (study of the object), the ratio of prose to verse poems is eighteen to twenty-eight; in his fourth collection, *Napis* (inscription), fourteen to twenty-six; and in his fifth, *Mr. Cogito*, five to thirty-five. The choice to use one form or the other was always highly deliberate with Herbert, depending on his attitude toward the subject of the poem, his distance from it, and his tone, as well as the rhythms he used. The more reflective poems, especially those that assume considerable distance from the subject and those that use strong irony, were frequently written in prose. The various modulations of these two basic forms were always carefully worked out. This is only one of the ways, but an important one, in which the form of Herbert's poetry is related to its content, and the resulting range of forms is astonishingly broad.

INANIMATE OBJECTS

Herbert's many poems about inanimate objects should be seen in the context of his attempt to explore the relationship between experience and reality. Herbert wrote fine poems (and again, his practice has been imitated by many younger Polish poets) about a pebble, a stool, a watch, armchairs, a clothes wringer; indeed, the title of one of Herbert's collections of poems means "study of the objects." Some readers have wondered why a poet such as Herbert, who was so consistently concerned with life and human experience, should write about lifeless objects. The poems were part of Herbert's attempt to separate what is subjective from what is objective and to see clearly. In "I Would Like to Describe," Herbert wrote: ". . . so is blurred/ in me/ what white-haired gentlemen/ separated once and for all/ and said/ this is the subject/ and this is the object." Herbert was always interested in inanimate objects but not because they are inhuman. On the contrary, he tended to find human traits in objects (rather than vice versa) and to discover a community of interest between humans and objects. In a conversation in 1969, Herbert said that he was fascinated by objects because

they are so completely different from us, and enigmatic. They come from a totally different world from ours. We are never sure that we understand them; sometimes we think so, other times we don't, depending on how much of ourselves we project on them. What I like about them is their ability to *resist* us, to be silent. We can never really conquer them or tame them, and that is good.

Thus, while Herbert humanized objects, he also respected their fundamental opacity. At the same time, there was no abyss between humans and inanimate objects—on the contrary, there is a sense of identity with them, based on the realization of human fallibility and imperfection. Herbert was engaged in breaking down the barrier between the human and the inanimate and in extending the limits of the human.

ENDURING THEMES

Herbert's first volumes contain most of the themes that interested him throughout his career; certainly, his enforced silence during the Stalinist decade in Poland, from 1946 to 1956, contributed to the ultimate strength of these poems. Others of his generation, such as Różewicz and Szymborska, adapted to the Stalinist demands and were permitted to publish; as a result, their books that appeared during this period are inferior to their later work. Herbert wrote for a long time without a public audience, but his poems assumed a firm core of consistency and strength as he developed his themes. First among them was the imperative to resist, to listen to the individual conscience; he was willing to suffer for his ideals. The moral demand to direct one's gaze at reality itself is present in Herbert's first volume, as is his gift for infusing the past with life. Some of these early poems are about the difficulty of writing after the war, about the loss of ideals; at a profound level, they reflected Herbert's formal training in philosophy—not because the poems are explicitly "philosophical" but because they are informed by an intense, overriding concern for truth and clarity. Herbert consistently directed his attention outward, at the world as it exists. It was this stance that also makes it possible to consider Herbert as a "public" poet. The lines in these early poems are relatively short; they often seem to follow the rapidity of thought, and they already display the great agility that is typical of Herbert's style.

HERMES, PIES I GWIAZDA

Herbert's second volume, *Hermes, pies i gwiazda*, is marked by the sudden infusion of prose poems in the second section. Irony becomes more prominent, and the poet's tone is increasingly mordant. The individual lines of poems are sometimes longer in this volume, although there is the same agility and rapid spontaneity of association that marked the first volume.

STUDIUM PRZEDMIOTU

Herbert's third volume, *Studium przedmiotu*, carried his dialogue with objects to its furthest point. The volume is also among his most critical, taking aim at contemporary social and political reality. As he did

this, however, Herbert evidently felt the need to assume a greater distance—critical distance—from the reality he sought to describe, and thus he adopted a variety of personas in this volume, giving his critique greater depth and historical reverberation.

NAPIS

Herbert's fourth book, *Napis*, shows a greater concern for textures, and the lines have become somewhat longer. This volume has been called Herbert's "expressionist" volume; in it, he gave full rein to his delight in dramatic metaphor. He developed further many of his previous themes, but the reader senses that there is a shift in the target of Herbert's sense of revolt. Focusing less on immediate social and political realities, the poet was increasingly concerned with the universal and the archetypal, extending back into the past and into the subconscious.

MR. COGITO

In Herbert's fifth collection of original poems, *Mr. Cogito*, the dominant theme is the identity of the self, explored through the title figure. Sometimes the persona of Mr. Cogito is entirely playful; at other times, he allows the poet to confront painful personal matters without obtrusive emotion. The volume contains a number of poems of striking philosophical depth, among them "Georg Heym—the Almost Metaphysical Adventure" and "Mr. Cogito Tells About the Temptation of Spinoza." Many poems in this book have longer lines than those of earlier volumes and are more meditative. They require a longer, deeper breath to read aloud, and some are very close to prose. A few are quite long and have a highly developed logical structure.

REPORT FROM THE BESIEGED CITY, AND OTHER POEMS

Report from the Besieged City, and Other Poems marks a sharp return to topicality and contemporary events—in this case, the coup d'état of General Wojciech Jaruzelski and the imposition of martial law. Again, events are seen in the context of a broad historical framework, but they are observed in the present, taking place under one's very eyes, as the title indicates. There are two major themes in this new collection. The first is the necessity to "bear witness" to the truth. Herbert assumed the role of chronicler of the "siege," and although he said this role is secondary to that of the people who are fighting, it is really of the utmost importance. Knowledge of the true nature of the war, the reality of the lives of those who take part in it, and even their very identity depend on the chronicler, the poet. The second major theme is suffering and the need for suffering, never presented fatalistically but rather combined with the imperative to revolt no matter how hopeless the situation. Rarely in contemporary literature has the need for resistance been stated so clearly, so forcefully, and with so few illusions.

The collection begins where "The Envoy of Mr. Cogito," the last poem in Herbert's previous volume, ended. In that poem, Herbert wrote that even if "the informers executioners cowards . . . will win," the individual must still revolt:

go upright among those who are on their knees
among those with their backs turned and those
    toppled in the dust
you were saved not in order to live
you have little time you must give testimony

. . . .

go because only in this way will you be admitted to
    the company of cold skulls
to the company of your ancestors: Gilgamesh Hector
    Roland
the defenders of the kingdom without limit and the
    city of ashes
Be faithful Go

ELEGY FOR THE DEPARTURE, AND OTHER POEMS

Elegy for the Departure, and Other Poems is made up of a translation of poems from *Elegia na odejście* (1990) as well as translations of works uncollected in English from throughout Herbert's career. Its four sections draw chronologically from his writing, and a less politicized Herbert is evident in the selected poems. Darkness was certainly pouring into Herbert's poetry and possibly into his life around the time when most of the poems from the 1990 collection were composed, but it was present in his verse from the beginning, especially in his early poems, in which he bid farewell to the ghosts of his friends fallen during the war.

The English volume opens with one such poem, called "Three Poems by Heart," which originally appeared in *Struna światła*. The first of its three move-

ments is a search for a person, or rather for a language, in which the memory of that person can be extracted from among horrifying images of wartime destruction:

I can't find the title
of a memory about you
with a hand torn from darkness
I step on fragments of faces
soft friendly profiles
frozen into a hard contour.

Readers will discern that here Herbert's voice is growing more personal, his irony more astringent. His stoicism seems to falter in the face of very human and basic fear, as in "Prayer of the Old Men," that ends on a mournful, pleading note:

but don't allow us
to be devoured
by the insatiable darkness of your altars
say just one thing
that we will return later

The book's last section, focused on Herbert's late poetry, contains some of his most spacious work, a groundspring of vitality and variety. There is a tarantella of a poem about Leo Tolstoy fleeing family and keepers at the end "with great bounds/ his beard streaming behind." There is a somber, perfectly tuned image of Emperor Hirohito, history's wildness departed, laboring over a *tanka* (a genre of Japanese poem) about the state railroad. There is the unsparingly registered loss of "Prayer of the Old Men":

when the children women patient animals have left
because they can't bear wax hands
we listen to sand pouring in our veins
and in our dark interior grows a white church
of salt memories calcium and unspeakable weakness.

The book ends with the expansive "Elegy for the Departure of Pen Ink and Lamp," in which Herbert laments the three objects presented in the poem both as companions of studious childhood and as symbols of the three ideas most often associated with "the Herbertian" vision: the critical mind, a "gentle volcano" of imagination, and "a spirit stubbornly battling" the darker demons of the soul. The tone of the poem is cryptic, and readers are unable to discern the nature of the personal catastrophe that seems to lie at its center. One learns only that the departure of the objects was caused by an unspecified "betrayal" on the part of the speaker and that it leaves him feeling guilty and power-less. The book ends with last words of the poem: "and that it will be/ dark." With that, the door closed on the work of Herbert.

OTHER MAJOR WORKS

PLAYS: *Jaskina filozofów*, pb. 1970 (wr. 1950's; *The Philosophers' Den*, 1958); *Dramaty*, 1970 (collection of four plays).

NONFICTION: *Barbarzyńca w ogrodzie*, 1962 (*Barbarian in the Garden*, 1985); *Martwa natura z wędzidłem*, 1993 (*Still Life with a Bridle: Essays and Apocryphas*, 1991); *The King of the Ants: Mythological Essays*, 1999.

BIBLIOGRAPHY

Anders, Jaroslaw. *Between Fire and Sleep: Essays on Modern Polish Poetry and Prose*. New Haven, Conn.: Yale University Press, 2009. Contains a chapter on Herbert that provides extensive analysis and notes the exploration of darkness in his poetry.

Barańczak, Stanisław. *A Fugitive from Utopia: The Poetry of Zbigniew Herbert*. Cambridge, Mass.: Harvard University Press, 1987. A useful introduction, one of the first book-length studies published in English.

Carpenter, Bogdana. "*The Barbarian in the Garden*: Zbigniew Herbert's Reevaluations." *World Literature Today* 57, no. 3 (Summer, 1983): 388-393. Excellent coverage in English by Herbert's translator.

Carpenter, Bogdana, and John Carpenter. Afterword to *Selected Poems*, by Zbigniew Herbert. 1977. Reprint. Kraków: Wydawnictwo Literackie, 2007. The translators' afterword to a reprint of *Selected Poems* provides a biography and some analysis of the works.

Hacht, Anne Marie, and David Kelly, eds. *Poetry for Students*. Vol. 22. Detroit: Thomson/Gale, 2005. Analyzes Herbert's "Why the Classics." Contains the poem, summary, themes, style, historical context, critical overview, and criticism. Includes bibliography and index.

Kraszewski, Charles. *Essays on the Dramatic Works of the Polish Poet Zbigniew Herbert*. Lewiston, N.Y.: E. Mellen Press, 2002. Five essays on Herbert as playwright, comparing his drama with his poetry.

Nizynska, Joanna. "Marsyas's Howl: The Myth of Marsyas in Ovid's *Metamorphoses* and Zbigniew Herbert's 'Apollo and Marsyas.'" *Comparative Literature* 53, no. 2 (2001): 151-170. Compares the Roman and Polish uses of the myth, emphasizing Herbert's "translation" of the story.

Shallcross, Bozena. *Through the Poet's Eye: The Travels of Zagajewski, Herbert, and Bridsky*. Evanston, Ill.: Northwestern University Press, 2002. Analyzes Herbert's *The Barbarian in the Garden*, focusing on the poet as traveler and observer.

Wood, Sharon. "The Reflections of Mr. Palomar and Mr. Cogito: Italo Calvino and Zbigniew Herbert." *Modern Language Notes* 109, no. 1 (1994): 128-142. Compares the two writers' creations of alter egos.

Zagajewski, Adam. Introduction to *The Collected Poems, 1956-1998*, Zbigniew Herbert. Translated and edited by Alissa Valles. New York: Ecco, 2007. Informative introduction that provides background and critical analysis.

John Carpenter
Updated by Sarah Hilbert

HESIOD

Born: Ascra, Greece; fl. c. 700 B.C.E.
Died: Ozolian Locris, Greece(?); date unknown

PRINCIPAL POETRY

Erga kai Emerai, c. 700 B.C.E. (*Works and Days*, 1618)
Theogonia, c. 700 B.C.E. (*Theogony*, 1728)
Works of Hesiod and the Homeric Hymns, 2005

OTHER LITERARY FORMS

Hesiod (HEE-see-uhd) is remembered only for his poetic works. A number of poems are erroneously attributed to Hesiod, among them *Shield* (c. 700 B.C.E.) and *Catalogue of Women* (c. 700 B.C.E.).

ACHIEVEMENTS

Hesiod was respected, next to Homer, as a leading poet-teacher of the early Greeks, and his reputation stood all but unchallenged throughout Greco-Roman antiquity. For lack of a better term, he is sometimes described as a didactic poet, although neither of his poems follows the strict definition of a genre that took shape more than four centuries later in the Hellenistic age. Hesiod adapted the formulaic style, meter, and vocabulary of the Homeric epic to two ancient genres from the Near East. The *Theogony* is Hesiod's version of the type of creation epic found in the opening chapters of the biblical Genesis, and it had a formative influence on the great classical poets from Aeschylus to Ovid, similar to the hold that the book of Genesis has had on poetic imaginations in the Christian era. The *Works and Days* springs from an equally ancient genre, the protreptic "wisdom literature" that influenced several books of the Old Testament and that can be traced back as far as the third millennium B.C.E. In Greece's more secular civilization, Hesiod's works never attained the status of holy writ; it was never supposed that the *Theogony* or the *Works and Days* was divinely inspired (save in a general way by the Muses) or that the myths contained in them were canonical. Hesiod's writings have a religious and moral fervor, however, and his version of Greek mythology, although far from complete, remains the most important systematic account of the Olympian deities to the present day.

BIOGRAPHY

Most of the available information about Hesiod's life comes from his own poetry. In the *Works and Days*, he says that his father came from Cyme, an Aeolian Greek town on the west coast of Anatolia about thirty miles southeast of Lesbos, and worked as a merchant seaman until hard times forced him to relocate to a homestead across the Aegean, in poor country northeast of Mount Helicon, in Boeotia. Hesiod was born and reared on his father's farm in Ascra, which he describes as "nasty in winter, disagreeable in the summer, and never good." In the *Theogony*, he describes his in-

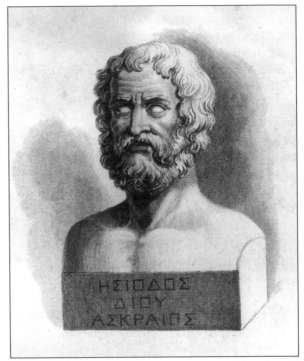

Hesiod (Hulton Archive/Getty Images)

vesture as a poet by the Muses while he was herding sheep at the foot of Mount Helicon. The parallels to this scene are Eastern, recalling the shepherd Moses, called by God away from his sheep, and Amos, summoned from his herds to prophesy. Another passage in the *Works and Days* tells of winning a trophy for a hymn at a festival in Chalcis on the nearby island of Euboea. Several references to a dispute with his brother Perses in the *Works and Days* indicate that Perses bribed the authorities when their father's estate was divided and took more than his share, but squandered his ill-gotten gain and came begging to his brother. In the *Works and Days*, Hesiod uses the occasion of Perses' unjust behavior as the context for his discussion of *Dikē* (justice) and *Hybris* (violence).

The traditional belief that Homer and Hesiod once met in a poetry contest and a supposed text of the contest (the *Agon*) are rejected by modern scholars. Thucydides adds that Hesiod was killed in Ozolian Locris, just west of Delphi, by local inhabitants in the precinct around the temple of Nemean Zeus; Hesiod was taken off guard because an oracle had told him he would suffer this fate at Nemea, a prophecy that he had interpreted literally as meaning the city itself. Pausanias and other sources say that a tomb of Hesiod could be seen at Orchomenos, in northwest Boeotia.

Much of this, even the autobiographical passages in Hesiod's works, must be approached with reservations. Greek and Roman tourists would pay well to see "Hesiod's tomb," and the story of his death conforms to standard features of the cult of the poet-hero (such as the death of Orpheus). The dispute with Perses is impossible to reconstruct clearly, although its literary function is easily understandable. That Perses was an actual individual living in Hesiod's day has sometimes been questioned; his name may be fabricated from the root *perth-, pers-* to suggest "waster" or "spoiler." The meeting with the Muses of Mount Helicon speaks for itself, and even the name "Hesiod" may be a generic nom de plume, "he who emits the voice" (as "Homer" may be interpreted as "he who fits [the song] together").

What remains of the life of Hesiod is probably better founded in truth. One of the few ancient poets who came from humble origins, Hesiod grew up in poverty; it is speculated that he adopted the trade of a rhapsode, reciting and composing poetry in central Greece. Unlike his fellow Boeotian Pindar, Hesiod never embraced the values of the nobility with their contempt for the peasant, although in the *Theogony*, he acknowledges the Muses' scorn of rustics. Throughout his two masterpieces, Hesiod retained the little man's distrust of corrupt "kings," the peasant's grim view of life's realities, and a democrat's belief in an abstract justice that is indifferent to social rank.

ANALYSIS

Judged purely as literature, Hesiod's work falls short of the highest rank. His writing is rambling and structurally undisciplined; his values are sometimes quaint, his lists of gods or seasonal farm chores tedious. Hesiod was more than a compiler of myth and wisdom, however; his lofty ideals, connecting justice with a vision of growing divine order, break through the catalog form with striking force; his unsentimental view of life, in which just behavior and hard work are the chief determinants of every person's destiny, is forceful and intentionally inspirational. Hesiod's writing is less graceful than robust; much of its power is derived from a

vision that made it a cornerstone of Greek thought and an influential component in the classical reading of neoclassical poets from the Renaissance through the Romantic era.

Because nothing is known of Hesiod's immediate literary context, it is hard to say how much is new in his two poems. It is sometimes rashly said that he was the first Greek to make a systematic account of divine mythology, the first to introduce Eros as a divinity, the first to engage in philosophy, and the like. There is no evidence for such claims, and although it may be reasonable to speculate with scholar G. S. Kirk that Hesiod came "near the beginning of a Boeotian poetical renaissance," it is hard not to see him as the culmination of a long oral tradition in Greece. His adeptness with formal battle pieces, tales of giants and monsters, and catalogs (a form often linked to Boeotia in particular), his self-consciousness in his vocation as a poet and his emphasis on the Muses and the poet's craft mark him as the practitioner of an already well-established and popular art. Attempts to link him with the subsequent development of philosophy in Ionia should be qualified by the fact that Hesiod's thought is still more theological and mythical than rational. Indeed, it fits the character of his thought better to study him as a theologian, although it is a matter of speculation that theological constructs are uniquely his.

It is also appropriate to perceive Hesiod as an essentially oral poet in the sense that (like Homer's) his style is formulaic to a high degree and his manner of organizing material is paratactic, "being often based" as Kirk says, "on the exploitation of casual associations rather than on the principle of strictly logical development." In *The Winged Word: A Study in the Technique of Ancient Greek Oral Composition as Seen Principally Through Hesiod's "Works and Days"* (1975), Berkley Peabody explores the ramifications of the allegedly oral composition of Hesiod's poems, but because the rigid distinctions that Milman Parry and A. B. Lord attempted to draw between oral and literary compositions have been found inapplicable in other traditions, it is no longer considered possible to define orality with absolute rigor. Hesiod's tradition and style are undeniably oral, but he may have used writing, and, as Eric Havelock has long since argued, the permanence of the written word (introduced to Greece in about 750 B.C.E.) may well have inspired him to compose the kind of works he left behind.

THEOGONY

The earlier of Hesiod's poems, the *Theogony* (genealogy of the gods) gives an account in about one thousand lines of dactylic hexameter of the origin of the world and the forces that control it: gods, Titans, monsters, and personified abstractions, down to the establishment of Zeus's world order. Although the original shape of Hesiod's poem has been confused by later additions to the text, it was clearly his intention to represent as his main theme the progressive emergence of order from disorder. Kirk states that through a rambling and digressive narrative, the reader can detect "some idea of a gradual progress, not only from more abstract cosmogonical figures to more concrete and anthropomorphic ones, but also from cruder and more violent gods to cleverer and more orderly ones." The core around which Hesiod's divine order forms is the succession of three generations: the first parents Uranus (sky) and Gaea (earth), then Cronus, then Zeus. Friedrich Solmsen has suggested an additional theme:

> The series of events which make up the history of the divine dynasty from the birth of Uranus and Gaea to Zeus's advent to power has been determined by, and owes its intrinsic unity to, the idea of guilt and retribution. It forms one great conception.

After a long poem in the form of a hymn to the Muses, Hesiod starts his account with a brief cosmogony beginning with Chaos (void) and after him Gaea, Tartarus, and Eros (the primal generative force). Here and throughout his poem, Hesiod does not distinguish clearly between places (Tartarus), conditions (Chaos), physical entities (Gaea), and forces (Eros). Following a common instinct of Greek thought, Hesiod admits them to his narrative as characters first and in addition whatever else that their names, genealogy, or actions might imply. Cosmogony therefore quickly fades into theogony as the process of generation takes over. Chaos gives birth to Erebus and Night, who in turn couple and beget Aether and Day. Gaea gives birth to Uranus, the Hills, and Pontus (the sea) before coupling with her son Uranus (in the primordial union of earth and sky) to

produce six male and six female Titans, three Cyclopes, and three Hundred-Handers. As Uranus tries to prevent the birth of these last three, Gaea conspires with Cronus, the youngest of her Titans, who cuts off his father's genitals as Uranus attempts to couple once more with Gaea. The blood from this mutilation falls to earth to beget the Furies, the Giants, and the tree nymphs. Cronus hurls his father's severed genitals into the sea, where the foam that spreads around them produces Aphrodite (the foam-, or *aphro-*, born goddess), who steps ashore at Cyprus attended by Eros and Himeros (longing).

There follows a catalog of some three hundred gods descended in two separate lines from Chaos and Gaea: from the former, the troublesome children of Night; from the latter, the three sons and three daughters of Pontus, who, in turn, spawn some fifty nymphs and a variety of other gods, sprites, and monsters. The catalog culminates in the birth of Zeus, son of the Titans Cronus and Rhea. Fearing a predicted overthrow by one of his children, Cronus swallows his offspring until their mother contrives to feed him a stone in the place of her youngest child, Zeus, who is kept safe in a Cretan cave. When Zeus comes of age, he forces Cronus to disgorge his three sisters Hestia, Demeter, and Hera and his brothers Hades and Poseidon. He also frees his uncles the Cyclopes, who in gratitude give him the thunder and lightning with which to win and maintain his rule.

Hesiod's genealogy concludes with an account of the progeny of the Titan Iapetus, with particular attention to the story of Prometheus, an etiological myth, explaining first, why the gods are served the bones and fat of a sacrifice rather than the good meat; second, how Prometheus stole fire for man; and third, how Zeus contrived woman for mortals as a curse to offset the Promethean blessing of fire. The general lesson of the Prometheus myth, with the chaining of the trickster-Titan who dares to match wits with Zeus, is the impossibility of escaping the wrath of Zeus. This intimation of Zeus's knowledge and power leads to an account of the great battle by which Zeus established his power in the world, the Titanomachy, a showpiece of action poetry that became the prototype of John Milton's War in Heaven. As earlier in the poem Zeus had freed the three

Cyclopes, so he now frees the Hundred-Handers to fight as his allies against the Titans. The blazing, crashing, thundering battle that ensues has a Wagnerian quality and may well have been a great crowd pleaser at Hesiod's recitations. It is followed by an equally impressive vision of the underworld to which Zeus consigns the conquered Titans. In a final battle (perhaps composed as a kind of encore to the Titanomachy), Zeus overcomes the last challenge to his power, the monster Typhoeus, a storm god who is defeated and, like the Titans, thrown into Tartarus. The poem concludes with Zeus's dispensation of titles and privileges to the Olympian gods and a series of seven marriages that consolidate his regime. In this genealogical coda, numerous younger gods are born, including the motherless Athena and the fatherless Hephaestus. At some point after this, perhaps with the list of goddesses who have lain with mortal men, the genuine work of Hesiod is believed to give way to the work of post-Hesiodic redactors intent on grafting the *Catalogue of Women* onto the *Theogony*. Although it is not agreed exactly where the break comes, the composition becomes looser near the end, and scholar Kurt Von Fritz states: "The text constantly deteriorates, till at the end it just dissolves."

LITERARY AND MYTHIC INFLUENCES

It is likely that theogonic poetry was well established in Greek oral tradition for generations before Hesiod, possibly as early as the Mycenaean age. Accounts of the origin of the world, the birth of the gods, and the establishment of the present order occur in archaic cultures from Iceland to the Pacific. More specifically, according to M. L. West, Hesiod's "succession myth," tracing the transfer of power from Uranus to Cronus to Zeus, "has parallels in Oriental mythology which are so striking that a connection is incontestable." A Hurrian succession myth, preserved in Hittite texts four centuries before Hesiod, and the Akkadian *Enuma Elis* (early second millennium B.C.E.), the official theogonic text used in the Babylonian New Year festival, provide mythic parallels so close as to justify the conclusion that the core of Hesiod's *Theogony* is a synthesis of Eastern stories known to the Greeks since the Minoan-Mycenaean period or somewhat later. This is not to say that Hesiod merely imitated Eastern poetry; like everything else that the Greeks borrowed, it was refashioned into a document of Greek culture.

WORKS AND DAYS

The same is true of the *Works and Days*, which might be called "The Wisdom of Hesiod" because of its affinity with works of exhortation and instruction attested in Sumeria as early as 2500 B.C.E., with Akkadian and Babylonian texts from c. 1400 B.C.E. and with Egyptian Middle Kingdom "instruction" texts from about the same time. In fact, "wisdom literature" is nearly as widespread in world cultures as is theogonic poetry. Hesiod's *Works and Days* shows a particular affinity with Eastern parallels: The myth of the five races of man has counterparts in Persia, India, and Mesopotamia; instruction in Hesiod's poem comes from a victim of injustice, as in a number of Egyptian wisdom texts, one of them more than one thousand years earlier than Hesiod; and the fable of the hawk and the nightingale points to the Near East, where the animal fable goes back to the Sumerians. These affinities, among others, argue that the *Works and Days* is not only cognate with Near Eastern poetic themes but was actually influenced by them.

The *Works and Days* is not narrative in outline, as is the *Theogony*. Instead, it is presented as a miscellany of advice and instructive stories to Perses, the poet's wastrel brother, who had bribed the "kings" and cheated him in the division of their father's estate. Its two themes are justice and work, and Hesiod makes it his business to show how they are intertwined in the life of a successful man. After a short poem to Zeus, Hesiod corrects what he had said in the *Theogony* about Eris, or Strife, daughter of Night. There are not one but two types of strife—one evil, the other good. Good strife is the healthy competition that urges men on to greater efforts in their work. Hesiod repeats the story of Prometheus to explain why humans have to work for their livelihood, elaborating the account of Pandora as if to imply that woman is the ultimate and definitive curse upon humanity.

As an alternative explanation of the wretched lot of humanity, Hesiod next offers the myth of the five races of man. This entropic version of human history, each generation being of a baser metal than its predecessor, contrasts significantly with the progressive history of the divine world in the *Theogony* and emphasizes the sense of hopeless distance between humans and gods that runs through much Greek poetry, especially tragedy. The fable of the hawk and his helpless victim, the nightingale, points to the supremacy of force in the animal world; as for the human world, Perses is asked to consider how justice wins out over violence because of the actions of Zeus. The role of Zeus as a punisher of injustice can be seen early in Homer's *Iliad* (c. 750 B.C.E.; English translation, 1611), and a passage in Homer's *Odyssey* (c. 725 B.C.E.; English translation, 1614) contains the idea that good crops and abundant livestock are rewards given to a just ruler. What is remarkable in Hesiod is the forcefulness with which he links justice, prosperity, and the role of Zeus as the embodiment of a just providence. It is justice that separates human life from that of the beasts: This *nomos*, or sacred law, is the decree of Zeus, and the success or failure of a person's life is the final proof that nothing escapes the eye of Zeus.

If this assertion seems more a statement of religious belief than an observation of fact, it is tempting to look anachronistically forward to some of the teachings of Calvinism, especially those that associated virtue with prosperity. A significant comparison can also be made with biblical wisdom literature, where the association of virtue with prosperity is standard, as in Proverbs 13:22, 13:25, and 14:11, for example. The next section of the *Works and Days* may seem a step closer to such a comparison: Hesiod preaches a work ethic in his famous exhortation to Perses, which represents hard work as the virtue that brings prosperity and idleness as the vice that brings ruin (see Proverbs 6:6-11). In the world that Hesiod depicts, therefore, justice and hard work are the route to success, violence and idleness the guarantors of disaster.

Obviously, the latter precept concerning work versus idleness is less religious than pragmatic, and the poem perceptibly shifts its emphasis at this point from the mythical, moral, and metaphysical to the practical. The lines that follow are a series of proverbs on how to keep what you have, beginning with moral and religious maxims and ending with prudent social and personal advice, such as that against sweet-talking women who are after a man's barn. The rest of the poem consists of specific advice to the farmer, a sketchy kind of

almanac telling when to plow and reap and what equipment to use, Hesiod outlining farming techniques, winter procedures, and other seasonal chores. He offers advice to the farmer who goes to sea to sell his goods; on when and how to marry; and on social, personal, and ritual hygiene. Finally, there is a list of good and bad days of the month.

Judged as a purely literary performance, the *Works and Days* is uneven, especially in the latter sections containing advice on farming, but students of the poem see a unity of conception and a dour kind of vigor that offsets some of its literary shortcomings. Occasioned by an act of injustice, the poem adheres to a single theme: Good farming is as much a part of justice as good statecraft would be for Plato in the *Politeia* (fourth century B.C.E.; *Republic*, 1701). Moreover, Hesiod's qualified pessimism and the vividness with which he reveals the harsh life of the farmer are an essential background to the stern values he preaches; there is little of the "pastoral" here. Hesiod lacks the aristocratic magnanimity of Homer and never achieves the smooth, leisurely expansiveness of Homeric narrative. In this respect, Hesiod's curt style is suited to the bleak life he represents. On the other hand, the explicit force of Hesiod's ethical vision surpasses anything in Homer. This is partly because the political context is more real to the modern reader: Instead of the "feudal" society of warrior-kings and their dependents, whose chief virtues lie in loyal service, Hesiod depicts independent men whose dignity lies in their ability to take care of themselves, their households, and their farms. The *Works and Days* is a moral and political tract that contrasts the justice of work not only with the idleness of fools but also with the corruption of "gift-devouring kings" who enjoy indolence at the expense of others. The poem is thus more than an interesting glimpse of eighth century B.C.E. Boeotian farm life; it is a valuable cultural document. Its significance for the Hellenic civilization then taking shape lies in the assertion of a divine and impersonal justice working for the common person as well as for the great. The ideal of a universal, evenhanded law was essential not only to the political life of the Greeks but also to the idea of early Greek tragedy, where *Dikē* is as inevitable as the other workings of nature.

BIBLIOGRAPHY

Clay, Jenny Strauss. *Hesiod's Cosmos*. New York: Palgrave Macmillan, 2003. A scholarly study of Hesiod's works and their expression of early Greek religious thought.

Edwards, Anthony T. *Hesiod's Ascra*. Berkeley: University of California Press, 2004. Edwards examines how Hesiod depicted Ascra in *Works and Days*, finding the village to be autonomous and recasting the dispute between Hesiod and Perses as a disagreement over the inviolability of the community's external border.

Gotshalk, Richard. *Homer and Hesiod: Myth and Philosophy*. Lanham, Md.: University Press of America, 2000. A study of the nature and function of the poetry of Homer and Hesiod when their work is considered in historical context as developments of poetry as a distinctive voice for truth beyond religion and myth.

Hunter, Richard, ed. *The Hesiodic Catalogue of Women: Constructions and Reconstructions*. New York: Cambridge University Press, 2005. A team of scholars attempt to explore the meaning, significance, and reception of a poem formerly attributed to Hesiod.

Lamberton, Robert. *Hesiod*. Fort Lauderdale, Fla.: Hermes Books, 1988. An accessible introduction to Hesiod's works. Historical background of the poems and problems of dating them are discussed. Major subsidiary works are analyzed.

Marsilio, Maria S. *Farming and Poetry in Hesiod's "Works and Days."* Lanham, Md.: University Press of America, 2000. Demonstrates how Hesiod and Vergil viewed the farming lifestyle as a system of belief unto itself. Includes a translation of *Works and Days* by esteemed translator David Grene.

Montanari, Franco, Antonios Rengakos, and Christos Tsagalis, eds. *Brill's Companion to Hesiod*. Boston: Brill, 2009. A collection of essays about Hesiod and his writings, including an analysis of poetry and poetics in his works and a look in to ancient scholarship on Hesiod.

Nelson, Stephanie A. *God and the Land: The Metaphysics of Farming in Hesiod and Vergil*. New York: Oxford University Press, 1998. Shows how Hesiod as well as Vergil viewed the farming lifestyle as a religion unto itself.

Penglase, Charles. *Greek Myths and Mesopotamia: Parallels and Influence in the Homeric Hymns and Hesiod*. New York: Routledge, 1997. Examines how Mesopotamian ideas and themes influenced Greek religious mythological works, including the Homeric hymns to the gods and the works of Hesiod.

Stoddard, Kathryn. *The Narrative Voice in the "Theogony" of Hesiod*. Boston: Brill, 2004. Looks at the narrative voice in *Theogony*, discussing whether it is autobiographical and who the implied author is.

Daniel H. Garrison

HERMANN HESSE

Born: Calw, Germany; July 2, 1877
Died: Montagnola, Switzerland; August 9, 1962

PRINCIPAL POETRY

Romantische Lieder, 1899
Hinterlassene Schriften und Gedichte von Hermann Lauscher, 1901
Gedichte, 1902
Unterwegs: Gedichte, 1911
Aus Indien, 1913
Musik des Einsamen: Neue Gedichte, 1915
Gedichte des Malers, 1920
Ausgewählte Gedichte, 1921
Verse im Krankenbett, 1927
Krisis, 1928 (*Crisis: Pages from a Diary*, 1975)
Trost der Nacht: Neue Gedichte, 1929
Jahreszeiten: Zen Gedichte mit Bildern, 1931
Besinnung, 1934
Leben einer Blume, 1934
Vom Baum des Lebens, 1934
Das Haus der Träume, 1936
Jahreslauf: Ein Zyklus Gedichte, 1936
Stunden im Garten: Eine Idylle, 1936
Chinesisch, 1937
Der lahme Knabe: Eine Erinnerung aus der Kindheit, 1937

Neue Gedichte, 1937

Orgelspiel, 1937

Ein Traum Josef Knechts, 1937

Föhnige Nacht, 1938

Der letzte Glasperlenspieler, 1939

Zehn Gedichte, 1939

Fünf Gedichte, 1942

Die Gedichte, 1942

Krankennacht, 1942

Stufen: Noch ein Gedichte Josef Knechts, 1943

Der Blütenzweig, 1945

Friede 1914; dem Feieden, 1945

Späte Gedichte, 1946

In Sand geschrieben, 1947

Drei Gedichte, 1948

Jugend-Gedichte, 1950

Zwei Gedichte, 1951

Rückblick, 1952

Zwei Idyllen, 1952

Alter Maler in der Werkstatt, 1954

Klage und Trost, 1954

Wanderer im Spätherbst, 1956

Zum Frieden, 1956

Das Lied von Abels Tod, 1957

Gedichte, 1958

Treue Begleiter, 1958

Freund Peter, 1959 (also known as *Bericht an die Freunde: Letzte Gedichte*)

Vier späte Gedichte, 1959

Stufen: Alte und neue Gediochte in Auswahl, 1961

Die späten Gedichte, 1963

Buchstaben, 1965

Poems, 1970

Stufen: Ausgewählte, 1972

Poems by Hermann Hesse, 1974

OTHER LITERARY FORMS

Though Hermann Hesse (HEHS-uh) is best known among English-speakers for his novels—especially *Demian* (1919; English translation, 1923), *Der Steppenwolf* (1927; *Steppenwolf*, 1929), *Siddhartha* (1922; English translation, 1951); *Narziss und Goldmund* (1930; *Death and the Lover*, 1932; also known as *Narcissus and Goldmund*, 1968), and *Das Glasperlenspiel: Versuch einer Lebensbeschreibung des Magister Ludi Josef Knecht samt Knechts hinterlassenen Schriften* (1943; *Magister Ludi*, 1949; also known as *The Glass Bead Game*, 1969)—he wrote a significant volume of work in other genres. He began composing poems as a precocious child, and despite his output in other literary forms, he continued writing verse throughout his long life. Many of his novels, in fact, contain rhymes, and since the 1950's much of his poetry has been adapted for musical pieces, especially in Europe. In addition to numerous collections of poems, Hesse wrote volumes of short stories, fairy tales, essays, articles, lectures and other nonfiction. He also edited several periodicals and served as editor for dozens of books, particularly from 1910 to 1926.

ACHIEVEMENTS

Hermann Hesse authored millions of words including hundreds, perhaps thousands, of poems. Much of his verse from the mid-1930's onward was self-published in small private editions featuring his hand-painted watercolors as gifts for friends and remains uncollected. Hesse first achieved recognition in 1904, winning the Wiener Bauernfeld Prize for his novel *Peter Camenzind* (English translation, 1961). He received the Fontane Prize for *Demian* in 1920, but returned it because the award was intended for new writers. In 1936, he was honored with Zurich's Gottfried-Keller Prize for Literature. In 1946, he received both the Nobel Prize in Literature and the Goethe Prize. He added the Wilhelm Raabe Prize (1950) and the Peace Prize of the German Book Trade (1955) to his laurels and was made a Knight of the Order of Merit in 1955. More than forty years after his death and eighty years since he adopted Swiss citizenry, Hesse continues to be one of the best-selling German-language authors in the country of his birth.

BIOGRAPHY

Hermann Hesse was born in Calw, a picturesque village in the Black Forest. He was the grandson of a publisher of religious tracts and the son of devout missionaries from the Pietists, an evangelical Protestant sect. His father, Johannes Hesse, was a German, born the son of a physician in Estonia (then part of the Russian Empire), and his mother Marie Gundert Hesse, a widow with two sons, was also of German heritage, though she had been born in India, where her father Hermann Gundert, a scholarly linguist, had preached.

A precocious child, young Hesse was difficult to handle and particularly acted out during the five years (1881-1886) when the Hesse family lived in Basle, Switzerland. After they returned to Calw, Hesse attended preparatory Latin school in Göppingen and did well in his studies. However, when his parents enrolled him in the Maulbronn Seminary, assuming he would follow them into the religious life, he rebelled and ran away. He contemplated suicide for the first but not the last time. He briefly attended a series of other schools before enrolling at the gymnasium at Cannstadt, but he was expelled in 1893, effectively ending his formal education at the age of sixteen.

Hesse apprenticed at a steeple clock factory before working in a bookshop in Tübingen, where he published his first collection of poetry in 1899. For four years thereafter, he worked in a bookshop in Basle. In 1904, he achieved his first literary success with the publication of *Peter Camenzind*, which convinced him to become a full-time freelance writer. That same year, he married Maria Bernoulli and fathered three children—Bruno, Heiner, and Martin—between 1905 and 1911 while living in Gaienhofen, Germany. Hesse frequently contributed to literary journals; regularly published fiction, nonfiction, and poetry; and traveled often, lecturing in Italy, Switzerland, Germany, and India.

In 1912, Hesse moved with his family to Berne, Switzerland. When World War I broke out, he attempted to enlist in the German military but was turned away because of vision problems, so he worked through the German consulate in Switzerland, editing journals and books for German prisoners of war. In 1916, Hesse underwent Jungian psychoanalysis, and during the 1920's, he visited spas for his health. In 1919, the same year that he published *Demian*—he left his family to live alone in Montagnola, where he would reside for the rest of his life. When he became a Swiss citizen in 1923, he divorced his first wife, and the following year, he married Ruth Wenger. They would divorce in 1927, the same year that *Steppenwolf* was published.

Hesse wed for a third time in 1931, to Ninon Aus-

länder Dolbin, and this marriage lasted. The author continued to publish collections of poetry until the end of his life, although he did not write another novel after *The Glass Bead Game*, considered his fictional masterpiece. During his final years, he divided his time between writing poetry and conscientiously answering the hundreds of letters he received daily. Afflicted with leukemia, he died of a brain hemorrhage shortly after his eighty-fifth birthday.

ANALYSIS

Virtually all of Hermann Hesse's fiction and poetry is autobiographical, even confessional to some degree. Although his major novels have been translated into English and many other languages—and to this day are the primary focus of study and critique—much of his nonfiction, short fiction, and poetry remains available only in German.

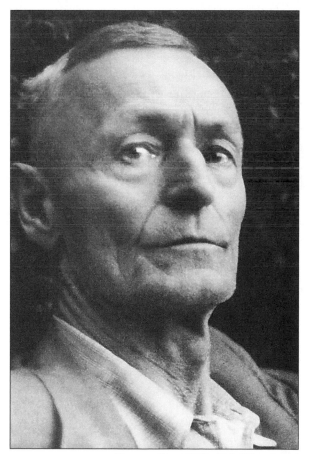

Hermann Hesse (©The Nobel Foundation)

Hesse's early poems are lyrical. Regular in meter and rhyme, they revolve around typical subjects of youthful inspiration: expressions of longing for women, insightful studies of nature, observations made while traveling, considerations of the self, and as might be expected from someone of his religious upbringing, reflections on the meaning of spirituality, faith, and belief. His charming hometown of Calw comes under frequent scrutiny; such poems are replete with realistic, telling details surrounding the honest, cheerful burghers who struggle for survival, and lines are crowded with fond memories. Hesse's career as a poet was given a boost at the turn of the twentieth century by a sympathetic critique of his *Romantische Lieder* (romantic songs) from fellow poet Rainer Maria Rilke, who, while praising his contemporary's use of metallic imagery, complained that Hesse's verbiage was too abstract. Rilke pronounced the collection "unliterary," which was considered a compliment, a contrast to the usual poetry of the time.

Even from the beginning, Hesse's poetry is more downbeat than exuberant. From an early age, he considered himself an outsider, an observer rather than a participant in the stream of life; a loner, he never felt he belonged anywhere. *Romantische Lieder*, although demonstrating conscious control of rhythm, rhyme, and the acoustic effect produced by combinations of words, is laden with images of unhappiness, depression, and uneasiness. Although Hesse would move between rhyme and free verse throughout his career, he would continually revisit these themes in his poems.

CRISIS

Crisis, an aptly named collection of poems, evolved when Hesse was writing *Steppenwolf*, one of his most influential novels. The poems reflect the latest and most catastrophic in a series of major turning points in his life. Individual pieces revolve around the mid-life crisis many aging men experience. They incorporate his feelings about the breakup of his first marriage, his realization that his second marriage was doomed, bouts of illness and insomnia and extreme depression, and a complete change in his philosophical outlook. Tired of life, out of balance physically and psychologically, weary of pursuing spiritual answers in his quest for self-knowledge, and fed up with his usual preoccupa-

tion with asceticism and intellectuality, he immersed himself completely in the sensual and emotional. For two years in the mid-1920's, Hesse caroused nightly, drinking himself into oblivion, experimenting with drugs, consorting with prostitutes, and visiting nightclubs to listen to live jazz.

The poems of *Crisis*, written mostly in straightforward rhyming quatrains, are brutally frank. They speak of the author—the lone wolf of the steppes, as depicted in *Steppenwolf*—saturating himself with whiskey, dancing the shimmy, cavorting with girls named Fanny and Adelaide, waking up alone with painful hangovers, and feeling overwhelming self-pity. The titles alone of many of the forty-five verses indicate his mood and temperament: "Poet's Death Song," "Growing Old," "After an Evening at the Stag," "To John the Baptist from Hermann the Drunkard," "The Seducer," "Schizophrenia," "The Debauchee," "Still Tipsy," "The Drunken Poet," and "Poor Devil on the Morning After the Masked Ball." However, despite sinking into the depths for a time, the experience had a cathartic effect on Hesse's psyche. His mind and body cleansed, he was able to resume a productive and satisfying career, using the insight gained from his exploration of the vulgar side of his nature.

POEMS

One of the first collections of Hesse's poems in English, *Poems* presents translator James Wright's selections, in both German and English, from the poet's earlier work, published between 1899 and 1921. The seventy-eight mostly brief rhyming poems are linked by a common thread: the theme of longing for home. This was an important consideration for Hesse at the time that he wrote these poems because he was alienated from his religious parents, physically removed from his birthplace, and as a nonparticipant in the military efforts of Germany during World War I, an outcast in his own country. The selections in *Poems*—particularly "I Know, You Walk," "Lonesome Night," "The Poet," "At Night on the High Seas," "Ode to Hölderlin," and "In a Collection of Egyptian Sculptures"—provide a good introduction to Hesse's recurring subject matter: loneliness, the inevitability of death for all living things, and the exploration of the self and the soul.

OTHER MAJOR WORKS

LONG FICTION: *Peter Camenzind*, 1904 (English translation, 1961); *Unterm Rad*, 1906 (*The Prodigy*, 1957; also known as *Beneath the Wheel*, 1968); *Gertrud*, 1910 (*Gertrude and I*, 1915; also known as *Gertrude*, 1955); *Rosshalde*, 1914 (English translation, 1970); *Knulp: Drei Geschichten aus dem Leben Knulps*, 1915 (*Knulp: Three Tales from the Life of Knulp*, 1971); *Demian*, 1919 (English translation, 1923; also known as *Demian: The Story of Eric Sinclair's Youth*, 1965); *Klingsors letzter Sommer*, 1920 (*Klingsor's Last Summer*, 1970; includes the three novellas *Klein und Wagner*, *Kinderseele*, and *Klingsors letzter Sommer*); *Siddhartha*, 1922 (English translation, 1951); *Aufzeichnungen eines Herrn im Sanatorium*, 1925 (also known as *Haus zum Frieden: Aufzeichnungen eines Herrn im Sanatorium*, 1947); *Der Steppenwolf*, 1927 (*Steppenwolf*, 1929); *Narziss und Goldmund*, 1930 (*Death and the Lover*, 1932; also known as *Narcissus and Goldmund*, 1968); *Die Morgenlandfahrt*, 1932 (*The Journey to the East*, 1956); *Das Glasperlenspiel: Versuch einer Lebensbeschreibung des Magister Ludi Josef Knecht samt Knechts hinterlassenen Schriften*, 1943 (*Magister Ludi*, 1949; best known as *The Glass Bead Game*, 1969; also known as *Magister Ludi: The Glass Bead Game*, 1970).

SHORT FICTION: *Eine Stunde hinter Mitternacht*, 1899; *Diesseits: Erzählungen*, 1907; *Nachbarn: Erzählungen*, 1908; *Umwege: Erzählungen*, 1912; *Aus Indien*, 1913; *Anton Schievelbeyns ohn-freiwillige Reiss nachher ost-Indien*, 1914; *Der Hausierer*, 1914; *Am Weg*, 1915 (also known as *Am Weg: Erzählungen*; also known as *Am Weg Frühe Erzählungen*); *Hans Dierlamms Lehrzeit*, 1916; *Schön ist die Jugend*, 1916; *Alte Geschichten: Zwei Erzählungen*, 1918; *Zwei Märchen*, 1918; *Märchen*, 1919 (*Strange News from Another Star, and Other Tales*, 1972); *Im Presselschen Gartenhaus: Eine Erzählung dem alten Tübingen*, 1920; *In der alten Sonne*, 1921; *Die Officina Bodoni in Montagnola*, 1923 (English translation, 1976); *Psychologia balnearia oder Glossen eines Badener Kurgastes*, 1924 (also known as *Kurgast: Aufzeichnungen von einer Badener Kur*, 1925); *Die Verlobung: Erzählungen*, 1924; *Piktors Verwandlungen: Ein*

Märchen, 1925; *Die Nürnberger Reise*, 1927; *Der Zyklon und andere Erzählungen*, 1929; *Weg nach Innen*, 1931; *Hermann Hesse*, 1932; *Kleine Welt: Erzählungen*, 1933; *Fabulierbuch*, 1935; *Stunden im Garten: Eine Idylle*, 1936; *Tragisch*, 1936; *Der Lateinschüler*, 1943; *Der Pfirsichbaum: Und andere Erzählungen*, 1945; *Traumfährte: Neue Erzählungen und Märchen*, 1945 (*The War Goes On*, 1971); *Kurgast; die Nuernberger Reise: Zwei Erzählungen*, 1946; *Geheimnisse*, 1947 (also known as *Geheimnisse: Letzte Erzählungen*, 1955); *Heumond; aus nach Innen: Vier Erzählungen*, 1947; *Weg nach Innen: Vier Erzählungen*, 1947; *Der Zwerg*, 1947; *Frühe Prosa*, 1948; *Kinderseele*, 1948; *Kinderseele und Ladidel*, 1948; *Zwei Erzählungen: Der Novalis; Der Zwerg*, 1948; *Der Bettler*, 1949; *Hermann Hesse*, 1949; *Bericht aus Normalien*, 1951; *Späte Prosa*, 1951; *Die Verlobung und andere Erzählungen*, 1951; *Weihnacht mit zwei Kindergeschichten*, 1951; *Diesseits, Kleine Welt, Fabulierbuch*, 1954; *Beschwörungen: Späte Prosa, Neu Folge*, 1955; *Der Dichter: Eine Märchen*, 1955; *Flötentraum*, 1955; *Der Wolf und andere Erzählungen*, 1955; *Zwei jugendliche Erzählungen*, 1956; *Augustus, Der Dichter; ein Mensch mit Namen Ziegler*, 1957 (also known as *Drei Erzählungen: Sugustus, Der Dichter; ein Mensch mit Namen Ziegler*, 1960); *Gesammelte Schriften*, 1957; *Klein und Wagner*, 1958 (also known as *Klein und Wagner: Novelle*, 1973); *Tessiner Erzählungen*, 1962; *Tractat vom Steppenwolf*, 1964 (*Treatise on the Steppenwolf*, 1975); *Prosa aus dem Nachlass*, 1965; *Der vierte Lebenslauf Josef Knechts*, 1966; *Aus Kinderzeiten und andere Erzählungen*, 1968; *Stories of Five Decades*, 1972; *Iris: Ausgewählt Märchen*, 1973; *Tales of Student Life*, 1976.

PLAY: *Heimkehr*, pr. 1958 (wr. 1919).

NONFICTION: *Boccaccio*, 1904; *Franz von Assisi*, 1904; *Faust und Zarathustra*, 1909; *Kriegslektüre*, 1915; *Zum Sieg*, 1915; *Lektüre für Kriegsgefangene*, 1916; *Zarathustras Wiederkehr: Ein Wort an die deutsche Jugend von einem Deutschen*, 1919; *Blick ins Chaos*, 1920 (*In Sight of Chaos*, 1923); *Wanderung, Aufzeichnungen: Mit farbigen Bildern vom Verfasser*, 1920 (*Wandering: Notes and Sketches*, 1972); *Elf Aquarelle aus dem Tessin*, 1921; *Erinnerung an*

Lektüre, 1925; *Betrachtungen*, 1928; *Eine Bibliothek der Weltliteratur*, 1929; *Magie des Buches*, 1930; *Zum Gedächtnis unseres Vatres*, 1930; *Beim Einzug ins neue Haus*, 1931; *Gedenkblätter*, 1937; *Der Novalis*, 1940; *Kleine Betrachtungen*, 1941; *Gedenkblatt für Franz Schall*, 1943; *Erinnerung an Klingsors Sommer*, 1944; *Nachruf auf Christoph Schrempf*, 1944; *Zwischen Sommer und Herbst*, 1944; *Zwei Aufsätze*, 1945; *Ansprache in der ersten Stunde des Jahres 1946*, 1946; *Dank an Goethe*, 1946; *Danksagung und moralisierende Bertrachtungen*, 1946; *Der Europaeer*, 1946; *Feuerwerk*, 1946; *Krieg und Frieden: Betrachtungen zu Krieg und Politik seit dem Jahr 1914*, 1946, 1949 (*If the War Goes On . . . Reflections on War and Politics*, 1971); *Statt eines Briefes*, 1946; *Antwort auf Bittbriefe*, 1947; *Eine Konzertpause*, 1947; *Stufen der Menschwerdung*, 1947; *Berg und See: Zwei Landschaftsstudien*, 1948; *Traumtheater: Aufzeichnungen*, 1948; *Über Romain Rolland*, 1948; *Begegnungen mit Vergagenem*, 1949; *Gedenkblatt für Adele*, 1949; *Gedenkblatt für Martin*, 1949; *Stunden am Schreibitisch*, 1949; *Wege zu Hermann Hesse*, 1949; *Erinnerung an Andre Gide*, 1951; *Gedanken über Gottfried Keller*, 1951; *Über "Peter Camenzind,"* 1951; *Herbstliche Erlebnisse*, 1952; *Lektüre für Minuten: Ein paar Gedanken aus meinen Büchern und Briefen*, 1952; *Kaminfegerchen*, 1953; *Nachruf für Marulla*, 1953; *Die Dohle*, 1954; *Notizblätter um Ostern*, 1954; *Über das Alter*, 1954; *Abendwolken: Zwei Aufsätze*, 1956; *Hilfsmaterial für den Literaturunterricht*, 1956; *Der Trauermarsch: Gedenkblatt für einen Jugendfreund*, 1957; *Eine Bodensee-Erinnirung*, 1961; *Ärzte: Ein paar Erinnerungen*, 1963; *Ein Blatt von meinem Baum*, 1964; *Neue deutsche Bücher: Literaturberichte für Bonniers Letterära Magasin, 1933-1936*, 1965; *Hermann Hesse: Essays*, 1970; *Politische Betrachtungen*, 1970; *Mein Glaube: Eine Dokumentation*, 1971; *Autobiographical Writings*, 1972; *Eigensinn: Autobiographische Schristen*, 1972; *Mein Glaube*, 1972; *Schriften zur Literatur*, 1972; *Die Kunst des Mussiggangs: Kurze Prosa aus dem Nachlass*, 1973; *My Belief: Essays on Life and Art*, 1974; *Reflections*, 1974.

EDITED TEXTS: *Der Lindenbaum: Deutsche Volkslieder*, 1910 (with Emil Strauss); *Eichendorffs Gedichte und Novellen*, 1913; *Gedichte*, 1913 (by Christian Wagner); *Des Knaben Wunderhorn*, 1913 (with Ludwig Achim von Arnim and Clemens Bretano); *Morgenländische Erzählungen*, 1913; *Der Zauberbrunnen*, 1913; *Lieder deutscher Dichter*, 1914; *Gesta Romanorum*, 1915; *Der Wandsbeker Bote: Eine Auswahl aus den Werken von Matthias Claudius*, 1915; *Alemannenbuch*, 1919; *Ein Schwabenbuch für die deutschen Kriegsgefangenen*, 1919; *Ein Luzerner Junker vor hundert Jahren*, 1920 (by Xaver Schnyder von Wartensee); *Dichtungen*, 1922 (by Salomon Gessner); *Märchen und Legenden aus der Gesta Romanorum*, 1926; *Dreissig Gedichte*, 1932 (by Johann Wolfgang von Goethe); *Geschichten aus dem Mittelalter*, 1976 (with others).

MISCELLANEOUS: *Der Junge Dichter: Ein Brief an Viele*, 1910 (also known as *An einen jungen Dichter*, 1932); *Kleiner Garten: Erlebnisse und Dichtungen*, 1919; *Aus dem "Tagebuch eines Entgleisten,"* 1922; *Sinclairs Notizbuch*, 1923 (by Emil Sinclair); *Bilderbuch*, 1926; *Kurzgefasster Lebenslauf*, 1929 (Erwin Ackerknecht, editor); *Mahnung: Erzählungen und Gedichte*, 1933; *Heiroglyphen*, 1943; *Bildschmuck im Eisenbahnwafen*, 1944; *Rigi-Tagebuch*, 1945; *Brief an Adele: Februar 1946*, 1946; *Ein Brief nach Deutschland*, 1946; *Indischer Lebenslauf*, 1946 (exerpts from *Das Glasperlenspiel: Versuch einer Lebensbeschreibung des Magister Ludi Josef Knecht samt Knechts hinterlassenen Schriften*, 1943); *An einen jungen Kollegen in Japan*, 1947; *Der Autor an einen Korrektor*, 1947; *Beschreibung einer Landschaf: Ein Stück tagebuch*, 1947; *Spaziergang in Würzburg*, 1947; *Zwei Briefe über das Glasperlenspiel*, 1947; *Blätter vom Tage*, 1948; *Legende von indischen König*, 1948; *Musikalische Notizen*, 1948; *Der Stimmen und der Heilige: Ein Stück Tagebuch*, 1948; *Versuch einer Rechtfertigung*, 1948 (with Max Brod); *Alle Bücher diesert Welt: Ein Almanach für Bücherfreunde*, 1949 (K. H. Silomon, editor); *An einem jungen Künstler*, 1949; *Aus vielen Jahren: Gegichte, Erzählungen und Bilder*, 1949; *Auszüge aus zwei Briefen*, 1949; *Gerbersau*, 1949; *Eine Arbeitsnacht*, 1950; *Ein Brief zu Thomas Manns 75 Geburstag*, 1950; *Das Lied des Lebens*, 1950; *Zwei Briefe: An einen jungen Künstler; das junge Genie*, 1950 (also known as *Das junge Ge-*

nie: Brief an einen Achtzehnjährigen, 1950); *Glück-wunsch für Peter Suhrkamp*, 1951; *Eine Handvoll Briefe*, 1951; *Nörgeleien*, 1951; *Eine Sonate*, 1951; *Ahornschatten, ein Brief*, 1952; *Allerlei Post: Rund-brief an Freunde*, 1952; *Aprilbrief*, 1952; *Dank für die Briefe und Glückwünsche zum 2 Juli 1952*, 1952; *Geburstag Ein Rundbrief*, 1952; *Gesammelte Dich-tungen*, 1952 (six volumes); *Letzer Gruss an Otto Hartmann*, 1952; *Das Werk von Hermann Hesse: Ein Brevier*, 1952 (Siegfried Unseld, editor); *Engadiner Erlebnisse: Ein Rundbrief*, 1953; *Regen in Herbst*, 1953; *Der Schlossergeselle*, 1953; *Doktor Knolges Ende*, 1954; *Die Nikobaren*, 1954; *Rundbrief aus Sils-Maria*, 1954; *Aquarelle aus dem Tessin*, 1955; *Knopf-Annähen*, 1955; *Ein paar Leserbriefe an Hermann Hesse*, 1955; *Tagebuchblatt: Ein Maulbronner Seminarist*, 1955; *Über Gewaltpolitik, Krieg und das Böse in der Welt*, 1955; *Cesco und der Berg*, 1956; *Gedichte und Prosa*, 1956; *Magie des Buches: Betrachtungen und Gedichte*, 1956; *Weihnachtsgaben und anderes*, 1956; *Wiederbegegnung mit zwei Jugendgedichten*, 1956; *Ein Auswahl*, 1957 (Reinhard Buchward, editor); *Gute Stunde*, 1957; *Malfreude, Malsorgen*, 1957; *Welkes Blatt*, 1957; *Antworten*, 1958; *Chinesische Legenge*, 1959; *Ein paar indische Miniaturen*, 1959; *Sommerbrief aus dem Engadin*, 1959; *An einen Musiker*, 1960; *Aus einem tagebuch des Jahres 1920*, 1960; *Ein paar Aufzeichnungen und Briefe*, 1960; *Rückgriff*, 1960; *Dichter und Weltburger*, 1961; *Schreiben und Schriften*, 1961; *Zen*, 1961; *Der Beichvater*, 1962 (selections from *Das Glasperlenspiel: Versuch einer Lebensbeschreibung des Magister Ludi Josef Knecht samt Knechts hinterlassenen Schriften*, 1943); *Prosa und Gedichte*, 1963 (Franz Baumer, edi-tor); *Erwin*, 1965; *Hermann Hesse: Eine Auswahl, für Ausländer*, 1966 (Gerherd Kirchhoff, editor); *Kindheit und Jungend vor Neunzehnhundert: Hermann Hesse in Briefen und Lebenszeugnissen, 1877-1895*, 1966 (Ni-non Hesse, editor); *Briefwechsel: Hermann Hesse—Thomas Mann*, 1968 (Anni Carlsson, editor; *The Hesse-Mann Letters: The Correspondence of Her-mann Hesse and Thomas Mann, 1910-1955*, 1975; Carlsson and Volker Michels, editors); *Briefwechsel, 1945-1959*, 1969 (with Peter Suhrkamp; Unseld, edi-tor); *Gesammelte Werke*, 1970 (twelve volumes);

Hermann Hesse, Helene Voigt-Diederichs: Zwei Autorenporträts in Briefen, 1897 bis 1900, 1971 (also known as *Zwei Autorenporträts in Briefen, 1897 bis 1900*, 1971); *Briefwechsel aus der Nähe*, 1972 (Magda Kerenyi, editor); *D'une rive a i'autre: Hermann Hesse et Romain Rolland*, 1972; *Lectüre für Minuten*, 1972 (Volker Michels, editor); *Die Erzählungen*, 1973 (Volker Michels, editor); *Gesammelte Briefe*, 1973 (Volker Michels and Ursula Michels, editors); *Glück, Späte Prosa: Betrachtungen*, 1973; *Reflections*, 1974.

BIBLIOGRAPHY

Cornils, Ingo. *A Companion to the Works of Hermann Hesse.* New York: Camden House, 2009. This work consists of essays from a number of different contri-butors, dealing with Hesse's novels and poetry. The book explores the author's interest in psychoanaly-sis, music, and Eastern philosophy, and the influ-ences of politics, painting, and other writers on his work.

Helt, Richard C. *". . . A Poet or Nothing At All": The Tübingen and Basel Years of Hermann Hesse.* Prov-idence, R.I.: Berghahn, 1996. A study of Hesse's for-mative years as a writer, particularly the period between 1899 and 1903, when he persevered to be-come a poet despite the disapproval of his family, health issues, and financial woes.

Hesse, Hermann, and Thomas Mann. *The Hesse-Mann Letters: The Correspondence of Hermann Hesse and Thomas Mann, 1910-1955.* Edited by Anne Carlsson and Volker Michels. New York: Jorge Pinto Books, 2005. This book presents the corre-spondence between two giants of German litera-ture—both Nobel Prize winners—who commiser-ate about the ravages of war and speculate about the fate of their native country.

Stelzig, Eugene L. "The Aesthetics of Confession: Hermann Hesse's *Crisis* Poems in the Context of the Steppenwolf Period." In *Hermann Hesse*, edited by Harold Bloom. Philadelphia: Chelsea House, 2002. Essay examines the poems of *Crisis* and re-lates them to the Steppenwolf period.

Tusken, Lewis W. *Understanding Hermann Hesse: The Man, His Myth, His Metaphor.* Columbia: Uni-versity of South Carolina Press, 1998. An overview of Hesse's life and literary significance, with particular attention paid to the themes, images, and metaphors in his novels, which often also were used in his poetry.

Ziolkowski, Theodore. *Modes of Faith: Secular Surrogates for Lost Religious Beliefs*. Chicago: University of Chicago Press, 2007. An examination of how writers in the early twentieth century—including James Joyce, Hesse, Thomas Mann, and H. G. Wells—treated the erosion of religious belief and the ascent of secular philosophies in their work.

Jack Ewing

HUGO VON HOFMANNSTHAL

Born: Vienna, Austro-Hungarian Empire; February 1, 1874
Died: Rodaun, Austria; July 15, 1929

PRINCIPAL POETRY

Ausgewählte Gedichte, 1903
Die gesammelten Gedichte, 1907 (*The Lyrical Poems of Hugo von Hofmannsthal*, 1918)
Loris, 1930
Nachlese der Gedichte, 1934
Gedichte und lyrische Dramen, 1946 (*Poems and Verse Plays*, 1961)
The Whole Difference: Selected Writings of Hugo von Hofmannsthal, 2008

OTHER LITERARY FORMS

The outstanding poetry of Hugo von Hofmannsthal (HOHF-mahn-stahl) forms only a very small portion of his literary legacy. During the 1890's, when his best poems were written, editions of his early lyric plays also appeared. They include *Gestern* (pb. 1891), *Der Tor und der Tod* (pb. 1894; *Death and the Fool*, 1913), *Die Hochzeit der Sobeide* (pr., pb. 1899; *The Marriage of Sobeide*, 1913), and *Theater in Versen* (1899). After 1900, he devoted most of his creative energy to the stage and published more than twenty additional books of dramatic writings before his death. Such works as

Elektra (pr. 1903; *Electra*, 1908), *Jedermann* (pr., pb. 1911; *Everyman*, 1917), *Der Schwierige* (pb. 1920; *The Difficult Man*, 1963), and *Das Salzburger Grosse Welttheater* (pr., pb. 1922; *The Salzburg Great Theatre of the World*, 1958) became very popular. Hofmannsthal achieved his greatest theatrical success, however, as librettist for the operas of Richard Strauss. Because of his lyric virtuosity, *Electra*, which he revised for Strauss, *Der Rosenkavalier* (pr., pb. 1911; *The Cavalier of the Rose*, 1912; also known as *The Rose Bearer*), and *Arabella* (pr., pb. 1933; English translation, 1955) received lasting acclaim. Hofmannsthal also wrote a few excellent short stories, parts of a novel, scenarios for several ballets, and more than two hundred essays, all of which have been published. Since his death, his notebooks and diaries have been edited, as have some twenty volumes of his extensive correspondence.

ACHIEVEMENTS

Unlike most poets, Hugo von Hofmannsthal did not go through a period of gradual literary development leading to eventual mature control of his art. Rather, he emerged at the beginning of his career as an accomplished lyricist and immediately became an enigma to the Austrian literary establishment. His earliest poems quickly caught the attention of critics and writers alike, especially the young Viennese moderns. His combination of youth and poetic genius was unparalleled in German letters, and many of his contemporaries found it very hard to reconcile the artistic power of his works with the teenage poet who had written them.

Among those most impressed with the young Hofmannsthal's creative facility was Stefan George. Much of Hofmannsthal's poetry appeared for the first time in *Blätter für die Kunst*, the literary organ of George and his circle. As a result, Hofmannsthal is often associated with the German Symbolists. Although he shared with George the desire to achieve the greatest possible perfection and purification of literary language and expression, his own lyrics are far more closely related to those of his friends Hermann Bahr, Arthur Schnitzler, and Richard Beer-Hofmann. As a part of this group, Hofmannsthal mediated ideas and prosody from a broad range of European models and traditions, created some of the most sensitive poems in modern German literature, and received acclaim in his own time as the greatest of the German Impressionists.

Hofmannsthal resisted the idea of compiling his poetry until years after he had turned his creative attention almost exclusively to drama. Only two collections were published in his lifetime, yet during a brief decade he had contributed to Austrian literature poems of beauty unequaled in the German language since the time of Johann Wolfgang von Goethe. The wider recognition that he later enjoyed as a dramatist and librettist came in no small measure as a result of his utter mastery of poetic language and lyric technique.

BIOGRAPHY

The only son of a Viennese bank director, Hugo Laurenz August Hofmann Edler von Hofmannsthal came from a mixed heritage of Austrian, Italian, and German-Jewish elements that were vitally important to his cultural and intellectual development. He was educated by private tutors until he was ten; then he entered secondary school in Vienna. An avid reader, he assimilated an astounding amount of knowledge in a very short time. His precocious intellect set him apart from the young people around him, contributing to a sense of loneliness that remained with him throughout his life.

In 1890, Hofmannsthal published his first poem, "Frage," under the pseudonym Loris Melikow. That summer, he became acquainted with the actor Gustav Schwarzkopf, who introduced him to Bahr, Schnitzler, and Felix Salten. Within the next few months, Hofmannsthal published additional poems, his first essay, and his first lyric play, *Gestern*, in periodicals in Vienna and Berlin.

One of three important friendships that strongly influenced Hofmannsthal's creative career began in December, 1891, when he met George, who had come to Vienna to seek him out. A productive, if often stormy, relationship with George lasted for fifteen years and generated a correspondence that in its significance for German literature has been compared to that between Goethe and Friedrich Schiller. Although Hofmannsthal initially felt comfortable in George's group, differences in temperament and creative outlook caused severe tension. Hofmannsthal soon removed himself from active participation in George's literary ventures,

even though their association did not break off completely until 1906.

During the 1890's, Hofmannsthal traveled extensively, met a variety of people, and set patterns that informed the remainder of his life. His first trip to Venice in 1892 was of special importance for his work as a whole. Venice became his second home and the setting for some of his later dramas. In 1892, he enrolled at the University of Vienna, where he briefly studied law. Between 1895 and 1899, he successfully completed a doctoral program in Romance philology. The late 1890's were especially productive years. While in Italy in 1897, he composed more than two thousand lines of poetry and lyric drama in one two-week period. By 1900, he had already written and staged several plays.

After marrying Gertrud Schlesinger in 1901, Hofmannsthal moved to Rodaun. During the years that followed, he devoted his time to mastering the drama, entering into enormously productive relationships with producer Max Reinhardt and composer Strauss. In

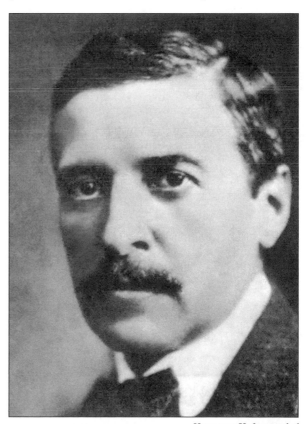

Hugo von Hofmannsthal

1903, Reinhardt encouraged him to create a free rendition of Sophocles' *Ēlektra* (418-410 B.C.E.; *Electra*, 1649), the production of which brought Hofmannsthal his first major theatrical success. After the play attracted the attention of Strauss, Hofmannsthal revised it, creating a libretto that when set to music was even more successful than the original drama. During the next twenty-three years, the two artists collaborated in the creation of five additional operas and several ballets.

For Hofmannsthal, World War I and the death of the old Austrian regime were a personal disaster from which he never recovered. After the war, he dedicated himself to the revival of Austrian and German culture. In 1917, he participated in the founding of the famous Salzburg Festival, and in the early 1920's, he edited and published several collections of writings by earlier authors. Beginning in 1920, however, his health began to fail, and he suffered recurring illness until his death. He died of a cerebral hemorrhage two days after the tragic suicide of his older son Franz.

ANALYSIS

In the essay "Der Dichter und diese Zeit" ("The Poet and This Time"), written in 1907, Hugo von Hofmannsthal outlined the key concepts that informed his poems. From his perspective, the principal responsibility of the modern poet was to provide the reader with access to the whole spectrum of human experience. If nothing else, Hofmannsthal's poetry reflects his overriding desire to participate in and become a part of everything that he saw, felt, or dreamed, and to share with others the intensity of his impressions of life. He envisioned the poet as one who unites past, present, and future into an eternal "now," recording, preserving, and analyzing everything that moves his era. A human seismograph that responds to living realities, the poet awakens his audience to the inner meaning of their own unexamined experience.

Hofmannsthal's view of the poet's relationship to his times explains the diversity of his lyric creations and the complexity of themes, moods, and ideas that inform his literary art. His poems are like fragments of a vast mosaic, in which each carefully positioned element exposes the beholder to a small yet powerful aspect of the human condition. Hofmannsthal sought to reveal the broad range of possibilities to be found or generated within the individual, while moving people in the direction of cogent answers to basic existential questions: What is a human? How can humans perceive their own nature and actively create, refine, and perfect the features of their unique inner world? He did not wish to impose on the reader a finished worldview but rather to offer raw materials, tools, and stimuli that might enable others to awaken, expand, and mold their own perceptions. While giving direction to those searching for meaning, he sounded the abyss of his own soul, exposing to the public eye the sensitive observations, the multicolored dreams, and the speculative visions that constituted his innermost self. The poems thus engendered reflect his encounters with beauty and loneliness interwoven with feelings of love and defiance, with landscapes, people, and the material things of external reality.

As an Impressionist, Hofmannsthal sought a faithful reproduction of subjective sensual experience and precisely noted mood. His lyrics are remarkable for their acute awareness of the incidental, the transitory, and the matchless spiritual state in all its peculiarities and narrow differentiations, nuances, shades, and halftones. His treatment of visual themes was especially effective; he wrote with a painter's eye. He saw mastery of language as the essence of poetic creation and systematically cultivated an elevated literary diction.

THE LYRIC DECADE

During his so-called lyric decade, Hofmannsthal capsulized in verse the most important aspects of his philosophy of life. His poems contain in embryonic form all the major ideas that he later expanded, modified, and refined in his dramas, librettos, and prose fiction. In combinations of vision and interpretation of the world and its phenomena, he developed a unified view of the internal harmony of present, past, and future reality, basing his approach on a concept he called preexistence. According to Hofmannsthal, existence has two points of reference: mortal life and preexistence. Preexistence is the human state when people are removed from mortal life. It is the state from which people come at birth, to which they go at death, and to which they travel temporarily in dreams or similar experiences. In this system, preexistence is absolute existence, while mortality is a transitory situation with little meaning outside the framework of preexistence.

The idea of preexistence is central to Hofmannsthal's explorations of basic human problems such as death, transitoriness, and the search for personal identity. Filtered through the lens of preexistence, life itself becomes an infinite process of creative transformation and refinement through which the person achieves oneness with all reality by concretely and spiritually experiencing an endless series of modes of being. In one of his earliest poems, "Ghaselen II" ("Ghazel II"), written in 1891, Hofmannsthal captured the essence of his notion of preexistence in lines that describe life as a wandering of the spirit through the hierarchy of beings, a process of changing and growing. While the course of transformation is one of purification, it does not always proceed upward. The transition may be from worm to frog or from poet to vagabond.

METAPHORS FOR THE MORTAL STATE

In harmony with the representation of life as a realm of continually changing roles, Hofmannsthal developed three poetic metaphors for the mortal state, each of which—the dream, the drama, and the game—represents a brief, sharply framed, experience. Although these metaphors are certainly not original and reflect a clear bond to a broad range of models in European literary tradition, Hofmannsthal's treatment of them is especially characteristic for his lyric poems. He used the dream to explore life as a creative process occurring completely within the person. Mortality perceived as drama, a direct outgrowth of the preexistence concept, allowed him to portray humans as actors passing through a series of external identities that in turn emerge as Faustian aspects of the individual spirit. Hofmannsthal was especially fond of the drama metaphor. He styled himself a spectator and from that perspective wrote the poems that most powerfully illuminate life as a stage production. The game metaphor is the least emphasized of the three and is less fully developed in his poetry. Later, Hofmannsthal centered dramas and stories around adult games, highlighting the figure of the adventurer/gambler. His lyrics, however, focus on the child's game as an aspect of the created inner self. His representations of the internal world are often populated with game-playing children who are at once formed in the image of the poet and subject to him as their creator.

"STANZAS IN TERZA RIMA"

In 1894, almost at the midpoint of his lyric decade, Hofmannsthal wrote a series of four poems in iambic tercets. He labeled them simply "Terzinen" ("Stanzas in Terza Rima"). Collectively, they provide excellent illustrations of his treatment of the basic human experiences of transitoriness and death, clearly elucidating his approach to these problems in the light of the theory of preexistence. A year later, in "Ballade des Äusseren Lebens," he would stress the emptiness of a world unaware of preexistence, questioning the relevance of mortality and dwelling on the transience, absence of coherence, and consequent lack of enduring value of earthly things. In "Stanzas in Terza Rima," however, he affirmed the permanence of all things perceived in absolute spiritual terms, providing a positive alternative for the person who is conscious of preexistence.

The first of the four poems, subtitled "Über Vergänglichkeit," questions the idea that the past can be borne away and lost forever without a trace. Central to the poet's deliberation is the stark awareness that his own essence is in a state of change and that it has metamorphosed from its former existence as a child. Consciousness of the past, however, also extends before childhood, in the realization that the poet existed before his mortal birth as an elemental part of his ancestors. Within the absolute realm of preexistence, his dead forebears are likewise a living part of the poet.

Hofmannsthal's approach to death is an extremely important facet of the doctrine of preexistence. In his poetry, he illuminated two clearly defined aspects of death as a basic experience of the individual spirit's eternal progression. The poem "Erlebnis" ("An Experience"), which he wrote two years before the "Stanzas in Terza Rima," focuses on death as a vehicle of transfer from mortality to preexistence. In beautifully vivid imagery, filled with powerful sensual impressions of light and sound, the poet describes death as a drowning in a translucent, light-weaving ocean, followed by an immediate longing for the mortal life that has been lost. The yearning itself is compared to that of a ship's passenger who sails past his hometown, unable to cross to the land that represents his childhood.

In "Stanzas in Terza Rima II," as in "An Experience," death is presented not as a feared unknown, but as something that is clearly understood. In the terza rima poem, however, stress is placed on the second aspect of the death experience, the flow of life from one form to another. In harmony with the notion of a continual passing through a hierarchy of beings, as developed in "Ghazel II," the poet points to the conveying of vital energy from one entity to another in the image of life fleeing from pale little girls into trees and grass. Death is nothing more than an outward manifestation of the bond that pervades all existence, linking life into a great whole.

"Stanzas in Terza Rima III" is the first of Hofmannsthal's poems to employ his characteristic metaphor of life as a dream. This lyric emphasizes the creative power of dreams: Because the stuff of which people are made has properties like those of dreams, people are able to merge and become one with their dreams. Like death, then, the dream becomes a vehicle by which people attain ultimate definition within the sphere of absolute existence. "Stanzas in Terza Rima IV" expands the dream metaphor to its final dimensions by placing within its scope external relations with other people, internal longings, the structure and perception of the material world, and the conclusive penetration and understanding of life and self.

POEMS AND VERSE PLAYS

From the very beginning of his literary career, Hofmannsthal felt himself drawn to the theater. That fact is especially relevant to his amplification of the life-is-a-drama metaphor in his poetry. Although he employed stage-related imagery in a variety of lyric contexts, the most representative poems in this category appear in the volume *Poems and Verse Plays* under the collective heading "Prologe und Trauerreden" ("Prologues and Elegies"). This set of lyric creations reveals the deeply personal nature of the drama metaphor, clarifying Hofmannsthal's self-appointed role as spectator in the theater of life.

One of the most famous poems in the group is "Prolog zu dem Buch 'Anatol'" ("Prologue to the Book 'Anatol'"), which was written to introduce a work by Schnitzler. It begins with a powerful, seemingly directionless, heterogeneous array of impressions from the domain of the theater. Latticework, artificial hedges, escutcheons, sphinxes, creaking gates, and waterfalls are artistically jumbled together. Throughout the first section, props, backdrops, and scenery are interwoven with bits of plays, apparently unconnected actors and actresses, and fragments of color and mood. The result is a vivid mosaic of constituents related only through their mutual association with the stage.

The second portion of the poem presents the reasons for the visible turmoil and disorder. The theater stands for the multiformity of mortal existence. The dramas that are performed proceed from natural personal impulse without effort, premeditation, or constraint, arising from within the players themselves. Hofmannsthal enlarges the metaphor to encompass himself and the reader among the actors and summarizes their involvement by depicting life as "plays that we have fashioned" and "comedies of our own spirit." He thus gives his own version of William Shakespeare's "All the world's a stage."

"ZUM GEDÄCHTNIS DES SCHAUSPIELERS MITTERWURZER"

In the elegiac poems, Hofmannsthal presented more intensely the relation between the drama metaphor and his concept of preexistence. The elegies, some of which are dedicated to the memory of real people, focus on the actor as symbolic man. "Zum Gedächtnis des Schauspielers Mitterwurzer" (in memory of the actor Mitterwurzer) is very representative of the poet's development of this particular theme.

"Zum Gedächtnis des Schauspielers Mitterwurzer" examines the implications of the actor's death with respect to absolute existence. When the player dies, it is quickly apparent that something extraordinary has perished: With him have disappeared all the figures to whom he gave life. The characters no longer live because the special essence that this actor gave them could come only from him. Another actor playing the same part would somehow give a different nature to the role, and the character, in spite of mask and props, would be a new one. Because of the feeling of final loss, the poet seeks to penetrate to Mitterwurzer's true identity and learns that the dead actor is essentially one with the dreamer. He molds and forms the existence that surrounds him. Like the dreamer's world, the realm created by the actor comes from within himself. Hofmannsthal portrays Mitterwurzer's body as a magic veil that houses everything, a veil from which the actor could conjure up not only various animals and people, but also, more important, "you and me."

Briefly stated, the actor gives life. In Hofmannsthal's framework, the actor is a conduit through which individual souls can bridge the gap between preexistence and mortality. The death of Mitterwurzer represents the loss of such a conduit. More profoundly tragic, therefore, than the passing of characters already portrayed is the untimely preclusion of those as yet unborn. The substance of the poem's final lament is that Mitterwurzer's death has caused the departure of inhabitants from people's internal worlds and has prevented the arrival of others who might have had their birth within people. In dying, the actor has deprived those left behind of precious elements of their own being.

"DER JÜNGLING UND DIE SPINNE"

"Der Jüngling und die Spinne," a two-part existential work written in 1897, near the end of Hofmannsthal's lyric period, is one of a very few poems that develop in detail his representation of humans as game players. Like the metaphors of the dream and the drama, the metaphor of the game is important to the definition of the internally formulated world of the individual. Creating a self-contained world, the artist "teaches" the "citizens" of that world certain games that then characterize both them and their creator. In the first segment of "Der Jüngling und die Spinne," a young man reveals himself as a representative Hofmannsthal figure, aware of his place in the middle of a universe, of which fate's decrees have made him master. While observing his "subjects," he notes their peculiar relationship to himself. Many have his own features. More important, they play games that he, as their originator, has taught them. For the youth, the process of looking inward is one of learning to understand not only himself but also life in its absolute sense. The transformation that occurs in the dawning of awareness is Hofmannsthal's ultimate symbol for the kind of impact that he intended his poetry to have on the reader. The timeless role of the poet—a synthesis of dreamer, actor, and player of games—is to teach actively by pro-

viding others with the needed personal keys to themselves.

"WHERE I NEAR AND WHERE I LAND . . ."

In the famous poem "Wo ich nahe, wo ich lande . . ." ("Where I Near and Where I Land . . ."), a powerful example of depth in simplicity, Hofmannsthal describes in greater detail the rapport that he wished to achieve with his public. Unlike the young man of "Der Jüngling und die Spinne," the "I" of "Where I Near and Where I Land . . ." is completely cognizant of his responsibility to elevate his world's inhabitants to spiritual planes beyond their present state. The teacher who has the capacity to communicate with the deepest levels of the soul, causing such levels to unfold in inner comprehension of self, might achieve the goal of Hofmannsthal's poetry, uplifting both himself and the world around him.

OTHER MAJOR WORKS

LONG FICTION: *Andreas: Oder, Die Vereinigten*, 1932 (*Andreas: Or, The United*, 1936).

SHORT FICTION: *Reitergeschichte*, 1899 (*Cavalry Patrol*, 1939); *Erlebnis des Marschalls von Bassompierre*, 1900 (*An Episode in the Life of the Marshal de Bassompierre*, 1952); *Das Märchen 672: Nacht, und andere Erzählungen*, 1905 (*Tale of the Merchant's Son and His Servants*, 1969); *Lucidor*, 1910 (English translation, 1922); *Drei Erzählungen*, 1927; *Das erzählerische Work*, 1969.

PLAYS: *Gestern*, pb. 1891; *Der Tor und der Tod*, pb. 1894 (*Death and the Fool*, 1913); *Das kleine Welttheater*, pb. 1897 (*The Little Theater of the World*, 1961); *Die Frau im Fenster*, pr., pb. 1898 (*Madonna Dianora*, 1916); *Der weisse Fächer*, pb. 1898 (*The White Fan*, 1909); *Der Abenteurer und die Sängerin*, pr., pb. 1899 (*The Adventurer and the Singer*, 1917); *Die Hochzeit der Sobeide*, pr., pb. 1899 (*The Marriage of Sobeide*, 1913); *Theater in Versen*, pb. 1899; *Der Kaiser und die Hexe*, pb. 1900 (*The Emperor and the Witch*, 1961); *Elektra*, pr. 1903 (*Electra*, 1908); *Das gerettete Venedig*, pr., pb. 1905 (*Venice Preserved*, 1915); *Kleine Dramen*, pb. 1906; *Ödipus und die Sphinx*, pr., pb. 1906 (*Oedipus and the Sphinx*, 1968); *Vorspiele*, pb. 1908; *Christinas Heimreise*, pr. 1910 (*Christina's Journey Home*, 1916); *König Ödipus*, pr., pb. 1910; *Alkestis*, pb. 1911; *Jedermann*, pr., pb. 1911 (*Everyman*, 1917);

Der Rosenkavalier, pr., pb. 1911 (libretto; *The Cavalier of the Rose*, 1912; also known as *The Rose Bearer*); *Ariadne auf Naxos*, pr., pb. 1912 (libretto; *Ariadne on Naxos*, 1922); *Der Bürger als Edelmann*, pr., pb. 1918; *Die Frau ohne Schatten*, pr., pb. 1919 (libretto; *The Woman Without a Shadow*, 1957); *Dame Kobold*, pr., pb. 1920; *Der Schwierige*, pb. 1920 (*The Difficult Man*, 1963); *Florindo*, pr. 1921; *Das Salzburger Grosse Welttheater*, pr., pb. 1922 (*The Salzburg Great Theatre of the World*, 1958); *Der Unbestechliche*, pr. 1923; *Der Turm*, pb. 1925 (*The Tower*, 1963); *Die ägyptische Helena*, pr., pb. 1928 (libretto; *Helen in Egypt*, 1963); *Arabella*, pr., pb. 1933 (libretto; English translation, 1955); *Das Bergwerk zu Folun*, pb. 1933 (*The Mine at Falun*, 1933); *Dramatische Entwürfe*, pb. 1936; *Silvia im "Stern,"* pb. 1959.

NONFICTION: *Gespräch über Gedichte*, 1904; *Unterhaltungen über literarische Gegenstände*, 1904; *Die Briefe des Zurückgekehrten*, 1907; *Der Dichter und diese Zeit*, 1907 (*The Poet and His Time*, 1955); *Wege und die Begegnungen*, 1913; *Reden und Aufsätze*, 1921; *Buch der Freunde*, 1922 (*The Book of Friends*, 1952); *Augenblicke in Griechenland*, 1924 (*Moments in Greece*, 1952); *Früheste Prosastücke*, 1926; *Richard Strauss und Hugo von Hofmannsthal: Briefwechsel*, 1926 (*Correspondence of Richard Strauss and Hugo von Hofmannsthal*, 1927); *Ad me ipsum*, 1930; *Loris: Die Prosa des jungen Hugo von Hofmannsthal*, 1930; *Die Berührung der Sphären*, 1931; *Briefwechsel zwischen George und Hofmannsthal*, 1938 (letters); *Festspiele in Salzburg*, 1938; *Selected Prose*, 1952; *Selected Essays*, 1955; *The Lord Chantos Letters and Other Writings*, 2005.

EDITED TEXTS: *Deutsche Erzähler*, 1912 (4 volumes); *Die österreichische Bibliothek*, 1915-1917 (26 volumes); *Deutsches Epigramme*, 1923 (2 volumes); *Schillers Selbstcharakteristik*, 1926.

MISCELLANEOUS: *Gesammelte Werke in Einzelausgaben*, 1945-1959 (15 volumes); *Selected Writings of Hugo von Hofmannsthal*, 1952-1963 (3 volumes); *Hofmannsthal: Gesammelte Werke*, 1979 (10 volumes).

BIBLIOGRAPHY

Bangerter, Lowell A. *Hugo von Hofmannsthal*. New York: F. Ungar, 1977. A critical analysis of selected works by Hofmannsthal. Includes an index and a bibliography.

Beniston, Judith. *Welttheater: Hofmannsthal, Richard von Kralik, and the Revival of Catholic Drama in Austria, 1890-1934*. Leeds, England: W. S. Maney, 1998. This study of Catholic drama in Austria compares and contrasts the works of Hofmannsthal and Richard von Kralik. Bibliography and index.

Bennett, Benjamin. *Hugo von Hofmannsthal: The Theaters of Consciousness*. 1988. New York: Cambridge University Press, 2009. A critical analysis and interpretation of Hofmannsthal's literary works. Bibliography and index.

Broch, Hermann and Michael P. Steinberg, trans. *Hugo von Hofmannsthal and His Time: The European Imagination, 1860-1920*. Chicago: University of Chicago Press, 1984. Examines the writer as a product of his time, placing him within it.

Del Caro, Adrian. *Hugo von Hofmannsthal: Poets and the Language of Life*. Baton Rouge: Louisiana State University Press, 1993. Del Caro argues that Hofmannsthal was an early opponent of aestheticism and was an heir of Friedrich Nietzsche in his search for a legitimate source for values. Includes bibliographical references and index.

Kovach, Thomas A. *Hofmannsthal and Symbolism: Art and Life in the Work of a Modern Poet*. New York: Peter Lang, 1985. A biographical and critical study of Hofmannsthal's life and work. Includes bibliographic references and an index.

_____, ed. *A Companion to the Writings of Hugo von Hofmannsthal*. Rochester, N.Y.: Camden House, 2002. Contains essays on all aspects of Hofmannsthal's life and works, including one on his poems and lyric drama. An introduction by the editor provides biographical information.

Vilain, Robert. *The Poetry of Hugo von Hofmannsthal and French Symbolism*. New York: Oxford University Press, 2000. Vilain suggests that Hofmannsthal's early interest in the works of the French Symbolists had an inhibiting effect on his own poetry. Includes bibliographical references and indexes.

Lowell A. Bangerter

FRIEDRICH HÖLDERLIN

Born: Lauffen am Neckar, Württemberg (now in
    Germany); March 20, 1770
Died: Tübingen, Württemberg (now in Germany);
    June 7, 1843

PRINCIPAL POETRY

Nachtgesänge, 1805
Gedichte, 1826 (*Poems*, 1943)
Selected Poems, 1944
Poems and Fragments, 1966
Selected Poems and Fragments, 1998
Odes and Elegies, 2008

OTHER LITERARY FORMS

The deep love for Greek culture that marked the lyric
poetry of Friedrich Hölderlin (HURL-dur-leen) also had
a profound impact on his other literary endeavors. Aside
from his verse, he is most remembered for the epistolary
novel *Hyperion: Oder, Der Eremit in Griechenland*
(1797, 1799; *Hyperion: Or, The Hermit in Greece*,
1965). In the story of a disillusioned Greek freedom
fighter, the author captured in rhythmic prose much of
his own inner world. The novel is especially notable for
its vivid imagery and its power of thought and language.
Fascination with the legend of Empedocles' death on
Mount Etna moved him to attempt to re-create the
spirit of the surrounding events in the drama *Der Tod
des Empedokles* (pb. 1826; *The Death of Empedocles*,
1966), which exists in three fragmentary versions. After 1800, he began translations of Sophocles' *Oidipous
Tyrannos* (c. 429 B.C.E.; *Oedipus Tyrannus*, 1715) and
Antigonē (441 B.C.E.; *Antigone*, 1729); his highly successful renderings were published in 1804. Among the
various essays on philosophy, aesthetics, and literature written throughout his career, his treatises on the
fine arts in ancient Greece, Achilles, Homer's *Iliad* (c.
750 B.C.E.; English translation, 1611), and the plays of
Sophocles are especially significant. Only a small portion of his correspondence has been preserved.

ACHIEVEMENTS

Unlike the great German lyricists with whom he is
compared, Friedrich Hölderlin did not attain substantial literary recognition in his own time. This lack of
recognition was in part a result of his own misperception
of his audience. While he directed his poems to the
broad following of the spiritual and intellectual renewal engendered by the French Revolution, his contemporaries, excepting a special few, did not penetrate
beyond the surface of his particular revelation of the rebirth of idealism's golden age.

Friedrich Schiller's early patronage gave Hölderlin
access to influential editors and other promoters of
mainstream literature, enabling him to publish in important journals and popular collections of the time. His
work appeared in Gotthold Stäudlin's *Schwäbisches
Musenalmanach auf das Jahr 1792* (1792) and *Po-
etische Blumenlese* (1793), as well as Schiller's *Thalia*
and other periodicals. Neither Schiller nor Johann
Wolfgang von Goethe, however, fully recognized Hölderlin's true gifts as a writer. Eventually, they distanced themselves from him, and Hölderlin fell into
obscurity.

After his death, Hölderlin remained forgotten until
his work was rediscovered by Stefan George and his
circle. George acclaimed him as one of the great masters of the age, pointing especially to the uniqueness of
his language and the expressiveness of his style. In the
modern poets whose works reflect a keen inner struggle
with the meaning of existence, he at last found a receptive audience, capable of appreciating his contribution
to the evolution of the German lyric. Among those
whose writings give strong evidence of his productive
influence are Georg Trakl, Rainer Maria Rilke, and
Hugo von Hofmannsthal.

For his special mastery of form, his naturalization of
classical Greek meters and rhythms in the German language, and his unique ability to clothe prophetic vision
in verse, Hölderlin now stands alongside Goethe as one
of the great poets of German idealism.

BIOGRAPHY

The untimely deaths of both his father and his stepfather determined the course of Johann Christian Friedrich
Hölderlin's childhood and youth. His mother, a devoutly
religious Lutheran, insisted that he prepare for a career
in the clergy. While attending monastery schools at
Denkendorf and Maulbronn, he began writing poetry

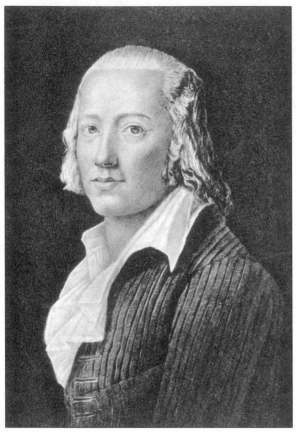

Friedrich Hölderlin (Hulton Archive/Getty Images)

that reflected the suffering of a sensitive spirit under the rigors of traditional discipline and an inability to reconcile the demands of practical reality with his inner sense of artistic calling. Youthful love affairs with Luise Nast (the "Stella" of his early poems) and Elise Lebret exacerbated the tension between the two poles of his existence.

In 1788, Hölderlin entered the theological seminary at the University of Tübingen. Although he completed his studies and received a master's degree that titled him to ordination, the years spent in Tübingen eased him away from any desire to become a pastor. With his friends Christian Ludwig Neuffer and Rudolf Magenau, he founded a poetry club patterned after the Göttinger Hain. He also joined a secret political organization with Georg Wilhelm Friedrich Hegel and Friedrich Schelling and openly advocated social reforms inspired by the ideals of the French Revolution. The true key to his rejection of a life of service in the

church, however, was neither purely artistic inclination nor political commitment but rather deep spiritual conflict within himself. Concentrated exposure to the literature, art, and philosophy of classical antiquity caused him to develop a worldview that placed the ancient Greek gods, as vital natural forces, next to Christ in importance for the dawning of a new, humane era of enlightenment and harmony. The tension between the old pantheon and Christian dogma made it impossible for him to feel comfortable in total dedication to institutionalized religion.

Among his contemporaries, Hölderlin's most important role model was Schiller, whose poetry had a strong impact on both his early Tübingen hymns and his later classicistic creations. In 1793, Hölderlin met Schiller for the first time. Their friendship remained rather one-sided; Schiller did not reciprocate the warmth and devotion of his awestruck protégé. Through Schiller's mediation, Hölderlin obtained the first of a long series of positions as a private tutor. These situations, despite their repeated failure, enabled him to avoid the necessity of accepting an appointment as a pastor.

Hölderlin's most significant assignment as a tutor began in 1795, when he entered the service of a wealthy banker in Frankfurt. A love affair with his employer's wife, Susette Gontard, provided the stimulus for a newfound sophistication in his poetry. Much of the substance that he treated in verse while in Frankfurt was later refined and presented in more perfect form in the exquisite odes, elegies, and hymns of his late period. Susette herself became the model for Diotima in his novel *Hyperion* and the poems related to it.

After an unpleasant scene with Susette's husband in 1798, Hölderlin fled to Homburg, where he remained until 1800 with his friend Isaak von Sinclair. Hölderlin continued to see and correspond secretly with Susette, but he was unsuccessful in establishing himself in a permanently meaningful way of life. An endeavor to edit a new journal and make his living as a freelance writer foundered. Plagued by an increasing inner isolation, he was compelled to return home to his mother.

From an artistic point of view, the years immediately after 1800 were the most important of Hölderlin's career; emotionally and spiritually, they were years of progressive devastation. New tutorial positions in Switzerland and France collapsed rapidly. In 1802, Hölderlin left Bordeaux and traveled home on foot. He arrived in Nürtingen mentally and emotionally disturbed after learning of Susette's death. In 1804, temporarily recovered from his nervous breakdown, he returned to Homburg, where Sinclair arranged for him to work as a librarian. When Sinclair was arrested for subversive political activities, Hölderlin's mental condition deteriorated drastically, and he was placed in a sanatorium. In 1806, he was declared incurably ill and given into the care of a carpenter and his wife. He spent the remainder of his life living in a tower room overlooking the Neckar, where he wrote occasional, strangely simple lyrics, played the flute and the piano, and received visitors.

ANALYSIS

In the final stanza of his famous poem "Die Heimat" ("Homeland"), Friedrich Hölderlin captured the essence of his personal artistic calling and its lyrical product. The pairing of love, the divine fire that stimulates creativity, with suffering, the holy reward that the gods give to their poet-prophet, defines the poles of existential tension that were a primary focus of his life and works. A peculiar mixture of the poetry of experience and that of ideas, his early hymns and his mature odes, elegies, and hymns in free rhythms are at once the offspring of intense adoration—of beauty, nature, Greek antiquity, an idealized world of tomorrow—and profound spiritual pain resulting from recognition of the abyss between the poet and the things that he cherishes. The result is a constant duality of mood: on one hand, deeply elegiac longing for the elements of a lost golden age; on the other, overwhelming joy in the message of love that is the joint legacy of the Greek world and the Christian tradition. Oscillating between hope and despair, anticipation and resignation, tragic darkness and powerfully prophetic vision, his verse documents the continuing struggle of a spirit that needs to belong to society yet remains alone as a priest who serves no church, a singer of a people no longer or not yet there.

Despite the concentrated projection of the deeply personal strivings of his own soul into his writings, Hölderlin's lyrics were based firmly in an age-old and broadly recognized tradition to which he gave new life. At the same time, they represent a mating of impulses from the German classical and Romantic movements that dominated the literary mainstream of his own time. His interpretation of models ranging from Plato to Spinoza, from Homer and Hesiod to Schiller and Goethe, and including Friedrich Gottlieb Klopstock, Johann Jakob Wilhelm Heinse, Christian Friedrich Daniel Schubart, and Ludwig Christoph Hölty generated a multisided literature that mixes a glowing sense of freedom with enthusiastic, unfettered pantheism and celebration of the highest human ideals with *Weltschmerz*.

INFLUENCE OF SCHILLER AND KLOPSTOCK

The influence of Schiller upon Hölderlin's early creations is especially noticeable. Scholars often point to the melancholy longing for the beauty and glory of Greece, the lost spiritual homeland, as a defining characteristic of Hölderlin's early verse. His various elaborations of this theme, particularly his emphatic presentations of the ancient gods as living elemental forces, give remarkable evidence of having been motivated directly by Schiller's well-known poem "Die Götter Griechenlands" ("The Gods of Greece"). Moreover, his acclaim of a new humanistic age in hymns to freedom, humanity, harmony, friendship, nature, and other abstract concepts was clearly inspired not only by his infatuation with the ideas of the French Revolution but also by a deep reverence for Schiller, whose treatments of those same subjects are key building blocks in the poetry of German idealism. Even the meter and syntax of Hölderlin's first lyric efforts are obvious products of his familiarity with Schiller's language and forms.

Hölderlin's Alcaic and Asclepiadean odes on nature, landscape, and love, written in Denkendorf and Maulbronn, are strongly subjective and self-oriented, weighed down by an almost oppressive intensity of reflection. The moods of Storm and Stress are clearly visible, as is Klopstock's basic tone, in which personal experience is raised into a suprapersonal religious sphere. Amid trivial occasional verse, sentimentally broad discourses on life, and curiously sad love poems written to Nast, there are already glimmerings of the elements that eventually informed Hölderlin's more characteristic lyrics. For example, "Die Unsterblichkeit der Seele" ("The Immortality of the Soul"), an ode that bears all the marks of Klopstock's manner, anticipates in direction and perception the later "Hymne an die Unsterblichkeit" ("Hymn to Immortality"), which was written in Tübingen. In the long hexameter poem "Die Teck" ("The Teck"), a glorification of a local mountain area, important themes of the late hymns appear: the Dionysian festival of the grape harvest, the sublime nature of dead heroes, the magnificence of the forested landscape saturated with the traditions of the fatherland, and the celebration of friendship.

A MISSION AND A SPIRITUAL HOMELAND

An important focus of the works created in Tübingen is Hölderlin's growing preoccupation with the awareness of a personal poetic mission. From the rejection of seminary life's inhibiting restrictions in "Zornige Sehnsucht" ("Angry Longing") to the magnification and praise of Greece, the Muses, and his personal gods in a first formal cycle of hymns, Hölderlin's formulations stress his belief in a calling to reinterpret Christian and classical ideals within the framework of his own era. He saw himself as a kind of prophet in a time of special revelation that needed poetic amplification. Accordingly, in the hymns, he presented aspects of a holy message based on the eternal example of antiquity. A pantheistic view of nature as a complex of ethical and emotional forces unified by a grand, divine essence charges the poems with living, vital myth in the creation of an ideal, harmonious realm that is the final goal of the poet's longing, both for himself and for all humankind.

The evocation of Greece as Hölderlin's spiritual homeland, which begins in earnest in the Tübingen hymns, is fleshed out, solidified, and given its ultimate direction in the verse that emerged alongside *Hyperion* in Frankfurt. Peculiarly combined with the reincarnation of the ancient Greek spirit in Diotima (Susette Gontard), the poet's priestess of love and embodiment of eternal beauty, is a new, no longer effulgent picture of Hellas that contains sorrow, suffering, and tragic elements. Intense passion is intertwined with philosophical thoughtfulness in poetry characterized by its hearty enthusiasm, expression that is still youthfully immature, and fantastic, sensitive landscapes that are painted with fine feeling. Special emphasis is placed on quiet loveliness and the constancy of nature in a worldview

that perceives life as originating in and striving toward childlike harmony. The most representative poems of this period are "Diotima," the first lyric fruit of a newly gained perception of love as a power that can suspend the continuity of time and bring to pass the rebirth of man, and "Hyperions Schicksalslied" ("Hyperion's Song of Destiny"), a penetrating treatment of the fathomlessness of existence that calls to mind Plato's separation of the realm of ideas from the world of phenomena.

DARK THEMES OF LATER YEARS

To a large extent, the significant poetic works that were written prior to Hölderlin's hasty departure from Frankfurt in 1798, and even those created shortly thereafter in Homburg, served as preliminary studies in language, form, and theme for the magnificent odes, elegies, and hymns that he wrote after 1800. It is somewhat ironic that his most sublime and deeply profound poems are the darkly mythological, prophetically intuitive visions of a mind on the brink of insanity. The ever-increasing emotional strain and existential pressure of his life without Susette served as a catalyst for the final refinement of ideas and structures that are the very essence of the night ode "Chiron," the wonderful elegy "Brot und Wein" ("Bread and Wine"), and the richly mysterious hymn "Patmos." In these and other masterworks of his final productive years, Hölderlin revealed more than ever before his quiet sensitivity, his pure and free view of nature, his precise sense of landscape saturated with the spirit of a creative life force.

Despite their diversity, the mature poems are linked together in a fusion of classical and Christian traditions that places the gods of ancient Greece and Christ on nearly equal footing. The twofold experience of the proximity of the divine and humanity's difficulty in understanding it forms the core of a poetry that is remarkable for its combination of tangible and ethereal elements. Important aspects of the integral system that is perfected and presented in these late writings include a hierarchical chain of genius-beings who govern absolute existence—Christ, the gods of Olympus, biblical prophets and patriarchs, apostles, Greek Titans, heroes, philosophers, great contemporary figures, spirits of nature and love; stress on the relationship of humans with Mother Earth; a poetic landscape that is saturated with powers that point toward the divine origins of life; and constant awareness of the prophetic task of the singer's art and of the conflict between suffering and joy. All these are expressed in language and rhythms that are pregnant with expectation, careful preparation, and unspoken faith. In many respects, it is not so much the imparted vision as the clarity, musicality, and exactness of diction and the expressive perfection and beauty of form that elevate the lyric works of Hölderlin's last creative surge to the level of true greatness.

THE TÜBINGEN HYMNS

A mélange of the revolutionary spirit of the times and interpretation of the basic Christian humanist tradition as mediated by Klopstock and Schiller, Hölderlin's Tübingen hymns are all variations on the same feeling: an endless willingness of heart to accept eternal values. The celebration of inalienable human rights—freedom, equality, friendship, honor—is filled with the youthful impetuousness of the poet's faith blended with a certain naïve tenderness and grace. Although not especially original in vocabulary, meter, and imagery, clearly influenced by models such as Schiller's "An die Freude" ("Ode to Joy"), these early poems convey the charm of their creator's exuberant enthusiasm, the animating tension that is central to his later works, and the love-oriented metaphysical basis of his worldview.

While the hymns do not belong to the poetry of experience, they can be described only loosely as idea poems. To be sure, they are thematically abstract, but their focus is not thought and allegory, as in Schiller's philosophical lyrics. Rather, it is a kind of fundamentally religious perception of the universe in which theoretical principles are given semidivine status. Various common symbols are employed with significant frequency. The mountain typically represents freedom or pride; the eagle stands for courage. Humility and the eternal flow of life appear as valley and river respectively. All nature thus becomes a boundless ideal whole that is the object of intense longing and the source of repeated spiritual ecstasy.

In each of the hymns, the glorification of a concept that has been elevated to godhood is presented in a clearly defined structure. First, the poet approaches the chosen divinity. A central portion of the poem then elaborates the abstract deity's sphere of operation. A triumphant view of the addressed entity's power and domain is climaxed by the poet's humble retreat into recognition of his own inadequacy.

Especially representative of the Tübingen songs are "Hymn to Immortality" and "Hymne an die Freiheit" ("Hymn to Freedom"). The former begins with the flight of the prophet-singer's spirit, powered by love, to the divine realm of endless life. The first stanza evokes two of the major themes of Hölderlin's oeuvre: the poet's godly mission as a seer who penetrates the revelation of creation, and love as the driving force, sacred center, and unifying essence of the world. The joyful intoxication of the vision, however, gradually recedes, leaving in the final lines only emptiness in the realization that human mortality makes it impossible for people to grasp and describe in song the unspeakable fulfillment of the immortal soul. "Hymn to Freedom" develops the idea that people can be completely free within the context of their intended holy life only if they remain true to the blessed laws of love that govern pure existence. By falling away from these divine ideals, humans subject themselves to the shame of hell. Anticipating the hope-filled resolution of the late hymns, the poem ends with the suggestion of a final attainment of freedom in the eternity beyond death.

NACHTGESÄNGE

In 1805, Hölderlin published a small collection of nine poems under the title *Nachtgesänge*. Although this group constitutes less than a third of his mature odes, it forms the core of his late production of Alcaic and Asclepiadean forms. The individual lyric creations are carefully refined renderings of Hölderlin's characteristic themes: the eternal existence of the Greek soul that still governs human action; the glorious mission of poets as magi ordained by the gods to be mediators of divine truth; the pain of separation and the never-ending tension between humans and the deity; spiritual reconciliation of the homeless singer's sorrow; and anticipation of the dawning of a new age in the gods' return. Accentuation of formal precision dominates a presentation that varies musically between lightly melodic language and dynamically passionate rhythms with heavily resounding vowels. Although love still appears as the binding force of extended nature, the motivating principle that gives these poems their special depth and flavor is an awareness of the tragic dominance of night.

Symbolically, night is the time of God's absence. It is the predominant feature of the entire era following the decline of classical civilization and the appearance of Christ. Ordained by the gods, it is endowed with sacred meaning and purpose, yet the poet longs for it to end in a bright revelation of light and for that reason faces its darkness with feelings that fluctuate between humble resignation and profound distress and pain.

Especially notable in the development of key odes is Hölderlin's tendency to frame his ideas in less demanding works, then to allow them to evolve in more complex versions that give full substance and direction to his message. Significant examples include "Der blinde Sänger" ("The Blind Singer") and its reinterpretation in "Chiron" and "Der gefesselte Strom" ("The Chained Stream"), rewritten as "Ganymed." "The Blind Singer" is an Alcaic ode that couches the theme of night in the problem of the poet's loss of sight. In the darkness, his creations lack inspiration, regained only when the gods restore his vision in new revelation. In "Chiron," the sightless singer-seer is transformed into a different symbol, the centaur Chiron, a healer who is struck by the arrow of the gods. The product of his wound is at once torment and ecstasy in apocalyptic visions of the cosmos. Like the blind poet, he is visited by the gods in a storm and sees a strong light break forth that gives everything order and harmony. "The Chained Stream," one of Hölderlin's most powerful celebrations of natural forces, is comparable to Goethe's "Mahomets Gesang" ("Mahomet's Song") in its vibrant imagery and pure musicality. The icebound stream, awakened from the night of winter by spring, arouses all nature to joy-filled life. In "Ganymed," the stream evolves into a symbol for the poet's feeling of aloneness in the world of mortals. It becomes the half-divine stranger Ganymed, whose only place of fulfillment and belonging lies in reconciliation with the gods in the arms of Zeus.

MOURNFUL ELEGIES

Hölderlin's most pronounced merging of classical Greek and Christian elements occurs in mournful elegies that combine lament for the passing of the golden age with deeply felt disappointment at the hollowness of contemporary reality. Overwhelming resignation is only partially offset by hope for the spiritual regeneration of humans. In tone, these poems are closely related to the mature odes, especially in their emphasis on night as the bridge between past and future. Their main thrust is to justify the poetic act in a dark age that destroys the very foundation of lyric art. Employing various approaches to the problem, Hölderlin examines the violent spiritual conflicts that characterize the situation of the modern lyricist. He is presented as being kept from fulfilling his divinely appointed mission by a cold era that needs his uplifting mediation more than ever. Notable is the acute awareness of the poet's homelessness in his own time; this condition is caused at least in part by his inability to forsake the Greek tradition in favor of pure belief in Christ as the only redeeming force in the world.

Two elegies stand out as representative examples of Hölderlin's mastery of this particular verse form. The most famous is "Menons Klagen um Diotima" ("Menon's Laments for Diotima"), a creation that is dominated by the experience of the author's separation from Susette Gontard. Equally powerful is the intensely mysterious "Bread and Wine," in which the figure of Christ is merged with elements of Greek gods and heroes and transformed into the wine god Bacchus at the center of a Dionysian vision of ancient Greece.

"Menon's Laments for Diotima" is a cyclical drama of the soul that begins with the separation of lovers, vacillates between the poet's resigned acceptance of the situation and longing for reunion, and ends with a prayer of thanksgiving for the hope of fulfillment in a new union beyond death. As the poem crescendos in the third section, the music of total isolation and loneliness gives way to harmonies of belief in an indissoluble relationship. The mystical conception that within the absolute context of existence true lovers can never lose each other leads in the final segments to the victory of a faith whose eternal beacon is Diotima.

In "Bread and Wine," Hölderlin comes to grips with night and emptiness in a deeply mystical revelation of the poet's role in bringing to pass the return of the gods. The invocation of darkness allows a hidden light to shine forth. From within its fire, a bright manifestation of Greece emerges, and the poet becomes a priest of Dionysus who prepares the way for a new encounter between humans and the divine. Special power arises from those parts of the poem in which concrete reality (images of evening in a small town) merges with images reflecting the fulfillment of the past and the promise of the future.

The tension between classical Greek and Christian traditions that animates all Hölderlin's mature lyrics is balanced in his Pindaric hymns by a strong mood of reconciliation and striving for harmony. Written in free verse but subject to complex structural rules, these poems are triadically arranged songs of prophetic awareness and dark, mythological, symbolic language. They treat the mysteries of life, death, and the gods in apocalyptic revelations of strange majesty that touch upon all of Hölderlin's major themes. Perhaps nowhere else in his work did he couch his view of the poet's relationship to eternity in such strong imagery of commitment, obedience, and worship.

EMPHASIS ON CHRIST

Especially significant in the late hymns is a more pronounced emphasis on Christ as the center of metaphysical contemplation. At this point in his life, Hölderlin's attitude toward the Messiah was extremely complex. The Savior figure of his poetic visions is therefore something of a composite of Germanic hero, Greek Titan, and embodiment of the eternal principle of love in which the everlasting presence of God is manifest anew. Particularly noticeable characteristics of the Christ who triumphs over suffering are a sensitive look of naïve piety, peaceful radiance of bearing, and a sense of mythic uniqueness.

In one of the crowning achievements of his artistic career, the profoundly beautiful hymn "Patmos," Hölderlin embarks on a haunting journey to the scene of Saint John's revelation in search of lingering evidence of the living Christ. The poem focuses on the stark tragedy of the Crucifixion as a symbol for the terror of divine absence that is overcome only in a process of sharing. The key concept is that of community, of the impossibility of grasping God alone. Musical cadences, forceful individual words, and rhythmic presentation of ideas are among the structural features that illuminate the landscape of the poet's spiritual universe.

Despite the victorious tone of most of the hymns, none of them documents total resolution of the dilemma generated by the poet's continuing allegiance to both the Greek gods and Christ. This fact is hammered home most dramatically in "Der Einzige" ("The Only One"), in which Christ's position of unique godhood clashes with the singer-prophet's desire to glorify all the gods because he cannot reconcile successfully their conflicting claims. By proclaiming Christ the brother of Bacchus and Hercules, Hölderlin attempts to make visible the painful conflict that arises from the very essence of the dual European heritage of his own origins. In so doing, he also creates a deeply personal symbol for a worldview that stands at the center of a lyric oeuvre that is matched in importance for the history of German poetry by the creations of few other writers.

OTHER MAJOR WORKS

LONG FICTION: *Hyperion: Oder, Der Eremit in Griechenland*, 1797, 1799 (*Hyperion: Or, The Hermit in Greece*, 1965).

PLAYS: *Antigone*, pb. 1804 (translation of Sophocles); *Oedipus Tyrannus*, pb. 1804 (translation of Sophocles); *Der Tod des Empedokles*, pb. 1826 (*The Death of Empedocles*, 1966).

MISCELLANEOUS: *Sämtliche Werke*, 1846 (2 volumes); *Sämtliche Werke: Grosse Stuttgarter Ausgabe*, 1943-1977 (8 volumes).

BIBLIOGRAPHY

Allen, William S. *Ellipsis: Of Poetry and the Experience of Language Ater Heidegger, Hölderlin, and Blanchot*. Albany: State University of New York, 2007. An examination of the poetry of Hölderlin, Martin Heidegger, and Maurice Blanchot with emphasis on poetic language.

Babich, Babette E. *Words in Blood, like Flowers: Philosophy and Poetry, Music and Eros in Hölderlin, Nietzsche, and Heidegger*. Albany: State University of New York Press, 2006. Compares and contrasts the works of Hölderlin, Friedrich Nietzsche, and Martin Heidegger. Contains topics such as philosophy and the poetic essence of thought.

Constantine, David. *Hölderlin*. Oxford, England: Clarendon Press, 1988. Substantial introduction to Hölderlin's life and work. The author seeks to write about Hölderlin chronologically and in an accessible way and to explore his life as a resource in the explication of his writing. Emphasizes Hölderlin as a poet of religious longing.

Fioretos, Arts, ed. *The Solid Letter: Readings of Friedrich Hölderlin*. Stanford, Calif.: Stanford University Press, 1999. Includes essays on philosophical and theological aspects of Hölderlin's work, his theory and practice of translation, and his poetry, ranging from early poems to uncompleted late hymns.

Heidegger, Martin. *Elucidations of Holderlin's Poetry*. Translated by Keith Hoeller. Amherst, Mass.: Humanity Books, 2000. Six essays on Hölderlin by the major twentieth century philosopher Heidegger, with an introduction by the translator. The goal is to be of use to the public as well as the scholar and includes the German as well as the English versions of the four poems to which Heidegger has devoted his essays. Emphasis is on the relationship of Hölderlin's poetry to modern European philosophy.

Henrich, Dieter, ed. *The Course of Remembrance, and Other Essays on Hölderlin*. Stanford, Calif.: Stanford University Press, 1997. A collection of essays on the ideas and the works of Hölderlin offering a glimpse of the early formation of German idealism. Contains a translation of Henrich's book devoted to Hölderlin's poem, "Remembrance." A vital resource for specialists and enthusiasts of the German Enlightenment and Romantic traditions.

Laplanche, Jean. *Hölderlin and the Question of the Father*. Edited and translated by Luke Carson. Victoria, B.C.: ELS Editions, 2007. Examines the life and works of Hölderlin with respect to his mental illness.

Lernout, Geert. *The Poet as Thinker: Hölderlin in France*. Columbia, S.C.: Camden House, 1994. A comprehensive historical survey of the reception of the poet's work by French critics and writers. Includes chapters on Heidegger's reading of Hölderlin, the French Revolution in Hölderlin's thought, and psychoanalytic theories about Hölderlin's illness. Also includes a chapter on the influence of Hölderlin on such important French authors as Albert Camus, Louis Aragon, and Philippe Sollers.

Ungar, Richard. *Friedrich Hölderlin*. Boston: Twayne, 1984. A basic and useful introduction to Hölderlin. Includes summaries and paraphrases of Hölderlin's poetry together with interpretations. Intended to assist readers who are encountering Hölderlin for the first time and to provide an understanding of the texts at the most elementary level. Includes chronology and annotated bibliography.

Lowell A. Bangerter

MIROSLAV HOLUB

Born: Pilseň, Czechoslovakia (now Czech Republic); September 13, 1923
Died: Prague, Czech Republic; July 14, 1998

PRINCIPAL POETRY
Denní služba, 1958
Achilles a želva, 1960
Slabikář, 1961
Jdi a otevři dveře, 1962
Kam teče krev, 1963
Tak zvané srdce, 1963
Zcela nesoustavná zoologie, 1963
Selected Poems, 1967
Ačkoli, 1969 (*Although*, 1971)
Notes of a Clay Pigeon, 1977
Sagittal Section: Poems New and Selected, 1980
Interferon: Or, On Theater, 1982
On the Contrary, and Other Poems, 1984
The Fly, 1987
Poems Before and After, 1990
Syndrom mizející plíce, 1990 (*Vanishing Lung Syndrome*, 1990)
Intensive Care: Selected and New Poems, 1996
The Rampage, 1997

OTHER LITERARY FORMS
The literary reputation of Miroslav Holub (HAW-loop) rests primarily on his poetry, but he also published several collections of prose as well as more than one hundred scientific papers and the monograph *Im-*

munology of Nude Mice (1989). He has also produced essays on mostly scientific, autobiographical, and cultural topics.

ACHIEVEMENTS

A widely renowned immunologist as well as an acclaimed literary figure, Miroslav Holub successfully combined the two seemingly disparate careers of scientist and poet. He is generally regarded as one of the most important poets of Eastern Europe to emerge after World War II and is widely praised for his ability to integrate scientific fact and human experience in his poetry. His poetry and his essay collections have been translated and published in many languages, and he has been widely acclaimed outside his homeland, especially in the English-speaking world.

During the 1960's and 1970's, Holub was a highly sought-after reader of his poetry, performing at such locations as the Spoleto Festival in Italy, the Lincoln Center Festival in New York, the Harrogate Festival in England, Poetry International in Holland, and the Cambridge Poetry Festival in England. He was a writer-in-residence at Oberlin College for a semester in 1979 and again in 1982 and was also awarded an honorary doctorate.

Because of his success as a scientist, Holub was able to travel widely even during the Cold War days of the Iron Curtain, conducting research and presenting papers at scientific conferences. His most notable scientific achievement was the development of a strain of nude (hairless) mice that were used to study various diseases.

BIOGRAPHY

Born in Pilseň, Czechoslovakia, Miroslav Holub was the son of Josef Holub, a lawyer who worked as a railway clerk, and Františka (Dvoráková) Holub, a language teacher. By the time Holub completed secondary school, Nazi occupation had closed down Czech universities. As a conscripted worker in a warehouse and at a railway station, he was writing and publishing poetry by the end of World War II.

In a national student competition in 1948, he was selected as winner of the third prize for poetry and fifth prize for prose, but the communist student leader dis-

solved the students' union rather than award the prizes. The only permissible poetry was in the Socialist Realist vein, a style that advocated communist ideals and adhered to narrow political and moral mores, which Holub viewed as a coverup of reality. As a result, Holub became silent for a period, devoting himself to science and receiving his M.D. in 1953 from Charles University. That year he also became editor of *Vesmír*, a popular science magazine, and he eventually returned to writing poetry as a kind of defense against the absurdity of the social order. In 1954, he became an immunologist on the staff of the Institute of Microbiology in Prague and also began work on his doctorate in immunology, completing the degree in 1958, the same year he published his first collection of poetry, *Denní služba*.

During the 1960's, Holub published several volumes of poetry in Czech that officials generally disregarded, but after he began to participate actively in the reformist movement by publishing essays in major Czech cultural and literary periodicals, he lost his job at the Institute of Microbiology in 1970. In addition, like many other Czech writers at the time, he was prohibited from publishing his work, and his books were removed from libraries. A new poetry collection ready for publication was destroyed, and Holub had to publish his compilation of selections by Edgar Allan Poe anonymously.

In 1973, the Czech press published a self-criticism in which Holub affirmed loyalty to the communist authorities. Although this action later caused negative reaction by fellow writers and the Czech public, freedom to work as a scientist was crucial to Holub. Subsequently he was allowed to continue his scientific research at the Institute for Clinical and Experimental Medicine in Prague, where he remained until his death in 1998. He was nevertheless unable to publish his poetry in Czechoslovakia except "under the table," where his works sold quickly. Meanwhile, Holub's work had been introduced to the English-speaking world in 1967 with the publication of *Selected Poems* by Penguin as part of its Modern European Poets series.

Although Holub spoke fluent English and read widely in it, he continued to write poetry in Czech. In periods of repression in Czechoslovakia, the English translations actually appeared before the Czech originals and brought him international acclaim. Despite his fame, Holub considered poetry a pastime. According to Holub in a 1967 interview by Stephen Stepanchev in *New Leader*, the Czech Writers Union offered him funding to be able to devote two years to poetry, but he refused, indicating his love for science and noting, "I'm afraid that, if I had all the time in the world to write my poems, I would write nothing at all." Though his literary friends were suspicious of his scientific profession and likewise his scientific colleagues questioned his poetic side, Holub himself disavowed a real conflict between science and poetry. He acknowledged, however, that for him science and poetry endured an "uneasy relationship," but he continued work in both until his death in 1998.

ANALYSIS

Beginning with his earliest poems, Miroslav Holub was clearly affected by what he viewed as the absurdities of life in a socialist regime. In his essay "Poetry Against Absurdity," he declared that following the communist takeover in Czechoslovakia there could be "No more words. Just sharp, concrete, viable, bleeding images, partly inherited from the surrealist imagery of the thirties." In an interview in *The Economist*, Holub indicated that lyrical poetry would have been impossible for him to write given the psychological conditions under which he lived:

> When you live in a time that forbids you to say anything that you wish to say, when you are obliged to conceal part of yourself, it is better not to speak about the self at all. It is better not to express inner feelings because, frankly, you cannot flow about your feelings. The conditions are so terrible that the only thing possible is plain statement.

Therefore, from his earliest days as a poet, Holub rejected the Czech lyrical and romantic tradition. He regarded American Imagist and physician William Carlos Williams, another scientist/poet, as a major influence, but most critics note that Holub moved beyond the simplicity of Williams's verse to write complex, intellectual poems with layers of meaning. Holub's poetry reflects his incisive mind, his scientific bent toward detailed examination, and his rational, analytical approach toward a subject. Scientific metaphors domi-

nate, even in Holub's definition of poetry as "some sort of infection."

Holub's poetic style, with its closeness to prose and with its terseness and objectivity, made his poems extremely well suited for translating into English, and these translations brought Holub international acclaim. Nevertheless, some critics have bemoaned the "nightmarish mesh of translations" that exists. In English, for example, significant variations occur in different translations of the same poems. Still, as readers repeatedly confirm, Holub's poetry communicates effectively even in translation.

DENNÍ SLUŽBA

In his first collection of poems, *Denní služba* (day duty), Holub set the tone, subject matter, and style that he was to follow with only limited expansions and variations throughout his career. Although this work has not been translated in English as a collection, many of the individual poems are available in one or more of the English collections.

"In the Microscope" functions as a metaphor for all his poetry, with its implicit comparison of the poet and the scientist and its emphasis on getting to the essence of life. Holub the poet chooses to examine life in the same way as Holub the scientist—through a microscope. Under the microscope, what first appear to be "dreaming landscapes,/ lunar, derelict" turn out to be full of "tillers of the soil" and "fighters/ who lay down their lives/ for a song."

Holub explores another of his major concerns in the form of a modernized version of the traditional fairy tale "Cinderella." The heroine spends her life dutifully, resignedly, solitarily carrying out her work of sorting peas, knowing that "she is on her own./ No helpful pigeons; she's alone./ And yet the peas, they *will* be sorted out." On one level Holub comments, as he so frequently does, on the repression of totalitarianism, but the poem moves on to comment on the mundaneness of life in general.

SAGITTAL SECTION

The first collection of Holub's poetry to be published in the United States, *Sagittal Section* had a bisected skull as its cover illustration. The illustration, as well as the poems themselves, emphasizes Holub's scientific point of view and his often expressed desire to lay things bare. The allusive, elliptical, ironic, and surrealist quality of his works is demonstrated repeatedly but nowhere better than in "The Fly." A female fly during the battle of Crécy mates with "a brown-eyed male," meditates "on the immortality of flies," lays "her eggs/ on the single eye/ of Johann Uhr,/ the Royal Armorer," and is then "eaten by a swift/ fleeing/ from the fires of Estrés."

INTERFERON

As David Young notes in his introduction to *Interferon: Or, On Theater*, this collection of poems functions through "two major metaphors, one from the world of immunological research that constitutes Holub's other profession, and one from the history of human attempts to understand the world by artificial and imaginative representations of it." Although the work is divided into four sections—"Biological Poems," "Towards a Theory of the Theater," "The Merry Adventures of the Puppets" and "Endgames"—both metaphors run throughout the work and are intermingled in various poems.

The ten-page title poem "Interferon" serves as a focal point for the collection by showing that the medical and theatrical metaphors are actually one. As Young says,

> Interference on the cellular level corresponds to the presence of theater in our lives; both are attempts to arrest and mesmerize destructive forces, disease and history, attempts that may succeed in the short run and fail in the long.

Clearly, the work reflects the experiences of postwar Eastern Europe with poetry that is impersonal, detached, and reduced to the basics; however, some personal elements emerge in love poems such as "Landscapes" and "United Flight 412." As forecast by the title, theater plays a significant role; in fact, some of the pieces might more aptly be called drama rather than poetry. Punch and Judy and Faust are major players, and myth and allegory predominate.

VANISHING LUNG SYNDROME

Perhaps Holub's finest collection of poetry translated into English, *Vanishing Lung Syndrome* covers vast areas of space and time with numerous historical, mythical, and contemporary references from a wide range of cultures. The poet moves rapidly from the Aztecs to Josef Bozek (one of the founders of Czech mechanics) in Bohemia in 1817 to a pedestrian who "slips into Wendy's" (the fast-food restaurant chain) in late twentieth century New York. Medical metaphors and ironic paradoxes abound as evidenced in the poem "Yoga": "What would they [poets] be without their disease./ The disease is their health." The opening poem, "1751," focuses on insane asylums and officious fools, while the concluding poem "The Fall from the Green Frog," presents "Mommy/ drowned in her lung edema" and Dad "cremated with ribbon of vomit in the corner/ of his mouth."

One of many overtly political poems written while Czechoslovakia was still under the constraints of communist rule, the 1988 poem "Wenceslas Square Syndrome" captures the sense of the poet on the tightrope. The poem opens in the dead of a winter's night while police patrol the square in the mists that hug the ground, the "smog of silence." Into this image of cold and "unreal" Holub inserts an image of the life-force, but one that is "schizophrenic" in the totalitarian cold:

> But from the linden that forgot
> to lose its leaves resounds a blackbird's mighty voice,
> . . . .
> song of the only December schizophrenic blackbird,
> mighty, everlasting song of the only
> schizophrenic blackbird,
> yes, of course,
> a song.

POEMS BEFORE AND AFTER

A valuable collection, *Poems Before and After* contains selected works from eleven of Holub's Czech volumes. Although most of the poems have been published in other English collections, such a large selection together in a single volume provides readers with an excellent overview of Holub's career. The "Before" and "After" of the title refer to poems written (though not necessarily published) before or after the 1968 Prague Spring, the liberal period of January-August, 1968, under the first secretary of the Czechoslovak Communist Party Alexander Dubček during which liberal reforms were instituted but that ended with the Soviet-led invasion of the country on August 20. The poems show Holub's development as poet both in complexity and in tone, and the "After" poems tend to reflect a darker, more pessimistic view of life, though not one without hope.

INTENSIVE CARE AND THE RAMPAGE

Holub's last two English-language collections, *Intensive Care* and *The Rampage* include poems from throughout his career interspersed with some new ones. The additions reflect how science, history, and myth continued to dominate Holub's poetry until his death. His tone remains skeptical and ironic, even reflecting a wariness about the newly gained freedom that came with the Velvet Revolution (the end of communist rule in Czechoslovakia). In "The Moth," Holub says,

> Freedom makes
> the moth tremble
> forever, that is,
> twenty-two hours.

In acknowledging the extreme brevity of the moth's life, Holub signifies his fears that freedom will also be short-lived.

Likewise his poem "At Last" celebrates newly gained intellectual and political freedom and expresses his anxieties about the future. He worries that "someone might cast/ a spell on us" or, perhaps worse, that, not knowing how to handle this freedom, "We might even/ be hostage/ to ourselves."

With poems like "Head-Smashed-In" and "The Slaughter-House," the final section of *The Rampage* suggests that life is violent, irrational, and full of paradoxes, but the poems are usually tempered with a sense of compassion and the slightest note of hope, as in "Landscape with Poets":

> and there will be
> either a new form of life
> or, possibly,
> nothing.

OTHER MAJOR WORKS

NONFICTION: *K principu rolničky*, 1987 (*The Jingle Bell Principle*, 1992); *Immunology of Nude Mice*, 1989; *The Dimension of the Present Moment: Essays*, 1990; *Ono se letelo: Suita z rodného mesta*, 1994 (*Supposed to Fly: A Sequence from Pilseó, Czechoslovakia*, 1996);

Shedding Life: Disease, Politics, and Other Human Conditions, 1997.

BIBLIOGRAPHY

Boxer, Sarah. "Miroslav Holub Is Dead at Seventy-four: Czech Poet and Immunologist." *The New York Times*, July 22, 1998, p. A17. Discusses the life and works of the poet, including his political stance and his scientific achievements.

Eagle, Herbert. "Syntagmatic Structure in the Free Verse of Miroslav Holub." *Rackham Literary Studies* 3 (1972): 29-49. Using a theory of free verse based on writings by the Formalists and Structuralists, Eagle provides a detailed, technical analysis of specific poems by Holub. Eagle uses the term "sytagmatic balance" to define the intonational principle that he believes unifies much of Holub's free verse.

Heaney, Seamus. "The Fully Exposed Poem." Review of *Sagittal Section* and *Interferon*. *Parnassus* 11, no. 1 (1983): 4-16. An excellent review that also discusses the effectiveness of Holub's poetry in translation.

Holub, Miroslav. "Poetry Against Absurdity." *Poetry Review* 80 (Summer, 1990): 4-8. Based on a lecture given by Holub at the Conference on Czech Literature, 1890-1990, at New York University in March of 1990, this essay effectively recalls the attempts by Holub and fellow Czech poets to record "the feeling of human responsibility in the overwhelming absurdity" of life following the Communist takeover in Czechoslovakia.

Walker, David, ed. *Poets Reading: The "Field" Symposia*. Oberlin, Ohio: Oberlin College Press, 1999. This collection of brief but excellent essays on Holub's poetry was originally published as a symposium on Holub in *FIELD* magazine. Dennis Schmitz's essay "Half a Hedgehog" and Tom Andrews's study "Hemophilia/Los Angeles" are particularly effective analyses of individual poems.

Wilde-Menozzi, Wallis. "Revising Miroslav Holub." *Southwest Review* 88, no. 4 (2003): 519-531. The author reflects on a 1994 interview with Holub, which he did not publish, partly because he found the poet to be elusive regarding his political stance.

Young, David. Introduction to *Interferon: Or, On Theater*, by Miroslav Holub. Oberlin, Ohio: Oberlin College Press, 1982. A brief examination of the role of science and theater in Holub's poems.

Verbie Lovorn Prevost

ARNO HOLZ

Born: Rastenburg, East Prussia (now Ketrzyn, Poland); April 26, 1863
Died: Berlin, Germany; October 26, 1929
Also known as: Bjarne P. Holmsen (with Johannes Schlaf)

PRINCIPAL POETRY
Klinginsherz, 1883
Buch der Zeit, 1885
Phantasus, 1898, enlarged 1916, 1925, 1929, 1961
Dafnis, 1904

OTHER LITERARY FORMS

Literary history recognizes Arno Holz (hawltz) as the cofounder and first important author and theorist of naturalism in Germany. In a sketch in *Papa Hamlet* (1889; coauthored with Johannes Schlaf, under the joint pseudonym Bjarne P. Holmsen), Holz contrasts the horrid living conditions and death of an unemployed Shakespearean actor and his family with the idealistic verses that the actor constantly recites. His play, *Die Familie Selicke* (pr., pb. 1890; with Schlaf), is a bleak tragedy, ridiculed by traditional critics as "primitive animal grunts of an ape theater," which presents the misery of an impoverished family, on Christmas Eve, bitterly awaiting the arrival home of the drunken father with his already spent paycheck, while the youngest child is dying.

Holz's significant theoretical writings are *Revolution der Lyrik* (1899), which rejects rhyme, meter, and all artificial stratagems of traditional poetry in favor of the natural rhythms of Holz's own *Mittelachsendichtung* (central-axis poetry), which is based "on the natural rhythms of things themselves"; and *Die Kunst: Ihr Wesen und ihre Gesetze* (1891-1893), which seeks to develop and present a new "natural-scientific" aesthetic.

Holz also wrote four monumental plays: *Sozialaristokraten* (pb. 1896), one of the few successful naturalistic comedies; *Die Blechschmiede* (pb. 1902; the sheet metal workshop), a 754-page satirical verse drama with a dramatis personae of more than 3,200 characters; *Sonnenfinsternis* (pb. 1908; eclipse of the sun), the tragedy of a naturalist painter who has mastered the "most complex precision-machinery of artistic technique" but cannot produce a masterpiece until his insight is heightened by the breakup of his marriage; and, finally, *Ignorabimus: Tragödie* (pb. 1913), an epistemological tragedy that pits natural-scientific positivism against Haeckelian cosmic monism.

ACHIEVEMENTS

In nonlyrical genres, Arno Holz is firmly established as the cofounder, with Schlaf, of naturalism or "consistent realism," which sought to reproduce reality with photographic precision, neutrally and without structure and emphasis; he was also the coinventor of the technique known as *Sekundenstil*, which meticulously registers every detail and change in an event "from second to second." On the stage, this technique is manifest in the seemingly unedited, undramatic dialogue, enabling dramatic time and performance time to coincide.

Holz's theoretical writings on lyric poetry have a certain permanent value insofar as he was the first theorist in Germany to break with the old notion of metrics; in a broader perspective, he pioneered the quest for the "essential" innate laws of artistic materials, a quest that Impressionism, expressionism, abstract art, Surrealism, and all modern art movements have pursued. He was wrong, however, in believing that his *Mittelachsenlyrik* (central-axis lyrics) would be the one universal form of all future poetry. Despite feeble attempts at imitation by other poets, including Rainer Maria Rilke, this central-axis poetry never became generally accepted, and today it is regarded as an interesting but merely idiosyncratic approach.

Recent critical appreciation has shifted from Holz's

naturalist contributions to the elaborate later versions of his great lyric masterpiece *Phantasus* (the short proto-*Phantasus*, 1898, although considerably less brilliant, has both intrinsic and hermeneutic value). This work did not, however, fulfill Holz's ambition to create a work that would be for the twentieth century what Homer's epics were for classical antiquity, or what Dante's *La divina commedia* (c. 1320; *The Divine Comedy*, 1802) was for the Middle Ages. *Dafnis*, written in the language and style of late-sixteenth century Baroque poetry, although generally acclaimed for its antiquarian virtuosity, seems thematically limited to a kind of naturalist pansexualism. *Buch der Zeit* expresses the new zeitgeist within traditional forms.

BIOGRAPHY

Arno Holz, the son of a druggist, was born on April 26, 1863, in Rastenburg, East Prussia. His family moved to Berlin when he was twelve. After his parents' divorce, he stayed in Berlin with his mother and attended high school but was not graduated. After a short period as an editor of a local newspaper, he spent the rest of his life in Berlin as a freelance writer, mostly in relative poverty. For about two years, he shared a room with Schlaf, and together they introduced naturalism into Germany. Gerhart Hauptmann dedicated his epochal *Vor Sonnenaufgang* (1889) to Bjarne P. Holmsen, their joint pseudonym. In the literary club Durch, they associated with the other leading naturalists. Later, Holz broke with Schlaf, and his dogmatic intransigence led him to engage in bitter disputes with Schlaf and others. For a time, Holz's plays enjoyed a limited success. He also earned some money from toy patents, but he never attained a secure financial existence. His complete works in ten volumes were published during his lifetime. He died in Berlin on October 26, 1929, a bitter and forgotten man.

ANALYSIS

Arno Holz's masterpiece in the lyric genre is *Phantasus*, a poem-cycle on which he worked for more than thirty years, and which developed from two tiny 50-page booklets (1898) to several successive expanded editions (1916, 1925, 1929), ultimately resulting in a final 1,600-page version (published posthu-

mously in 1961). In the first edition, the poems were short, only one being more than one page long, and so scantily developed as to be almost outlines rather than poems—the term "telegram poetry" has since been applied to them. By the 1916 edition, however, more by a process of internal germination and luxuriation than by cumulative addition, the book had reached monumental proportions. A single line could have as many as thirty-five words, and one poem in book 6 is 372 pages long and contains one of the longest sentences on record in the German language—a single sentence occupying 70 pages. Thus, an author who first became known as a cofounder of the naturalist movement in Germany climaxed his literary career with a work that, in its baroque virtuosity, at first sight seems to represent the very opposite of naturalism.

PHANTASUS, 1898

The poem-cycle *Phantasus* aims to be a modern *Divine Comedy*, a cosmic embodiment of the twentieth century "scientific" worldview, largely as understood in the evolutionary writings of the monist philosopher Ernst Haeckel. The Haeckelian conception of the embryonic repetition of phylogenetic evolutionary stages underlies Holz's self-interpretation: "Just as before my birth I passed through the entire physical development of my species, at least in its main stages, so since my birth through its psychic ones. I was 'everything' and the numerous and variegated residues of this [evolution] are stored up in me."

The lyrical technique by which the vast panorama of world reality is deployed in *Phantasus* is, basically, the detailed elaboration of introspective contents, whether from the real world or imaginary worlds, and the identification of the lyric self with each and all. In Holz's own words: "The ultimate secret of the . . . *Phantasus*-composition consists in my incessantly splitting myself up into the most heterogeneous things and forms." Many short poems of proto-*Phantasus*, which are lengthened only moderately in later editions, identify the lyrical self with particular beings: natural objects, such as a star ("I am a star, I shine") or a lake (". . . my heart is this lake. . . . Purple fishes swim through my dark water"); real human beings ("I am the richest man on earth"); mythical figures ("I am the dwarf Turlitipu"); imaginary creatures ("Every thousand years

I grow wings. Every thousand years my purple dragon body rushes through the darkness"); a cultural artifact, such as a Greek statue ("Corinth created me. I saw the sea") or an Oriental idol ("At night around my temple grove, seventy bronze cows stand watch"); or God himself, in caricature ("My silver cloud-beard floods the sky. I snore").

Holz's aesthetic dicta, "Art equals nature minus x," and "Art has a tendency to become nature again," are thus not meant in the sense of a meticulous naturalistic copying of external reality. For Holz, the location of detailed "nature" is in the inner experience, memory, thought, and aspirations of the individual consciousness, where all reality is concentrated. The Holzian postulate that makes it possible for the lyric consciousness to become coextensive with the entire universe and with each item in it is the phenomenological view that reality exists neither centrifugally in a transcendental realm beyond things nor centripetally in a quasi-substantial subjective self but on a middle ground in the phenomena themselves. One poem begins: "Do not listen beyond things. Do not brood over yourself. Do not seek yourself. You do not exist." The poem then identifies the self: "You are the dispersing smoke that curls from your cigar," "the raindrop on the window-sill," the "soft crackling" of a kerosene lamp. The subjective-objective dichotomy is overcome in the phenomena that are understood as the contents of consciousness, where the lyrical self and the universe coincide—which accords with the psychology of Ernst Mach.

In *Phantasus*, this self reaches to the outer limits of time and space, ranging from the infinite to the infinitesimal, open ended in either direction. The objects in space are, moreover, not static and inert but dynamic and changing: "tattered planet-systems" mark late stages of stellar development; "glacial primal suns" have not yet ignited to full life. An organic metaphor depicts the prolific genesis of new reality in the cosmos: beyond "red fixed-star forests which are bleeding to death" [that is, dispersing their energy] ". . . beyond worlds of night and nothingness, grow glimmering new worlds—trillions of crocus blossoms." An organic metaphor also succinctly affirms the paleontological antiquity of the lyric self in a "telegram-poem," which later became the first poem of the entire expanded cycle:

Seven billion years before my birth
I was a sword-lily.
My seeking roots
suctioned
into a star.
On its dark water
floated
my huge blue blossom.

Stylistically, this organic metaphor that structures Holz's cosmic imagination is made even more evident in the lexical and syntactical profusion of the 1925 *Phantasus* version. In that version, the genesis of the stars and galaxies is visualized in the metaphor of a plant scattering its sparkling spores into interstellar darkness. From a relatively static impressionistic snapshot, the poem has developed into a sinewy, twisting vine sprouting forth lexical tendrils out of its plant-like syntax. This is typical: In the later versions of *Phantasus*, the proliferation of verbs, adverbs, adjectives, and pages-long prepositional phrases destabilizes the images by inundating the nouns in a flood of less substantial parts of speech. In proto-*Phantasus*, Holz's central-axis poetry served to capture momentary static impressions; in the expanded versions, it evolves into a syntactic image of the pervasive organicism of all reality.

PHANTASUS, 1929

The idea of the cosmic universalism of the lyric self is developed in five very long poems of the 1929 *Phantasus*. In addition to the 2-page introductory "Seven Billion Years" poem, book 1 consists entirely of two very long cosmic poems totaling 180 pages. The first, "Machtmythus" (myth of power), which uses a seven-line poem from proto-*Phantasus* as its point of departure, describes with meticulous precision the gradual rise and ultimate decadence of a vast Asiatic empire under a mighty leader (symbolizing the lyric self). Built on deceit and cruelty, this empire nevertheless made Buddha a cultural possibility. Sometimes "at night in dreams" this monstrous "beast of power" that had overrun the whole earth like a deadly global catastrophe seeks to break free again. The second, "Pronunciamento," follows human history and evolution backward from the storming of the Bastille to the "tiny clump of protoplasm" that made the first hesitant transition from inanimate to animate reality. The "pro-nouncement" asserts the eternal recurrence of the self: "I have always existed" in the men and women of all cultures and in all living creatures, and so also "I will never die." Some stages along the journey backward in time—all experienced as a primary participant by the lyric self—are a seventeenth century witch-burning, the discovery of America by Christopher Columbus, the Children's Crusade, the raids of the Muslims and Vikings, the lascivious excesses of the Roman Empress Messalina, the crossing of the Alps by Hannibal, the survival of the Battle of Salamis by an oarsman, the fighting off of a huge python by a prehuman, and the engagement of dinosaurs in mortal combat in the Jurassic age on terrain that is now the bed of the Indian Ocean.

All book 3 is a single 467-page poem called "Das tausandundzweite Märchen," which developed from a fifteen-line poem in proto-*Phantasus*. The framework situation of the poet's attic room, his tobacco pipe, and his occasional drink of brandy, is recalled at intervals throughout the poem. The "story" falls into two parts. The first is a journey to Asia, partly on an imaginary zeppelin, partly on foot through a variety of wild landscapes and deserts, including the Himalayas. The second part is a surrealistic twelve-course banquet, a sequence of Herculean ordeals in which various repulsive figures present disgusting foods for the "lyric self" to eat. Each hideous presenter and each nauseating food is described most graphically, and the "lyric self" overcomes its revulsion and succeeds in downing each disgusting course by dwelling imaginatively on the charms and qualities of the Princess Gülnäre in twelve different dialectically positive elaborations that always begin with the words "She has thick, three-yard long, five-braided pigtails that weigh four pounds." Symbolically, the whole sequence represents physical revulsion for organic matter, which is then overcome by the great organic beauty and delight represented by the female body.

Comprising most of book 4, "Grosser Dichtermittwochnachmittag in meiner Feuerstuhlbude" is a complex literary satire based on a nineteen-line proto-*Phantasus* poem. Finally, a 109-page poem of book 5, titled "Die Hallelujawiese" ("The Alleluia Meadow"), grew from a ten-line "telegram-poem."

On its merry Alleluia Meadow
my joyous heart tolerates no shadow.
Red, laughing Rubens-saints
dance the cancan with Viennese laundry maids.
Under almost breaking liverwurst trees
Correggio kisses Io.
No one is embarrassed.
That ass Goethe lies aslant fat Caroline's lap.
Little winged rascals call "Prost,"
Jobst Sackmann [Johannes Schlaf], my darling, chugs
    down a caraway brandy.

The first phrase alone, "On its merry Alleluia Meadow," is expanded to more than three full pages (125 lines) by the addition of numerous adjectives and phrases in clusters that define Holz's realm of creative imagination, symbolized by the Alleluia Meadow. On one hand, it is naturalistic, seeking to embrace all reality without any moralistic scruples or condemnation; it is, among many other things, "wanton, hilarious, madcap," "pan-cosmic, ownspheric, kaleidoscopic, gigantic"; "this-earthly, Utopian, other-worldly, Atlantean"; "faunic, mischievous, phrynically bacchantic, orgiastic, fantastic, cynically corybantic"; "unrestrained, . . . unaffected, untrained, undegenerate, hyperanimalic"; in short, it is "unashamedly amoral." On the other hand, it is idealistic, embracing all the most subtle and sublime contents and aspirations of human subjectivity "in most exquisite . . . delicate, pure"; "most aetherial, legendary, chimeric"; "most prismatic, jubilatic [sic], ecstatic"; "most irridescent, rainbowlike heavenly colors . . . with Arcadian, El-Doradan, Scheherazadan Paradise-wonders"; and it longs for the "most phantasmagoric, hallucinatoric, fairytalesplendorifloric, . . . most seraphic, sublime, cherubic enchantments." In this poem, the poetic imagination "tolerates no shadow," in the sense that it exercises the utopian function of excluding all unhappiness and torments, whether inherent in life itself or inflicted by humanity and society, and endorses absolutely every desire of the human heart.

In the original short poem, this utopian vision is symbolized by disparate persons and cultural figures engaging in sexual activity or drinking together. In the vastly elaborated version, all men, animals, and birds participate in a vast cosmic orgy with the sex act represented by three and one-half large pages of three-word rapturous sexual exclamations in primitive dialect mingled with onomatopoeic bird calls to represent the satisfaction of a primary urge. The wellspring of all this activity is "every desire . . . every lust that ever was vibrant in man, Satan, God, or animal." The jungle of verbal-proliferations builds up to frenzied heights; copulation covers the whole earth; all languages and nationalities, all territories and dwellings are involved; countless historical figures and lesser persons are all engaged in a great sexual concatenation. Four of these long poems, "Machmythus," "Pronunciamento," "Das tausand-undzweite Märchen," and "The Alleluia Meadow," are among Holz's finest works.

PROTO-PHANTASUS BOOKLETS

The two small proto-*Phantasus* booklets supply the primary intuitive substratum on which the great sixteen-hundred-page *Phantasus* is built. This early version can be characterized as Impressionist, with *Jugendstil* and Symbolist motifs. This form of Impressionism works with little dabs of color, little strokes of intuited accuracy. In addition to the broad cosmic motifs, numerous small proto-*Phantasus* poems center on the Impressionist themes of the children's paradise, the small German town, exotic or mythical lands, dreams, love and sex, gods and demons, the poetic mode of existence—themes that provide the spark to ignite the volatile poetic imagination. One childhood poem specifically describes the Holzian process of poetic fantasizing: "I lie on the old herb-deck and 'simulate'"; Holz pictures two neighbors as "God" and the "devil." God is the baker Knorr, who wears a white hat and has liqueur bottles displayed in his window. When the sunlight shines through them, the pastry looks yellow, red and blue. The devil is the chimney sweep Killkant in his black cylinder hat and dirty shoes, who rolls his eyes—making them look white—whenever he passes by "God's" liqueur bottles. This kind of "simulation" on a boyish level gives an idea of the symbolic truth-structures in Holz's sensory images. The *tertium comparationis* here is the have/have-not category. The boy, the chimney sweep, and the devil are have-nots. An image of desire is portrayed without protest and with great economy, using color ciphers—the object of desire bathed in beautiful colors, the frustrated desire imaged in the empty white of the eyes—but the sensory

level also has beauty for its own sake, apart from any symbolic values, since reality resides in the phenomena as the content of consciousness.

Some of the childhood poems suggest that the move from East Prussia must have been traumatic for the young Holz. The sentence, "Far away on the island Nurapu blooms the tree Bo" combines the exotic with nostalgia for childhood; memory of the "other world" of Grandmother's porcelain figurines and tulips reminds the poet how bleak his present existence is: "Here no cuckoo-clock calls, no lavender-pot smells." Hearing a bird, the poet remembers what he had had as a child "and then—forgot." Small-town Germany is also linked with the childhood-paradise motif: "Red roofs! Out of the chimneys here and there, smoke, up high in sunny air . . . now a hen cackles. The whole town smells of coffee." The exotic, the erotic, the childlike fantasy blend together in *Jugendstil* poems of palaces, temples, parks, and naked girls. Peering through a window of "a little palace in an old park" he sees "a rose-patterned tapestry, a blue divan, and a naked lady feeding a cockatoo." One poem describing a group of chic boarding-school girls ends with the narrator catching the most beautiful one by the waist and exclaiming in a *Jugendstil Marseillaise*: "Girls, disrobe and dance naked between swords." A similar sex-wish motif occurs in the mythical form of a shaggy faun catching a naked girl, or, comically, God himself snapping up "a little fin de siècle girl—black stockings, yellow silk waistcoat, and lily-underpants." In one dragon-demon poem, the creature observes the rabble's baseness and rapacious greed; without conjunction or transition the last line follows: "My claws glimmer, my eyes glow." The entire threat of retaliation by a violated moral order is contained in these luminous traces.

PHANTASUS, 1961

The later editions of *Phantasus* add little to the primary intuitive base. Despite its fifteen hundred additional pages, the final edition contains only about forty new poems; all the rest are expanded from the one hundred single-page poems of the 1898 proto-*Phantasus*. The additional length results not from the discovery of new basic motifs, but from the elaboration and explication of detail, from linguistic acrobatics and analytical cerebration, from the attempt—under the influence of

Walt Whitman—to inject ever more circumstantial reality into the discourse, often with cascades of synonyms and sentences that are thirty or forty pages long. The compact cultivated gardens of the originally impressionistic poems have been overtaken, as it were, by a linguistic tropical jungle of spoken rhetoric, an encyclopedic effort to capture every detail and nuance of external reality in a manner compatible with the modern "natural-scientific" worldview.

OTHER MAJOR WORKS

SHORT FICTION: *Papa Hamlet*, 1889 (with Johannes Schlaf; as Bjarne P. Holmsen).

PLAYS: *Die Familie Selicke*, pr., pb. 1890 (with Schlaf); *Sozialaristokraten*, pb. 1896; *Die Blechschmiede*, pb. 1902; *Sonnenfinsternis*, pb. 1908; *Ignorabimus, Tragödie*, pb. 1913.

NONFICTION: *Die Dichtkunst der Jetztzeit*, 1883; *Die Kunst: Ihr Wesen und ihre Gesetze*, 1891-1892; *Revolution der Lyrik*, 1899; *Die befreite deutsche Wortkunst*, 1921.

MISCELLANEOUS: *Das Werk von Arno Holz*, 1924-1925 (10 volumes).

BIBLIOGRAPHY

Burns, Rob. *The Quest for Modernity: The Place of Arno Holz in Modern German Literature*. Bern, Germany: Lang, 1981. A critical study of Holz's work. Includes bibliographic references.

Frish, Walter. *German Modernism: Music and the Arts*. Berkeley: University of California Press, 2005. In a chapter on German naturalism, Frish describes Holz's idea of revolutionary poetry and analyzes how it was evidenced in *Phantasus*.

Furness, Raymond, and Malcolm Humble, eds. *A Companion to Twentieth Century German Literature*. 2d ed. New York: Routledge, 1991. Contains a short biographical essay on Holz that describes his role in founding German naturalism and provides some analysis of his works.

Lessing, Otto Eduard. *Masters in Modern German Literature*. 1912. Reprint. Honolulu: University Press of the Pacific, 2005. Reprint of a classic work contains information on German literature in the early 1900's and contains a chapter on Holz.

Oeste, Robert. *Arno Holz: The Long Poem and the Tradition of Poetic Experiment*. Bonn, Germany: Bouvier, 1982. An analysis of the poetic works of Holz and the historical background of epic and experimental poetry. Includes an index and a bibliography.

David J. Parent (including original translations)

HOMER

Born: Possibly Ionia, Asia Minor (now in Turkey);
c. early eighth century B.C.E.
Died: Greece; c. late eighth century B.C.E.

PRINCIPAL POETRY

Iliad, c. 750 B.C.E. (English translation, 1611)
Odyssey, c. 725 B.C.E. (English translation, 1614)

OTHER LITERARY FORMS

Homer is noted only for his magnificent epic poems.

ACHIEVEMENTS

Homer's extant poetry consists of the *Iliad*, an epic of about sixteen thousand hexameter lines, and the *Odyssey*, a twelve-thousand-line poem in the same meter. A number of other poems attributed to Homer in late antiquity—the epigrams (twenty-six short poems contained in the *Life of Homer* that were attributed to Herodotus), *Margites, Batrachomyomachia* (battle of the frogs and mice), and the *Homeric Hymns* (thirty-three narrative hexameter poems in honor of various Greek divinities)—can be shown on the basis of style to postdate him. These latter poems may be either imitations or independent compositions in the general epic mode of the *Iliad* and the *Odyssey*.

Despite minor inconsistencies of detail—"even Homer nods," explained the Roman poet Horace—both the *Iliad* and the *Odyssey* give the impression of being complete compositions, unified in theme and elaborate in structure, which combine the powers of dramatic narrative poetry with the delicacy and nuance of lyric. Their aim is nothing less than to offer to posterity the world of the heroic past. This they accomplish with such force and conviction that the imaginative representation of the Trojan War and its aftermath becomes a kind of immortality: Just as the heroes of the *Iliad* and the *Odyssey* predict that they will become the subject of song, so Homer's song lives on. The supreme self-confidence of the genre, which exhibits heroes battling to gain the glory of being mentioned in epic poetry, must have been built on the facts of social life in a highly critical, reputation-conscious culture. Homer was the ultimate representative of that culture. More than anything else, literacy may have caused its decline. It was Homer's achievement, then, to have composed so well that his work survived the onset of a new order, in which the poet's status as arbiter of the heroic, repository of tradition, and sole source of history, was drastically reduced. In terms of intellectual history, Homer may have been the genius who translated what was essentially "oral poetry" into a new medium: the written word.

Although his art is on a much larger scale, Homer still resembles the bards whom he portrays: Demodocus, Phemius, and Odysseus himself in the *Odyssey* and Achilles in book 9 of the *Iliad*. Like Achilles, who sings the heroic deeds of the ancestral heroes while sitting in his tent, Homer produces commemorative poetry. The naming of all the combatants in the Trojan conflict, in book 2 of the *Iliad*, is a relic of the sort of "catalog poetry" that must have been predominant in the traditional poetry of Greece before Homer. Comparative study has shown that the long and detailed battle scenes of the middle books in the *Iliad* represent a poetic genre that is paralleled by the heroic verse of many other cultures. Who fought a particular battle, which side won, and what the exploits were that brought about victory—these are the main concerns of such epics. Homer surpasses these martial epics. In the *Iliad*, he produces a poem that, while commemorating the fall of Troy (a historical event well known to ancient Greeks), dwells more on the problem of human mortality and its ramifications than on national pride over victory. One senses a profound and sympathetic poetic intelligence at work as Homer portrays the deaths of Hector and Patroclus and prefigures the death of Achilles. This universal sympathy extends even to

the minutiae of the incessant killings in Iliadic battle scenes. There, no one dies without remark: One warrior is described as handsome, another's wife and children at home are mentioned, a third is an only son. It is difficult to judge Homer's achievement because nothing of his predecessors' poems survives, but it is clear from other epic verse, ancient and modern, that the *Iliad* is a masterpiece of the genre precisely because it goes beyond generic constraints and refuses to be mere praise of battle glory.

Like Odysseus, who narrates his adventures for the pleasure of the Phaeacian court in the *Odyssey*, Homer also delights his audience. In this, he surpasses comparable "adventure" narratives in both complexity and tone. His art lies in his ability to combine the themes of revenge, escape, initiation, and reunion in the *Odyssey*, in the same way that Demodocus, the Phaeacian bard, recounts epic tales (the Trojan Horse story) as well as amatory tales (the Ares and Aphrodite story). The *Odyssey*, then, shows that side of Homeric poetry that most resembles Odysseus himself, the "man of many turnings." It weaves multiple plots, centered on three major characters (Telemachus, Odysseus, and Penelope), whereas the *Iliad* concentrates on the single theme of Achilles' wrath and its consequences. The tone, also, of the *Odyssey* distinguishes it from the folktales, romances, and picaresque tales of travel with which it is often compared. The Odyssean sense of purpose gives moral value to the poem: Odysseus must return home to affirm the value of Greek culture. His slaying of the suitors, often criticized as excessive in Homer's rendering, is justified as divine retribution for the mistreatment of strangers (Odysseus himself being the "stranger" in his own land). Thus, the poem is aesthetically and culturally satisfying, although in a different mode from that of the *Iliad*: Odysseus, and by implication Greek intelligence, is seen to be invincible.

Versatility in approach, attention to detail, control and seriousness of tone, the ability to incorporate and exceed earlier generic elements of his tradition—these are only a small part of Homer's achievement. More than this, Homer may be credited with crystallizing for later generations of European poets the genre of epic, regardless of whether those poets imitated him. In fact, many did. His influence on later Greek, Latin, and vernacular literature is enormous, a fact well documented by such scholars as Gilbert Highet. Apollonius Rhodius, Ennius, Vergil, Dante, Ludovico Ariosto, Pierre de Ronsard, Edmund Spenser, John Milton, and Ezra Pound are among the epic poets in his debt. Drama from Aeschylus on, lyric poetry, history, and the modern novel often reflect the brilliance of Homer's creations. This is not surprising; Aristotle had seen that the poems exemplify certain universal tendencies of plot, which he classed in the *Poetics* (probably between 334 and 323 B.C.E.) as tragic (*Iliad*) and comic (*Odyssey*). A writer in any mode that touches these two views of life, therefore, could conceivably use Homer as a model.

In terms of his own culture, Homer's achievement is best illustrated by the paucity of epic poetry not contained in the *Iliad* or *Odyssey* that survives today. Various literary and critical sources, among them Attic tragedy and Alexandrian commentaries, make clear the existence in ancient Greece of a body of traditional epic concerning the Trojan War and surrounding events. Of this wealth of material, only fragments under the collective title of the Epic Cycle survive. Clearly, the prestige of Homer's compositions eventually effaced all other poetic treatments of the Trojan War story, leaving only hints in the works of some ancient authors that there had once been other stories told of Achilles, Odysseus, and the other heroes of Homeric epic.

BIOGRAPHY

Although the *Iliad* and the *Oydssey* are attributed to Homer, nothing is known for certain about the poet (or poets) who wrote these works. It should be noted that in ancient times, as well as in modern scholarship since the nineteenth century, opinion has varied on whether both epics were the creation of one poet. In Alexandria during the third and second centuries B.C.E., a group of critics known as the Chorizontes (separators) denied that one person composed both poems; at the same time, Aristarchus, one of the most influential editors of the text of the poems, maintained that the cross-references from the *Odyssey* to the *Iliad* do show the epics to be the work of one poet. It is not impossible that the works are by different poets, each a master; it is perhaps wiser to side with Aristarchus and the majority opinion of antiquity in attributing the *Iliad* and the *Odyssey* to

one composer. The British scholar D. B. Monro demonstrated in the nineteenth century that the *Iliad* and the *Odyssey* never describe the same minor incidents relating to the Trojan War but instead form a series of similar vignettes. "Monro's Law," as this phenomenon has come to be called, might indicate that Homer consciously sought to avoid repeating himself; on the other hand, one could argue that the two poems represent narrative traditions so well known in the world of early Greece that any composer, while working on one poem, would automatically avoid a topic that he knew to be in the other one. Thus, the question of authorship remains open to debate, part of the larger Homeric question that continues to fascinate students of these poems.

The dearth of biographical detail that might have explained the genesis of these remarkable works, although perplexing to scholars since antiquity, may actually have helped the poems to survive, for it enabled Greeks of all city-states to adopt them as their own "history"—one that clearly did not favor one region at the expense of another, or the traditions of one city-state exclusively, but rather attempted to integrate all the various versions of the Trojan War. Homer could never be dismissed as a biased observer whose local associations led him to trim the truth.

The anonymity of Homer is that of the epic genre itself. Evolving over generations of oral performance before an audience that knew poetry well, the art form that culminated in the *Iliad* and the *Odyssey* conventionally made no mention of its performers. It is not accidental that even the name of Homer soon became a subject of speculation among the Greeks. Some ancient sources equated *Homeros* (the Greek form of the poet's name) with a noun meaning "hostage" and appended a story about the poet's early life to support the etymology. Others said that the word meant "blind." There is no evidence to support either guess. Indeed, the traditional picture of the blind bard is exactly that: a tradition—which is to say that it is still important "evidence" but not an established fact. It may reflect an ideology that conceives of the poet as "blind" to all contemporary, external influence, one who depends instead on what he "hears" from the Muse whom Homer addresses in the prologues of both poems. The Muse (another obscure word, perhaps related to the Greek root meaning "to remind" or "to remember") embodies and transmits Greek traditional stories through the epic poet. In the final analysis, then, for both Greeks and moderns, who Homer was is not important; what he transmits, is. Freed from the biographical method of criticism, the student of Homer can concentrate on the poetry itself.

The tradition of Homer's blindness can also be interpreted on another level—the social. The composition and performance of poetry was perhaps one of the few crafts available to the sightless in early Greek society. The figure of the blind bard Demodocus in the *Odyssey* (sometimes taken to be Homer's "self-portrait") could reflect a real situation: Such poets may have sung for aristocratic courts. Therefore, a conventional picture of the blind bard or an actual description (in general terms) may lie behind the story of Homer's handicap.

The problem of convention versus actuality (or individual observation of reality) is the main critical problem of Homeric poetry. How much is actually Homer's "invention" and how much belongs to the long tradition that he inherited? To what extent does Homer defy the tradition? The question is partially unanswerable, since Homer's predecessors have not survived. Nevertheless, some light is shed on Homeric innovations in traditional motifs by the comparative study of epic poetry. Thus Albert B. Lord, in his *The Singer of Tales* (1960), is able to bring parallel motifs from modern Serbo-Croatian heroic songs to the interpretation of certain episodes in the *Iliad* and *Odyssey*. The absence and return of Achilles, for example, can be seen as a "story pattern" that Homer has conflated with another pattern, the "death of the substitute"—in this case, Patroclus.

Such studies have increasingly shown that the poems are almost entirely "traditional" in their themes and motifs; at the same time, they exhibit a distinctive dramatic control that has modified themes so as to de-

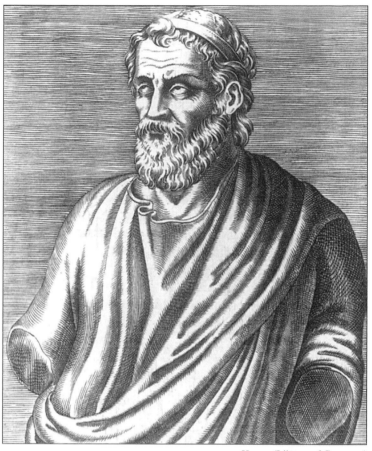

Homer (Library of Congress)

velop essential meanings. Thus, while Homer may have inherited the story of Achilles' wrath or Odysseus's wandering, only his own arrangement must be responsible for final narratives that, by a sophisticated counterpoint of themes—war and peace, life and death, fathers and sons—create complex worlds of significance. Although one knows nothing about the poet, his presence is immanent in the poems.

ANALYSIS

Before proceeding to analyze Homer's poems themselves, something must be said about the nature of the poetry. That the *Iliad* and the *Odyssey* bear the marks of oral traditional poetry is now generally admitted, although opinions differ concerning the way in which this "oral" poetry was transcribed and transmitted. An understanding of oral poetics helps one to appreciate certain features of Homeric epic, such as repetition, which might be faulted were the poetics of written literature applied to the texts.

The origin of Homeric verse in oral poetry, composed before the art of alphabetic writing was brought to Greece (probably in the eighth century B.C.E.), has been the subject of academic discussion since the time of German philologist Friedrich A. Wolf, whose *Prolegomena ad Homerum* of 1795 began the modern era of Homeric study. Scholarship in the century after Wolf, however, chose to mine the larger vein that Wolf had opened in his work—namely, the thesis that the Homeric poems, as they exist, represent a collection of shorter lays on simple themes such as the wrath of Achilles that were edited or expanded early in antiquity. Thus, following Wolf, "analyst" criticism (as it came to be known) developed in response to the bulk and complexity of Homer's poems.

A highly literate society's Romantic ideas of the "primitive," illiterate bard did not accord well with these elaborate epics, so it was denied that one masterful poet produced both the *Iliad* and the *Odyssey*, or even one of them, alone. It is true that about a third of the poems, taken together, are repeated lines. Nineteenth century analyst criticism explained these internal repetitions as "borrowings" done by a series of editor-poets who had read other parts of the poems when those parts existed as individual lays. In a way, analyst criticism foreshadowed modern work on oral poetics, which can show that individual themes develop distinctive phraseological patterns that are then repeated whenever the theme recurs (although sometimes in modified form): a scene of sacrifice, for example, or the launching of a ship; a scene of taking a bath or giving a gift—all contain similar language whenever they appear in the poem. Such occasions were nearly ritual or, often, were ritual; it is only to be expected that traditional language describes them repeatedly, and it is no artistic fault. Analyst critics, however, having no field experience of living oral traditions, did not realize that heroic poems of a great many verses are attributable to single poets (Kirghiz bards, for example, have produced 125,000-line epics), nor did they realize that repetition is a key element in the effects of heroic epic, where it produces a rhythm in the composition parallel to the rhythm of the audience's own world.

It was left to a young American philologist, Milman Parry, to explain the real significance of such Homeric phenomena as repeated whole verses, scenes, and phrases. His demonstration showed that one class of repeated elements, the "formulas" or "groups of words regularly used under the same metrical conditions to express an essential idea," formed a system. Parry made detailed comparisons of noun-epithet combinations ("wily Odysseus"; "swift-footed Achilles"). His classifications showed that adjectives with proper names were determined by the demands of Homeric meter rather than by sense in a particular passage. In other words, "cloud-gathering Zeus" differs from "Zeus who delights in thunderbolts" or "Zeus, father of men and gods" not because Homer, in any one line, intends a different picture of the supreme Olympian god, but because the three noun-phrases can fill up different positions in the highly complex dactylic hexameter verse. His system demonstrated that almost every major figure in the poems has a set of adjectives to modify its name (with minute exceptions), but that only one noun-adjective combination exists for any given metrical position.

Parry concluded that such a widespread but economical system must have evolved over a long period of time. A single poet in a literate culture—Vergil, for example—would have no need to devise such a system, even if he could, but oral poets, under the pressure of improvised composition, might be expected to create just such aids to their art. Parry, with help from his assistant, Albert Lord, was able to find modern analogies for his theory in the coffee houses of Muslim communities in Yugoslavia, where oral poets entertained. "Formulas" could be identified in the Serbo-Croatian songs that Lord and Parry heard; singers discussed their art with them. In short, the analogy with modern oral poetry, used with caution, adds immensely to a study of Homer. The ability of oral poets to transmit, combine, and modify inherited themes, as well as language, seems perfected in the poet of the *Iliad* and the *Odyssey*.

ILIAD

"Sing, goddess, the ruinous anger of Achilles, Peleus's son"—the *Iliad*'s opening lines contain in essence the plot of the following twenty-four books of the poem. It is Achilles' wrath at being deprived of the woman Briseis, his prize of war, by the Greek commander Agamemnon, which causes Achilles' withdrawal from the fighting before Troy and the subsequent death of many of his companions. Among these is his beloved friend Patroclus, who dies in Achilles' stead, attempting to ward off destruction from the Greeks while Achilles, defending his own standard of honor as a hero, waits for Agamemnon to make suitable recompense for the stolen woman. Only Patroclus's sacrifice is able to stir Achilles to fight. He proceeds to kill Hector, the mainstay of Troy and the slayer of Patroclus, and thereby chooses his own destiny: death at a young age, with undying fame.

The anger causes ruin, then, for thousands of Greek and Trojan warriors, for Patroclus (whom Achilles least expects to harm) and ultimately for Achilles himself. His death, though not described within the narrow time-limits of the *Iliad* (the main actions occur within the space of a few days), is rehearsed in the precisely delineated killing of his comrade. Apollo plays a supporting role in causing Patroclus's death in book 16, as he will when Achilles later is fatally wounded by Paris, whose abduction of Helen from Greece precipitated the Trojan War. Hector, in his own death speech, foretells the scene. Thus, the three deaths are inextricably linked: Anger kills the angered.

Achilles' anger might first be mistaken for youthful impetuosity or even childish resentment, but as Achilles' speeches to the entreating embassy of book 9 show, the hero's anger is fundamental to his nature as hero. Achilles rejects his society with an idealist's moral clarity—rejects that world in which a young man must war for an older man's stolen wife, under the command of an inferior man (Agamemnon) who takes "by right" the young man's own woman. This is the *Iliad*'s tragic irony. It is compounded by the irony that the wrath of the hero is sanctioned and justified by Zeus, who has agreed to further Achilles' request for compensatory honor; yet not even Zeus can save Achilles from the consequences of being born half divine and half human. His latter heritage ensures that Achilles must grieve and die.

Achilles, son of the divine sea-nymph Thetis and the mortal Peleus, is genetically unfit to live in either

world, and the *Iliad* depicts his magnificent attempt at integration. His heritage, in the form of the father-son theme, is prominent throughout the poem. The opening line, with its patronymic "son of Peleus" hints at the theme; the ending in book 24 makes the theme explicit. In this regard, the *Iliad* moves from the influence of the mother to that of the father. Thetis is the one who, in book 1, persuades Zeus to honor her son by making the Greek warriors feel his need as they are hard-pressed in the fight. Yet this possibility of winning the highest glory, of being recognized as best of the Greeks—the divine stature akin to Thetis's divinity—fails to take into account the hero's humanity. Once he realizes that it is time to die, Achilles is dominated by the remembrance of his father.

In this reading of the poem, fathers are the lowest common denominators of the human. With increasing insistence, the theme recurs in the *Iliad*: Book 6 contains two examples. First, Glaucus and Diomedes, despite opposite affiliations, can find in their fathers and grandfathers common friends. This inherited bond becomes their reason for avoiding the slaying of each other. Next, in the same book, the completely mortal Trojan counterpart of Achilles, Hector, meets his wife Andromache on the city wall. Hector's doomed infant son, Astyanax, is also present, and the poet arranges the scene so that the fate of Troy finds its symbol in the baby. He will not grow up to be "lord of the town" as his name signifies (and as his father is) but will be taken when the town falls, and both Hector and his wife know this. In this, their final conversation, the relationship of Hector with his son is placed in the wider context of paternal relations, as each partner recalls a father: Andromache mentions Eetion, killed in a raid by Achilles early in the war; Hector says that he is fighting not only for his own but also for Priam's glory, although he knows that the effort is in vain. This consciousness of genealogy and relation gives the *Iliad* much of its impression of depth, revealing as it does inherited motivations.

The heroic imperative, always to excel, is partly motivated by competition with fathers—filial piety is only part of the reason why heroes fight—and this side of the theme is not neglected. A father's example or instructions shame several heroes to join battle. Agamemnon goading Diomedes in book 4 and Odysseus goading Achilles in book 9 make use of the theme; Nestor, in book 11, unwittingly uses it to send Patroclus off to his death. In the final book of the poem, Priam also uses the common experience of fathers: On a night mission to the Greek camp to retrieve his son's corpse, the old man prompts Achilles to remember Peleus, his father. This time the purpose of the reminder is peaceful, and it succeeds; the poem ends in reconciliation, at least on the level of the individual. Achilles' new realization of his own mortality enables him humbly to accept a father's wish—in pointed contrast, no doubt intentional, to Agamemnon in book 1.

If the father-son theme emphasizes Achilles' mortal side, the theme of anger, from the poem's beginning, emphasizes the divine. The interaction of human and divine is one of the most important Homeric themes; Achilles is a paradigm for the way in which such interaction occurs. A Greek audience would have been attuned to the word that Homer uses to describe Achilles' state. *Mēnis* (the first word of the poem) is not ordinary anger; it connotes divine wrath. In fact, Achilles is the only mortal of whom it is used. There is, then, inherent antagonism between Achilles and the divine. Achilles, like any man, will inevitably lose in this contest because he must die. Gregory Nagy has shown that the theme of god-hero antagonism underlies the Greek concept of the hero in both poetic narratives and actual cult practices. Achilles' death, therefore, can be seen not only as the result of his human commitment but also as the logical result of his near-divine status, his encroachment on divine prerogatives when he indulges his ruinous wrath. This explains why Apollo joins Paris in the killing of Achilles (as Hector predicts in book 22).

For many readers, the role of the gods in both the *Iliad* and the *Odyssey* is problematic. If events are predetermined, as the poet seems at times to say, how can a hero such as Achilles choose his destiny? Again, there appear to be levels of divine necessity. The will of Zeus is carried out in the poem, according to the prologue in book 1; yet Zeus himself must bow to restraint in accepting the predetermined death of his son Sarpedon later in the poem. The great span of time that led to the crystallization of Homeric poetry could account for the variant notions in the poems, from meteorological gods

to moral forces: Zeus can thus without contradiction be both the "cloudgatherer" and the god who punishes the violators of guest-host relations. Then again, Homer is free to choose to emphasize whatever aspect of divinity best suits his poetic needs at a given point: He is not bound by a theology. In fact, the mention of "fate" can often be taken as the poet's way of saying "This is the way in which the plot goes"; the epic poet has Zeus's omniscience, thanks to the Muses.

Actually, the Homeric picture is remarkably consistent in one aspect: Gods act as mortals. They drink, deceive, laugh, love, hold grudges, have favorites; they merely do not die. Homer repeatedly develops the dramatic possibilities of this basic contrast, especially in "interlude" portions that do not significantly advance the plot. (The key plot-forwarding books are 1, 9, 11, 16, 19, 22, 23, and 24.) Thus, book 5 contains episodes of deadly serious fighting as Diomedes has his heroic hour at the Trojans' expense, but the book ends with the comic assaults on Ares and Aphrodite. The effect is only to underscore how much mortals stand to lose in war.

At times the parallelism of divine and human worlds means that many actions appear to be caused by both human desires and divine will. For Homer, this is not a contradiction; the gods play a part in the world of men, but human beings are still free to make up their own minds—these are self-evident facts to the poet. This "double-motivation," the dual point of view that perceives events from both divine and human perspectives, creates in the epic a sense of heightened pathos balanced by impersonal tragic resignation. In a way, the duality reproduces that of the divinely inspired and objective poet as he sings, again and again, the one-time, life-or-death crisis of his hero.

The special beauty, then, of traditional poetry like the *Iliad* emerges in even such a brief analysis as this, where it has been shown that even the first line of the poem plunges one into thematic depths. Because of the nature of the medium, the same could be said of almost any line in the epic.

ODYSSEY

Homer's *Odyssey*, when contrasted with the *Iliad*, might well appear to be the work of another poet. It represents another world, the world of peaceful existence.

In space and time it is the *Iliad*'s opposite, ranging widely over twenty years and dozens of locales, rather than describing only a few days. Its hero, Odysseus, is also the polar opposite of Achilles; a hero of intelligence rather than might, he survives the war and the homecoming, unlike Achilles or even Agamemnon. Whereas in the *Iliad* one manifestation of the hero's character predominates—his wrath—the *Odyssey* presents Odysseus as the possessor of a number of qualities and abilities. It is not accidental that more epithets beginning in the Greek word for "many" (*poly-*) attach to Odysseus than to any other figure in the epics. His "many turnings" are at one time essential to the plot of the poem (the many turns he takes) and to his disposition (as a man of much-turned thought) and so make a proper subject for the first line of the *Odyssey*: "Tell me, goddess, the man of many ways who was much buffeted after he sacked Troy."

The main plot of the poem   the return of the absent husband to his faithful wife, despite the odds—must have existed in folktale form before Greek epic appropriated it for the story of the homecoming Odysseus. The story can be paralleled in tales of many cultures, ancient and modern. Subplots, such as the encounters with the giant (Cyclops) and the witch (Circe), are also clearly from the common stock of popular narratives. Homer's fashioning of these materials is what makes the *Odyssey* unique.

First to be noticed is the small scope actually given such adventure motifs in the poem as a whole. They occur only in Odysseus's own narration of his experiences, books 9 through 12. His relationship with Calypso, the divine nymph who wished to detain him and make him immortal, is described not as a wonder-tale but in natural terms. The only unusual aspect of her island home, Ogygia, is its lush vegetation, symbolic of the excessive life she offers. The hints of Elysium in the description of the island (the land of the dead), and of her own darker nature (Calypso means "the hider" and connotes burial) are only undertones, subtly managed by the poet. Similarly, Scheria, the island of the Phaeacians who send Odysseus back to Ithaca on the last leg of his voyage, is described as a believable, realistic social setting—albeit for an unusual society. The reader is far from the nightmarish world of Cyclops,

Circe, the Lotus Eaters, Scylla, and Charybdis. The primary distinguishing mark is the absence of danger; Ogygia and Scheria pose more spiritual temptations, offers to abandon the centripetal voyage home. For Odysseus's temperament such dangers equally threaten extinction. Without establishing his place as ruler of his Ithacan home, the hero has no reason to live. He must keep in motion until that rest.

Another unique feature of the *Odyssey* is tied to the adventure tales: Odysseus, not the poet, tells them. As noted earlier, Odysseus acts as a bard in the poem about him, and in so doing he creates a curious doubling of narrators. Two effects follow: First, time is artfully disarranged, so that a composite picture of Odysseus—past and present—emerges; second, irony enters the poem. By distancing the events through a second narrator, the poet leaves open the possibility that the tales of Odysseus are tailored by him, a possibility that gains credibility when the reader sees Odysseus tell at least five lies during the tale-telling in the second half of the poem.

If the irony of the device is admitted, it can be seen to accord with other artful displacements in the structure of the *Odyssey*, such as the so-called *Telemacheia*, or "story of Telemachus" (books 1 through 4). Why, in a poem about Odysseus, does the hero not appear until book 5? Why does his son hold the stage? Again, the answer lies in Homer's desire for sophisticated and ironic narration. The reader sees Telemachus setting out on his own odyssey, starting the process of initiation into manhood; at the same time, one sees the final step in his father's voyage back. From the divine prologue to this tale of crossed paths, the audience knows that Athena has arranged both the miniature odyssey of the son to Pylos and Sparta to learn of his father, and the journey of Odysseus himself. Yet neither participant in the plan knows about it. What seems to them to be hazardous appears to the audience as divine providence. The technique is, in fact, comic.

The "happy" ending of the *Odyssey* also reminds readers of comedy: The bad are punished (the suitors killed), the good rewarded, and a wedding of sorts takes place. It might be noted that Homer once again uses the father-son theme to accomplish the poem's final reconciliation: Not only is Odysseus reunited with Telemachus (and thus the beginning of the poem is joined with the end), but also Laertes, Odysseus's father, joins in the final battle. There is no better definition of what survival meant to a Greek: the reintegration into a social setting of family and community. The *Odyssey* is thus aesthetically and culturally satisfying.

Although it is often compared unfavorably with the *Iliad*—one ancient critic compared the *Iliad* to the sun at midday and the *Odyssey* to sunset, claiming that the latter was composed in Homer's old age—the *Odyssey* is perhaps less restricted by the presuppositions of Homeric Greek culture. The *Iliad* has had few successors in outlook; the *Odyssey*'s are legion. Both poems present a complete view of life: one as tragic, one as transcending tragedy.

BIBLIOGRAPHY

Alden, Maureen J. *Homer Beside Himself: Para-Narratives in the "Iliad."* New York: Oxford University Press, 2001. Advises students and others new to the *Iliad* on how to read, understand, and absorb the poetry, and then offers an analysis.

Bloom, Harold. *Homer.* Rev. ed. New York: Chelsea House, 2007. A collection of critical essays, including one on the epic as a genre, that examine Homer and his works.

Brann, Eva. *Homeric Moments: Clues to Delight in Reading the "Odyssey" and the "Iliad."* Philadelphia: Paul Dry, 2002. A close and witty exploration of the experience of reading Homer.

Carlisle, Miriam, and Olga Levaniouk, eds. *Nine Essays on Homer.* Lanham, Md.: Rowman and Littlefield, 1999. This collection of essays offers insight into Homer's themes and style.

Dalby, Andrew. *Rediscovering Homer: Inside the Origins of the Epic.* Norton, 2006. Dalby speculates that Homer was a woman. Speculation aside, this is an excellent introduction to the history and historicity of the Trojan War and its companion epics.

Kim, Jinyo. *The Pity of Achilles: Oral Style and the Unity of the "Iliad."* Lanham, Md.: Rowman and Littlefield, 2000. An argument for the unity of the *Iliad* that surveys recent scholarship. Bibliography.

Lord, Albert B. *The Singer of Tales.* 2d ed. Cambridge, Mass.: Harvard University Press, 2000. This edition offers a new introduction and a CD-ROM containing audiovisual material from research in the Balkans by Milman Parry, who recorded and studied a live tradition of oral narrative poetry to find how Homer had composed his two monumental epic poems. Lord's book, based on Parry's research, intends to demonstrate the process by which oral poets compose.

Nagy, Gregory. *The Best of the Achaeans.* Rev. ed. Baltimore: The Johns Hopkins University Press, 1999. Sophisticated and stimulating analysis of the hero in Greek civilization and how the language of Greek epic defines his role.

Powell, Barry B. *Homer.* 2d ed. Malden, Mass.: Blackwell, 2007. A concise introduction by a professor of classics writing with students in mind. Considers the Homeric question by reference to recent scholarship. Good bibliography.

Reece, Steve. *Homer's Winged Words: The Evolution of Early Greek Epic Diction in the Light of Oral Theory.* Boston: Brill, 2009. Reece uses oral theory to examine the works of Homer.

Richard Peter Martin

HORACE

Born: Venusia (now Venosa, Italy); December 8, 65 B.C.E.

Died: Rome (now in Italy); November 27, 8 B.C.E.

PRINCIPAL POETRY

Satires, 35 B.C.E., 30 B.C.E. (English translation, 1567)

Epodes, c. 30 B.C.E. (English translation, 1638)

Odes, 23 B.C.E., 13 B.C.E. (English translation, 1621)

Epistles, c. 20-15 B.C.E. (English translation, 1567; includes *Ars poetica*, c. 17 B.C.E.; *The Art of Poetry*)

Carmen Saeculare, 17 B.C.E. (*The Secular Hymn*, 1726)

The Epistles of Horace, 2001 (David Ferry, translator)

OTHER LITERARY FORMS

Horace (HAWR-uhs) is noted for his poetry and the literary theory in *The Art of Poetry*.

ACHIEVEMENTS

Horace is the premier Roman lyric poet. He invented what was to become a particularly influential verse genre, the poetic autobiography. A transmitter and reshaper of early Greek poetry, he turned an essentially minor form (compared with epic and tragedy) into a vehicle for incisive and important political and philosophical statements, while retaining the melodic qualities of his Greek predecessors Sappho, Alcaeus of Lesbos, Anacreon, and Callimachus, among others. Horace's poetry stands at the midpoint between two conceptions of lyricism: the early Greek mode of socially oriented "occasional" verse, on one hand, and modern meditative poetic statement, on the other. Indeed, he did much to bring the latter into being.

Aside from the Horatian lyric stance, the poet bequeathed to Western literature a model technique, one often imitated though rarely equaled. The technique is painstaking; mosaic art is perhaps the best metaphor for it. Friedrich Nietzsche described its effects with wonder: "Every word, by sound, by position, and by meaning, diffuses its influence to right, to left, and over the whole." Again, Horace had illustrious Greek predecessors in using such verbal artistry, notably the Hellenistic poet Callimachus, whose insistence on brevity, exactness, and the "thin" Muse (as opposed to the inflated pseudo-epic style) is repeatedly alluded to by his Roman imitator two centuries later. Horace used the Callimachean aesthetic rule to measure and castigate earlier Roman poets, especially Gaius Lucilius, whom he made his model in the *Satires*. It is clear, moreover, that Horace made the artistic rule into a moral precept as well, a rule for pragmatic, practical behavior (as opposed to self-deceiving, "inflated" self-importance and its attendant vices). In this admirable synthesis, he again blended a typically Roman concern for morality with a Greek love of formal beauty.

In addition to these innovations by mediation of Greek and Roman elements, Horace appears to have been the first Roman poet—and perhaps the only one, next to Vergil—to have meditated on the role of rhetoric in verse. There is a constant tension in Horatian verse between communication, using all the devices of the long classical tradition of rhetoric, and contemplation, dwelling on image, sound, and ambiguity within the space of an individual poem, with little apparent concern to "persuade" a reader. The main lines of this opposition will be seen in Horace's poetic career: from writing *Epodes*, almost all of which address an audience explicitly, urging action or hurling insult, the poet proceeded to the composition of *Satires* or, as he called them, *sermones*, "conversations." Then, having experimented with public and semiprivate modes of discourse, his poetry turns inward to private concerns in the *Odes*; if Horace "reveals" himself at all in the four books of *Odes*, it is only behind a series of masks. Next, he turns to a communicative genre again in the *Epistles*, but here the ostensible "letter" form is still less revealing than one might expect: The poems pretend to be real missives when they are in fact artfully contrived peeks at a persona. Consequently, the "real" Horace is never seen; his image is fractured by a hall-of-mirrors display of poetic skill. It is significant, in fact, that the ancient "Life" of Horace tells how the poet arranged a gallery of mirrors around the sides of his bedroom; the same urge powers the life and the work of this enigmatic man.

Such a personality exerted a powerful attraction on succeeding generations of poets. Horace, unlike most ancient pagan authors, was read and studied during the Middle Ages (if only for his easily excerpted moral maxims), so that many manuscripts of his poems survived to the Renaissance, at which time his poetry could be appreciated in its fullness by such men as Pierre de Ronsard, Petrarch, Michel Eyquem de Montaigne, and, later, Ben Jonson, Andrew Marvell, Robert Herrick, and John Milton. Horace's *Odes* in particular became popular, sometimes to the disadvantage of the poetry, which was misunderstood as the offhand versifying of a jolly, rotund Epicurean, or distorted to read like the precepts of a Christian moralist. By early in the twentieth century, the *Odes* had been translated more than one hundred times in England and France and nearly as often in Germany and Italy. In short, Horace's own predictions of poetic immortality were fulfilled, for he had written at the conclusion of the first three books of the *Odes*: ". . . I have completed a memorial more lasting than bronze . . . not all of me will die; I shall avoid the goddess of death (most of me). . . ."

BIOGRAPHY

Quintus Horatius Flaccus gives more details about his own life, in writing intended for the public, than any other Roman author. His poetry, however, is not undiluted autobiography; even when he purports to tell the truth about his younger days, it can be shown that he is distorting facts slightly for effect. Thus, while it is probably true that Horace's father was a freed slave, as the poet reports in a touching tribute, it is probably not the case that he was "poor in a thin little piece of land," as Horace would have his reader believe. Horace's father must have had a greater income than that if he could afford to send his son to Rome for schooling alongside the offspring of Roman knights and senators, bypassing the local academy at which the sons of set-

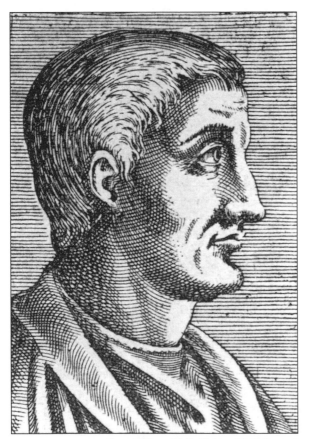

Horace (Time & Life Pictures/Getty Images)

tlers and centurions were taught. It appears that life as an auctioneer's agent (*coactor*) was sufficiently rewarding for the poet's father.

Horace's early education, then, resembled that of any upper-class Roman of the day: study of the Greek classics, primarily Homer, first in the antique translation of Lucius Livius Andronicus, later in the original. Unlike most freedmen's sons, Horace continued his education on the "university" level at Athens, where he studied moral philosophy; no doubt he also continued to read Greek poetry, since his earliest productions show wide acquaintance with the body of lyric verse from the seventh century B.C.E. on. Finally, it was in Athens that Horace began his education in a harder school. There Brutus, the slayer of Julius Caesar, came, eager for new recruits, a few months after the murder in 44 B.C.E.; Horace, along with other young Romans, such as Cicero's son Marcus, joined the campaign against the followers of Caesar in the civil war. As military tribune, Horace took part in the Battle of Philippi of 42 B.C.E., in which his leader, Brutus, met defeat.

On his return home, Horace evidently found that his father's land had been confiscated, to be given to veterans of the victorious army. In an autobiographical section of one epistle, Horace claims that the resulting poverty drove him to write poetry. One must see through Horace's artful irony once again: He cites this bit of personal history in the context of explaining why, at his advanced age, he has been slow to write; there is no pressing need, the poet says, since he is well-off now. Yet Horace could not have been poverty-stricken in his early years, since he was able to purchase the rather high post of scribe to the magistrates, an office that had responsibilities for keeping official records. This employment probably gave him time to write the *Epodes* and the early poems of the *Satires*, and this poetry, in turn, led to his greater fortune.

Horace had the good luck to become a friend of the poet Vergil, who was five years his senior and already a rising talent; Vergil introduced Horace to his own patron, Gaius Maecenas, and, nine months after the meeting, Maecenas invited the young Horace to join his circle of writers. Ironically, Maecenas, as well as being an amateur poet and patron of the arts, was a sort of minister of culture to Horace's former military enemy,

Octavian, soon to become the emperor Augustus and now nominal "first citizen" of the Roman state. Horace was eventually recognized by the emperor and was even offered a position as private secretary, which he refused; it seems the poet preferred the delights of the Sabine farm, a gift to him from Maecenas about 31 B.C.E., to the bustle of Rome and official business.

Horace remained obedient to the commands of Augustus in the literary sphere, however, composing the fourth book of *Odes* specifically at his request. Augustus as a greatly admired figure, savior of the Roman state, also plays a role in Horace's more political poems, in particular the so-called Roman odes. Horace was so successful in treading the line between personal and public commitments with regard to Augustus that he remained in the good graces of the emperor to his death; he named Augustus his heir, but the latter's true fortune was to inherit mention in Horace's poems.

Other details of Horace's life are often deduced from his poetry, but it has been sufficiently shown that this is a risky undertaking. Often, the "incidents" alleged to have taken place reflect Horace's reading of earlier poetry: He loses his shield in battle, for example, only because the Greek poets Archilochus and Alcaeus (and probably Anacreon) did the same, according to their poems; such was literary convention.

The most that one can say about Horace's later life is that it was comfortable; it included the refreshments of country living as well as the latest in Roman gossip and enabled the poet to nurture his muse while avoiding the frequent pressures to write anything other than what he wished—military epic, for instance.

Horace was buried on the Esquiline hill, near the grave of his friend and patron Maecenas, whose death preceded his by a few months.

ANALYSIS

Certain recurring themes and continuing preoccupations can be traced throughout Horace's work: the tendency, from the start of his writing career, to combine Greek and Roman motifs and techniques; his insistence, again from the very start, on a certain "Alexandrian" (or Callimachean) style; his increasing awareness of poetry as personal communication as well as public statement; and his concern with Roman politics of the day.

The seventeen poems that later grammarians and scribes called "epodes" (from the Greek word denoting the shorter line of a couplet) Horace called *iambi* (iambics), a title that would have carried several significant messages to an attentive literate audience. In a collection of iambic poetry, the contemporary reader of Horace's poems would expect savage invective verses. This had been the traditional content of *iambi* since the seventh century B.C.E., when the Greek poet Archilochus of Paros used the form to compose abusive satires of his contemporaries. Archilochus's verse was so effective that its victims, a prospective father-in-law among them, reportedly committed suicide. Horace's *iambi* do reflect this tradition—but only to a small degree. Epodes 4, 6, 8, 10, and 12 are surely Archilochean in inspiration: They exhibit the typical direct address to the victim (a degenerate rich man, an unnamed enemy, or lust-crazed hags, in Horace's poems); obscenity and colloquial speech (only here in Horatian verse); and the "animal persona" device often adopted by the Greek poet (such as the implicit equation of the poet with a wolf, and the ironic reversal in another epode, in which a formidable hag becomes wolf to Horace's lamb). Furthermore, Horace hints that he is adopting the Archilochean mode; he refers in epode 6 to the "spurned son-in-law" who had his revenge on "faithless Lycambes" (the name of Archilochus's victim), and in epode 10 he uses the very same motif that the Greek poet had employed, wishing horrible shipwreck on an enemy.

The reader who had expected to find pure invective in Horace's *iambi*, however, would be disappointed. In what was to become his typical fashion, Horace inserted elements of the traditional genre only to play with them in a sophisticated remodeling of tradition. So it is that the remaining epodes hint at invective poetry but then veer off into other generic types—praise poetry, love poetry, *recusatio* (refusal), pastoral, and variations of these. In this refashioning, Horace again had some precedent in Callimachus, the third century Greek poet, who had also written *iambi* but had used them for yet another prodigious display of esoteric mythical and historical allusion.

EPODES

What is most fresh in Horace's *Epodes* is the use of the form for direct address on current topics. Epodes 1,

7, 9, and 16 all touch on the civil war between Brutus and the followers of Caesar (and later, Antony and Octavian). The introductory poem, as is customary, is addressed to Horace's patron, Maecenas, and so was probably the last poem to be written. As in epode 9, here the topic of war is only background to the main theme of the poem: Maecenas is sailing off to Actium with Octavian; Horace, cleverly using military and political language, pledges his loyalty to the patron and adopts the stance of an *imbellis*, or "noncombatant," poet. Although it might appear to be a minor point, such a stance is crucial to Horace as poet of the *Epodes*. From the start, he is hinting that it will not be his chosen task to praise Maecenas or Octavian for military victories. Horace is, instead, to live a modest existence at home, viewing war only from a distance and being free to write humorously about anything he might like—as he proceeds to do in the remaining epodes. The poem is, then, introduction, apology, refusal, and praise of the patron. Even at this early point of his career, Horace is a master of *multum in parvo*, "saying much in a short space."

The prevalence of humorous poems in the *Epodes*, such as epode 2 (a mock pastoral put in the mouth of a Roman moneylender), epode 3 (a mock threat to Maecenas for a gift of garlic), and epode 5 (the baroque lament of a witch's victim), further emphasizes the serious intent of civil war poems such as epode 7, in which Horace berates the fratricidal citizens of the city of Romulus and Remus (a fratricidal pair). At the same time, even in the "serious" poems, Horace does not forget his role—he is a poet, not a social reformer. Thus, the final civil war poem, epode 16, resembles epode 7 in its refusal to offer solutions to the conflict. It might appear that the poet does come up with an answer in this address to an imaginary Roman assembly: He proposes an expedition to the Isles of the Blest and the abandonment of all of Rome's problems. The reader must see through Horace's dramatic setting, however: The assembly cannot have been Roman (and therefore the possibility of the proposal being accepted is rejected); the details of the Isles of the Blest are too obviously the stock motifs of impossible pastoral scenes, common from Hesiod on. Ending as it does with the word *fuga* (flight), the poem is better interpreted as Horace's

ironic reply to the escapist element at Rome: Civil war is in the blood, and there is no flight. This is invective in sheep's clothing.

A final indication of Horatian artistry in the *Epodes* arises from the deployment of the poems within the book. Scholars have noticed symmetry in theme between epodes 5 and 17 (both about Canidia the witch), epodes 6 and 15 (revenge warnings), epodes 8 and 12 (abuse of hags), epodes 9 and 13 (symposium settings), and epodes 11 and 14 (love elegies).

SATIRES

By 30 B.C.E., Horace had published another carefully arranged collection of poems, the *Satires*, consisting of two books, each containing about one thousand dactylic hexameter verses and dealing with an astonishing array of topics, from the history of the genre (which Horace traced to Greek Old Comedy) to travel narrative to imaginary conversations in the Underworld. The title *Satires*, in fact, is misleading: There is little abuse here, no invective directed against historical personages (the names all being stock characters), and little, if any, serious intent to correct morals. The poet seems to have referred to his work as *sermones* (conversations); this title far better describes the content and style of the poems.

Although the *Epodes* follows a principle of opposite arrangement, those near the beginning of the book being echoed symmetrically by poems near the end, the *Satires* can be read in sections that form a clear progression, from moralizing harangue through autobiographical essays to anecdotes of Roman life; then, after an "apology" poem, the second book presents a new strategy of poetic setting: All eight poems are somehow dialogues, with named or imaginary interlocutors. The now-familiar Horatian device of variety in content subjected to strict formal control appears not only on the level of arrangement. Within individual poems, Horace strives for the effect of random conversation, yet this "talk" is not merely transcribed street speech. It is artistically abbreviated and modified to fit smoothly into the difficult hexameter meter. The ability to overcome such technical difficulties marks Horace as a master. A few examples might illustrate this achievement.

First, Horace does not claim for himself the honor of having invented the "conversation" genre, although this is surely his innovation in the history of *satura* (satire). Instead, he names the earlier Roman poet Lucilius as his model. Satire 1.4, in which he discusses his debt, however, also contains the specific objections that Horace makes to Lucilian style, and these form a sort of poetic creed for the later poet. Lucilius (whose huge output survives only in fragments) "used to recite two hundred verses an hour, standing on one foot, as a grand performance," says Horace; there would be much to excise from such versifying. For Horace, brevity is art. Again, Horace sees poetry as hard work; Lucilius, he alleges, was "lazy at bearing the labor of writing correctly."

In true ironic fashion, Horace proceeds to undercut his assertions by claiming that he is not a "real" poet himself, but only someone who enjoys enclosing talk in meter. He makes the statement to avoid being called a savage satirist by the industrious, greedy Romans: His "work" is only play, Horace says, and not the dangerous occupation that many consider it.

To diminish further the threat of his satire, Horace makes the famous claim that, whereas epic, high-poetic diction is instantly recognizable, if one were to subtract meter from his own poems, there would not be even "the limbs of a sundered poet" left over. At times, as in the nine-line parenthetical remark embedded in the *Satires*, Horace goes to extremes to prove that his poetry is more like conversation. The conceit adds all the more irony to these compositions, as it is clear from such poems as the programmatic satire 1.10 on which side of the stylistic question Horace really stands. Here, in the final poem of the first book (as traditional as opening poems for the placing of poetic credos), he provides the most concise rationale for his own style:

And so it's not enough to make the hearer laugh;
(Yet this is also a virtue of some sort)
One needs conciseness, so that the thought runs on,
Doesn't tangle itself up with words that burden tired ears.
And talk should have now a sad, often a happy cast,
Doing the part now of an orator, now again a poet.

This creed, at least, is one Horace follows. Poet and rhetorician, in the *Satires* he merges low style (stemming from the commonplace style of third century Greek popular moral sermons) with high (that of earlier Greek and Roman epic, tragic, and lyric verse). Carefully chosen diction jostles home truths in the poems, making the *Satires* an authentic image of Rome itself, where all types of humanity could be seen. As the English Augustan poets knew, satire is the urban genre *par excellence*; Horatian satire, in its gently teasing pretense of "talking" to the city, is central to later examples of this poetic mode.

ODES

If the *Satires* is still fresh after two thousand years, that fact is partly the result of Horace's completely original choice of tone, a strength that sustains the *Odes* as well. In this collection of eighty-eight poems in various meters, supplemented by a later fifteen poems, the poet most often speaks in the first person to another. Maecenas, Vergil, Augustus, and other actual contemporaries are among the addressees; so are various divinities and inanimate objects (a boat, a wine jar, a spring). Yet these are far from being simple poetic letters—Horace would experiment with the epistle form a few years later. Rather, they use the convention of an addressee to proceed in one of two directions: Either the topic changes abruptly from the person addressed to what is really the subject of the poem, or the addressee becomes the topic. An example of the first type is *Odes*, book 1, in which Maecenas, addressed in the first two lines as "defense" and "pleasing source of pride" (*dulce decus*) for the poet, drops out of sight for the next thirty lines while Horace develops his contrast between the poet and other occupations; the poet is humble by comparison but also free and secluded:

As for me, ivy on literary brows
Transports me to gods' company; the cool wood grove,
Light choruses of Nymphs with Satyrs
Keep me from the crowd. . . .

Only in line 35 does Maecenas reappear: "If *you* count me with lyric's inspired bards, head held high I'll hit the stars," the poet concludes. Thus, the poem defines the poet (or at least that "I" that is Horace's poetic personality) instead of focusing on communication with the addressee.

In the second type of ode, the poems in which the addressee becomes the topic, Horace pays most attention to creating dramatic and often humorous situations by means of unexpected words, mere hints about time, place, and background, and artfully withheld information about the character of the speaker. Even though he appears to offer us slices of his own life, Horace is at the farthest possible remove from confessional poetry in the *Odes*. The second type integrates the addressee into the poem more completely; it contains examples of Horace's better poems. One such, *Odes*, book 1, deals with love (as about one-third of the odes do), but in a typically oblique way, as part of a short moralizing discourse in the words of an unnamed narrator. The first word of the poem puts the reader into the scene. "*You see how Mt. Soracte stands, white in deep snow. . . .*" Outside, all is ice-jammed; trees and rivers freeze over; inside, by contrast, warmth rules, as the speaker orders "Thaliarche" (a slave?—the Greek name, "festival ruler," has significance) to pile more logs on the fire and pour more wine. Once allowed to eavesdrop on the domestic conversation, the reader is lured into imagining details that Horace slyly keeps concealed: The speaker must be an older man, since he takes the role of adviser ("Leave the rest to the gods; don't seek to know tomorrow's fate"). Ending his bland dismissals in a tightly worded vignette, he specifies what activities the young man beside him should be pursuing: "Now, go after the whispers in the evening, the welcome laugh that gives away the girl hiding in an intimate nook, the pledge-ring snatched from a wrist, or a finger barely resisting." The shift in what occupies the speaker's mind is enough to characterize him for any reader, and one rereads the poem with a fresh eye. Is it the snow ("white," line 1, like his description of "white-haired old age," line 17) that reminds the poem's persona of death? Is the frozen world somehow to be reconciled with the melting girl? Thirty nouns, eighteen adjectives, and almost no exposition, in Horace's hands, can prompt such larger questions. If the *Odes* approaches philosophic concerns, it is solely through such intense viewing of the physical world in all its contrasts, not through the obvious (and often ironically placed) moral platitudes that one also finds in Horace.

The two forms of address, then—self-reflective poems to real persons and dramatic, self-concealing poems to imaginary ones—between them utilize all the old lyric themes, of love, death, wine, and mythology.

As in the poetry of one of his Greek models, the sixth century Alcaeus, the seemingly unpoetic theme of politics also finds a place in Horace's poetry. Horace lacks Alcaeus's direct involvement in local affairs, yet his lyrics allow the public voice of the *Epodes* and *Satires* to emerge, as it does most clearly in book 3 of the *Odes*. Ironically, this public poetry cycle begins with a reassertion of the poet as master of esoteric art: "I hate and shun the uninitiated crowd." He calls himself "priest of the Muses." Like the distancing achieved by masks in drama, or by animal personas in fables, this withdrawal enables Horace to speak his mind more plainly. In theme, these "Roman Odes" cover the Roman ethical vocabulary: *paupertas* (a noble small means); *virtus* (courage and incorruptibility); *justitia* (the rule of law); *imperium* (the rule of appointed power).

Horace inevitably associates the last mentioned with Augustus, whom he praises as equal to the divinized heroes of Greek myth, but in the same poem he also advises against too ambitious a campaign in the East. It is worth noting how Horace can give advice without becoming dangerously offensive. First, he places the warning in the veiled words of the goddess Juno, who speaks within the poem in a mythological excursus. Second, he employs the technique of *recusatio* to avoid getting deeply into the subject. The poem ends: "Muse, where are you heading? Don't go telling the talks of gods; attenuate in small music the great affairs." More than in the *Epodes*, where the technique first appears, the poet of the *Odes* restricts his topics by this Callimachean device; his subject is love affairs, not statecraft.

Horace innovates further, using this lyric device, by turning the stylistic call for "small" (*tenuis*, or "thin") themes into a moral imperative, most clearly in *Odes*, book 2, to Grosphus. Because neither riches nor political power give personal peace or stop anxiety, the solution, says Horace, is good-humored resignation in rustic seclusion. "*Small* fields" and the "*thin* breath of a Greek rustic Muse" (Greek because Horace in the *Odes* imitates the meter and often the content of Sappho and Alcaeus)—these are the poet's fated gifts. The implied "seclusion" is only part of Horace's poetic strategy, and it need not have been actual: A true recluse does not write verse like this or attempt to justify his personal integration of life and style.

EPISTLES

In the *Epistles*, both the ironic tension and the philosophical tone of the Grosphus ode find expression as Horace returns to humorous hexameter verse. The twenty poems of the first book show the poet applying the combined lessons of his earlier work. As in the *Odes*, each poem is addressed to someone, ensuring tonal control; as in the *Satires*, each pretends to instruct the reader on some moral point. The persona adopted now is that of an eclectic philosopher, "sworn to no one school." The letter form allows a joking, rapid, conversational style, and the style, in turn, disguises Horace's serious pronouncements on subjects ranging from the psychology of the Roman practical mind, to Stoicism, to the client-patron relationship. Some of the scattered short poems resemble actual letters; the longer poems, meanwhile, read like an epistolary novel in their gradual creation of character: that of a gentleman-farmer-poet of small means but rich in insight (especially into his fickle nature: "At Rome I want Tibur, at Tibur, Rome. . . .").

Although Horace, in the introductory poem of the first book, claims to have abandoned lyric verse, this does not mean that he has forgotten his high standards of craftsmanship. In a gibe at his imitators, he shows that he prides himself on the pioneering achievement of the *Epodes* and *Odes*, particularly the latter, in which he still has confidence despite the poor public reception. A final example of his craftsmanship appears as the last epistle in the book, where Horace addresses the collection as he would caution a recently freed slave eager to participate in the life of the city. It is an extended metaphor; the poet warns that "you will be loved while you are still young—then you'll end up teaching small boys in a small town somewhere" (a common occupation for old slaves as well as old books). What the book will teach is Horace himself, "who stretched his wings out bigger than his nest . . . a slight man, tanned and graying, quick to anger but easy to calm down."

Only with this exhibition of the unique Horatian combination of humor with precise literary estimation in mind should one read the most famous and most imitated epistle, the *Ars poetica*, which forms the finale to the second book. That work, also, is a letter; it purports to instruct the sons of Piso about poetry. Many attempts have been made to detect various technical theories behind the work, but it is, rather, an amusing and eclectic virtuoso piece. After four hundred lines of animated, veering argumentation, its primary message comes to this: Write verse the way I have done, with clarity, wit, and flair, learnedly, laboriously, and playfully. So one returns, again, to the Horatian corpus, not to any one statement about poetry, but to learn how to write verse. It is a good principle in reading Horace and, indeed, all literature.

BIBLIOGRAPHY

Commager, Steele. *The Odes of Horace*. Reprint. Norman: University of Oklahoma Press, 1995. Commager's book is widely regarded as the most substantial, incisive commentary on Horace's verse in English. He approaches Horace as a "professional poet," one committed to art as a vocation. Horace's distinctive characteristic is that he writes poetry about poetry, as if he wants to define the idea and demonstrate verbal craftsmanship at the same time.

Harrison, Stephen, ed. *The Cambridge Companion to Horace*. New York: Cambridge University Press, 2007. Provides orientation and coverage for those new to the study of Horace as well as new perspectives on the poet for those more advanced.

Highet, Gilbert. *The Classical Tradition: Greek and Roman Influences on Western Literature*. New York: Oxford University Press, 1985. Through judicious use of the index, the curious student can survey European attitudes toward Horace's poetry since the Renaissance. Highet is an opinionated and lively critic who inspires a return to primary texts.

Levi, Peter. *Horace: A Life*. New York: Routledge, 1998. Biography of the poet intended for general readers with little understanding of classical life or literature. Emphasizes the personal relationships that inspired his poetry; provides insight into the historical events that shaped Horace's thought. Offers close textual analysis of key works, including an extensive discussion of *The Art of Poetry*.

McClatchy, J. D., ed. *Horace, The Odes: New Translations by Contemporary Poets*. Princeton, N.J.: Princeton University Press, 2002. McClatchy collects new interpretations of Horace's works by today's preeminent poets.

McNeill, Randall L. B. *Horace: Image, Identity, and Audience*. Baltimore: The Johns Hopkins University Press, 2001. The author explores how Horace used technique to write about his personal existence in his poetry.

Oliensis, Ellen. *Horace and the Rhetoric of Authority*. New York: Cambridge University Press, 1998. This introduction to Horace covers the poet's entire career and all the genres in which he wrote.

Putnam, Michael C. J. *Artifices of Eternity*. Ithaca, N.Y.: Cornell University Press, 1986. Putnam presents a detailed analysis of Horace's last work, the final book of *Odes*. Traditionally the fourth book is considered not unified and is said to show Horace bowing to Augustus's influence. Putnam argues that Horace remakes Augustus as the poet sees him. The approach has interesting biographical implications for interpreting Horace's last years.

Woodman, Tony, and Denis Feeney, eds. *Traditions and Contexts in the Poetry of Horace*. New York: Cambridge University Press, 2002. Distinguished scholars present essays on various aspects of Horace, some of them examining a single poem in great detail.

Richard Peter Martin

VICTOR HUGO

Born: Besançon, France; February 26, 1802
Died: Paris, France; May 22, 1885

PRINCIPAL POETRY

Odes et poésies diverses, 1822, 1823
Nouvelles Odes, 1824
Odes et ballades, 1826
Les Orientales, 1829 (*Les Orientales: Or, Eastern Lyrics*, 1879)
Les Feuilles d'automne, 1831
Les Chants du crépuscule, 1835 (*Songs of Twilight*, 1836)
Les Voix intérieures, 1837
Les Rayons et les ombres, 1840

Les Châtiments, 1853
Les Contemplations, 1856
La Légende des siècles, 1859-1883 (5 volumes; *The Legend of the Centuries*, 1894)
Les Chansons des rues et des bois, 1865
L'Année terrible, 1872
L'Art d'être grand-père, 1877
Le Pape, 1878
La Pitié suprême, 1879
L'Âne, 1880
Les Quatre vents de l'esprit, 1881
The Literary Life and Poetical Works of Victor Hugo, 1883
La Fin de Satan, 1886
Toute la lyre, 1888
Dieu, 1891
Les Années funestes, 1896
Poems from Victor Hugo, 1901
Dernière Gerbe, 1902
Poems, 1902
The Poems of Victor Hugo, 1906
Océan, 1942

OTHER LITERARY FORMS

Besides his rather prolific output in the field of poetry, Victor Hugo (YEW-goh) achieved prominence in two other genres as well. His novels, for which he is best known in the United States, span most of his literary career and include such recognizable titles as *Le Dernier Jour d'un condamné* (1829; *The Last Day of a Condemned*, 1840), *Notre-Dame de Paris* (1831; *The Hunchback of Notre Dame*, 1833), and *Les Misérables* (1862; English translation, 1862). Hugo was a successful playwright in his time, but only *Hernani* (pr., pb. 1830; English translation, 1830) has received sustained attention. The preface to his play *Cromwell* (pb. 1827; English translation, 1896), however, is frequently studied by scholars because of its attack on the three unities, so long observed by French classical writers, and because of Hugo's elaboration on his theory of the union of the grotesque and the sublime. His other plays are a *mise en oeuvre* of the dramatic principles found in the *Cromwell* preface.

Although less well known as an essayist, Hugo did write in the genre. His better-known essay collections include *Le Rhin* (1842; *The Rhine*, 1843), *William Shakespeare* (1864; English translation, 1864), *Choses vues* (1887; *Things Seen*, 1887), and *En voyage: Alpes et Pyrénées* (1890; *The Alps and Pyrenees*, 1898). Hugo also wrote and delivered a number of political speeches in the Chambre des Pairs. Among these are the "Consolidation et défense du littoral," which was delivered in the summer of 1846, "La Famille Bonaparte," which was delivered the following spring, and "Le Pape Pie IX," which was presented in January, 1848.

ACHIEVEMENTS

"Ego Hugo": This was the inscription emblazoned on the Gothic armchair that stood in the dining room in the Hugos' Guernsey home. Dubbed an ancestral chair by the poet, it remained conspicuously empty at mealtime. For Victor Hugo's critics, this motto became a symbol of an oversized ego. For his admirers, the empty chair symbolized the greatness of Hugo the poet, if not Hugo the man. Indeed, his place in literature is unquestioned, and no other French poet since has been able to match his production and influence.

Hugo excelled in a wide variety of verse forms: ode, lyric, epic, satire, and heroic narrative. His versatility in mode was matched by variations in tone, from the eloquence and rhetorical precision found in *Les Châtiments* (the chastisements), for example, to the simplicity and grace of *Les Contemplations*. Conventions that were in vogue at the time, such as the marvelous and the fantastic, the medieval and the Oriental, were translated by Hugo into verse. The poet also found inspiration in the imagery of dreams, spiritualism, and metempsychosis. His poetry set the tone and the style for Romantic verse; his choice of subjects and his novel uses of stylistic devices influenced the Parnassians and the Symbolists.

The sheer volume of Hugo's production would have assured him a place in literary history even if the strength and character of the man had not assured his celebrity. Hugo's resiliency allowed him to overcome personal tragedy and to express his grief in verse. He championed causes such as free, compulsory education, universal suffrage, the right to work, and the abolition of the death penalty, before such political postures

were popular. In all, Hugo was a man of deep convictions, of great sensibility, and of tremendous ego whose poetic creation reflected all these aspects of his complex personality.

BIOGRAPHY

Victor-Marie Hugo was born at Besançon, the third son of Joseph Léopold Sigisbert Hugo and Sophie Trébuchet. His father, a career military man, served with distinction in the postrevolutionary army. He later became a general and viscount, as well as a close associate of Joseph Bonaparte, Napoleon's brother. Though gifted with military tenacity, the elder Hugo unfortunately was not capable of such steadfastness on the home front. Madame Hugo soon tired of his lusty nature and infidelities, finding relief in the arms of General Victor Fanneau LaHorie, an opponent of Napoleon, who was Victor Hugo's godfather. Shortly after Hugo's birth,

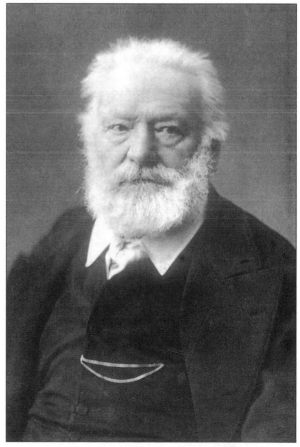

Victor Hugo (Hulton Archive/Getty Images)

Madame Hugo moved her children to Paris to be near LaHorie. After LaHorie became an enemy of Napoleon's regime, she hid him in her quiet house with a large garden in the rue des Feuillantines. During those eighteen months, the gentle "M. le Courlandais" taught the eight-year-old Hugo to read and translate Tacitus, and he impressed the young boy with the ideal of liberty; indeed, Hugo was to have a lifelong sympathy for the oppressed. In later years, he would fondly remember those days spent playing in the garden with his brother and with a girl named Adèle Foucher. Madame Hugo somehow provided a tranquil environment for her children, unembittered by constant marital strife.

Though LaHorie had provided some formal training, the education of the Hugo brothers remained spotty because of the family's frequent moves. The family took two trips to visit the boys' father: to Italy in 1809 and to Spain in 1811-1812. During that last trip, the boys were enrolled at the Collège des Nobles in Madrid. The year in Spain was to provide Hugo with much material for his later works. The Spanish hero Ernani would become the hero of his play, with the Masserano palace as one of its settings; the hunchback Corcova at the seminary would become the inspiration for Quasimodo; the street Ortoleza reappears in the play *Ruy Blas* (pr., pb. 1838; English translation, 1890).

In 1814, General Hugo insisted that his sons be enrolled at the Pension Cordier, where they spent four years studying the sciences. To relieve the drudgery, the brothers wrote poems and plays during their leisure hours. Soon, this pastime became a successful enterprise. At the age of fifteen, Hugo entered the French Academy's poetry contest, receiving an honorable mention. In 1819, he won two prizes from the Académie des Jeux Floraux of Toulouse. Hugo and his brother Eugène entered law school to please their father but spent most of their efforts in the founding of a magazine called *Le Conservateur littéraire*. Among the early contributors to the venture was Alfred de Vigny, who was to become one of Hugo's closest friends. In this magazine, Hugo published his "Ode sur la mort du duc de Berry" and the first version of what was to become his second novel, *Bug-Jargal* (1826; *The Noble Rival*, 1845). The ode placed Hugo in the favor of

the Royalists, among them his idol François-René de Chateaubriand, in whose presence the poet was received shortly after the publication of his ode. Soon, the Hugo brothers were admitted into the Société des Bonnes Lettres, an ultra-Royalist group; by this time, Hugo had adopted his mother's Royalist views.

With the death of his mother in 1821, Hugo entered a period of extreme poverty. He abandoned *Le Conservateur littéraire* and strove to make a living. In 1822, Hugo published the *Odes et poésies diverses*. Conservative and Royalist in content, these odes earned for Hugo a royal pension. He was able to marry his childhood sweetheart, Adèle Foucher, and continue with his literary career.

The years between 1822 and 1828 were filled with creative and literary activities. In 1823, Hugo published the second edition of *Odes et poésies diverses* as well as his first novel, *Han d'Islande* (1823; *Hans of Iceland*, 1845). The following year, Hugo's *Nouvelles Odes* were published. In 1825, Hugo was named, along with Alphonse de Lamartine, to the Legion of Honor "for his noble efforts . . . to sustain the sacred cause of the altar and the throne." The year 1826 saw the publication of Hugo's *Odes et ballades*, as well as his second novel, *The Noble Rival*. The publication the following year of the bold preface to *Cromwell* established Hugo as the spokesperson for the new Romantic school. Hugo's father, Léopold, died in 1828, an event that greatly grieved the poet. Since the death of his mother, Hugo and his father had achieved a rapprochement. This friendship rendered the poet more sympathetic to the Bonapartist cause and served to counterbalance the Royalist fervor that he had received from his mother. In that same year, Hugo's play *Amy Robsart* (pr. 1828; English translation, 1895) was presented.

During these years, the Hugo home had become the focal point for the gathering of literary young men caught up in the Romantic revolution against the formalism of the seventeenth and eighteenth centuries, men such as Charles Augustin Sainte-Beuve, Alfred de Vigny, Alfred de Musset, Théophile Gautier, Gérard de Nerval, and Émile and Antoine Deschamps. This group, which became known as the *cénacle*, sought to break the bonds of the dramatic unities, of poetic versification, and of the choice of subject matter, and rallied to expand the imaginative and aesthetic field. Hugo was the unquestioned head of the group. From his ideas and from the discussions that took place in his home during those years sprang new branches of Romanticism, including the Parnassian school.

The next few years were emotionally difficult ones for Hugo. Though he continued to receive acclaim for his new collection of poems *Les Orientales*, striking because of their exoticism; for his play *Hernani*, which heralded a decisive victory for Romantic drama; and for *The Hunchback of Notre Dame*, which established Hugo as a great writer of the historical novel, the security of his home life had begun to crumble. In 1829, Hugo's best friend, Sainte-Beuve, had revealed to the poet his love for Hugo's wife, Adèle. In spite of this revelation, Hugo tried to maintain the friendship, made more difficult by Sainte-Beuve's assertion that his love was reciprocated. In his distress, Hugo found comfort in a relationship with an actress, Juliette Drouet. It was an affair that would last fifty years and that was eventually accepted by Adèle Hugo. Drouet was transformed through her love for the poet into a devoted companion who remained virtually cloistered in her quarters, content to read and to copy his books.

These personal afflictions and affections found expression in the poetic works that followed: *Les Feuilles d'automne* (the leaves of autumn), *Songs of Twilight, Les Voix intérieures* (the interior voices), and *Les Rayons et les ombres* (the rays and shadows). These collections contrasted markedly with Hugo's previous poetic works in both tone and style. Unlike the exotic and colorful *Les Orientales*, for example, these poems sought to express the more intimate relationships found in love, childhood, and friendship, as well as in humankind's association with nature. In 1843, two other disasters, the death of his daughter Léopoldine and the failure of his play *Les Burgraves* (pr., pb. 1843; *The Burgraves*, 1896) caused Hugo to put down his pen for some time. As always, tragedy accompanied success in the poet's life.

Meanwhile, Hugo's political involvement intensified. In 1841, he was elected to the French Academy. As his prominence grew, it followed that he should be raised to peerage, and this indeed occurred in 1845. From this position, Hugo addressed the parliament on

such matters as capital punishment and the plight of the poor, subjects on which he had already written in *The Last Day of a Condemned* and *Claude Gueux* (1834), and which would be fully exploited in a work already in progress at this time, *Les Misérables*. Because of his concern for the ordinary man and the unfortunates, he was elected a "representative of the people" in 1848 and a year later became a Parisian delegate to the Assemblée Nationale. During the 1848 Revolution, Hugo published his opinions in his journal *L'Événement*, and though he was aligned with no particular political party, the periodical was suppressed. He grew increasingly suspicious of Louis Napoleon's ambitions, and though Hugo had originally supported him for the presidency, he delivered a scathing address before the Assemblée in July of 1851 in which he called the president "Napoleon the Little." As a consequence of this attack, Hugo fled France shortly after the coup d'état of December, 1851. This event marked another change in the poet's political stance: Having been a Royalist and then a Bonapartist, Hugo next became a Republican.

Hugo went first to Belgium, where he stayed only for a short time, then moved to the Channel Islands of Jersey and then Guernsey, where he finally settled with his family and with Juliette Drouet from 1855 to 1870. These were to be very productive years for Hugo. After a long silence, the poet's voice was again heard in 1853 with the publication of *Les Châtiments*, in which he vehemently denounced Louis Napoleon and his empire. In 1856, Hugo published *Les Contemplations*, in which he integrated lyrics, meditative poems on his daughter's death, and more visionary and mystical verses. In large measure, these poems would influence the Symbolists. With the publication of the first *The Legend of the Centuries* in 1859, an extensive epic that detailed humankind's progress from slavery to freedom, Hugo achieved the unquestioned reputation of "poet-seer."

It was as if Hugo's long silence had caused him to relish his renewed literary voice, for his productivity during the 1860's remained substantial. In 1862, his great novel *Les Misérables* appeared, succeeded by *Les Chansons des rues et des bois* (the songs of the streets and the woods) in 1865. These were followed in 1866 by another novel, *Les Travailleurs de la mer* (1866; *The Toilers of the Sea*, 1866). As always, his literary acclaim was accompanied by personal sorrow. Adèle Hugo died in 1868 in Brussels of apoplexy. Her wish had been to be buried beside her daughter Léopoldine. Hugo accompanied her body as far as the French frontier. The following year, Hugo's next novel, *L'Homme qui rit* (1869; *The Man Who Laughs*, 1869), was published. It received little acclaim at the time, and it has been only rarely studied since.

The fall of the Second Empire on September 3, 1870, ended Hugo's long exile from France. He returned during turbulent times: The war with Prussia and the civil war that ensued left Hugo disillusioned. During this time, his son Charles died, his daughter Adèle was confined to an asylum, and his son François became gravely ill. Once more, the poet returned to Guernsey, this time not so much to escape political forces as to seek solace. He recorded his feelings in *L'Année terrible* (terrible year).

Hugo returned to Paris in 1873 after finishing his novel *Quatre-vingt-treize* (1874; *Ninety-three*, 1874), which was published the following year. Then seventy-one years old, he found great consolation in his grandchildren, spending long hours with them and sharing childhood delights. For his age, his productivity was amazingly constant. In 1877, there appeared the second volume of *The Legend of the Centuries*, as well as *L'Art d'être grand-père* (the art of being a grandfather). These were followed by *Le Pape* (the pope), *La Pitié suprême* (the supreme pity), *Religions et religion* (1880), *L'Âne* (the ass) and a play, *Torquemada* (pb. 1882; English translation, 1896). On May 11, 1883, Juliette Drouet died of stomach cancer; her death was a terrible blow to Hugo. He published nothing else during his lifetime except the final volume of *The Legend of the Centuries* in 1883. His health steadily declined, and he died of pneumonia on May 22, 1885. He was buried in the Panthéon beside Voltaire and Jean-Jacques Rousseau.

In 1875, Hugo had written his literary will, which specified that after his death all his manuscripts without exception should be published. This testament was faithfully executed, allowing for the appearance of the following posthumous publications: *Théâtre en liberté*

(pb. 1886), *La Fin de Satan* (the end of satan), *Toute la lyre* (all of the lyre), *Dieu* (God), *Les Années funestes* (the fatal years), and *Dernière Gerbe* (last sheaf). A portion of his letters, *Correspondence* (1896-1898), and his travel books, *The Alps and Pyrenees* and *Things Seen*, were also published.

ANALYSIS

Victor Hugo's poetry took many forms, from the lyric to the epic to the elegiac. Along with this variety of form, the range of the poet's ideas expanded during his long career. From poems with political overtones, Hugo's poetry grew to exhibit the tenets of Romanticism. He wrote of more personal and intimate subjects, such as family and love. He also wrote about humankind's relationship with nature and with the Creator. As Hugo matured, his themes became more philosophical and humanitarian, and his self-appointed role became that of a poet-seer attempting to understand the mysteries of life and creation.

ODES ET BALLADES

Hugo's shift toward Romanticism and away from political themes first became apparent in *Odes et ballades*. In this collection, the poet makes copious use of the fantastic, the uncanny, and the horrifying, a popular style of the time, exemplified by the German ballads of Gottfried Burger, Christoph Wieland, and Johann Wolfgang von Goethe. Hugo's inspiration was drawn also from contemporary translations of Spanish, English, and French ballads, a diversity of sources that infused his own ballads with eclecticism.

In the preface to *Odes et ballades*, Hugo compares the sculptured gardens of Versailles with the primitive forests of the New World. The artificiality of the former, Hugo claims, stands in opposition to the laws of nature, whereas in the untouched forests, "everything obeys an invariable law." The true poet, then, must look to nature as his model, forsaking the contrived in favor of the natural. This was the new precept that Hugo sought to follow in this work.

Hugo received praise from his contemporaries for his imaginative use of his subject matter and for his great technical versatility. He used not only the classical Alexandrine but also other forms of versification, such as the octosyllabic line in the poem "La Fiancée du timbalier" ("The Cymbaleer's Bride") and the little-used Renaissance seven-syllable line in "À Trilby." Though original and clever, these poems are devoid of the philosophical intent that characterizes the poet's later work. They were pronounced excellent, however, by a young critic for *Le Globe* by the name of Charles-Augustin Sainte-Beuve.

LES ORIENTALES

Les Orientales marks Hugo's departure from neoclassical rhetorical forms and inaugurates his bolder, more colorful style. Hugo's use of metaphor gains precision and originality; he employs verse forms drawn from the Renaissance Pléiade, to which he had been led by Sainte-Beuve.

The most famous poem of *Les Orientales* is "Les Djinns" ("The Djinns"), which exhibits Hugo's technical virtuosity. There is exoticism in the choice of both subject and form; in this, the poem is representative of the entire collection. The djinns are identified as evil spirits who sweep into a town and leave just as quickly. Their anticipated arrival is marked by a mounting from a two-syllable line to a decasyllabic line, while their departure is signaled by a parallel decrescendo. In this manner, Hugo is able to create an atmosphere of mystery and terror, with a contrasting feeling of relief. The poem won the plaudits not only of Hugo's contemporaries, but also of later poets and critics; Algernon Charles Swinburne was to comment that no other poet had "left a more exquisite piece or one more filled with delicate lyricism."

LES FEUILLES D'AUTOMNE

In *Les Feuilles d'automne*, Hugo's lyrical voice achieves maturity. The central themes are those of childhood, nature, and love. Although the style is less spectacular than that of *Les Orientales*, Hugo achieves a profound poetic effect through greater simplicity. His treatment of domestic themes is reminiscent of William Wordsworth, whose works Hugo may have known through the influence of Sainte-Beuve.

The opening poem is a tribute to the poet's mother's love and devotion. This is followed by a warm acknowledgment of his father, in which Hugo recalls the General's house at Blois and mourns his father's death. These panegyrics to his parents set the tone for the entire collection.

Less than a handful of poems deal with the topic of childhood, yet Hugo was the first to introduce this subject into French verse. The masterpiece of the collection is one such poem, "Lorsque l'enfant paraît" ("Infantile Influence"), touching in its description of the young child whose presence signifies a blessed household. Hugo concludes with a prayer imploring God to preserve family and friends from a home without a child. Such a sentimental ending would not have been found in *Les Orientales*, and it manifests a further development in the poet's style.

Another development, but on a different plane, establishes the poet's concern for the correspondences between people and nature, as in the poem "Ce qu'on entend sur la montagne" ("What Is Heard on the Mountain"). The role of the poet becomes significant in such an interchange; he becomes an interpreter in this dialogue, as Hugo announces in "Pan." These assertions were manifest again in later poetic works.

LES RAYONS ET LES OMBRES

In *Les Rayons et les ombres*, Hugo conceives of a social mission for the poet. The poet becomes a sacred dreamer, an impartial observer of his time, seeking inspiration from humankind, nature, and God. This collection is, therefore, rather diverse in its subject matter. There are love poems, poems devoted to nature, verses inspired by a search for religious significance, childhood memories, and poems with greater social content.

Two celebrated poems are to be found in *Les Rayons et les ombres*. The first is "Tristesse d' Olympio," in which the poet is presented as a keeper of the secrets of the universe. The tone of sadness that pervades the piece is in large measure a reflection of the unhappy events of 1837, the year it was written. Sainte-Beuve had published a story titled "Mme de Pontivy," in which he described a love affair similar to his alleged affair with Adèle Hugo. Hugo's daughter Léopoldine had been seriously ill that year. At the same time, the poet himself had been afflicted with an eye disorder. In that same year also, Hugo's brother Eugène died after spending many years in an asylum, his illness caused in large part by Hugo's marriage with Adèle, whom he had also loved. The inspiration for the poem is, therefore, overwhelmingly personal. The mood of the poem reflects Hugo's disillusionment with the mutability of nature. In striking contrast with poems of this same genre, such as Alphonse de Lamartine's "Le Lac" ("The Lake"), Hugo asserts that, though nature may forget, humankind will not.

The second important poem in this collection is "Oceano Nox." Though it is much shorter and less complicated than "Tristesse d'Olympio," it nevertheless successfully introduces the sea into Hugo's poetic corpus. The poet chose the elegiac form to describe the force of the ocean and the tragedy of men who are engulfed in the sea, remembered only for a short time by their loved ones. The final stanza is powerful in its description of the desperate voices contained in the roar of the sea at night.

"L'EXPIATION"

It was during his stay in Jersey in 1853 that Hugo published *Les Châtiments*, a volume of satiric poetry. The work is a ceaseless diatribe against the Second Empire and Louis Napoleon. Hugo's indignation against the emperor was inexhaustible. He believed Napoleon to be a tyrant, a ruler who had compromised the liberty of the French people. Hugo evokes every imaginable vituperative image in his denunciation of "Napoleon the Dwarf." Though these pages are replete with a succession of ingenious epithets and metaphors, one poem in this collection is particularly noteworthy, "L'Expiation."

The poem combines both epic and satiric styles; its structure is particularly ingenious. Opening with an account of the glorious reign of Napoleon I, it develops the concept of the crime that the poet must expiate: the coup d'état on the *Dix-huit Brumaire* of the revolutionary calendar. Hugo then details the emperor's retreat from Moscow, his army's struggle in the blinding snow, the loss of countless men to the elements. Napoleon wonders at this point whether this is his punishment. A voice replies: *No*.

The second part of the poem recounts the Battle of Waterloo. Hugo describes the conflict at its height. Napoleon witnesses the fall of the French army, and this time he knows that his defeat will be total. Once more the question is asked: Is this the punishment? Once more, the voice answers: *No*.

The third segment of the poem concerns Napoleon's exile on Saint Helena. Hugo ably contrasts the prisoner Napoleon with the formerly glorious emperor. The latter is now preoccupied with the memories of Moscow, with his wife's infidelity, and with the constant surveillance of his jailer, Sir Hudson Lowe. As the fallen emperor lies dying, he once more raises the question: Is this the punishment? This time, the voice replies: *Not yet*.

Thirty years later, Napoleon I is awakened in his tomb by a familiar voice. It is the voice of his nephew, who has debased the name of Napoleon. Now the punishment is clear: The name of Napoleon is to be remembered not in glory but in ignominy.

Though it is known that Hugo researched his subject carefully, the tension and the concentration of events that make this poem so remarkable are his own distinctive contributions. The ingenuity of the threefold intervention of the voice sustains the dramatic movement, while the portrait of Napoleon is a powerful study in contrast.

LES CONTEMPLATIONS

Published in two volumes, titled *Autrefois* (former times) and *Aujourd'hui* (today), *Les Contemplations* has been called by the critic Ferdinand Brunetière "the most lyrical collection in the French language." The dividing line between the two volumes was the death of Hugo's daughter Léopoldine, in 1843. Consequently, the poems in this collection are very personal, yet the poet generalizes his experiences to include the experiences of all people. Central to the work is the relationship of God and humankind, of humankind and external nature, and of life and death.

In this collection, there are two groups of poems that are particularly significant. The first is "Pauca meae," comprising seventeen poems composed between 1841 and 1855. They were inspired by Hugo's daughter, Léopoldine. The best-known poem in this series is "A Villequier," which expresses the poet's deep despair at the loss of his beloved daughter. It treats the poet's attempt to submit to the will of God and to resign himself to a life without his child. Though he is able to achieve the former, complete resignation is something that eludes him. Unable to restrain his emotion, he claims the right to weep. The grief of a father dominates the rest of the poem, which concludes on a note of extreme sadness.

The second important series in *Les Contemplations*, "Au bord de l'infini," comprises twenty-six poems containing a statement of Hugo's philosophical ideas. The poet aspires to penetrate the unknown, perhaps through prayer. His search for truth will be as a winged dreamer or as a startled wise man. The crowning piece of this series, "Ce que dit la bouche d'ombre" ("What the Mouth of the Shadow Says"), deals with such concepts as Pythagoreanism (in particular, the metempsychosis of souls), Platonism, and pantheism.

"What the Mouth of the Shadow Says" is set at the dolmen of Rozel. There the poet meets a specter with whom he discusses the unity of the universe and the essential vitality of all that is in it. Everything in creation has a soul and a consciousness, but how is this universe to be explained? If God is in everything and everything is in God, then how can one reconcile the imperfections of the world with the perfection that is God? It is here that Hugo introduces the notion of evil. If evil is caused by the absence of light, then the resulting darkness and heaviness can only be associated with matter. Because humans are conscious of the difference between darkness and light, then humans choose to do evil by their own free will. Moreover, humans choose their own punishment. An evildoer's soul will be metamorphosed into something degrading; the soul of Judas, for example, is to be found in the spit of men. Ultimately, however, there is hope for humankind, a hope that the dualism between light and darkness, between goodness and evil, will be reconciled. It is on this thought that the poem ends.

THE LEGEND OF THE CENTURIES

Considered by many to be the greatest epic poem since the Middle Ages, *The Legend of the Centuries* differs from other epics in its humanitarian concerns. Hugo states in the preface that he is interested in showing the human profile "from Eve, the mother of men, to the Revolution, the mother of peoples." This is to be accomplished with the notion of progress foremost in his mind. This is not a historical collection, but rather, as Charles Baudelaire put it, a collection of those things that are poetic, that is, legend, myth, and fable, those things that tap the deep reservoirs of humanity.

Among the many subjects presented are the following: "Le Sacre de la femme" ("The Crowning of Women"), which opens the volume and which treats the story of Eve, not from the perspective of Original Sin, but from the perception of idyllic beauty; "La Conscience" ("Conscience"), which is the story of Cain's attempt to flee from the Eye that follows him everywhere, even to his grave; "Booz endormi" ("Boaz Asleep"), which was inspired by the Book of Ruth and in which Hugo attributes to the patriarch Boaz a dream in which he sees a great oak leading from himself to David and finally to Christ; "Le Mariage de Roland," which is considered by critics to be the prototype of the little epic and which presents the four-day struggle between Roland and Olivier, ending with the proposal that Roland marry Olivier's sister; "La Rose de l'infante" ("The Infanta's Rose"), which deals with the destruction in 1588 of the Spanish Armada and describes a great gust of wind that scatters the fleet and simultaneously arrives in the royal garden of Aranjuez, stripping the petals of the rose held by the infanta and scattering them in the nearby fountain; "Le Satyr" ("The Satyr"), which is considered to be the most important philosophical poem of the collection and treats the double nature of humankind, beings at once allied with the gods because of their spirit, but who now have their feet in the mud; and two poems, "Pleine mer" ("Out at Sea") and "Plein ciel" ("Up in the Sky"), which together constitute "Vingtième siècle," contrasting the evils of old-world war symbolized by the steamship Leviathan with the vision of goodness symbolized by the airship.

LA FIN DE SATAN

Although *La Fin de Satan* was not published until after Hugo's death, it was conceived of during his stay in Guernsey. Hugo's treatment of the fallen angel differs greatly from the Miltonic version. Whereas the fall of Satan in Milton's work is precipitous, in Hugo's version Satan's fall takes thousands of years, while the feathers from his wings fall even more slowly. Furthermore, while Milton's Satan reigns over a host of other devils, Hugo's Satan is alone until he is able to engender a daughter, the veiled Isis-Lilith. It is she who brings evil into the world. After the great Flood, she returns to Earth the three weapons with which Cain had slain Abel: a bronze nail, a wooden club, and a stone. For Hugo, these instruments symbolically represent war, capital punishment, and imprisonment. These three representations determine the structure of the work.

In the first section, "Le Glaive," Hugo illustrates the evils of war through the symbolic character of Nimrod. Hugo's Nimrod is arrogant and bellicose, and his attack on the kingdom of God is doomed to failure. The most remarkable section of this first part concerns another Hugoesque creation. One of the feathers from Lucifer's wings had not fallen into the abyss, landing instead on the edge of a precipice. The angel, Liberty, engendered from this feather is a creation of God rather than of Satan, and together with Lilith, she represents the dual nature of Lucifer-Satan.

The second section, centering on an earthly drama, is titled "Le Gibet" ("The Cross"). It is divided into three parts: "La Judée," "Jésus-Christ," and "Le Crucifix." Hugo's attack on capital punishment takes the form of a contrast between the innocent Christ, who is crucified, and the guilty Barabbas, who is set free. Hugo adds an effective scene not found in the biblical narration, wherein Barabbas comes to the foot of the Cross after the Crucifixion.

In the meantime, Liberty beseeches God to allow Lucifer to return to the light. Before putting Lucifer into a peaceful sleep, she receives his blessing to undo the work of Lilith on Earth. The final section of the poem, dealing with imprisonment, was not complete at Hugo's death. Hugo, however, did write a conclusion to the work, titled "Satan pardonnée" ("Satan Pardoned"). Liberty is able to gain the salvation of both humankind and Lucifer.

Dieu

Composed in large part during Hugo's stay in Guernsey in 1855, *Dieu* was left unfinished for many years. Hugo returned to it in 1875, and it was published posthumously in 1891. The poem concerns Hugo's search for God. Twenty-one voices warn the poet of the futility of his search for a complete understanding of God; nevertheless, the poet continues on his journey. He meets a series of symbolic birds, for he himself is winged. These birds are emblems of various understandings of the godhead: atheism, skepticism, Manichaeanism, paganism, Judaism, and Christianity. Finally, the poet achieves the light in "La Lumière" ("The Light"), although he is denied complete understanding,

for a veil falls before him. Humankind is to know the secrets of the infinite only in death.

Together with *La Fin de Satan*, *Dieu* represents a synthesis of Hugo's religious and philosophical ideas, revealing the poet as a privileged seeker of truth. Hugo shows himself to be not only a master of versification but also a man consumed by the desire to comprehend the deeper mysteries of existence and of the universe.

Other major works

LONG FICTION: *Han d'Islande*, 1823 (*Hans of Iceland*, 1845); *Bug-Jargal*, 1826 (*The Noble Rival*, 1845); *Le Dernier Jour d'un condamné*, 1829 (*The Last Day of a Condemned*, 1840); *Notre-Dame de Paris*, 1831 (*The Hunchback of Notre Dame*, 1833); *Claude Gueux*, 1834; *Les Misérables*, 1862 (English translation, 1862); *Les Travailleurs de la mer*, 1866 (*The Toilers of the Sea*, 1866); *L'Homme qui rit*, 1869 (*The Man Who Laughs*, 1869); *Quatre-vingt-treize*, 1874 (*Ninety-three*, 1874).

PLAYS: *Cromwell*, pb. 1827 (verse drama; English translation, 1896); *Amy Robsart*, pr. 1828 (English translation, 1895); *Hernani*, pr., pb. 1830 (verse drama; English translation, 1830); *Marion de Lorme*, pr., pb. 1831 (verse drama; English translation, 1895); *Le Roi s'amuse*, pr., pb. 1832 (verse drama; *The King's Fool*, 1842; also known as *The King Amuses Himself*, 1964); *Lucrèce Borgia*, pr., pb. 1833 (*Lucretia Borgia*, 1842); *Marie Tudor*, pr., pb. 1833 (English translation, 1895); *Angelo, tyran de Padoue*, pr., pb. 1835 (*Angelo, Tyrant of Padua*, 1880); *Ruy Blas*, pr., pb. 1838 (verse drama; English translation, 1890); *Les Burgraves*, pr., pb. 1843 (*The Burgraves*, 1896); *Inez de Castro*, pb. 1863 (wr. c. 1818; verse drama); *La Grand-mère*, pb. 1865, pr. 1898; *Mille Francs de Recompense*, pb. 1866; *Les Deux Trouvailles de Gallus*, pb. 1881; *Torquemada*, pb. 1882 (wr. 1869; English translation, 1896); *Théâtre en liberté*, pb. 1886 (includes *Mangeront-ils?*); *The Dramatic Works*, 1887; *The Dramatic Works of Victor Hugo*, 1895-1896 (4 volumes); *Irtamène*, pb. 1934 (wr. 1816; verse drama).

NONFICTION: *La Préface de Cromwell*, 1827 (English translation, 1896); *Littérature et philosophie mêlées*, 1834; *Le Rhin*, 1842 (*The Rhine*, 1843); *Napoléon le petit*, 1852 (*Napoleon the Little*, 1852);

William Shakespeare, 1864 (English translation, 1864); *Actes et paroles*, 1875-1876; *Histoire d'un crime*, 1877 (*The History of a Crime*, 1877-1878); *Religions et religion*, 1880; *Le Théâtre en liberté*, 1886; *Choses vues*, 1887 (*Things Seen*, 1887); *En voyage: Alpes et Pyrénées*, 1890 (*The Alps and Pyrenees*, 1898); *France et Belgique*, 1892; *Correspondance*, 1896-1898.

MISCELLANEOUS: *Oeuvres complètes*, 1880-1892 (57 volumes); *Victor Hugo's Works*, 1892 (30 volumes); *Works*, 1907 (10 volumes).

BIBLIOGRAPHY

Bloom, Harold, ed. *Victor Hugo*. New York: Chelsea House, 1988. Essays on all aspects of Hugo's career. Includes introduction, chronology, and bibliography.

Frey, John Andrew. *A Victor Hugo Encyclopedia*. Westport, Conn.: Greenwood Press, 1999. A comprehensive guide in English to the works of Victor Hugo. Includes a foreword, a biography, and a bibliography. Frey addresses Hugo as a leading poet, novelist, artist, and religious and revolutionary thinker of France. The balance of the volume contains alphabetically arranged entries discussing his works, characters, and themes as well as historical persons and places. Includes a general bibliography.

Ionesco, Eugène. *Hugoliad: Or, The Grotesque and Tragic Life of Victor Hugo*. New York: Grove Press, 1987. This uncompleted work of Ionesco's youth—written in the 1930's in Romanian—is a sort of polemical antibiography, intended to dethrone its subject. The reader must take responsibility for separating fact from fiction, to say nothing of judging the aptness of the playwright's cheerless embellishments of anecdotal material. Postscript by Gelu Ionescu.

Ireson, J. C. *Victor Hugo: A Companion Guide to His Poetry*. New York: Clarendon Press, 1997. A detailed critical study dealing with Victor Hugo's verse in its totality, showing how each work was composed, how the themes evolved, and the consid-

erations that dictated the sequence of his publications. Includes bibliographic references.

Maurois, André. *Olympio: The Life of Victor Hugo*. Translated by Gerard Hopkins. New York: Harper & Row, 1956. Originally published in French in 1954. This is probably as close an approach as possible to an ideal one-volume biography dealing with both the life and the work of a monumental figure such as Hugo. Of the sparse illustrations, several are superb; the bibliography, principally of sources in French, provides a sense of Hugo's celebrity and influence, which persisted well into the twentieth century.

_____. *Victor Hugo and His World*. London: Thames & Hudson, 1966. The 1956 English translation of Maurois' text noted above was edited to conform to the format of a series of illustrated books. The result is interesting and intelligible, but rather schematic. In compensation for the vast cuts in text, a chronology and dozens of well-annotated illustrations have been added.

Peyre, Henri. *Victor Hugo: Philosophy and Poetry*. Translated by Roda P. Roberts. University: University of Alabama Press, 1980. A study of Hugo's philosophy as evidenced by his poetry. Contains translations of selected poems with an index and bibliography.

Porter, Laurence M. *Victor Hugo*. New York: Twayne, 1999. A basic biography of Hugo that covers his life and works. Bibliography and index.

Richardson, Joanna. *Victor Hugo*. New York: St. Martin's Press, 1976. A well-written, scholarly biography divided into three sections, "The Man," "The Prophet," "The Legend." With detailed notes and extensive bibliography.

Robb, Graham. *Victor Hugo*. New York: W. W. Norton, 1998. Thorough biography of Victor Hugo reveals many previously unknown aspects of his long life and literary career. Includes detailed notes and bibliography.

Sylvie L. F. Richards

I

GYULA ILLYÉS

Born: Rácegrespuszta, Hungary; November 2,
1902
Died: Budapest, Hungary; April 15, 1983

PRINCIPAL POETRY

Nehéz föld, 1928
Sarjúrendek, 1931
Hősökről beszélek, 1933
Szálló egek alatt, 1935
Rend a romokban, 1937
Külön világban, 1939
Összegyüjtött versei, 1940
Egy év, 1945
Szembenézve, 1947
Egy mondat a zsarnokságról, 1956 (*One Sentence
on Tyranny*, 1957)
Kézfogások, 1956
Új versek, 1961
Nem volt elég, 1962
Dőlt vitorla, 1965
A költo felel: Válogatott versek, 1966
Poharaim: Összegyujtött versek, 1967
Fekete-fehér, 1968
Abbahagyott versek, 1971
*Haza a magasban: Összegyüjtött versek, 1920-
1945*, 1972
Minden lehet, 1973
Teremteni: Összegyüjtött, 1946-1968, 1973
Különös testamentum, 1977
Összegyüjtött versei, 1977 (2 volumes)
Nyitott ajtók: Összegyüjtött versforditások, 1978
(2 volumes)
Közügy, 1981
What You Have Almost Forgotten: Selected Poems,
1999
Charon's Ferry: Fifty Poems, 2000

OTHER LITERARY FORMS

Although principally a poet, Gyula Illyés (IHL-
yays) was also the author of significant prose and
drama. Two of his most important prose works appeared in the 1930's: *Puszták népe* (1936; *People of the
Puszta*, 1967), widely translated, is partly an autobiographical documentary and partly a sociography of
Hungary's poverty-stricken peasantry; *Petőfi* (1936;
English translation, 1973) is both a personal confession
and a scholarly analysis of the great nineteenth century
poet, Sándor Petőfi. Published late in Illyés's life, the
essays collected in *Szellem és erőszak* (1978; spirit and
violence), officially banned but published in the West
in a facsimile edition, reflects his concern about the
mistreatment of four million Hungarians living as minorities in countries neighboring Hungary. His principal plays deal with a search for lessons in Hungary's
history.

Illyés also excelled as a translator of Louis Aragon,
Ben Jonson, Robert Burns, Paul Éluard, Victor Hugo,
Jean Racine, François Villon, and others; a collection
of his translations was published in 1963 as *Nyitott ajtó*
(open door).

ACHIEVEMENTS

Gyula Illyés is internationally recognized as one
of the leading poets of the twentieth century. French
poet and critic Alain Bosquet wrote about him: "Only
three or four living poets have been able to identify themselves with the soul of the century. Their genius burns in the Hungarian poet Gyula Illyés." The
International Biennale of Poets in Knokke-le-Zoute,
Belgium, awarded him its Grand Prix in 1965, and
the University of Vienna awarded him the Herder
Prize in 1970. He received two literary prizes in France:
the Ordre des Art et Lettres in 1974 and the Grand Prize
in 1978 from the Société des Poètes Français. In 1981,
he was awarded the Mondello literary prize in Italy.
In 1969, he was elected vice president of the International PEN Club. In Hungary, among many other
awards, he was three times the recipient of the Kossuth
Prize.

Apart from the highest critical acclaim, Illyés
achieved the status of a national poet and an intellectual
leader in Hungary and in Europe. His unbending loy-

alty to the downtrodden and his contributions in clarifying the most important issues of his times earned him an extraordinary moral authority.

BIOGRAPHY

Gyula Illyés was born into a family of poor farm workers on one of the large estates of a wealthy aristocrat. His grandfather was a shepherd and his father a mechanic; the joint efforts of his relatives were needed to pay for his schooling in Budapest. At the end of World War I, the Austro-Hungarian monarchy collapsed, giving way to a liberal republic, which was taken over by a short-lived Communist regime. Illyés joined the Hungarian Red Army in 1919. After the old regime defeated the revolution, he fled to Vienna in 1920, then went to Berlin, and a year later to Paris. He attended the Sorbonne, studying literature and psychology, and he supported himself by tutoring and by working in a book bindery. His earliest poetry appeared in Hungarian émigré periodicals. During those years, he made the acquaintance of many young French poets, some of whom later became famous as Surrealists: Aragon, Éluard, and Tristan Tzara. In 1926, the political climate became more tolerant in Hungary, and Illyés returned. He worked as an office clerk and joined the circle connected with the avant-garde periodical *Dokumentum*, edited by Lajos Kassák. Some of his early poems caught the eye of Mihály Babits, a leading poet and senior editor of the literary periodical *Nyugat*, and in a short time, Illyés became a regular contributor to that outstanding modern literary forum.

Illyés's first collection of poems was published in 1928, followed by twelve other books of poetry and prose, resulting in literary prizes as well as critical and popular recognition during the next ten years.

Another decisive event in Illyés's life is best described by him:

> I have arrived from Paris, being twenty-three-and-a-half years old. My new eyes saw a multitude of horrors when I looked around my birthplace. I had a deep and agonizing experience, I was outraged, shocked and moved immediately to action upon seeing the fate of my own people.

The result of this experience was *People of the Puszta*, a realistic personal account of the hardships and injus-

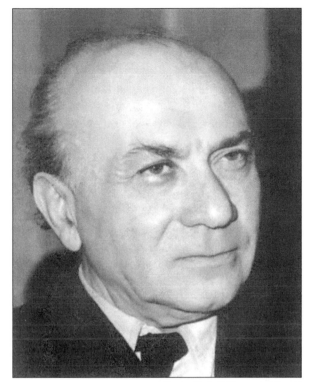

Gyula Illyés (©Hunyady József)

tices that the poorest estate-servant peasants suffered. With this book, Illyés had joined the literary/political populist movement, which fought between the two world wars for the economic, social, educational, cultural, and political interests of the peasantry and, later, the working class as well.

In 1937, Illyés became one of the editors of *Nyugat*, and, after its cessation, he founded and edited its successor, *Magyar Csillag*. After World War II, Illyés was offered leading literary and political positions and edited the literary periodical *Válasz* from 1946 to 1949, but as the Stalinist Communist Party, with the help of the occupying Soviet army, enforced totalitarian control over the country, Illyés withdrew from public life. He continued to write, however, and his poems and plays created during these years of dictatorship address the issues of freedom, power, morality, and hope. His monumental poem *One Sentence on Tyranny*, written in the early 1950's but not published until 1956, was officially banned in Hungary; it became the emblem of the 1956 revolution. After the revolution was crushed by the Soviet army, Illyés went into passive resistance, not publishing anything until the government's release, in 1960, of most jailed writers.

In the 1960's and 1970's, Illyés published some thirty books, including poems, plays, reports, essays, and translations. In his old age, his themes became increasingly universal, and he died at the height of his creative powers, addressing issues of vital concern not only to his nation but also to humanity at large.

ANALYSIS

Gyula Illyés's immense prestige and world renown were largely the result of his ability to integrate the philosophies and traditions of Eastern and Western Europe, the views and approaches of the rational intellectual and of the lyric dreamer, and the actions of *homo politicus* and *homo aestheticus*. In a 1968 interview, Illyés confided, "With all the literary genres with which I experimented I wanted to serve one single cause: that of a unified people and the eradication of exploitation and misery. I always held literature to be only a tool." Five sentences later, however, he exclaimed, "I would forgo every single other work of mine for one poem! Poetry is my first, my primary experience and it has always remained that." André Frenaud has remarked of Illyés that he is a poet of diverse and even contradictory impulses: a poet who can be "violent and sardonic, who lacks neither visions coming from deep within, nor the moods of sensuality. He knows the cowardice of man and the courage needed for survival. He knows the past and interrogates the future."

Illyés began his literary career in the 1920's under the influence of Surrealism and Activism. He found his original style and tone at the end of the 1920's and the beginning of the 1930's. Lyric and epic qualities combined with precise, dry, objective descriptions (whose unimpassioned tone is occasionally heated by lyric fervor) determine the singular flavor of his poetry.

NEHÉZ FÖLD AND SARJÚRENDEK

Illyés's first book of poems, *Nehéz föld* (heavy earth), strongly reflects his intoxication with Surrealism and other Western trends. His next collection, *Sarjúrendek*, represents a turning point in his art; in this volume, Illyés turned toward populism and *engagé* realism, although he still retained many stylistic features of the avant-garde.

Illyés's tone became increasingly deep and bitter, his themes historical, and his style more and more intellectual during the 1930's and 1940's. In this period, he wrote many prose works, most of which reflected on historical, social, and political themes. He did not publish any significant collection of new poetry between 1947 and 1956. During this time of harsh political repression, he wrote historical dramas in which he sought to strengthen his people's national consciousness by the examples of great patriots of the past.

KÉZFOGÁSOK

Illyés's poetic silence ended in 1956 when he published a volume of poems titled *Kézfogások* (handshakes). This volume initiated another new phase for the poet: His style thereafter was more intellectual, contemplative, dramatic, and analytical. He never lost the lyric quality of his poetry, however, and the passionate lyricism of his tone makes the moral, ethical, and historical analysis of his poems of the next twenty-five years glow with relevance, immediacy, and urgency.

DŐLT VITORLA

A good example of this style is found in his collection *Dőlt vitorla* (tilted sail), published in 1965. This book contains a number of long poems—written in free verse—about his fellow writers and artists, amplifying their messages, identifying with their visions, and offering Illyés's conclusions. The volume also contains a number of prose poems. In his preface, Illyés gives his reasons for using this genre: He states that he wants "to find the most common everyday words to express the most complicated things. . . . To concentrate into a piece of creation all that is beautiful, good and true without glitter and pretention but with innovation and endurance."

Written in the middle 1960's to another writer, "Óda a törvényhozóhoz" ("Ode to the Lawmaker") analyzes the role of poets. The poet is "the chief researcher" who uncovers the future, "the progressive, the fighter, the ground breaker," a destroyer of surface appearances "who separates the bad from the good," who shows when the ugly is beautiful and when the virgin is a harlot. Such experimenters, such researchers, are the writers he celebrates: "They are the ones I profess as examples! They are the ones who signal the direction towards a tomorrow!" The tomorrow that these exemplary researcher-poets promote is one of pluralism and tolerance. In this poem, a passionate lyricist evokes a future that the rational intellectual already knows—a future that requires freedom combined with order. "Make laws, but living laws so that we [can] stay human." The poet demands recognition of shadings and nuances, of the "exception, which may be the rule tomorrow."

How can the individual relate to the modern powers of his world as well as realize his individual goals of freedom and humanity? The title poem of *Dőlt vitorla* offers a clue. "Look—when do mast and sail fly forward most triumphantly? When tilted lowest." The ancient Aesopian parable, about the reed that bows to the wind and survives while the proud oak tree breaks and dies, is given a new dimension in this poem: The boat flies forward while it heels low. The issue of relating to the ruling power structure—of surviving sometimes unbearable dictatorial pressures and of being able to realize oneself in spite of authoritarian inhumanities—has been a perennial problem in Hungary. Illyés's sailboat offers a possible solution to the dilemma of whether one should compromise or perish: It sways, bows, and bends, but using, instead of opposing, the forces of the wind, it dashes ahead.

ONE SENTENCE ON TYRANNY

Sometimes such a solution is not possible: The wind may be a killer hurricane. In totalitarian dictatorships, there is no escape. This is the conclusion reached by Illyés in *One Sentence on Tyranny*. This 183-line dramatic sentence is a thorough and horrifying analysis of the nature of such total oppression. Tyranny permeates every minute of every hour. It is present in a lover's embrace and a wife's goodbye kisses; it is present not only in the torture chambers but also in the nursery schools, the churches, the parliament, and the bridal bed; it is in everything, so that, finally, man becomes tyranny himself. He creates it, and it stinks and pours out of him; it looks at him from his mirror. Where there is tyranny, all is in vain. In Illyés's poem, the metaphors of Franz Kafka have become dehumanizing and annihilating realities.

STRENGTH AND WEAKNESS

The opportunity of people to be happy and free, to be able to fulfill themselves, should not depend on power or brute force. What chance do the weak have? Illyés the lyric poet and the concerned humanist is at his best when he redefines strength and weakness in several long poems written in the 1960's.

In "Ditirambus a nőkhöz" ("Dithyramb to Women"), he contrasts the hard, sharp, strong and proud forms of being with the fragile, yielding, and soft forms, and he finds the latter ones stronger: "Not the stones and not the metals, but grass, loess, sedge became the protest." Not the fortresses but the twig, wax, and pen have carried humans so far. Not the weapons and the kings but the clay, the fur, the hide have become the leaders. Not the armored soldiers storming to victory but the loins and breasts, the singing and the spinning, the everyday-working and humanity-protecting women have become the strongest. "Good" strength is defined here not as the strength of force, weight, uncompromising boldness, and pride, but as the strength of flexibility, endurance, resilience, beauty, and love. The contrast is masterfully woven not only between the forceful and softly enduring but also between the boastfully heroic and the gray, everyday, silent endeavor. As Illyés emphasizes in the concluding lines of another poem, "Hunyadi keze" ("The Hand of Hunyadi"): "Cowardly are the people who are protected by martyrs alone. Not heroic deeds but daily daring, everyday, minute-by-minute courage saves men and countries."

This motif of quiet everyday work and courage gives new dimensions to Illyés's theme of strength in weakness; it provides depth to the idea, further developed in "Az éden elvesztése" ("The Loss of Paradise"), a modern oratorio, a moral-political passion play about the chances of the average weak and powerless human individual to avoid the impending atomic cataclysm. After repudiating those who, because of naïveté, blind faith, fatalism, or determinism, accept the inevitability of an atomic war, Illyés argues with those who would capitulate to the threatening powers because of their feelings of weakness and powerlessness.

In his "Hymn of the Root," Illyés emphasizes that "Leaf and tree live according to what the root sends up to them to eat" and that "from the deepest depths comes everything that is good on this Earth." In a "Parable of the Stairs," he offers a concrete program of "everyday, minute-by-minute courage," by which the seemingly weak and powerless can win over the powerful, over dehumanization, over evil.

Whenever we correct a mistake, that is a step. Whenever we dress a wound: one step. Whenever we reprimand a bossy person: one step. Whenever we do our job right without needing a reprimand: ten steps. To take a baby in one's arm, to say something nice to its mother. . . .

In the final lines of this oratorio, the prophet urges his people:

> When the day of fury comes,
> when the atom explodes,
> on that final day,
> before that terrible tomorrow,
> people let us dare to do
> the greatest deed:
>
> . . . . . .
>
> let us begin here, from the depths
> by the strength of our faith,
>
> . . . .
>
> let us begin life anew.

OTHER MAJOR WORKS

LONG FICTION: *Hunok Párizsban*, 1946.

PLAYS: *Ozorai példa*, pb. 1952; *Fáklyaláng*, pb. 1953; *Dózsa György*, pb. 1956; *Malom a Séden*, pb. 1960; *Kegyenc*, pb. 1963; *Különc*, pb. 1963; *Tiszták*, pb. 1969; *Testvérek*, pb. 1972; *Sorsválasztók*, pb. 1982.

NONFICTION: *Petőfi*, 1936 (English translation, 1973); *Puszták népe*, 1936 (*People of the Puszta*, 1967); *Magyarok*, 1938; *Ebéd a kastélyban*, 1962; *Kháron ladikján*, 1969; *Hajszálgyökerek*, 1971; *Szellem és erőszak*, 1978; *Naplójegyzetek, 1977-1978*, 1991.

TRANSLATION: *Nyitott ajtó*, 1963 (of various poets).

BIBLIOGRAPHY

Berlind, Bruce. Introduction to *Charon's Ferry: Fifty Poems*, by Gyula Illyés. Evanston, Ill.: Northwestern University Press, 2000. Berlind's introduction to this work from the Writings from an Unbound Europe series, provides information on Illyés's life and his poetry.

Kolumbán, Nicholas, ed. *Turmoil in Hungary: An Anthology of Twentieth Century Hungarian Poetry*. St. Paul, Minn.: New Rivers Press, 1982. A collection of Hungarian poetry translated into English with commentary.

Serafin, Steven, ed. *Twentieth-Century Eastern European Writers: Third Series*. Vol. 215 in *Dictionary of Literary Biography*. Detroit: Gale Group, 1999. Contains a brief essay on Illyés.

Smith, William Jan. Introduction to *What You Have Almost Forgotten*, by Gyula Illyés. Willimantic, Conn.: Curbstone Press, 1999. The well-known poet provides a substantial introduction to Illyés and his poetry.

Tezla, Albert. *An Introductory Bibliography to the Study of Hungarian Literature*. Cambridge, Mass.: Harvard University Press, 1964. Contains publication information and some commentary on Illyés's work.

_____. *Hungarian Authors: A Bibliographical Handbook*. Cambridge, Mass.: Harvard University Press, 1970. Extension of *An Introductory Bibliography to the Study of Hungarian Literature*, and is to be used in conjunction with that work.

Károly Nagy

J

JUAN RAMÓN JIMÉNEZ

Born: Moguer, Spain; December 23, 1881
Died: San Juan, Puerto Rico; May 29, 1958

PRINCIPAL POETRY

Almas de violeta, 1900
Ninfeas, 1900
Rimas, 1902
Arias tristes, 1903
Jardines lejanos, 1904
Pastorales, 1905
Elegías puras, 1908
La soledad sonora, 1908
Elegías intermedias, 1909
Elegías lamentables, 1910
Baladas de primavera, 1911
Pastorales, 1911
Laberinto, 1913
Estío, 1916
Diario de un poeta recién casado, 1917 (*Diary of a Newlywed Poet*, 2004)
Poesías escojidas, 1917
Sonetos espirituales, 1917 (*Spiritual Sonnets*, 1996)
Eternidades, 1918
Piedra y cielo, 1919 (*Sky and Rock*, 1989)
Segunda antolojía poética, 1922
Belleza, 1923
Poesía, 1923
Canción, 1936
La estación total, 1946
Romances de Coral Gables, 1948
Animal de fondo, 1949
Libros de Poesía, 1957
Tercera antolojía poética, 1957
Three Hundred Poems, 1905-1953, 1962
Dios deseado y deseante, 1964 (*God Desired and Desiring*, 1986)
Selected Poems, 1974

Le realidad invisible, 1983 (*Invisible Reality (1917-1920, 1924)*, 1986)
Naked Woman = La mujer desnuda, 2000
The Poet and the Sea, 2009

OTHER LITERARY FORMS

Somewhat ironically perhaps, Juan Ramón Jiménez (hee-MAY-nuhs) is probably best known for his *Platero y yo* (1914, enlarged 1917; *Platero and I*, 1956), a collection of sketches in prose largely about his native Moguer. As always in Jiménez's noncritical work, however, his poetic vision and lyric expression are most apparent.

ACHIEVEMENTS

In 1903, Juan Ramón Jiménez revealed himself as a prolific poet, and by 1916, no one could surpass Jiménez's position and influence as a poet in the Hispanic world. His twenty-two years spent in the United States, Puerto Rico, Cuba, and South America from 1936 to his death indicated no overall diminution of his creativity as a writer or of his authority as a critic. Appropriately, both for the excellence of his work and the half century devoted to it, he received the Nobel Prize in Literature in 1956, the first Spaniard to win it since 1920.

BIOGRAPHY

Juan Ramón Jiménez was born in Moguer, a typical town in Andalusia, Spain, steeped in tradition, colorful but slow-moving. His father, Victor, had come from north-central Spain to make his fortune in viniculture, acquiring extensive vineyards and numerous wineries in Moguer. Purificación, Jiménez's mother, was a native Andalusian and a very good mother, although perhaps too indulgent toward her youngest child, Juan Ramón. The future poet had a comfortable and happy early childhood in the family's new home on the Calle Nueva. Later, he learned to ride and, on horse or donkey, developed his love of nature in the beautiful countryside, which offered some compensation for the scant cultural stimulation of the town. After four or five years of elementary education in Moguer, Jiménez, then eleven years old, was sent with his brother to a Jesuit school near Cádiz, where he completed his secondary studies at age fifteen.

The *colegio* offered the best education available in the region, and Jiménez was a good, well-behaved student. Although somewhat homesick and averse to the school's regimentation, he was alert, imaginative, and intellectually curious, enjoying a variety of subjects, especially drawing and literature. His meditative mind and love of nature inclined him to religion and, despite later aversion to the Roman Catholic Church, among the six schoolbooks that he kept permanently were the Bible and Thomas à Kempis's *Imitatio Christi* (c. 1427; *The Imitation of Christ*, c. 1460-1530). Upon graduation, Jiménez went to Seville to study painting and to develop his passion for poetry. His father had wanted him to study law at the university, but he had no interest in prelaw studies and neglected them for the arts. The family's prosperity made it possible for Jiménez to indulge himself and choose between two financially unpromising careers. Some early paintings show that he

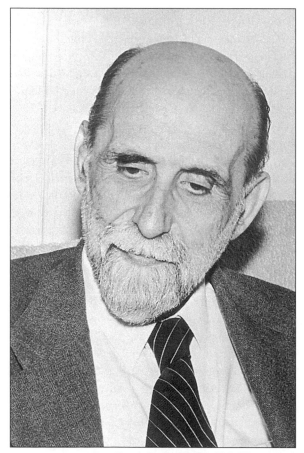

Juan Ramón Jiménez (©The Nobel Foundation)

might have become a fine painter, but the publication of his first poems evoked favorable criticism and turned him to poetry.

Fatigue and emotional strain in Seville put Jiménez under the care of doctors in Moguer, yet he continued to write feverishly, sending poems to magazines in Madrid and establishing contacts with poets there. Somewhat capricious and unreasonable, he shunned social events in Moguer and, despite two or more youthful love affairs, preferred to be alone. The poems sent by Jiménez to *Vida nueva* met with such favor that the magazine's editor, Francisco Villaespesa, and Rubén Darío, the Nicaraguan poet and leader of *Modernismo* who had been in Spain since 1899, invited the young poet to visit Madrid to help them reform Spanish poetry. Life in Madrid was exciting. Jiménez became close friends with Darío and other contemporary poets, and despite some excesses criticized by the academicians, his first collections were hailed as the work of a promising newcomer. His father's sudden fatal heart attack in 1900 caused Jiménez's nervous illness, which had recurred during the stimulating sojourn in Madrid, to worsen to the point that he required care in a sanatorium in Bordeaux.

In France, Jiménez read Charles Baudelaire and the Symbolist poets and continued to write, expressing his grief, sometimes in the excessively sentimental manner of the nineteenth century, sometimes in a more dignified, authentic style. Returning to Madrid rather than Moguer in 1901, the young poet continued his sheltered, privileged life in the Sanatorio del Rosario. Surrounded by tranquillity and beauty, Jiménez entertained friends and relatives more than ever before, and his retreat became a literary salon and social center. His work soon became known in the New World, and his popularity and influence grew with each volume. In 1903, Jiménez and a number of other young poets began to publish the literary journal *Helios*, the eleven issues of which exercised great influence—so much so that Miguel de Unamuno y Jugo, certainly not identified with *Modernismo*, was willing to be a contributor. While Darío gave Spanish poetry new subtlety, beauty, and music, Unamuno's influence deepened and intensified it. Later in 1903, Jiménez went to live with his physician and friend, Luís Simarra, with whom he remained for two years. With Simarra's encouragement and that of other scholars, Jiménez expanded his knowledge in several fields by reading and attending lectures at the Institución Libre de Enseñanza. The liberal views at this institution further eroded Jiménez's already weakened traditional religious convictions.

Unlike most of his colleagues, Jiménez felt less comfortable in Madrid than in a more rural setting. In 1905, ill again and homesick, he returned to Moguer, where he remained for six years, not with his family but in a house at Fuentepiña owned by them. There he rested and wrote, avoiding society for the most part. In 1910, at the age of twenty-eight, Jiménez was elected to the Royal Spanish Academy, but he declined membership, not only then but also on two subsequent occasions under different political regimes. With his sisters' marriages and other changes, including financial ones, the family's situation declined. Although Jiménez preferred solitude and nature, there were periods of tedium and depression for him, especially as he continued to suffer sporadically from ill health. Occasional amorous interludes were followed by disenchantment, bitterness, and remorse. In 1912, it seemed time to return to Madrid, where, except for brief visits to Moguer, the poet remained until 1936.

In four years at the Residencia de Estudiantes, the heart of intellectual and literary activity in Madrid, in the company of celebrated thinkers and writers, Jiménez completed two volumes of poetry and his prose masterpiece, *Platero and I*. His experimentation in content and form continued, and he gave evidence of increasing maturity in every way. In 1912, too, Jiménez had met Zenobia Camprubí Aymar; they soon became engaged and were married in 1916. Zenobia, who was part American, was lovely—as had been other women in the poet's life—and intelligent, interested in the same things that interested Jiménez. Above all, Zenobia was lively, a quality that proved very helpful for the sober, moody Jiménez. After a trip to New York and his wedding, Jiménez published his *Diary of a Newlywed Poet*, a work marking his entrance to full maturity and long considered his best by the critics and author alike. He continued to grow in all respects, producing more significant poetry in the years from 1916 to 1923 than during any other period in his life, and might have be-

come the "grand old man" of poetry had his temperament permitted.

Like so many other Spanish refugees from the Civil War, Jiménez headed for the United States in 1936, first visiting Washington, D.C., briefly as a cultural emissary of the Spanish Republic, then visiting Puerto Rico and Cuba for three years, finally settling for six years in Coral Gables, Florida, and later in Washington, D.C. His fame as a poet and critic was great, especially in Hispanic circles, and he lectured, read his poetry, and wrote numerous critical essays but produced no new poetic works for a time. Between 1942 and 1951, however, he published four major works and began a fifth that he was not to complete. Despite numerous invitations, Jiménez and his wife rarely left the United States. In 1956, Jiménez won the Nobel Prize in Literature, two days before Zenobia's death from cancer. He died in 1958 and is buried in Moguer with his wife.

ANALYSIS

The Spanish intellectuals and writers of the Generation of '98 saw the need to arouse the national conscience and envisioned a vigorous, creative Spain in every aspect of life. The presence of Darío in Madrid had drawn many to the city and to *Modernismo*, the literary movement of which he was the chief exponent. Both the French Symbolists, who had largely inspired *Modernismo*, and Darío himself strongly influenced Juan Ramón Jiménez's poetry for more than a decade. In 1903, Jiménez published a collection of lyric poems, *Arias tristes*, which revealed that he had abandoned the excessive sentimentality and random experimentation and imitation of his earlier collections for a more mature position based on firmer understanding of his talents.

ARIAS TRISTES

Arias tristes is divided into three "movements," each prefaced by the score of a *Lied* by Franz Schubert and dedicated to a friend. In addition, the second part has an epigraph taken from Paul Verlaine, and the third, one from Alfred de Musset. The second part is further prefaced by Jiménez's commentary on his own work, which is "monotonous, full of moonlight and sadness," and concludes with an evocation of Heinrich Heine and Gustavo Adolfo Bécquer as well as of Verlaine and

Musset and an entreaty to all kindred spirits to weep for those who never weep. A vague, subdued sadness prevails here as in much Symbolist poetry. Avoiding novelty for the sake of novelty, Jiménez employs the verse of the romance exclusively and with a versatility that remains unmatched. Seemingly artless in its simplicity, the verse reveals great mastery in the use of enjambment to give it fluency and grace and in its diction, chosen for maximum musicality as well as meaning. Among the best poems in the collection are those that capture Jiménez's love of his native Andalusian landscape in delicate and original imagery.

JARDINES LEJANOS AND PASTORALES

In part under the influence of Unamuno, who wrote for Jiménez's journal, *Helios*, but favored exploiting traditional Spanish inspiration, but more so under the influence of his doctor and close friend Simarro, who introduced him to the principles of liberal education of the Institución Libre de Enseñanza, the poet began to explore sources other than Symbolism and *Modernismo*, and in 1904 and 1905, respectively, produced two collections of verse, *Jardines lejanos* (distant gardens) and *Pastorales*. The former is full of musical allusions that convey Jiménez's emotional, often sad responses to music, and it has a new, conventional, and superficial eroticism that separates it from his earlier work. The second volume, like *Arias tristes* and *Jardines lejanos*, is prefaced with musical notations (from Christoph Gluck, Felix Mendelssohn-Bartholdy, and Robert Schumann), and its verse is chiefly that of the romance (usually four-line stanzas, odd lines unrhymed, even lines assonanced), but it is less introverted, less morbid, and less sorrowful than its predecessor. Jiménez's prolonged stay in the Guadarrama Mountains had completed his cure and brought him back to an appreciation of nature, albeit in solitude and mystery.

BALADAS DE PRIMAVERA

For Jiménez, the years from 1906 to 1912, spent in his native Moguer, represented both a physical and a spiritual renewal, as well as a return to *Modernismo*. In no less than nine books of poetry, he again emulated Darío in his experimentation with forms, fascination with the music of words, and joyous eroticism in nature. *Baladas de primavera* (ballads of spring) exem-

plifies this phase of Jiménez's development. In *Baladas de primavera*, he eschews the exotic figures and decor so typical of the Parnassians, Symbolists, and modernists; here, his sensuality is simpler, more tender, and closer to that of Musset, Verlaine, and Francis Jammes, experienced more personally than vicariously. Again, there is the inspiration from the heritage of popular Spanish poetry, evident both in form—as in the use of a rhythmic line as a musical refrain, conveying no particular meaning but with an appealing lilt—and in content, where ingenuous and simple expression belies profound thought or poignant emotion.

LA SOLEDAD SONORA

Jiménez's trilogy of elegies—*Elegías puras*, *Elegías intermedias*, and *Elegías lamentables*—marked a return to the Baudelairean Decadence of some earlier volumes. These poems have little of the spontaneity and musicality of the pastorals and ballads, largely because of the poet's efforts to adapt his material to the fourteen-syllable Alexandrine, usually in four-line stanzas with assonance in the even lines, not Jiménez's best poetic medium. The poet continued to modify and perfect the Alexandrine as well as other forms in four more volumes, *La soledad sonora* (the sonorous solitude) being the most representative. This collection articulates with particular clarity the poet's personal view of the world.

The epigraph of *La soledad sonora* is taken from Saint John of the Cross, reinforcing the link with the sixteenth century mystical poet suggested by the title of the collection. The apparent paradox in the antithetical "sonorous solitude" disappears when the reader becomes aware that solitude here does not mean withdrawal from the world but rather intimate communion with it. Moreover, this work contains much more auditory imagery, along with the characteristic range of visual and other sensuous images, than found in earlier works, a change made possible for Jiménez by his solitude. The poet's normal tendency to Impressionism extends here to synesthesia, a common feature of *Modernismo* and one to which Jiménez's keen sensory perception easily adapted. The poet's skill in prolonging the perfect instant to render it infinite, occasionally disturbed by thoughts of the passage of time and death, is epitomized in his contemplation of the pine tree by his house at Fuentepiña. Jiménez's perceptions of the odor and sounds of the tree that best characterizes the Andalusian scene are transformed from sensations of the moment into a mystical experience in which he finds himself attuned to the eternal.

SPIRITUAL SONNETS

Back in Madrid until his exile from Spain, Jiménez associated with many prominent artists and intellectuals, but by this time in his career, he was less open to stylistic influences. His *Spiritual Sonnets* are unique in his oeuvre in that they are composed almost exclusively of classic eleven-syllable sonnets with the traditional *abba* rhyme scheme. The discipline of these poems, which are characterized by a high degree of technical perfection, is matched by great emotional restraint. Here, Jiménez achieves a balance between thought and feeling. Despite the great mastery of form and the structural and verbal precision of these poems, genuine emotion prevents exclusive concern with intellectual subtlety, formal perfection, and verbal agility for its own sake. The introductory "Al soneto con mi alma" ("To the Sonnet with My Soul"), with its physical images translated in each case into ideal images and arranged in pairs, contains the essence of the volume.

ESTÍO

Estío (summer) marks further Jiménez's maturation in terms of emotional and poetic authenticity; most notable in *Estío* are the variety, flexibility, and verbal economy of the verse. Jiménez's treatment of love in this volume, inspired by his love for his fiancé, is in marked contrast to the immature eroticism of earlier works.

DIARY OF A NEWLYWED POET

Less than a year after his wedding, Jiménez published *Diary of a Newlywed Poet*, a combination of free verse and brief prose pieces generally recognized as a key work, his best, in the poet's own opinion. This collection is composed of six groups of poems, each with a title that identifies its theme. The principal themes of the volume are married love and the poet's metaphysical reflections on his ocean voyage to the United States and return voyage to Spain. This was not only his first contact with America but also his first experience of the sea. The expanse, monotony, and solitude of the gray ocean and gray sky immediately gripped him; he was

most impressed by the endless, restless motion of the sea, like the beating of a huge, cosmic heart, giving the ocean a kind of immortality that he had never perceived before. Jiménez's awareness of the sea as an image of the entire physical world, changing constantly yet remaining fundamentally the same, gave *Diary of a Newlywed Poet* a metaphysical dimension previously lacking in his verse. The collection marked the mature poet's search for more universal values in poetry and life at a time when the vogue of *Modernismo* had passed. *Diary of a Newlywed Poet*, followed by *Eternidades* (eternities), *Sky and Rock*, *Poesía*, and *Belleza* (beauty), set a new direction for Spanish poetry and established decisively Jiménez's position and influence.

EXPLOITING SPANISH HERITAGE

Like Unamuno and Antonio Machado, Jiménez continued to keep abreast of the latest movements in literature and the arts yet sought inspiration primarily in Spanish traditions. Although it cannot be said that, either by age or temperament, Jiménez had become the "grand old man" of Spanish poetry, he did not recommend novelty for novelty's sake to his fellows, and he began to find fault not only with imitations of foreign works but also with the innovations of the Spanish vanguard poets. (Indeed, he had grown somewhat crotchety and, except for his wife, more solitary than ever.) His own originality was no longer achieved in defiance of tradition, but rather in a harmonious blend of change with the traditional. The *romancero*, Saint John of the Cross, Luis de Góngora y Argote, and Bécquer exemplify the vital heritage that Jiménez and the greatest of his contemporaries would continue to exploit. In fact, the Generation of '27 indirectly took its name from Góngora, whose tricentenary was celebrated in that year and to the admiration of whose virtuosity Jiménez had contributed. The Mexican essayist Alfonso Reyes, Jiménez's longtime friend, compared him physically and spiritually to Góngora as well as to the tortured figures in many of El Greco's paintings.

POETRY FROM THE NEW WORLD

During the first part of Jiménez's life in the New World, spent in Puerto Rico and Cuba, the poet wrote many articles for newspapers and magazines published in every country of Latin America. For several years, however, he wrote no new poetry, publishing several volumes that were no more than anthologies or rearrangements of old materials, perhaps because he thought that his American readers would find them new. Finally, in Florida, his inspiration returned and, before a trip to Argentina and Uruguay in 1948, he produced *La estación total* (total season) and *Romances de Coral Gables*. Although the former also contains some of his earlier work, Jiménez added much that was a distillation of all his poetic experience and a reaffirmation of the values of *Diary of a Newlywed Poet*. *La estación total* not only acts as a summation, but also points the way to the joyous sense of fulfillment of *Animal de fondo* (animal of depth).

In the collections immediately preceding *La estación total*, Jiménez had expressed the fundamental tension in his being—both a source of inspiration and a soul-wearying affliction. Torn between light and shadow, truth and falsehood, hope and doubt, he would be whole only when these opposites were united, perhaps only in death. In contrast, "Desde dentro" ("From Inside"), the first poem of *La estación total*, is positive and confident; in this collection, Jiménez finally attains the transcendent reality that he had grasped imperfectly and fleetingly in earlier work. "Plenitude" might well be the title of the volume, which reveals the poet's awareness of plenitude in three dimensions: the "eternal," seen in nature; the "external," experienced through the senses; and the "inner reality," discovered intuitively. Communicating a sincere, intensely personal religious experience through language alone, these poems are inevitably marked by a certain obscurity and ambiguity, desirable if readers are to be permitted their own interpretations.

ANIMAL DE FONDO

Animal de fondo was to be the first part of *God Desired and Desiring*, a much larger work that Jiménez never completed. The twenty-nine poems of the collection were not intended to be read as individual pieces but rather as links in a continuous chain. A dynamic rhythm, strongly suggestive of the motion of the ship on which Jiménez sailed to South America, prevails throughout the sequence. Soothed by the gentle movement of the sea, the poet is as satisfied as a child rocked and comforted in his mother's arms, attaining at last the complete sense of fulfillment that he has sought since childhood and to which he has aspired throughout his long, arduous efforts as a poet. Contrary to the tradition of Spanish mysticism, which expresses the divine through the language of human love, Jiménez uses religious metaphors to deify his sensitivity to the beautiful, for poetic creation is also a religious experience, an intimate union, although not, as in the customary mystical sense, a union with God. The theme of "La transparencia Dios, la transparencia" ("Transparency, God, Transparency") is that of the whole collection, expressing the struggle between the poet and his personal god to achieve successful union in art and love, "as a fire with its air" in its ardor. There is some ambiguity in the poems that follow, as Jiménez attempts to distinguish his god from God, often in paradoxical and contradictory terms. Among the several attributes of his god, Jiménez discovers love, found in all the elements but not solely spiritual or divine. "En mi tercero mar" ("On My Third Sea") reveals his god to be one of human love also, that of the poet for his wife, as much physical as spiritual. The poet's "great knowledge" is his awareness of being complete when, as perceiver, he merges with that which is perceived. On the sea, his god is the "mirror" of himself, but in "La fruta de mi flor" ("The Fruit of My Flower"), the imagery becomes more abstract, and Jiménez's vision turns inward. The sensibility that has been like a halo about him through life now enters his being, and the flower of promise bears the fruit of fulfillment. Whether Jiménez's mysticism is orthodox or not, the joyous yet humble religious attitude, the flexible meter and other aspects of prosody, and the novel imagery of *Animal de fondo* often remind one of the *canciones del alma* (songs of the soul) of Saint John of the Cross.

It is neither as theologian nor as philosopher but as a great lyric poet that the author of *Animal de fondo* is remembered. Unfortunately, recurring depression prevented Jiménez from maintaining in his last poems the optimism of *Animal de fondo*. In more than fifty years of poetic production, however, Jiménez's aesthetic and spiritual vision remained clear and his creative ability vigorous. Constant renewal kept his work from becoming dated, although his roots were always deep in the Spanish traditions that sustained his entire poetic creation.

OTHER MAJOR WORKS

SHORT FICTION: *Historias y cuentos*, 1979 (*Stories of Life and Death*, 1985).

NONFICTION: *Platero y yo*, 1914, enlarged 1917 (*Platero and I*, 1956); *Españoles de tres mundos*, 1944; *Monumento de amor*, 1959; *El trabajo gustoso*, 1961; *La corriente infinita*, 1961.

MISCELLANEOUS: *Tiempo y espacio*, 1986 (*Time and Space: A Poetic Autobiography*, 1988).

BIBLIOGRAPHY

Fogelquist, Donald F. *Juan Ramón Jiménez*. Boston: Twayne, 1976. An introductory biography and critical analysis of Jiménez's major works. Includes a bibliography of the poet's works.

Jiménez, Juan Ramón. *The Complete Perfectionist: A Poetics of Work*. Edited and translated by Christopher Maurer. New York: Doubleday, 1997. Maurer, who has written widely on Spanish literature, has collected and categorized the thoughts and aphorisms recorded by Jiménez in his quest for perfection in life and his work. Maurer provides context for the maxims set down by Jiménez, allowing the reader to begin to know Jiménez as a person and a poet as well as a philosopher.

_____. *Time and Space: A Poetic Autobiography*. Translated by Antonio T. de Nicolás. New York: Paragon House, 1988. Nicolás provides some excellent translations and a detailed introduction to the prose work *Tiempo* and the prose and poetry of *Espacio*. His well-documented presentation is supported by analysis in a historical context.

Predmore, Michael P. Introduction to *Diary of a Newlywed Poet: A Bilingual Edition of "Diario de un poeta reciencasado,"* by Juan Ramón Jiménez. Translated by Hugh A. Harter. Selinsgrove, Pa.: Susquehanna University Press, 2004. The extensive, multipart introduction contains information about the life of the author as well as critical analysis that examines the nature of the work, its use of the prose poem and free verse, the European influence on the author, and its autobiographical nature.

Wilcox, John C. *Self and Image in Juan Ramón Jiménez*. Chicago: University of Illinois Press, 1987. Examines the evolution of the poetry from pre-modern origins through modernism and its endurance through the postmodern era. Focuses on the work as process and reader interpretations from various perspectives, including formalist, structuralist, and poststructuralist readings as well as other critical readings of the enigmatic poet's prolific corpus.

_____. "T. S. Eliot and Juan Ramón Jiménez: Some Ideological Affinities." In *T. S. Eliot and Hispanic Modernity, 1924-1993*, edited by K. M. Sibbald and Howard Young. Boulder, Colo.: Society of Spanish and Spanish-American Studies, 1994. A discussion of Jiménez's connections with literary movements in England and the United States.

Young, Howard T. *The Line in the Margin: Juan Ramón Jiménez and His Readings in Blake, Shelley, and Yeats*. Madison: University of Wisconsin Press, 1980. This analysis demonstrates the influences upon the poet's work by English poets William Blake, Percy Bysshe Shelley, and William Butler Yeats. Jiménez had translated their poetry, and the Spanish poet's admiration is evident in his own poetry as he departed from his Spanish and French models. This investigation yields interesting biographical data as well as critical readings and literary analyses. The poet's affinity for British literature was evident in his life and work.

Richard A. Mazzara

SAINT JOHN OF THE CROSS
Juan de Yepes y Álvarez

Born: Fontiveros, Spain; June 24, 1542
Died: Úbeda, Spain; December 14, 1591

PRINCIPAL POETRY

"Vivo sin vivir en mí," wr. 1573 ("I Live Yet Do Not Live in Me")

"Adónde te escondiste," wr. 1577 ("The Spiritual Canticle")

"En el principio moraba," wr. 1577 ("Ballad on the Gospel 'In the Beginning Was the Word'")

"En una noche oscura," wr. 1577 ("The Dark
   Night")
"Llama de amor viva," wr. 1577 ("The Living
   Flame of Love")
"Que bien sé yo la fonte," wr. 1577 ("Although by
   Night")
"Encima de las corrientes," wr. 1578 ("Ballad on
   the Psalm 'By the Waters of Babylon'")
"Entréme donde no supe," wr. c. 1584 ("Verses
   Written on an Ecstasy")
"Tras de un amoroso lance," wr. c. 1584 ("A
   Quarry of Love")
The Complete Works of St. John of the Cross, 1864,
   1934, 1953
Poems, 1951

OTHER LITERARY FORMS

Saint John of the Cross wrote several prose works
that use methodologies of Scholastic criticism to expli-
cate themes in his poetry: *Cántico espiritual* (c. 1577-
1586; *A Spiritual Canticle of the Soul*, 1864, 1909), *La
subida del Monte Carmelo* (1578-1579; *The Ascent
of Mount Carmel*, 1864, 1922), and *Llama de amor viva*
(c. 1582; *Living Flame of Love*, 1864, 1912). Discussion
of them in the text is parallel with that of the poems.

ACHIEVEMENTS

With Saint Teresa of Ávila, Saint John of the Cross
carried out the reform of the Carmelite Order and defended the Descalced Carmelites' rights to self-determination within obedience. In addition to becoming
rector of the Carmelite College at Alcaláde Henares
and founder of the Descalced Carmelite College in
Baeza, John was vicar of the El Calvario Convent in
Andalusia and prior of Los Mártires in Granada and of
the Descalced Carmelite Monastery in Segovia. Moreover, he participated in the foundation of at least eight
Descalced Carmelite houses throughout Spain. John
was beatified in 1675 by Pope Clement X, canonized in
1726 by Pope Benedict XIII, and declared Doctor of the
Church in 1926 by Pope Pius XI.

In Spain, John is considered to be the most successful lyric poet of the sixteenth century because of his
harmonious resolution of popular and medieval traditions with the new learning and literary forms of the Re-

naissance. Beyond Spain, perhaps because of his singular dedication to one ideal and the strength of his vision,
his poetry continues to rank among the finest love poetry written in any language.

BIOGRAPHY

Saint John of the Cross was born Juan de Yepes y
Álvarez in 1542 in the town of Fontiveros in the kingdom of Old Castile. His father, Gonzalo de Yepes,
and his mother, Catalina Álvarez, had worked in that
small village for thirteen years as silk weavers and
merchants, aided by John's older brother, Francisco.
Gonzalo de Yepes's great-grandfather had been a favorite of King Juan II; one uncle was an Inquisitor in
Toledo; three others were canons; and one was the
chaplain of the Mozarabic Chapel in Toledo.

Because of her lower social status, Catalina Álvarez
was hated by her husband's family, so much so that on
Gonzalo's death they refused to help her support his
three children, forcing them to live in poverty. In 1548,
they moved to Arévalo, where Francisco was apprenticed as a weaver and John, without success, attempted
a variety of trades.

From Arévalo, the Yepes family moved to the town
of Medina del Campo, famous since the Middle Ages
for its annual three-month-long international trade fair.
There, John learned his letters and learned to beg for his
Jesuit school. His brother married, and his mother,
Catalina, in spite of their difficulties, took in a found-
ling. In 1556, when Emperor Charles V stopped at
Medina on his way to his retirement at the monastery at
Yuste, John saw the hero of European spiritual unity.
The great moment did not, however, contribute to
John's learning a trade. In 1563, he was taken to the
Hospital de la Concepción by Don Alonso Álvarez de
Toledo, where he became a nurse, working in that
profession until he was twenty-one years old.

In 1563, having rejected the offer to become the
hospital's chief warder, John left it to profess in the Order of Mount Carmel. The young Spaniard followed
the rule of the Order in perfect obedience, according to
contemporary accounts, but he spent hours searching
for the spirit of the primitive rule in *A Book of the Institutions of the First Monks* (reprinted in 1507). In this
fourteenth century work, John discovered the tradition

of the eremitical way, which leads through austerity and isolation to the experience of the Divine Presence. John received permission to follow the old rule when he made his final profession before Ángel de Salazar, who had recently allowed Teresa to found the Order of Descalced Carmelites in Ávila.

After professing in 1564, the young friar traveled to the University of Salamanca, to which the Spanish then referred as *Roma la chica* because of its large international student body and its superb reputation in theology. He spent the first three years at Salamanca as an *artista* and the fourth as a theologian studying, not with the famous Francisco Vitoria, founder of international law, nor with Luis de León, who taught there between 1565 and 1573, but with the more traditional Father Guevara and Father Gallo, who taught Thomas Aquinas's *Summa theologiae* (c. 1265-1273; *Summa Theologica*, 1911-1921) and Aristotle's *Ethica Nicomachea* (n.d.; *Nicomachean Ethics*, 1797). The effect of this study appears in John's later writing. Rather than posing a threat to his mystic contemplation, Scholasticism served to keep his mystic effusions within the confines of reality, fostering a clarity of language and logical development, a lyricism of thought, and a psychology of common sense that made his work accessible to all readers.

The faculty during those years at Salamanca longed for intellectual emancipation, and many, such as Luis de León, were cautioned and often jailed for years by the Inquisition. The debate was between the Scholastics, who authorized only the Latin Vulgate, and the Renaissance-inspired Scripturalists, who wished to translate the Hebrew and Koine Greek into modern languages. Typically, John did not involve himself in this intellectual turmoil but continued to seek the solitary spirit of Mount Carmel. His zeal was so great that in 1566, those Carmelite students who were entrusted to his tutelage by the vicar general of the Order, Juan Bautista Rubeo, complained of John's rigor, self-discipline, and near-constant state of contemplation. John's course was not the outward one. Instead of finishing his university career, he left Salamanca in 1567 for Medina del Campo, where he said his first Mass at the Church of Saint Anne in the presence of his brother, the latter's family, and his mother, Catalina Álvarez.

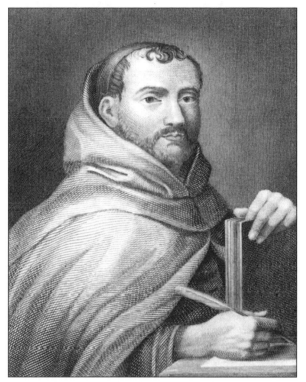

Saint John of the Cross (Hulton Archive/Getty Images)

Because it was permissible to do so among the Carmelites, John immediately decided to enter the Carthusian Order for a life of total silence, solitude, and contemplation. His decision was delayed, however, by his meeting Teresa, who had come to Medina del Campo, with Vicar General Rubeo's blessing, to establish a convent for Descalced Carmelite nuns. Teresa convinced John to follow the contemplative way within his own Order so that her nuns would have a confessor. Moreover, at the time of Teresa's visit, King Philip II wrote to Father Antonio Heredia, the prior of Saint Anne's, giving him permission to reform the Carmelite Order of Monks as well, telling him that a wealthy gentleman had donated a house in the hamlet of Duruelo for that very purpose.

In August, 1568, Teresa, three nuns, one Julián de Ávila, and John left Medina del Campo for the city of Valladolid and for Duruelo. Teresa taught John the old rule through example as she commanded his aid in establishing the Convent of El Río de los Olmos outside Valladolid. She then changed his name from Juan de San Matías to John of the Cross. She also persuaded him that recreation in the form of music, song, and dance were necessary (as well as taking long walks, which prevented the Carmelites from becoming surly) and sent him with one workman to prepare the house at Duruelo for the eventual arrival of Father Heredia from Saint Anne's.

During their five weeks of rigorous labor, John revived the mode of desert life of the original Carmelites, going barefoot, wearing serge vestments, fasting, praying, and doing penance. When Father Heredia arrived to take charge, John was careful to observe Vicar General Rubeo's dictates not to depart in principle from the Unmitigated Carmelite Order as already defined, so as to avoid antagonizing them. While Teresa's letters to Heredia reveal her concern regarding the severity of the brothers' penances and flagellations, John's mother, Catalina Álvarez, came to be their cook, his brother Francisco came to sweep their cells, and Ana Isquierda came to wash and mend their clothes.

From Duruelo, John went to establish religious houses in the towns of Mancera and Pastrana, and in 1570, he went to the University of Alcaláde Henares to found a college for the Order. At Alcalá, John tutored his charges in Thomist philosophy, heard their confessions and those of the nuns at the Imagen Convent, and directed the friars in their contemplative life.

In 1571, Teresa called John to be the confessor at the Convent of the Incarnation in Ávila. She relates that, during the months of December and January, she began to have access to the ineffable experience of *matrimonio* and that John was of immense help to her: "One cannot speak of God to Father John of the Cross because he at once goes into ecstasy and causes others to do the same," she writes. The practical-minded Teresa complained that John's desire to bring everyone to spiritual perfection was a source of constant annoyance. Moreover, testimony from his living companions, Father Germaine and Brother Franciso, claimed that John was tormented with frightful night apparitions and on one occasion was severely beaten by an enraged countryman—all of which he welcomed.

Suddenly, the reformed Order began to encounter difficulty on every level. In 1570, Philip II appointed visitors to examine the houses, an action that angered Vicar General Rubeo. He retaliated by appointing vari-

ous defenders, who were sent to each of the provinces. Teresa left the Convent of the Incarnation and met Father Gracián, who persuaded her to disregard Vicar General Rubeo's orders not to establish houses in Andalusia simply because the vicar general felt that the vitality of southern Spain was incongruent with the contemplative way. With Gracián's assurance that Philip II would support her, Teresa, then sixty-three years old, went ahead and established houses in Seville, Peñuela, and Granada. Rubeo accordingly declared the Descalced Order disobedient and ordered the immediate evacuation of the Andalusian convents in 1575. Gracián and Teresa refused; he was excommunicated, and she was ordered by the Council of Trent to pick a convent where she would spend the remainder of her days. She refused and decided to spend another year in Seville.

Meanwhile, John was still serving as confessor at La Incarnación in Ávila, until Gracián called him and other Descalced Carmelites to Almodóvar in 1576. Father Gracián proposed that the reformed Order name its own definitors and provincials, in effect making themselves independent of the Unmitigated Carmelites under Father Rubeo. At this meeting, John wished, as usual, to avoid conflict. In fact, he opposed the election of officers from among the reformed Order, since the Calced brothers already fulfilled these duties, leaving the followers of the reformed Order to their meditations. John's voice went unheard, and Gracián succeeded.

Rubeo reacted by sending Father Jerónimo Tostado to visit the Spanish Descalced houses to discourage their expansion. Supposedly, had Teresa and Gracián taken their case to Rome, the pope could have settled their differences with Rubeo. Philip II, however, was eager to maintain the traditional Spanish monarchical sovereignty over the Church Militant and impeded Gracián and Teresa's move in that direction.

In 1577, Teresa attempted to return to La Incarnación in Ávila, but Tostado excommunicated all the nuns who voted for her reinstatement as prioress. He evicted them from the convent and denied them access to their confessors. He then tried to persuade John to abandon Teresa and reenter the unreformed Order, promising him a priorship. John refused.

While visiting Teresa, who was living in secrecy in Toledo, John was arrested by the secular arm of the Roman Catholic Church, beaten, and locked in isolation. When he was led out for interrogation, he succeeded in escaping back to his cell to destroy letters, only to be recaptured and imprisoned within the Carmelite monastery in a closet at water level on the River Tajo. There he remained from December, 1576, until his escape in August, 1577. Teresa repeatedly wrote Philip II regarding the situation, but her letters went unanswered. Rubeo and Tostado considered Teresa's work finished and John to be a rebel who had disobeyed by serving as confessor to the Convent of the Incarnation in Ávila without Rubeo's express permission.

While he was imprisoned, John composed, among others, his poems "The Spiritual Canticle" and "The Living Flame of Love," which, according to nineteenth century Spanish critic Menéndez y Pelayo in his *Historia de los heterodoxos españoles* (1887), "surpass all that has ever been written in Spanish." John was fed bread and water only three times a week on the floor of the refectory, after which he was beaten by each of the friars, who verbally insulted his kneeling form. Occasionally, so that he would not collapse from hunger, he was given rancid sardines.

After loosening the bolts of his cell door during his jailer's absences, John lowered himself down a rope made of bedclothes to the monastery garden. There, a stray dog showed him a route of escape. Believing that the Virgin Mary was lifting him, he succeeded in scaling two walls to reach the street. By hiding in doorways of various houses, he made his way in full daylight to the Carmelite Convent of San José, where he found refuge for several days until the nobleman Don Pedro González de Mendoza arranged for his recuperation at the Hospital of Santa Cruz. During John's stay with the nuns of San José, he spoke of his captors in glowing terms as his benefactors who had brought him to an understanding of grace, to which he referred as "the dark light." He recited to the nuns the poems he had composed while in captivity, and one of the nuns wrote them down.

Because Tostado's persecution of the Order had abated, John was soon appointed vicar of the El Calvario monastery in Andalusia. John customarily led the thirty monks into the mountains for evening meditations. According to tradition, they ate only salads made from wild herbs that were carefully chosen by an expert, the cook's mule. On feast days, they dined upon *migajas*, bread fried in oil. At El Calvario, John wrote *The Ascent of Mount Carmel*.

One year later, in 1579, John was ordered by Father Ángel de Salazar to take three friars to the university town of Baeza and set up a monastery in an old house; this was to become the College of Our Lady of Mount Carmel. The college quickly became an object of intense curiosity among the faculty at the university, who, believing that John enjoyed infused wisdom, respected his insight into the mysteries of the faith and attended his lectures on morals and religious questions. John, however, prudently sent his charges to the university to study theology.

In 1581, John and his companion, Brother Jerome, established a convent of four nuns in Granada. The following year, John was elected prior of the Carmelite monastery there, Los Mártires. The revolt of the Alpujarras, in which Moorish converts to Christianity had elected a king and rejected their new religion, had been suppressed by Philip II ten years prior to John's arrival. Consequently, many of the children born to apostate families now served as slaves or protected servants in the homes of wealthy Old Christian families. Moreover, during those years there lived in Granada a ninety-year-old woman remembered as La Mora de Ubeda, who had gained a reputation among contemporary Muslim theologians for mystic wisdom acquired through the *faqir* tradition. The young *moriscos* drawn to their fathers' faith were threatened with years of rowing in the king's galleys should they wear Moorish clothes; carry Moorish weapons; speak, read, or write Arabic; bathe too frequently; dance the zambra; or play Moorish instruments. John served as confessor to *moriscos* and Old Christians alike, and to those seduced by the splendors of the city crowned by the Alhambra and the Generalife, he taught that "we travel not in order to see but in order not to see."

In Granada, John wrote the books *A Spiritual Canticle of the Soul* and *Living Flame of Love* to distinguish the contemplative way to unity according to the Divine Will from both natural and Muslim mysticism, which often took the form of possession and madness. According to John, these states were outwardly nearly indistinguishable from the transports of the dark light of grace; they occurred, he said, not only among Christians drawn to the Illuminist movement but also among the young *moriscos*, on whom he was often called to perform exorcisms.

While John was still at Baeza, a wealthy young Genoese, Jesús María Doria, professed within the Descalced Order and quickly found favor with Teresa through Philip II's recommendation. Doria was to be John's nemesis. Teresa, well aware of the Italian's keen mind, sent him to her friend Gracián, who in turn sent him as their representative to Rome. In 1582, Doria returned to Spain with special papal privileges, determined to reorganize the Order of Descalced Carmelites according to the *machina* of the Italian houses. In order to do so, he succeeded in having himself elected vicar general of the Order and unsuccessfully tried to send his former superior and continual rival, Gracián, to Mexico. In 1588, through a general conference, he revamped the Order's governing structure. Meanwhile, John, while founding monasteries and convents in Córdoba, Segovia, and Málaga, sought to mediate between Doria's missionary zeal to send Carmelites throughout all Christendom and beyond and Gracián's equal determination to keep the Order small and confined to Spanish soil. At a general meeting in Almodóvar, John actually spoke out against the hunger for power he saw invading the Order in the guise of worthy projects—but to no avail.

In 1588, John was appointed prior to the convent in Segovia, which became the seat of government of the Order during Doria's frequent trips abroad. Philip II learned of John's able administration and commended him for it. John's companions, however, attested that he scourged himself regularly, was sickly, wore spartograss undergarments and chains that drew blood, fasted almost continuously, and refused to wear anything but the heaviest clothing the year round. He slept only three hours each night and still heard confessions and ministered to the sick while trying to reconcile Gracián and Doria. His inner life was such that on occasion he was incapable of carrying out the simplest task, so frequent and overwhelming were his raptures. The last time he saw his brother Francisco, whom he claimed to have loved more than anyone else, John told him of a vision in which Christ asked him his desire. To Christ, John replied, "Suffering to be borne for Your sake and to be despised and regarded as worthless." His prayer was to be answered.

In 1589, the nuns of the Order, convinced that Doria was determined to abolish the reforms initiated by Teresa, petitioned Gracián and John to be separated from the Brothers over whom Doria ruled. Doria learned of the conspiracy from Luis de León and, suspecting that both Gracián and John were supporting the feminine rebellion against him, denounced the two to Philip II, who intervened directly with an order that the nuns remain.

At the next chapter meeting, John was denied any post whatsoever. First the council accepted and then rejected his offer to lead twelve Carmelites to Mexico. He and Gracián were to learn the extent of Doria's anger. In Seville during the chapter meetings, there was such fear of Doria that no one dared to oppose him. John bravely spoke out, accusing Doria of destroying charity, free discussion, and the right to self-determination within the rule. Doria reacted by sending John into exile, to the solitude of the desert monastery of Peñuela in Extremadura. Gracián suffered a worse fate, being stripped of his habit, expelled from the Order, and sent begging justice to Rome. The accusation against him was disobedience.

In Peñuela, John became seriously ill with an infection and went to Úbeda seeking aid. There, the prior treated him badly because, years earlier, John had scolded him for his manner of preaching. John's ecstatic prayer in Segovia, as reported by his brother Francisco, was answered in Úbeda: "not to die a superior, to die where he was unknown and to die after great suffering."

ANALYSIS

The work of Saint John of the Cross, although not copious, presents a synthesis of medieval learning and Renaissance form, couched in the tradition of Spanish realism. He sought through his poems and books to explain to his Order the nature of the three steps through contemplation to union with the Divine Presence: the *via purgativa*, the *via iluminativa*, and the *via unitativa*. The poem "The Dark Night" and the poet's book-length explication *The Ascent of Mount Carmel* address the beginner or novice, revealing the two spiritual revolutions he will experience; the poem "The Spiritual Canticle" and its book-length explication *A Spiritual Canticle of the Soul* address the *aprovechantes*, who intermittently see their aspirations fulfilled; the poem "The Living Flame of Love" and its explication *Living Flame of Love* address those perfect religious aspirants who seldom cease to experience the dark light of grace. The three poems were written during the imprisonment of John in Toledo in 1577, the first book during his priorship at El Calvario in 1578, and the remaining two while he was prior of Los Mártires in Granada in 1581. Although the works become clearer when read in the context of sixteenth century Spain, John's method of combining medieval, Renaissance, and popular traditions to explain the mysteries of the faith in terms of universal human experience frees his writing from its historical limitations.

John's prose explicates his poetry: *The Ascent of Mount Carmel*, *A Spiritual Canticle of the Soul*, and *Living Flame of Love* use the methodology of Scholastic criticism to explain the doctrine contained in his three major poems. The author readily admits that the intellect hinders rather than aids one's progress toward meditation, but he maintains that reason, in theology as well as in physics and psychology, is the only reliable guide. Reason and the concomitant qualities of simplicity and clarity are extolled as those values most to be esteemed in the religious life of prayer and discipline, so that the contemplative may avoid the danger of becoming attached to the intricate beauty of the ritual rather than to its spirit. The contemplative must present a tabula rasa—freeing his will from the self so that he may be charitable, his understanding from knowledge so that he may have faith, and his memory from continuity so that he may have hope—before he may receive grace.

Reason enables John to distinguish the contemplative's two passages through the "dark night," first from initiate to *aprovechante*, then to perfect, from the states of melancholy, *aboulia*, and possession that they closely resemble. The initiate's enthusiasm soon be-

comes anger in the form of the frustration experienced by a child denied the rewards he seeks, and he is then subject to pride, restlessness, boredom, envy, impatience, fetishism, and dishonesty until, when he least expects it, he "stand[s] alone in the bitter and terrible dark night of the senses" in which the world appears inverted. The initiate entering the first dark night manifests total distraction and fear that he is lost. All his attempts to regain the source of his former well-being are foiled. Some initiates attempt to begin their discipline again, to no avail. Most, on entering the first dark night, manifest madness in the form of extreme sexual desire, blasphemy, and vertigo.

Once they have overcome these trials, however, the *aprovechantes* may lose their humility and attack with too much confidence, to the point that their experience of grace is self-deceiving and they become blinded by hallucinations, voices, and transports. Since the *aprovechantes* have not completely overcome their former affections, they are in danger of becoming physically and psychologically ill.

According to John, the second passage through the dark night to perfection is even more difficult and may last many years. For the physically weak, it is unbearable. The *aprovechantes* experience spiritual poverty, helplessness, detachment, incomprehension, an absence of will, and anguish over losing mind and memory. They may by chance finally acquire wisdom in the form of the dark light of the fire described in *Living Flame of Love*. The perfect is then enjoined to make of his soul a hiding place where the beloved may live with gracious company in pleasure and ease.

Although John's psychology is limited to three faculties (the will, reason, and memory) and four interrelated emotions (pleasure, pain, fear, and hope), he provides a clear view of the spiritual adventure of a sixteenth century Spaniard who is not called to the territorial adventure of imperial expansion. In an interesting image, John compares the reluctant adventurer to a canvas that refuses to be still for the artist's brush.

"THE DARK NIGHT"

In "The Dark Night," John presents the momentary union of the novice's soul with God in terms of the fulfillment of the desires of two lovers who have been separated. Most directly, the poem re-creates the escape of the beloved at night from her house to a meeting with her lover outside the walls of the city, where they surrender themselves to the rapture of their passion. The beloved recalls her fear, her desire, the necessary deceptions and precaution, the shock of being found by her lover, and the joy of the encounter, with its consequential loss of self in a union with all and nothingness.

The simplicity of the poem gives it its strength and almost hypnotic power. The Spanish is rustic, although not uncultured, and it characterizes the beloved with a pastoral simplicity and innocence as she ventures forth to meet her lover. Morphologically and syntactically, the poet gives the beloved's words some features of that dialect between Gallego-Portuguese and Castilian that characterizes the standard literary form of rustic speech known as *sayagués*. Moreover, the poet employs a stanza that discourages elaboration in favor of simplicity, clarity, and precision. From the soldier-courtier Garcilaso de la Vega (1501-1536), who two decades earlier had revolutionized Spanish poetry by successfully adapting the softer Italian hendecasyllable to the more regularly accented and rigid medieval Spanish verse, John borrowed the *lira*. By alternating three heptasyllables and two hendecasyllables within a rhyme scheme that seals the lines by pairing them without regard to length, the poet using the *lira* directs his thought inward and inhibits elaboration. The inward direction of the poem, reflecting the recollection necessary for the beloved's escape, is reinforced by the poet's skillful use of repetition within and between the strophes. Through onomatopoeia, he re-creates with sibilants and voiceless fricatives the darkness, silence, secrecy, and softness of the adventure.

To overcome the temporal limitation of the language of the poem, the poet uses a series of apostrophes to the night. The poem is a re-creation of the encounter in which the beloved attributes to the night the same immediacy ascribed to the lover. Again, in response to the inward direction of the poem, the apostrophe culminates in the center of the poem, in which the metamorphosis of lover-beloved occurs on the morphological level: "amado con amada/ amada en el amado transformada." The fusion of the lovers becomes confusion,

and the sounds of the poem overwhelm the sense, so that the original gender distinction between the allomorphs "amado" and "amada" disappears into "transformada."

"THE SPIRITUAL CANTICLE"

"The Spiritual Canticle" enlarges the theme of "The Dark Night" to include mortification and illumination. The poem, comprising forty *liras*, is an eclogue, modeled on those of Garcilaso, in which John presents the lovers in a dialogue as shepherds who are now espoused. (In "The Dark Night," they had to escape in order to be united.)

The first stanzas present the beloved initiate moving through the *via purgativa* as a young shepherdess seeking her lover, who has abandoned her soon after revealing his love. Her sense of loss turns her life into an attenuated death and a desperate search for reunion. First, she tries to reach him through other shepherds. Then she abandons both her fears and her pleasures to look for him on her own. As she wanders, the beauty she discovers reminds her of his grace, until she is overwhelmed by longing. The shepherds who speak to her of him merely increase her pain, because she cannot understand the meaning of their words. As she has already surrendered her will to him, she believes her punishment is unjustified, yet she hopes that by his possession of her, she will regain the self she has lost and the reason for being that she lacks. When she least expects it, her lover's eyes appear to her, reflected in a fountain where she quenches her thirst. The *via purgativa* ends with the medieval motif of the maid at the fountain overtaken by a stag.

The next step toward union, the *via iluminativa*, begins with fear. The beloved flees in panic until the lover's words assure her that her flight merely attracts him more, and therefore her attempt to escape is futile. Since the beloved has not acquired perfection, the *via iluminativa* of the *aprovechante* and the *via unitativa* of the perfect become confused. The beloved may ascend to union and also descend to mortification on the secret ladder introduced by the poet in "The Dark Night." In the fourteenth and fifteenth stanzas, the beloved finds union with her lover, expressed as an ecstatic vision of mountains, valleys, strange islands, sweet melodies unheard, and sonorous silence. The vision is enriched by imagery reminiscent of the Old Testament Song of Songs and, because of the absence of verbs, is made to appear simultaneous.

The beloved must descend from union, presented as a garden in Zion, first to mortification in which she defends their vines from foxes; then to illumination in which she weaves their roses into garlands; then back to mortification in order to defend their solitude, to conjure the rain-laden western wind, to restrain the envious, and to hide her lover away in silence while distracting him with the delights of her raptures. To aid his beloved, the lover proudly commands his creation, through song, to abandon them to their rapture. He then proceeds to raise her again to union, regaling her with the fulfillment of her desire, healing her sorrow, defending her tranquillity with the controlled power of lions, the wealth of gold shields or coins, the luxury of purple hangings, and the peace derived from a social structure based on others' admiration and awe before the brilliance of their passion and the fragrance of their wine that, because of its age, gives delight without sorrow.

In stanzas 26 through 29, the beloved addresses those same admirers of her rapture in order to explain her distraction. She reveals that it derives from the wine that she shares with her lover and that consequently her only concern has become to learn to love well. She explains to them that she will no longer be among them on the commons, because she has become entranced with loving, losing herself only to be found by her lover. In the last ten stanzas, unconcerned that their admirers overhear, she addresses her lover and reveals to them the source of their love. His passion derives from one insignificant grace, presented as a single hair blown across her throat. Because of her humility and unworthiness, the continuation of that passion arises from the beauty that flows from his eyes, and is reflected in her, as her passion arises from discovering her reflection in him. The verbal tenses of these last eight stanzas refer not to chronology but to the fulfillment of the lover and beloved's purpose. The distinctions among past, present, and future disappear as the lovers explore profound and lofty mysteries. Accordingly, the eclogue ends not in the classical manner of the shepherd's departure with the setting sun, but with the image of horses descending a hill to drink water once the siege they had resisted is lifted.

"THE LIVING FLAME OF LOVE"

The third of the poems written by John while in the monastery prison of Toledo, "The Living Flame of Love," continues the allegory of "The Dark Night" and "The Spiritual Canticle." This work presents in four *liras* the song of the beloved to her lover's passion during their ecstatic union. The beloved is now perfect inasmuch as her grace is actual rather than potential. These *liras*, having six rather than five lines and deriving from Garcilaso's friend and immediate literary predecessor, Juan Boscán, are freer, less vacillating and inwardly directed than the first two poems.

The poem is one of the most intense moments in a powerful literary tradition. In it, the beloved sings of the lover's passion as a life-giving and living fire that consumes with fulfillment rather than destruction. The beloved rejoices in her total surrender and pleads to have the rapture made complete by his destruction of the barriers that still divide them. His passion captures, wounds, and subdues her with a gentleness that reveals to her the nature of eternity. The taste of this knowledge turns her heart from the sorrow of living an attenuated death apart from her lover to the joy that his presence infuses as she comes into being through his love. The dark light emanating from her lover's fire illuminates the entirety of her beauty when the poem ends abruptly with her lover's breath rousing her passion again as he awakens on her breast.

Three other poems written in Toledo at the same time do not achieve as perfect a synthesis of the eclogue, Song of Songs, and folk motifs derived from the tradition of the romances and courtly lyrics of the *villancicos* as do the three poems presented here. The *coplas de pie quebrado*, known as "Although by Night," present the medieval motif of the *fonte frida* in such a way that the night acquires at least thirteen different meanings through an equal number of contexts. In the nine *romances* that constitute the "Ballad on the Gospel 'In the Beginning Was the Word,'" the poet employs the same method as in his major poems, explaining the mysteries of the faith in terms of the varieties of human love. In "Ballad on the Psalm 'By the Waters of Babylon,'" the ascetic's sense of alienation and his consequent rejection of the world are presented in terms of the Babylonian captivity of Israel's people, who refuse to sing the jubilant songs of Zion.

OTHER MAJOR WORKS

NONFICTION: *Cántico espiritual*, c. 1577-1586 (*A Spiritual Canticle of the Soul*, 1864, 1909); *La subida del Monte Carmelo*, 1578-1579 (*The Ascent of Mount Carmel*, 1864, 1922); *Llama de amor viva*, c. 1582 (*Living Flame of Love*, 1864, 1912).

MISCELLANEOUS: *The Complete Works of St. John of the Cross*, 1864, 1934, 1953.

BIBLIOGRAPHY

Brenan, Gerald. *St. John of the Cross: His Life and Poetry*. 1973. Reprint. New York: Cambridge University Press, 1989. This biography includes a translation of John's poetry by Lynda Nicholson. Bibliography.

Gaylord, Mary Malcolm, and Francisco Marquez Villanueva, eds. *San Juan de la Cruz and Fray Luis de León: A Commemorative International Symposium*. Newark, Del.: Juan de la Cuesta, 1996. This collection of works from a symposium examines mysticism in literature, focusing on John and Luis de León. Includes index.

Hardy, Richard P. *John of the Cross: Man and Mystic*. Boston: Pauline Books and Media, 2004. This biography covers John's life from its start to end. Contains an appendix on how to read his works and one with selected texts.

_____. *Search for Nothing: The Life of John of the Cross*. New York, Crossroad, 1982. Hardy wrote this biography to explore John's humanity and make his personality accessible to the modern reader. Hardy provides a necessary corrective to more traditional accounts of John's life.

Herrera, Robert A. *Silent Music: The Life, Work, and Thought of Saint John of the Cross*. Grand Rapids, Mich.: W. B. Erdmans, 2004. This biography of John sees him as a man "whose life was a heroic attempt to assimilate and to be assimilated by the Divine." Places John in his contemporary world and examines his writings in context.

Kavanaugh, Kieran. *John of the Cross: Doctor of Light and Love*. New York: Crossroad, 1999. A study of John that reprints the poems and includes useful features such as a select bibliography. Illustrated.

Payne, Steven. *Saint John of the Cross*. New York: Continuum, 2005. This biography in the Outstanding Christian Thinkers series looks at the saint's life and works, in particular examining his mysticism.

_____, ed. *John of the Cross: Conferences and Essays by Members of the Institute of Carmelite Studies and Others*. Washington, D.C.: ICS, 1992. This collection of essays deals with John's thinking on a variety of theological topics, useful to the scholar as well as the general reader. Each essay includes bibliographical notes.

Perrin, David Brian. *For Love of the World: The Old and New Self of John of the Cross*. San Francisco: Catholic Scholars Press, 1997. This work examines the beliefs of John and places him within the history of the Roman Catholic Church. Includes index.

Ruiz, Federico, et al. *God Speaks in the Night: The Life, Times, and Teaching of John of the Cross*. Translated by Kieran Kavanaugh. Washington, D.C.: ICS, 1991. This book commemorates the fourth centenary of John's death with almost one hundred short essays authored by Spanish Carmelite scholars and is lavishly illustrated with beautiful color photographs and illustrations. Organized around the central events of John's life, this volume provides a wealth of information of use to the scholar as well as the general reader. Includes an index of names and places.

Kenneth A. Stackhouse

JUDAH HA-LEVI

Born: Tudela, Kingdom of Pamplona (now in
    Spain); c. 1075
Died: Egypt; July, 1141
Also known as: Abū al-Ḥasan; Yehuda ben Shemuel
    ha-Levi; Yehuda Halevi

PRINCIPAL POETRY
Dīwān, twelfth century
Selected Poems of Jehudah Halevi, 1924, 1925,
    1928, 1942, 1973
Die schönen Vermasse, 1930
Kol Shirei Rabbi Yehudah Halevi, 1955
Shirei ha-qodesh, 1978
Ninety-two Poems and Hymns of Yehuda Halevi,
    2000

OTHER LITERARY FORMS

Primarily famous as a poet, Judah ha-Levi (JEW-
duh haw LEE-vi) also wrote an apologetic religious
treatise, the *Kuzari* (twelfth century; English translation, 1947), and several letters, in the rhymed prose
characteristic of formal Hebrew and Arabic letters of
the Middle Ages, which have been preserved and are of
interest for their literary style. One of these is translated
in Benzion Halper's *Post-Biblical Hebrew Literature*
(1921) and reprinted in Franz Kobler's *Letters of Jews
Through the Ages*. Some important Judeo-Arabic letters were translated into English by S. D. Goitein,
"Judeo-Arabic Letters from Spain," in J. M. Barral,
editor, *Orientalia Hispanica*, 1974.

ACHIEVEMENTS

To understand Judah ha-Levi's position as one of the
foremost Hebrew poets not only of the medieval period
but also of all time, it is necessary to survey briefly the
"firmament" in which he is said to be one of the shining
stars—that is, medieval Hebrew poetry. Hebrew poetry
began with the Bible, and it would even be possible to argue that secular poetry began there as well, if such books
as the Song of Songs may be understood to be secular
rather than allegorical. In the Hellenistic period, Jewish
poets wrote some Greek verse, and apparently some

verse in Persian during the period of the post-Talmudic
era in Babylonia. It was the influence of Arabic poetry,
however, throughout the Muslim world—where the majority of Jews in the medieval period lived—that aroused
Jewish intellectuals to attempt a renaissance of the Hebrew language. Hebrew had long been relegated to religious poetry (*piyyut*) for recitation in the synagogue and
some few compositions on purely religious subjects.
Simply by composing Hebrew poetry on secular themes,
and using adaptations of Arabic meter, ha-Levi's predecessors were effecting a linguistic revolution. These
first efforts began in Muslim Spain in the tenth century,
and quickly reached a level of excellence in the eleventh century with the generation preceding ha-Levi.

Samuel ibn Nagrillah, born in Córdoba at the height
of the cultural flourishing of Muslim civilization in
Spain, rose to a position of power almost unheard of for
a Jew at that time and in that area; he became prime
minister and commander in chief of the armies of the
Muslim kingdom of Granada (there were other Jewish
ministers and even prime ministers in Muslim Spain
and elsewhere, but he was the first known Jewish general since the one who served Cleopatra). As an active
soldier, fighting battles against the enemies of his kingdom every year for eighteen years, he wrote virtually
the only Hebrew war poetry extant. In addition, he
found time to compose no less than three volumes of
Hebrew poetry on a variety of themes, as well as a work
on grammar and a book on Jewish law.

Solomon ibn Gabirol was the other outstanding Hebrew poet of that period. Although his life was marked
by frustration and suffering, his poetry can only be described as brilliant, often rising above whatever his
misfortunes may have been to sing the lyric themes of
love, nature, wine, and other topics. He began writing
while still a teenager and expressed the audacity and
hubris of youth in some of his early poems, praising his
own poetry and fame. He was a philosopher and a
mystic—more famous in the Christian world for his
Fons vitae (the Latin translation of his original work)
than among his fellow Jews. Both of these elements
are present in many of his poems, some of which reveal profound philosophical insights or are tinged with
mystical longings. Most famous of these is the lengthy
religious-mystical-philosophical poem *Keter malkhut*,

translated frequently into numerous languages (perhaps the best version in English is *The Kingly Crown*, translated by Bernard Lewis).

Contemporary with ha-Levi, although his senior and for many years his mentor and friend, was the great Moses ibn Ezra of Granada. Perhaps the finest of the Hebrew poets of medieval Spain and certainly the most complex, he has been the least understood and appreciated. His poetry is far from simple; it consists of an intricate filigree of biblical language, with allusions to the Talmud, the Midrash, and Arabic poetry and letters. This texture is characteristic of the other medieval Hebrew poets as well, but Ibn Ezra's style is particularly complex. A philosopher as well as a poet (his work in this field still has not been completely edited), he also wrote the only important medieval work on Hebrew poetics. This work details the history of Hebrew poetry and poets to his time, analyzing at length the various rhetorical devices and poetic embellishments employed over the years.

Ha-Levi thus came at the end of what could be termed the "classical period" of medieval Hebrew poetry, and the period in which he lived and wrote was by no means as conducive to creative production as that of the previous generations of poets. Following a civil war that led to the destruction in 1013 of the central caliphate of Córdoba, the Muslim part of Spain was divided into a series of *taifa* (city-state) kingdoms, such as that of Granada, of which the poet Ibn Nagrillah was prime minister. These were generally weak and divided among themselves, with constant fighting and quarreling, thus providing the opportunity for which the Christians had long been waiting. Ferdinand I was able to unite Leon and Castile and begin the "reconquest" of Muslim Spain. Alfonso VI succeeded in conquering Toledo in 1085; in response to this loss of territory, the Muslims invited the fanatic Almoravids of North Africa to invade Spain and help rid them of the Christian threat. In 1090, the Almoravid troops entered Granada, an event that came just after the massacre of many Jews there. The Christian reconquest itself had serious repercussions for the entire Jewish community, both in Christian and in Muslim Spain. Caught between invading Christian troops and Almoravid Muslim forces, Jews fought and suffered on both sides. The poet Moses

ibn Ezra was forced to flee from Granada, as were most of the Jews there, and he spent many years wandering in exile in Christian Spain, primarily in Navarre. During the same period, ha-Levi wandered from city to city in Muslim Spain, and it appears almost fruitless to try to trace these wanderings. In spite of this less-than-ideal situation, he managed to produce a very respectable body of poetry, both secular and religious in theme.

Even in his own time, or soon thereafter, ha-Levi was recognized as one of the greatest of the Spanish Hebrew poets. His contemporary and friend Ibn Ezra may not have shared this opinion, since in his work on poetics, he mentions ha-Levi only as a composer of some riddles, but this judgment may have been written before the poet had done most of his best work. Judah al-Harizi (who lived in the early thirteenth century) said of ha-Levi's poems that they are "sweeter than honey," adding that "he took all the treasures from the treasury of poetry and locked its gate after him." Abraham Bedersi of Provence (who also lived in the thirteenth century) said of ha-Levi, "He prevailed over his fellow-poets; to ha-Levy say: My perfection and my light." Nearly all the nineteenth century scholars who pioneered in the study of Hebrew poetry concurred. Heinrich Heine, who acquired his limited knowledge of Hebrew poetry from reading the German works of some of these scholars, joined in praise of ha-Levi. Heine, in his "Princezzin Sabbath" ("Princess Sabbath"), erroneously attributes to ha-Levi the famous *piyyut* "Lekha dodi" (actually written by Solomon Alkabes) recited at Friday evening services.

Heine dedicated four lengthy poems to ha-Levi. The first of these is a highly romantic and inaccurate picture of the poet's youth. The second, "Beiden Wassern Babels," one of Heine's finest poems, has a reference to "Ghaselen" as one of the various kinds of poems that ha-Levi wrote. This may puzzle some readers: The term is a transliteration of Arabic *ghazal* (erotic poetry), a form in which ha-Levi excelled. In the final poem, "Meine Frau ist nicht zufrieden," Heine explains to his wife that the three stars of Hebrew poetry were ha-Levi, Ibn Gabirol, and Ibn Ezra; he advises her to abandon her theaters and concerts long enough to devote some years to studying Hebrew so that she can read their poems in their original language.

BIOGRAPHY

Judah ha-Levi, in Arabic surnamed Abū al-Ḥasan, was born in Tudela, Spain. His father is referred to in a letter as a rabbi and great scholar, but this may have been merely a courtesy. Otherwise, nothing is known of him. There is absolutely no evidence to support the oft-repeated claim that ha-Levi studied either with the great Isaac Alfasi in Lucena or with his successor Joseph ibn Megash. It is true that ha-Levi composed a eulogy on the death of the former, but this was not unusual considering that Alfasi was the greatest rabbi in Spain, and many poets composed eulogies in his honor. At some time during his youth, certainly not later than 1089, ha-Levi left Christian Spain for Andalusia in Muslim Spain and sent a letter to Ibn Ezra in Granada, together with an imitation of one of Ibn Ezra's poems. Thus began a long friendship with Ibn Ezra and his brothers that lasted until their death.

Like many Jews in medieval Spain, ha-Levi was trained in medicine, and he practiced as a doctor at a later period in his life. Although he was probably wealthy and even engaged in commerce in his later years, in his younger life, he received financial support by writing poetry in praise of patrons.

Ha-Levi had one daughter, who is supposed to have written at least two poems and who was married to Isaac ibn Ezra (the son of the great biblical commentator Abraham ibn Ezra, himself a poet but not related to Moses ibn Ezra). Isaac ibn Ezra, also a poet of note in later years, accompanied his father-in-law on his famous journey, when, at about the age of fifty, ha-Levi decided to leave his beloved Spain and go to the Holy Land. He and his companions arrived in Egypt in 1140. He remained in Egypt for a year, and died there in July, 1141.

ANALYSIS

Judah ha-Levi may not entirely deserve his reputation as the greatest of medieval Hebrew poets, a reputation that is based largely on nineteenth century scholarship, when little was known of the work of other Hebrew poets of the period; certainly, however, he is one of the four greatest. He mastered most of the themes typical of Hebrew poetry: wine, love (both of women and of boys), nature, friendship, panegyric, complaint, and humor. Ha-Levi wrote a number of religious or "liturgical" poems as well. Like most of the religious poems that come from the Spanish school, they are far simpler in style and vocabulary than the secular verse. His secular poetry, which constitutes the largest part of his work, is often difficult and at times stiff, but he can move the modern reader with his emotions; he can arouse a smile and even a laugh. Some of his love poetry, dealing with both sexes, ranks among the finest in Hebrew verse. There is no doubt, however, that the poetry for which he is most famous and was best remembered is his "Zion" poetry. The poet came to the conclusion that, like the rabbi in his religious treatise, the *Kuzari*, he had to abandon his "temporary home" in the Exile and go to the land scared to his people: "My heart is in the East [Zion] and I am in the ends of the West [Spain]; How can I taste what I eat, and how can it be sweet?"

Leaving his home was not easy, however, and one of ha-Levi's most poignant poems describes his emotions about leaving his daughter and his grandson and namesake, Judah:

> I do not worry about property or possessions
> nor wealth nor all my losses—
> Except that I foresake my offspring,
> sister of my soul, my only daughter.
> I shall forget her son, a segment of my heart,
> and I have, except for him, nothing to discuss—
> Fruit of my womb and child of my delights;
> how can Judah forget Judah?

"ODE TO ZION"

Of all the poems that ha-Levi wrote while contemplating his trip and during the perilous sea voyage that he so well describes (the meter of one poem makes the reader "feel" the motion of the sea during a storm), none is more famous than the "Zionide" ("Ode to Zion"), which has been translated into numerous languages in many versions. Of all the poems ever written by Jew or Gentile in praise of Zion, this is surely the best known and the most stirring.

The poem opens with the poet's plaintive query to Zion concerning the scattered Jewish people who daily seek the welfare of Zion: "Do you inquire of the welfare of your captives?" There follows the famous line in which the poet says that in his dreams of the return of the people to Zion, he is "a lute for [their] songs." He mentions his desire to wander in the now-desolate land, and all the places that he names are places where God appeared to Jacob; thus, they are symbolic of the holiness of the land and also reflect ha-Levi's interest in revelation, an interest that is central also in the *Kuzari*. "There," in Jerusalem, "your Creator opened facing the gates of heaven your [Zion's] gates," he says, reflecting the rabbinic allegory, borrowed in turn by Christian writers, indicating that there is a heavenly city of Jerusalem corresponding to the earthly one, the gates of which are the gates of Heaven. In Jerusalem, the poet says, he shall prostrate himself "and delight in [the city's] stones exceedingly and favor [its] dust," a reference to Psalm 102:15.

From his ecstatic vision of himself walking barefoot in the land, verging on allegory ("the life of souls is the air of your land, and of flowing myrrh the dust of your earth, and flowing honey your rivers"), the poet turns to polemics against the Muslims, who had conquered and inhabited the land, profaning, in his eyes, the sacredness of the place. The reader must remember that this poem was written while the poet was still in Muslim Spain, and—almost as if he were afraid to express anti-Muslim sentiment openly, even in Hebrew—he hides behind allusions; for example, "How can the light of day be sweet to my eyes while I see in the mouths of crows the corpses of your eagles?" becomes fully intelligible only when the reader realizes that the Hebrew word for ravens (or crows), *orvim*, is almost identical in sound to the Hebrew word for "Arabs," *Aravim*.

From the pit of captivity, he says, the exiled people are longing for return: "the flocks of your multitude which have been exiled and scattered/ from mountain to hill and have not forgotten your folds." These lines echo Jeremiah 50:6: "My people hath been lost sheep, their shepherds have caused them to go astray . . . they have gone from mountain to hill, they have forgotten their resting place." Because the Jews of medieval Spain knew the Old Testament books almost by heart, such allusions would not have been lost on them.

Another significant allusion is found in the line "Shinar and Pathros—can they compare to you in greatness, or their vanity be likened to your perfection and enlightenment?" Shinar and Pathros are biblical terms for Babylonia and Egypt, but the reader cannot help

feeling that there is yet another meaning: the medieval Muslim lands that represented the culture with which the Jews of Spain, at least, were trying to compete.

From praise of Jerusalem, the poet turns, prophet-like, to consolation, declaring that God longs once again to make the city a habitation for his glory. The poem concludes in a mood that is both a challenge and a litany of praise: "Happy he who waits, and arrives, and sees the ascendancy of your light, and upon whom breaks your dawns—/ To see the goodness of your chosen and to rejoice in your happiness in your return to your former youth!"

LEGACY

"Ode to Zion" became almost an anthem of the Jewish people in the Middle Ages and for centuries afterward, although astonishingly few know it in the twenty-first century. It entered into the liturgy and was recited in synagogue services throughout the world. No other Hebrew poem was so frequently imitated by so many poets in different lands.

In the late twentieth century, the revival of Hebrew as a living language prompted renewed interest in the entire corpus of Hebrew poetry, and several excellent anthologies were published, ranging from biblical verse to modern Hebrew poetry written in Israel. In this renaissance of Hebrew poetry, the works of ha-Levi were discovered by a new generation of readers.

OTHER MAJOR WORK

NONFICTION: *Kuzari*, twelfth century (English translation, 1947).

BIBLIOGRAPHY

Brener, Ann. *Judah Halevi and His Circle of Hebrew Poets in Granada*. Boston: Brill/Styx, 2005. Part of the Hebrew Language and Literature series, this volume looks at the lives of Judah ha-Levi and the other Hebrew poets in Spain. Includes translations of selected poems.

Halkin, Hillel. *Yehuda Halevi*. New York: Schocken, 2010. This biography notes the importance of poetry to Andalusian Jews and provides in-depth analysis of it in telling the story of Judah ha-Levi's life.

Judah ha-Levi. *Ninety-two Poems and Hymns of Yehuda Halevi*. Translated by Thomas Kovach, Eva

Jospe, and Gilya Gerda Schmidt. Edited by Richard A. Cohen. Albany: State University of New York Press, 2000. Provides translations of Judah ha-Levi's hymns and poems, including "Ode to Zion." Also includes an introductory essay.

Menocal, Maria Rosa, Raymond P. Scheindlin, and Michael Sells, eds. *The Literature of Al-Andalus.* New York: Cambridge University Press, 2000. Part of the Cambridge History of Arabic Literature series, provides a biographical look at the literature of Judah ha-Levi in Arabic Andalusia.

Scheindlin, Raymond P. *The Song of the Distant Dove: Judah Halevi's Pilgrimage.* New York: Oxford University Press, 2008. Examines Judah ha-Levi's pilgrimage, using the poems as one of the sources of information.

Silman, Yochanan. *Philosopher and Prophet: Judah Halevi, the Kuzari, and the Evolution of His Thought.* Translated by Lenn J. Schramm. Albany: State University of New York Press, 1995. Explores the whole range of Judah ha-Levi's philosophical and religious thought, from Aristotelianism, to form and matter, divinity, theology, anthropology, god and world, and more.

Yahalom, Joseph. *Yehuda Haveli: Poetry and Pilgrimage.* Jerusalelm: Hebrew University Magnes Press, 2009. Follows the poet from Muslim Spain to Zion. To describe the journey, uses his *Dīwān* as well as autobiographical letters and correspondence from the Cairo Geniza collections.

Norman Roth (including original translations)

JUVENAL

Born: Aquinum (now in Italy); c. 60 C.E.
Died: Place unknown; c. 130 C.E.

PRINCIPAL POETRY
Saturae, 100-127 C.E. (*Satires*, 1693)

OTHER LITERARY FORMS
Juvenal is known only for his poetry.

ACHIEVEMENTS

Humanities instructor Gilbert Highet called Juvenal (JEW-vuhn-uhl) "the greatest satiric poet who ever lived." In his own time, Juvenal seems to have been largely ignored; of his contemporaries, only Martial refers to him. He was first appreciated by Christian writers, who found his strictures on pagan Rome congenial. Tertullian (c. 155-160 to after 217) borrowed phrases from him. Lactantius (c. 240-c. 320) praised the satirist. Decimius Magnus Ausonius (c. 310-c. 395) imitated his work, as did Ausonius's pupils, Saint Paulinus of Nola (c. 352 or 353 to 431) and Aurelius Clemens Prudentius (c. 348-after 405). Saint Jerome (between 331 and 347-probably 420) in his treatise against marriage draws on Satire 6.

Non-Christian authors also began to appreciate Juvenal some 250 years after his death. Ammianus Marcellinus (c. 330-c. 395) claimed that among aristocrats of the late fourth century, Juvenal and the third century biographer Marius Maximus were the only two authors read. Servius (fourth century), in his commentary of Vergil, quotes Juvenal about seventy times. The Egyptian satirist Claudian (c. 370-c. 404) wrote two satires in imitation of Juvenal. Dante placed Juvenal among the righteous pagans in limbo, in the company of such other classical writers as Homer, Ovid, and Lucan.

Juvenal's popularity increased during the Middle Ages. Aimeric's *Ars lectoria* (1086; art of reading), which divided authors into categories of gold, silver, copper, iron, tin, and lead, placed Juvenal among nine writers in the highest category. In medieval florilegia (collections of excerpts), Juvenal was cited more often than any other classical writer.

The first printed edition of Juvenal appeared about 1470 in Rome. By 1501, some seventy editions of the satirist's works had been printed in Italy alone, exceeding the number of editions of the works of any other classical author except for Cicero, Vergil, and Ovid. In his attack on Cardinal Thomas Wolsey, *Why Come Ye Nat to Courte* (1522), John Skelton credits Juvenal as serving as his poetic model. Skelton quotes Juvenal in *Speke, Parrot* (1521) as well. Desiderus Erasmus included more than fifty of Juvenal's epigrams in the *Adagia* (1500; *Proverbs or Adages*, 1622). Ben Jonson's *Sejanus His Fall* (pr. 1603; commonly known as *Sejanus*) opens with courtiers quoting Juvenal. Hamlet in his eponymous play (William Shakespeare's *Hamlet, Prince of Denmark*, pr. c. 1600-1601) is probably reading Juvenal's tenth satire when he encounters Polonius.

John Dryden and friends translated Juvenal into English in 1693, and Dryden's satires are Juvenalian. John Oldham (1653-1683) adapted Juvenal's Satires 3 and 13. Jonathan Swift quotes Juvenal about twenty times, and the fierce indignation of his writing echoes that of the Romans. Samuel Johnson adapted Satire 3 as *London* (1738) and Satire 10 as *The Vanity of Human Wishes* (1749), his two major poems. In 1775, Edmund Burke, urging the House of Commons not to blockade the American colonies, warned "spoliatis arma supersunt" (plundered, they still have weapons), quoting from Satire 8. Victor Hugo's *Les Châtiments* (1853), attacking Napolean III, is based on Juvenal; one of the satires is even addressed to him. Highet lists Aldous Huxley, Arthur Koestler, and George Orwell among twentieth century heirs of the Roman satirist.

BIOGRAPHY

Little is known about the life of Decimus Junius Juvenalis, commonly known as Juvenal. In Satire 3, Umbricius, who is retiring to Cumae, says that he hopes to see Juvenal occasionally in the poet's native Aquinum, indicating Juvenal's birthplace. Martial, in Epigram 7.91 (93 C.E.), calls Juvenal "facundus" (eloquent), a term equally appropriate for speakers and poets. Since Juvenal had not yet published any verse, Martial probably is praising Juvenal's rhetorical ability. In Epigram 12.18 of about a decade later (c. 102), Martial imagines Juvenal sweating as he walks through Rome courting a patron, indicating that his friend was poor. The early satires also seem to reflect a writer in straitened circumstances. Juvenal began publishing about 110, when, he writes, he had passed middle age, indicating a birth date of about the year 60.

Satire 7 praises Hadrian for patronizing writers, and Juvenal's circumstances seem to have improved after that emperor's accession in 117. In Satire 11, he invites a friend to his house in Rome for a frugal dinner, with food from his farm in Tivoli. In Satire 15.45, he claims to have observed Egypt. His last book of satires was published about 130, and he probably died soon afterward.

Later commentaries embellished his life, maintaining that he was the son or stepson of a well-to-do freedman, though Juvenal repeatedly mocks such men. According to these accounts, he indulged in rhetoric for amusement. In about 93, an epigram (7.90-92) angered Domitian, who exiled him to Egypt and confiscated his property. After Domitian's assassination in 96, Juvenal returned to Rome but now was poor, a condition he endured until about 117.

ANALYSIS

The word "satire" derives from the Latin *sat*, which means "sufficient" or "full." Satire is a miscellany, dealing with a variety of subjects in a range of metrical forms. Juvenal inherited a Roman satiric tradition dating at least as far back as Quintus Ennius (239-169 B.C.E.; commonly known as Ennius), whose works in this genre dealt with daily life. Cicero and Aulus Gellius refer to the third century B.C.E. Greek Cynic philosopher Menippus of Gadara, who in serio-comic prose ridiculed the pseudo-philosophers of his day. Marcus Terentius Varro (116-27 B.C.E.; commonly known as Varro) imitated Menippus in prose and poetry, treating a wide range of subjects. Horace, Persius, and Juvenal credited Gaius Lucilius (c. 180-103 B.C.E.) as the true creator of satire. Using dactylic hexameter, the meter of epic, Lucilius attacked individuals by name. Lucilius focused on social and moral vices and follies rather than on political matters.

In Satire 1.85-86, Juvenal says that he takes as his province all human activity, people's pledges, fears, anger, lusts, joys, and bustling about. While modeling his meter and subject matter on Lucilius, he recognized that naming living people could prove dangerous. Therefore, he chose to cite the dead as exemplars of contemporary misbehavior. Also, condemning previous rulers such as Nero and Domitian would please the current emperor. Seeking to elevate the status of satire above that of epic and tragedy, Juvenal claims that whereas those genres deal with fiction, satire treats reality. Like Lucilius, he relies heavily on the epic meter of dactylic hexameter. His verses contain 3,600 of these, compared to Horace's 2,400 and Persius's 650. To elevate his diction, he employs periphrasis. Instead of naming Pluto in Satire 10.112, he calls the god the son-in-law of Ceres. At

16.6, he refers to Juno as the mother of the Muses who delights in the sandy shore of Samos. Juvenal is memorable because of his aphoristic quality. Thus, he writes that honesty is praised and neglected (1.74). At 10.356, he advocates praying for a healthy mind in a healthy body. In Satire 6 at Oxford fragment 31-32, he denies that appointing sentries over a wife will guarantee her chastity, for who will guard the guards? The oft-repeated phrase "bread and circuses" is his (10.8).

Juvenal's style is rhetorical. His first satire begins with four rhetorical questions, implying that his audience shares his view. The third and fourth of these questions employ anaphora (repeating the same opening word for emphasis). These are two of his favorite devices throughout his writing. Other rhetorical elements that he frequently employs are anadiplosis (repeating at the beginning of a clause a word or words that end or appear prominently in the preceding one, such as in 2.135-136, 6.34-35, 7.213-214) and epanalepsis (using the same word or clause after an interval, as in his lines 9.67-68, 10.365-366, 12.48). Like the rhetorician, the satirist argues a viewpoint and seeks to persuade an audience. Juvenal offers proof to support his position and refutes opposing arguments. For example, in Satire 7, he maintains that writers, including rhetoricians, must eke out a living. He acknowledges that Marcus Fabius Quintilianus (c. 35-after 96 C.E.; commonly known as Quintilian), the most famous of all Roman practitioners of the art of rhetoric, was rich, but he notes that Quintilian was an exception. In the midst of his attack on Lateranus in Satire 8 for his wild behavior, he introduces an apologist who says that youth must have its fling. Juvenal then responds that Lateranus is too old to benefit from that excuse.

Juvenal's satires exemplify rhetorical types. Satires 5 and 6, for instance, seek to dissuade. In the former, he urges Trebius to abandon the degrading life of a client to a rich man; in the latter, he warns Postumus against marriage. Satire 8 conversely argues for two propositions: that virtue rather than birth confers true nobility and that a provincial governor should not exploit the populace. Other standard forms he uses are the invitation to dinner (Satire 11) and the mock-epic (Satire 4). Though Juvenal sometimes relies on logical persuasion, he most frequently applies exempla drawn from

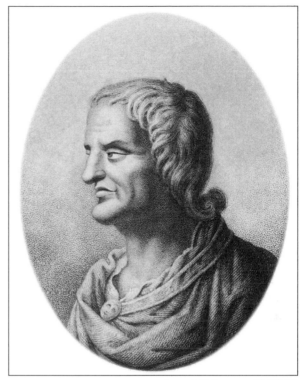

Juvenal (©Bettmann/CORBIS)

history, mythology, or invented character types, such as the insolent patron Virro of Satire 5.

Two themes that recur in his work are the viciousness of the rich and the decline of Rome from its ancient virtue. Satire 5 condemns the rich for selfishness. The women he criticizes in Satire 6 all have money. Eppia, who leaves her husband to run off with a gladiator, is married to a senator. Censennia torments her husband with impunity because she has brought him a dowry of a million sesterces. The licentious Tullia and Maura are carried about in litters, which were reserved for the families of senators. The parents who set bad examples for their children in Satire 14 are all upper-class. Money for Juvenal is the great corrupter of sexual relationships, friendship, the entire social order.

A conservative, Juvenal contrasts the vices and follies of the present with the golden age of the past, the farther back the better. His sharpest attacks are directed toward innovators, upstarts, and those who fail to adhere to the established code of behavior. At the beginning of Satire 6, Juvenal writes that Chastity once resided on earth, but that was before Jupiter had grown a beard. The third century B.C.E. soldier and consul Manius Curius Dentatus would serve home-grown vegetables for dinner; now even a slave rejects such fare (Satire 11). In those early times, people knew their place in the social order, and Romans were not influenced by Greek, Jewish, and Egyptian tastes and practices. Among Juvenal's less attractive traits is his xenophobia. In the process of showing what he regards as Rome's decadence, he presents a vivid portrait of the city and its inhabitants.

SATIRE 3

As Juvenal's friend Umbricius prepares to leave Rome for rural retirement at Cumae, he explains his decision to the poet, painting a nightmare picture of the city in his argument for leaving. After the opening twenty-one lines that set the scene at the Porta Capena on the Appian Way, Umbricius begins his attack. He observes that an honest person cannot earn a living in Rome (lines 21-189). Only lying is valued (lines 21-57). Moreover, foreigners have displaced natives (lines 58-125), and honest poverty is scorned (lines 126-189). Moreover, Rome is dangerous. Umbricius presents the perils that beset the urban dweller through the course of a day, from predawn fires and collapsing buildings (lines 190-231) to crowded streets and overloaded carts (lines 232-267), to ruffians who prey on pedestrians at night (lines 233-314). The poem ends with Umbricius's farewell (lines 315-322). Through Umbricius, Juvenal articulates his recurring themes of the corrupting influence of wealth, the pernicious effect of foreigners and foreign manners, and the difficulties facing the honest poor like Umbricius and himself.

SATIRE 10

Published some fifteen years after Satire 3, in the mid-120's, this later poem adopts a less damning tone. It still argues, in this case against what Johnson called the vanity of human wishes. Juvenal maintains that people pray for the wrong things (lines 1-11): wealth (lines 11-55), power (56-113), eloquence (114-132), military prowess (133-187), long life (188-288, aptly the longest section), and beauty (289-345). Using selected examples from history and mythology, a typical device of the poet, he shows how none of these desired traits brings happiness. Better to trust to the gods and not ask for anything. If one does pray, one should re-

quest a healthy mind in a healthy body and courage (lines 346-366). This stoical, reflective conclusion reflects the diminished bitterness in many of Juvenal's poems in books 3-5 (Satires 7-16).

BIBLIOGRAPHY

Braund, S. H. *Beyond Anger: A Study of Juvenal's Third Book of Satires*. New York: Cambridge University Press, 1988. Though he focuses on Satires 7-9, Braund discusses all the poems, and his insights into book 3 illuminate Juvenal's work.

Courtney, E. *A Commentary on the Satires of Juvenal*. London: Athlone Press, 1980. A substantial introduction discusses Juvenal's life, themes, style, meter, and text. Courtney provides a useful introduction to each poem, followed by detailed analysis for individual words and lines.

Friedländer, Ludwig. *Friedländer's Essays on Juvenal*. Translated by John R. C. Martyn. Amsterdam: Adolf M. Hakkert, 1969. Consists of five chapters from Friedländer's introduction to his 1895 edition of Juvenal. Still an excellent source for information about the satirist's life, poetry, influence, and text.

Highet, Gilbert. *Juvenal the Satirist: A Study*. Oxford, England: Clarendon Press, 1954. An accessible introduction to the life, work, and influence of the Roman satirist. Highet devotes a separate chapter to each satire.

Jones, Frederick. *Juvenal and the Satiric Genre*. London: Duckworth, 2007. Part of the Classical Literature and Society series, this work looks at Juvenal and the genre in which he wrote.

Juvenal. *Juvenal: The Satires*. Translated by Niall Rudd. Oxford, England: Clarendon Press, 1991. A good modern translation with useful notes and introduction by William Barr.

_____. *Juvenal: The Sixteen Satires*. Translated by Peter Green. 3d ed. New York: Penguin, 1998. An idiomatic rather than literal translation, with an extensive (sixty-seven-page) introduction and helpful notes.

Plaza, Maria, ed. *Persius and Juvenal*. New York: Oxford University Press, 2009. A collection of essays on Persius and Juvenal. A number discuss Juvenal and the genre of satire.

Joseph Rosenblum

K

NIKOS KAZANTZAKIS

Born: Iraklion, Crete, Ottoman Empire (now in
Greece); February 18, 1883
Died: Freiburg, West Germany (now in Germany);
October 26, 1957

PRINCIPAL POETRY

Odysseia, 1938 (*The Odyssey: A Modern Sequel*,
1958)
Iliad, 1955 (modern version; with Ioannis Kakridis)
Odysseia, 1965 (modern version; with Kakridis)

OTHER LITERARY FORMS

Although Nikos Kazantzakis (ko-zont-ZO-kees)
himself always regarded *The Odyssey* as his crowning
achievement, he has received international acclaim primarily as a novelist; in addition, he is recognized in his
own country and to a lesser extent throughout Europe
as a playwright, essayist, translator, and writer of travel
books. His travelogues of Russia, Spain, and Great
Britain combine vivid description with political and
cultural commentary. A prolific translator, he has provided his countrymen with modern Greek renditions
of many Western writers, including Friedrich Nietzsche, Jules Verne, Charles Darwin, Henri Bergson, and
Dante. Kazantzakis collaborated on a modern Greek
translation of Homer's *Odyssey* (c. 725 B.C.E.; English
translation, 1614) and *Iliad* (c. 750 B.C.E.; English
translation, 1611). Kazantzakis's published novels include *Toda Raba* (1929; English translation, 1964);
De tuin der Rotsen (1939, better known as *Le Jardin
des rochers*; *The Rock Garden*, 1963); *Vios kai politeia
tou Alexe Zormpa* (1946; *Zorba the Greek*, 1952); *Ho
Christos xanastauronetai* (1954; *The Greek Passion*,
1953, also known as *Christ Recrucified*); *Ho Kapetan
Michales* (1953; *Freedom or Death*, 1956; also known
as *Freedom and Death: A Novel*); *Ho teleutaios
peirasmos* (1955; *The Last Temptation of Christ*, 1960;

also known as *The Last Temptation*); and *Ho phtochoules tou Theou* (1956; *Saint Francis*, 1962; also known
as *God's Pauper: Saint Francis of Assisi*).

ACHIEVEMENTS

Though for English-speaking readers, Nikos Kazantzakis's achievements as a novelist may continue to
overshadow his performance as a poet, anyone wishing
to understand the success of the novels both as literary
masterpieces and as philosophical documents must
turn to *The Odyssey* to discover the roots of Kazantzakis's genius.

Readers who become acquainted with Kazantzakis
in translation cannot fully appreciate one of the most
significant aspects of his work. Modern Greek is actually two languages: demotic, or spoken Greek, which is
highly colloquial, and *Katharevousa*, or purist Greek,
which is much more formal, containing many words
not used in everyday speech. Among partisans of demotic, Kazantzakis was a member of the most radical
group. He campaigned to have it adopted as the official
language of the nation—the language used in schools.
He wrote educational materials in demotic, as well
as essays and popular articles advocating its use; he
intransigently employed words and constructions rejected by all but the most extreme demoticists.

Nowhere is Kazantzakis's passion for demotic
demonstrated more clearly than in *The Odyssey*. He
composed this masterwork over a period of fourteen
years, during which he spent much time traveling the
back roads of his own country, gathering words in the
way a more traditional scholar might gather old letters
or documents. Indeed, *The Odyssey* has been described
by author Peter Bien as a repository of demotic words
and phrases, an encyclopedic compendium of the spoken language gathering the pungent idioms of Greek
fishermen and shepherds, country people and common
folk.

Hence, at its best, *The Odyssey* has an immediacy
and a freshness in its imagery that truly makes it a rival
of its classical forebear. At its worst, however, as many
critics have been quick to point out, the language of the
poem violates the very principles that it is supposed to
embody, for Kazantzakis's extreme demoticism led
him to employ many rare words—words that the Greek

reader is unlikely to have encountered anywhere else, either in speech or in writing. Nevertheless, the popularity of *The Odyssey* with the general public in Greece attests the overall success of Kazantzakis's project. The English-speaking reader is fortunate to have Kimon Friar's gifted translation, which preserves the simple, colloquial nature of Kazantzakis's original Greek. Friar also mirrors Kazantzakis's meter in English by using iambic hexameter in his translation.

The ability to synthesize the apparently conflicting philosophical views of Nietzsche and Bergson and to transform this new view of humanity into art is Kazantzakis's unique achievement as a writer. Nowhere does that synthesis become more apparent than in *The Odyssey*, where these two opposing philosophies appear almost at war in a plethora of images that vivify abstract philosophical principles. In the poem, one can see the idea of the human existential struggle to assert individuality and importance in a world without meaning portrayed with insight and technical skill. Kazantzakis's Odysseus, like the heroes of his later novels, appears larger than life, for Kazantzakis believed that the truly great man always rises above the limitations of the flesh and works toward a state of complete spirituality, setting himself apart from the masses, who are content to live without questioning the meaning of their existence. Like other great writers of the twentieth century, Kazantzakis has been able to mine the events of his own life, the history of his nation, and the myths of Western culture with equal success to produce poetry that strikes the reader with its penetrating insight into universal human problems.

BIOGRAPHY

Nikos Kazantzakis was born in 1883, in a land that had for centuries been the site of bitter struggles for independence from the Turks. One of his first memories was of a night when, at the age of six, while with his family hiding from the Turks, his father made him swear to help kill the women of their family rather than let the marauders have their way with them. Fortunately, Kazantzakis did not have to carry out the promise.

In 1902, Kazantzakis left Crete to study at the University of Athens. Upon graduation in 1906, he de-

parted for Paris, where he was introduced to the works of Nietzsche and Bergson. Kazantzakis returned to Athens, where he presented his dissertation on Nietzsche to the faculty of the university to gain a teaching position there. A proponent of "positive nihilism," Kazantzakis saw himself as a prophet who would use his art to "save" the world. Until 1921, he remained in Greece, writing (primarily plays) and taking an active part in business and government. For a brief period, he was a member of the Greek government under prime minister Eleftherios Venizelos, but when Venizelos fell from power, Kazantzakis, disillusioned, left for Paris.

Kazantzakis spent much of the remainder of his life in restless travel. Even when he was relatively settled on the island of Aegina, he often went away, either to the mainland of Greece or to other parts of Europe. His 1907 marriage to Galatea Alexiou lasted only briefly, and he enjoyed a succession of female companions in the various places he visited. His relationship with Helen Samiou, which began in 1924, finally culminated in marriage in 1945.

In the mid-1920's, Kazantzakis traveled in France, Germany, Austria, and Italy, and later to the Middle East and Egypt, living on the scant revenues from works submitted to Greek magazines. His professed communism caused him some trouble at home but secured for him an invitation to the tenth anniversary of the Russian Revolution in Moscow in 1927. His experiences there provided the material for a book in which he explained his theory of "metacommunism."

During the 1920's, Kazantzakis decided to embody his own beliefs about the role and destiny of modern humanity in a long sequel to Homer's *Odyssey*. In 1924, Kazantzakis began the first draft of the poem. For the next fourteen years, he worked on this project diligently, carefully revising and shaping the work he was to consider his masterpiece. The poem went through numerous revisions—including seven major drafts— but always Kazantzakis had in mind his goal of re-creating in the Homeric character a concrete representation of modern humanity's struggle to give meaning to life. During these years, Kazantzakis's own life was something of a struggle. He spent part of the time in Gottesgab, Czechoslovakia, part in other areas of Europe, especially Spain, constantly engaged in other works to support himself and Helen Samiou so that he could continue with his poem.

The experiences garnered during these years of travel found their way into *The Odyssey*, too, as Kazantzakis himself pointed out in letters to numerous friends. In 1938, an American patron was so moved by the beauty of the poem that she offered to fund the publication of a limited edition. Kazantzakis accepted, and in that year a press run of three hundred copies was issued under the supervision of Helen Samiou. Though the poem was slow to gain critical acceptance, the young people of Greece and Crete found much to like in Kazantzakis's epic.

Kazantzakis's personal odyssey took him to Great Britain in 1939, then back to Aegina, where he spent the war years writing and translating and quietly supporting the resistance movement against the German occupation force. Although in 1941 he had said that he was not comfortable working as a novelist, in 1943, Kazantzakis turned to that form to portray a part of his personal history; the result was his most famous work, known to English-speaking readers as *Zorba the Greek*.

In 1946, the Greek Society of Men of Letters proposed Kazantzakis for the Nobel Prize in Literature. That nomination was repeated several times in succeeding years, and men such as Thomas Mann and Albert Schweitzer supported Kazantzakis's candidacy. Though he never received the Nobel Prize, Kazantzakis seemed unaffected. The postwar years saw him resume his travels on the Continent and in Great Britain, and in 1947, he was appointed director of UNESCO's Department of Translation of the Classics. During the final years of his life, he resurrected old manuscripts and returned to subjects that had haunted him for years, producing a series of novels. He continued to write plays as well and planned several major dramas that never materialized. During the 1950's, sponsorship by literary figures such as Max Tau in Germany, Borje Knos in Sweden, and Max Schuster in America provided opportunities for Kazantzakis's works to reach audiences throughout Europe and the English-speaking world.

By 1952, Kazantzakis's health had begun to fail,

and in 1954, he enrolled in a clinic in Freiburg, where he was diagnosed as suffering from a form of leukemia. Undaunted, he continued to write and travel, returning to Freiburg for treatment when necessary. On a tour of Japan and China in 1957, he received a bad vaccination; though he returned immediately to Freiburg for medical attention, he died in the clinic there on October 26.

ANALYSIS

It has been said that Nikos Kazantzakis tells one story and that his novels, plays, and poems merely provide different historical backdrops to a single universal theme: the struggle of humans to learn the truth about themselves and about God. There is little doubt that humankind's search for God is at the center of all of Kazantzakis's writings, and his early philosophical tract, *Salvatores Dei: Asketike* (1927; *The Saviors of God: Spiritual Exercises*, 1960), provides a gloss for his entire life's work. Initially a follower of Nietzsche, who had proclaimed the death of God, Kazantzakis adopted the belief that the God of the Christian and Jewish traditions was indeed dead, that the hard facts of evolution had proven conclusively that traditional beliefs were inadequate to explain or justify the human condition. Nevertheless, Kazantzakis did not abandon the notion of God altogether; rather, for him the term "God" represented a kind of omega point, a teleological focus for all of humankind's endeavors toward self-fulfillment. In a curious twist of logic, Kazantzakis saw God as needing humans as much as humans need him, for God is created by humans as the embodiment of all that humans hope to be. Ultimately, though, humans must come to the realization that life is essentially meaningless and that whatever meaning they give to their existence is purely self-imposed. It is the fate of the truly heroic individual to pursue the quest for meaning in spite of his knowledge that the quest is futile, to raise a cry against this horrible fact that the only end for humans is the abyss of nothingness that awaits them at death. It should not be surprising, then, to find that the poem Kazantzakis considered his greatest literary achievement deals with religious and philosophical questions, and that his hero wrestles with metaphysical issues.

THE ODYSSEY

The reader first confronting Kazantzakis's *The Odyssey* is most often struck by its length; twice as long as its Homeric namesake, the poem is consciously epic both in scope and in structure. Kazantzakis employed traditional conventions, but he did so in a way that was distinctly modern. The hero's voyage and quest provide the structural framework in which dozens of seemingly disparate adventures reveal character and illuminate themes. The diversity of action and the cast of characters are exceptionally great, as is the geographical sweep of the poem: Odysseus begins his second great voyage in Greece, travels across the Mediterranean Sea and the African continent, and ends his wanderings in the Antarctic.

The Odyssey can best be classified as part of a tradition started soon after Homer composed his *Odyssey*, that of the "continuation" epic. The poem relates the further adventures of Odysseus, who as early as the fifth century B.C.E. was considered by readers of Homer's epic to be ill suited to a life of leisure on Ithaca after twenty years of wandering about the Mediterranean basin. From his classical source, Kazantzakis has taken not only his main character, but also others whose stories he chooses to complete (Telemachus, Laertes). Kazantzakis has also gone to the *Iliad* for a handful of other Homeric figures (Helen of Troy, Menelaus, Idomeneus). Figures from Greek mythology such as Heracles, Tantalus, and Prometheus figure prominently in the work as well.

Following the long-standing tradition of Homeric continuations, Kazantzakis begins *The Odyssey* with his hero already returned to power in Ithaca, having killed Penelope's suitors. Odysseus's wanderlust leads him to reject quickly the domestic life on his island (his people, including Telemachus, find him unbearable as well). Odysseus assembles about him a band of adventurers with whom he departs on a journey he knows will end in death. In succession, he travels to Sparta, where he abducts a willing Helen, languishing at home with Menelaus; to Knossos, where he helps topple a society that, though once the cradle of Western civilization, is now hopelessly corrupt; to Africa, where he fights to overthrow the ineffectual and decadent Pharaoh and his court; and through the African desert and up the Nile to its source, where he constructs a city for his followers, a band that now numbers in the hundreds. His utopian city is destroyed by an earthquake, however, and at that point Odysseus abandons all his followers and becomes a great ascetic, wandering alone about Africa until he reaches the ocean. There, he embarks on a ship built in the shape of a coffin, sailing south to the Antarctic; in that southern clime, he has one last brush with civilization, in an Eskimo-like village whose inhabitants are all killed by a natural disaster just as Odysseus leaves them. The hero then sails alone until he meets his death on an iceberg.

This short summary hardly does justice to the wide variety of incidents that make up the poem. Throughout, however, Kazantzakis gives his work unity through a series of images that constantly remind the reader that the poem is more than mere adventure. As Kimon Friar points out in the introduction to his translation, "sun, flame, fire, and light compose the chief imagery" in the poem; these symbolize for Kazantzakis pure spirit—the real goal of Odysseus's search. Perhaps almost as important is Kazantzakis's use of birds to suggest both the various qualities of human characters and the constant struggle of humanity to emerge from the physical world and enter the realm of the purely spiritual. Most important among these references are those that associate human characteristics with specific species. Odysseus's mind is described on more than one occasion as a "hovering hawk" or a "hunting hawk"; the hero calls himself a "black crow" patiently waiting to wreak destruction; on another occasion, he speaks of his mind as "an eagle, grasping Africa in its claws." Helen is a "decoy-bird"; Odysseus's heart is like a "caged bird"; he is told by a wise craftsman in Knossos that freedom makes one's soul soar like "a giddy bird." On numerous occasions, bird imagery is used to explain the nature of God himself. One example is particularly illustrative. Speaking with a fellow prisoner in Egypt, Odysseus says that God "spreads the enormous wing of good from his right side,/ the wing of evil from his left, then springs and soars./ If only we could be like God, to fly with wayward wings!"

THE NATURE OF ODYSSEUS AS HERO

Perhaps the best way to appreciate both the poetry and the philosophy of Kazantzakis's epic is to examine the nature of his hero. Though modeled closely on Homer's Odysseus, Kazantzakis's Odysseus carries a greater symbolic load than his classical predecessor. First, he is a representative of the author himself. During the years when Kazantzakis was first composing the poem, he once referred to himself as Don Odysseus, and indeed the experiences Kazantzakis gleaned from a lifetime of travel are embodied in his hero. Furthermore, Odysseus is presented as a type of Everyman—or better, of the existential person. His external travels are paralleled by the internal struggle he constantly faces within himself as he tries to free himself from the entanglements of the flesh and "ascend to God." Odysseus is constantly reminding himself and others that nothing in life has any real meaning, but the struggle to establish meaning (even while knowing that the attempt will end in failure) motivates him and gives him real stature among men.

Always fond of adjectives, Kazantzakis uses them lavishly to describe Odysseus. The epithets that characterize Kazantzakis's hero reveal similarities with his Homeric predecessor and establish his position as a Kazantzakian seeker for God and truth. At times, he is the crafty, ruthless warrior of Homer's *Odyssey*, called by various sobriquets, such as "archer," "fox-minded man," "much-traveled man," "worldwide roamer," "double faced," "resourceful," "sly," and "swifthanded." He is, unlike the classical Odysseus, also a "soul seizer," "soul leader," "deep-sighted man," the "man of seven souls," often a "heaven baiter" and a "mind battler." He takes on the characteristics of other famous characters, or meets with them in various guises in the course of his wanderings. In the crucial books of the poem immediately preceding the construction of his ideal city (books 12 through 15), he shares many characteristics with the biblical Moses, leading his people out of Egypt, communing with his "God" atop the mountain, entering into a promised land and establishing a utopian community. Later, he meets with Captain Sole (Don Quixote) and the black fisher boy (Christ), with whom he debates about the right way to face the trials of life.

Face them he does, directly and uncompromisingly, in a fashion distinctly Kazantzakian. Odysseus at times indulges almost to excess in the pleasures of the flesh; at other times, he eschews such activity with intensity

and sincerity. In him, perhaps more than in any other character in the canon of Kazantzakis's works, one can see the twin tendencies toward asceticism and sensuality that Kazantzakis perceived to be the essence of the human condition.

Odysseus's clear vision of the human condition causes him to act ruthlessly at times, even with his God. For him, humans' greatest task is to defy their fate and assert their independence: "I drink not to the gods," he tells his people upon returning to Ithaca, "but to man's dauntless mind!" "The awesome ancient gods are now but poor bugbears," he says on another occasion. When Menelaus tells him that humans become a kind of god by following their fate, Odysseus replies: "I think man's greatest duty on earth is to fight his fate,/ to give no quarter and blot out his written doom./ This is how mortal man may even surpass his god!" Clearly, Odysseus's "God" is not the traditional Christian deity; rather he is the God Kazantzakis conceived of early in his own life, described in *The Saviors of God* as a deity dependent on humanity for his existence as much as humanity is traditionally thought to depend on God.

Thus, Odysseus proclaims a new set of commandments for the existential world. The "ten command ments" he chisels in stone in his new city in Africa provide a capsule of Kazantzakis's own philosophy: "God groans, he writhes within my heart for help"; God "chokes" in the ground, and "leaps from every grave"; God "stifles" all living things, and all living things "are his cofighters." Man himself must "love wretched man at length, for he is you, my son." Additionally, he must "love plants and beasts . . . the entire earth." Man must each day "deny [his] joys, [his] wealth, [his] victories, all" because "the greatest virtue on earth is not to become free/ but to seek freedom in a ruthless, sleepless strife."

Beside his commandments, Odysseus carves an arrow shooting toward the sun, symbolizing man's ascent toward the special God that Kazantzakis conceives of as one with man in the struggle to make meaning of his existence. By these rules, Kazantzakis's hero lives his own life; by them, Kazantzakis suggests that modern humans may come to give meaning to their lives, not because life has meaning, but because the struggle to achieve human perfectibility will itself provide joy (the Bergsonian élan vital) in the midst of the tragedy that Kazantzakis, following Nietzsche, sees at the root of the human condition.

OTHER MAJOR WORKS

LONG FICTION: *Ophis kai krino*, 1906 (*Serpent and Lily*, 1980); *Toda Raba*, 1929 (English translation, 1964); *De tuin der Rosten*, 1939 (better known as *Le Jardin des rochers*; *The Rock Garden*, 1963); *Vios kai politeia tou Alexe Zormpa*, 1946 (*Zorba the Greek*, 1952); *Ho Kapetan Michales*, 1953 (*Freedom or Death*, 1956; also known as *Freedom and Death: A Novel*); *Ho Christos xanastauronetai*, 1954 (*The Greek Passion*, 1953; also known as *Christ Recrucified*); *Ho teleutaios peirasmos*, 1955 (*The Last Temptation of Christ*, 1960; also known as *The Last Temptation*); *Ho phtochoules tou Theou*, 1956 (*Saint Francis*, 1962; also known as *God's Pauper: Saint Francis of Assisi*); *Hoi aderphophades*, 1963 (*The Fratricides*, 1964).

PLAYS: *Xemeronei*, pr. 1907; *Melissa*, pr. 1939; *Kouros*, pr. 1955; *Christophoros Kolomvos*, pr. 1956; *Three Plays: Melissa, Kouros, Christopher Columbus*, 1969.

NONFICTION: *Salvatores Dei: Asketike*, 1927 (*The Saviors of God: Spiritual Exercises*, 1960); *Ispania*, 1937 (*Spain*, 1963); *Ho Morias*, 1937 (serial; 1961, book; *Journey to the Morea*, 1965); *Iaponia-Kina*, 1938 (*Japan/China*, 1963); *Anghlia*, 1941 (*England*, 1965); *Anaphora ston Greko: Mythistorema*, 1961 (autobiography; *Report to Greco*, 1965).

BIBLIOGRAPHY

Bien, Peter. *Kazantzakis: Politics of the Spirit*. Princeton, N.J.: Princeton University Press, 1989. This study focuses on the evolution of Kazantzakis's personal philosophy up to the point of his publication in 1938 of *The Odyssey*. Properly documented with a rich international bibliography, a detailed chronology, and an index of names and titles.

_____. *Nikos Kazantzakis*. New York: Columbia University Press, 1972. A reliable scholarly introduction to Kazantzakis's life and work, with a useful bibliography.

Dombrowski, Daniel A. *Kazantzakis and God*. Albany: State University of New York Press, 1997. Contains chapters on the Bergsonian background, transubstantiation, eating and spiritual exercise, the new Middle Ages, theism, mysticism, method and purpose, and panexperientialism and death. Dombrowski also has an appendix on Friedrich Nietzsche's place in Kazantzakis's thought. Includes notes, bibliography, and an index of names.

Kazantzakis, Helen. *Nikos Kazantzakis: A Biography Based on His Letters*. New York: Simon & Schuster, 1968. A valuable collection of letters and photographs arranged chronologically. The letters are only lightly annotated.

Lea, James F. *Kazantzakis: The Politics of Salvation*. University: University of Alabama Press, 1979. Presents an overview of the writer's career; closely examines his use of language; studies his poetry, prophetic style, and political philosophy; and discusses his search for order in chaos. Chapter 5 concludes with his vision of freedom and hope. With detailed notes and bibliography.

Middleton, Darren J. N. *Broken Hallelujah: Nikos Kazantzakis and Christian Theology*. Lanham, Md.: Lexington Books, 2007. An examination of Kazantzakis's religious beliefs and how they affected his writings.

Newton, Rick M. "Homer and the Death of Kazantzakis' Odysseus." *Classical and Modern Literature* 9, no. 4 (Summer, 1989): 327-338. This study contrasts Homer's Odysseus with Kazantzakis's more extensive treatment of the hero's voyage. Provides insights into Kazantzakis's poetics.

Stanford, W. B. *The Ulysses Theme: A Study in the Adaptability of a Traditional Hero*. 2d ed. Oxford, England: Basil Blackwell, 1963. This book contains some valuable insights into Kazantzakis' poem, particularly with reference to his concept of the hero. Only some twenty pages are given to his work, however, mostly in comparison with Joyce.

Laurence W. Mazzeno

KARL KRAUS

Born: Gitschin, Bohemia (now Jičin, Czech
    Republic); April 28, 1874
Died: Vienna, Austria; June 12, 1936

PRINCIPAL POETRY

Worte in Versen, 1916-1930 (9 volumes)
Poems, 1930
Dicta and Contradicta, 2001

OTHER LITERARY FORMS

Karl Kraus (krows), widely regarded as one of the
greatest mid-twentieth century satirists, is not known
primarily as a poet. His powerful cultural criticism took
several forms, and poetry was but one of them. Kraus
was most effective as a writer of prose, producing thousands of essays and aphorisms. He is also important as a
dramatist, his greatest work in that form being his pacifist play *Die letzten Tage der Menschheit* (pb. 1922;
The Last Days of Mankind, 1974), written during
World War I. Most of Kraus's writings first appeared in
his own journal, *Die Fackel*.

ACHIEVEMENTS

The vitriolic Karl Kraus, who hauled the powerful
and the pitiful alike before a tribunal of total satire, was
a legend in his lifetime, both adored and vilified by his
contemporaries. Following a decade of desuetude, his
work was rediscovered and reissued in Germany and
Austria after World War II. Numerous editions, studies, and translations have focused critical attention on
this satirist, whose dictum (*Spruch*) or contradiction
(*Widerspruch*), "I have to wait until my writings are ob-
solete; then they may acquire timeliness," seems to be
coming true. As literary critic and historian of German
literature Erich Heller has put it,

> Karl Kraus did not write "in a language," but through him
> the beauty, profundity, and accumulated moral experi-
> ence of the German language assumed personal shape
> and became the crucial witness in the case this inspired
> prosecutor brought against his time.

Kraus's timeliness and, at long last, his relative ex-
portability derive at least in part from certain parallels
between his age and the early twenty-first century, which
has need of his vibrant pacifism; his principled defense
of the spirit against dehumanizing tendencies; and his
"linguistic-moral imperative," as literary critic and expert
of German literature J. P. Stern puts it, which equates
purity of language with purity of thought, a return to the
sources of spiritual strength, and steadfastness of moral
purpose. Kraus lived a life that oscillated between love
and hate. "Hatred must make a person productive," he
once wrote; "otherwise one might as well love."

The thirty-seven volumes of *Die Fackel* represent a
gigantic effort to fashion the imperishable profile of an
age from such highly perishable materials as newspaper reports. The journal was an enormous pillory, a running autobiography, a uniquely personal history of
Austria-Hungary (an empire that Kraus regarded as a
"proving ground for the end of the world"), and a world
stage on which Kraus dramatized himself and his satiric mission. His markedly apocalyptic stance as a
"late" warner derives from his epoch's Zeitgeist: transitoriness, disintegration, and inner insecurity.

Kraus's unremitting satirical warfare against the
press (and in particular the influential *Neue freie Presse*
of Vienna) was motivated by his view of journalism as
a vast switchboard that concentrated and activated the
forces of corruption, dissolution, and decay. Recognizing a disturbing identity of *Zeit* and *Zeitung*, the age
and the newspapers it spawned, with *Worte* ("words")
usurping and destroying *Werte* ("values"), he had apocalyptic visions of the world being obliterated by the
black magic of printer's ink. Decades before Hermann
Hesse coined the phrase *das feuilletonistische Zeitalter*
("the pamphleteering period") in his utopian novel *Das
Glasperlenspiel: Versuch einer Lebensbeschreibung
des Magister Ludi Josef Knecht samt Knechts hinterlassenen Schriften* (1943; *Magister Ludi*, 1949; also
known as *The Glass Bead Game*, 1969), Kraus recognized his age as "the age of the *feuilleton*," in which
newspaper reports took precedence over events; form
eclipsed substance; and the style, the atmosphere, the
"package" were all-important. Excoriating the press,
that "goiter of the world," for its pollution of language
and its poisoning of the human spirit, Kraus anticipated
the judgments of contemporary critics of the media,
and his diagnosis still has relevance.

BIOGRAPHY

Karl Kraus was the son of a prosperous manufacturer of paper bags, and the family fortune supported him to a large extent for most of his life. In 1877, the family moved to Vienna, and Kraus spent the rest of his life in that city, with which he—like Sigmund Freud—had a love-hate relationship. After attending the University of Vienna without earning a degree, Kraus attempted a career on the stage. His failure as an actor irrevocably steered him to journalism and literature, though his talent for mimicry and parody as well as his penchant for verbal play found ample expression in his later public readings as well as in his writings. In 1892, Kraus began to contribute book reviews, drama criticism, and other prose to various newspapers and periodicals. In his twenties, however, his satirical impulse became too strong for any kind of accommodation, and

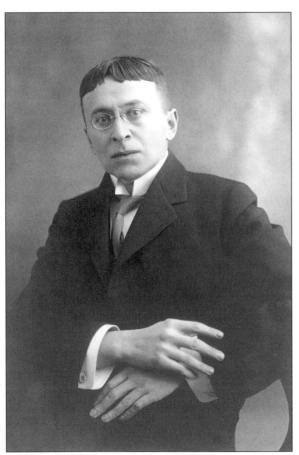

Karl Kraus (Hulton Archive/Getty Images)

Kraus rejected the prospect of becoming a sort of "culture clown" absorbed by a deceptively slack and effete environment and accorded, as he put it, "the accursed popularity which a grinning Vienna bestows."

Because work within the establishment seemed to be hedged in with multifarious taboos and considerations of a commercial and personal nature, Kraus rejected a job offer from the *Neue freie Presse* and founded his own journal, *Die Fackel*, the first issue of which appeared on April 1, 1899, and which from the beginning had an incomparably satiric *genius loci*. After 1911, the irregularly issued periodical contained Kraus's writings exclusively: "I no longer have contributors," he wrote. "I used to be envious of them. They repel those readers whom I want to lose myself." Kraus's periodical did continue to have numerous "contributors," albeit unwitting and unwilling ones: the people who were copiously quoted in its pages and allowed to hang themselves with the nooses of their own statements, attitudes, and actions.

Kraus's first major works were a literary satire titled *Die demolirte Literatur* (1897; the demolished literature), a witty diatribe about the razing of a Vienna café frequented by the literati, and an anti-Zionist pamphlet, *Eine Krone für Zion* (1898; a crown for Zion). (Kraus left the Jewish fold as early as 1898 and was secretly baptized as a Roman Catholic in 1911, but he broke with the Church eleven years later and thereafter remained unaffiliated with any religious group. He has been called everything from "an arch-Jew" and "an Old Testament prophet who pours cataracts of wrath over his own people" to "a shining example of Jewish self-hatred.") If Kraus's early writings were directed largely against standard aspects of corruption, the second period of his creativity may be dated from the appearance of his essay *Sittlichkeit und Kriminalität* (1902, reissued in book form in 1908; morality and criminal justice), in which Kraus concerned himself, on the basis of contemporary court cases, with the glaring contrast between private and public morality and with the hypocrisy inherent in the administration of justice in Austria. In turning a powerful spotlight on a male-dominated society with its double standard, shameless encroachments on privacy, and sensation-mongering press, Kraus dealt with many subjects and attitudes that are germane to present-day problems: education, women's rights, sexual mores, and child abuse. The gloomy, bitter wit of such essays gave way to lighter humor in Kraus's next collection, *Die chinesische Mauer* (1910; the Great Wall of China).

The outbreak of the war in 1914 marked a turning point in Kraus's life and creativity, and the outraged convictions of the pacifist and moralist inspired him to produce his most powerful and most characteristic work. Following several months of silence, Kraus delivered a sardonic public lecture on November 19, 1914. "In dieser grossen Zeit . . ." (in these great times) may be regarded as the germ of his extensive wartime output. Kraus set himself up as the lonely, bold, uncompromising chronicler of what he termed "the last days of mankind" and "the Day of Judgment" for the benefit of a posterity that might no longer inhabit the planet Earth. Kraus's mammoth and all-but-unperformable play *The Last Days of Mankind*, written between July, 1915, and July, 1917, first appeared in several special issues of *Die Fackel* and then in book form. Its 209 scenes, with prologue and epilogue, take place "in a hundred scenes and hells" and feature people who, in Kraus's view, had all the stature, substance, and veracity of characters in an operetta yet were bent on enacting the tragedy of humankind. The play is a sort of *phonomontage* in that the hundreds of real as well as fictitious persons reveal and judge themselves through their authentic speech patterns, with the satirist attempting to make language the moral index of a dying way of life as he uses actual speeches, newspaper editorials, war communiqués, and other documents.

The story of Kraus's postwar writings and polemics is basically the history of his disillusionment as his "homeland's loyal hater." The best that Kraus could say about the Austrian republic, a small country that was still bedeviled by "the parasites remaining from the imperial age and the blackheads of the revolution," was that it had replaced the monarchy and had rid Kraus of "that burdensome companion, the other K. K." (The reference is to the abbreviation of *kaiserlich-königlich*, "royal-imperial," the designation of many Austro-Hungarian institutions.) In the 1920's, Kraus engaged in extended polemics with the publicist Maximilian Harden (once an admired model), the critic Alfred

Kerr, and the poet Franz Werfel (one of several apostles turned apostates). He castigated the unholy alliance between a police chief, Johannes Schober, and a crooked press czar, Imre Békessy, and Kraus succeeded with his spirited campaign to "kick the crook out of Vienna." The literary harvest of the Schober-Békessy affair was another documentary drama, *Die Unüberwindlichen* (pb. 1928; the unconquerables). Another of the plays written in the 1920's was *Wolkenkuckucksheim* (pb. 1923; cloudcuckooland), a verse play based on Aristophanes and presenting a sort of Last Days of Birdkind but with a Shakespearean solo by the lark at the end promising conciliation and peace.

Beginning in 1925, Kraus used *Theater der Dichtung* ("theater of poetry," or "literary theater") as a designation for many of his public readings of his own works and those of others, spellbinding one-person shows in which he presented poetry, prose, and entire plays to large audiences. (By the end of his life, he had made seven hundred such presentations in various cities.) These readings must be regarded as an integral part of his creativity and perhaps even as the apogee of his effectiveness. Kraus may be credited with the revival of interest in the nineteenth century Viennese playwright and actor Johann Nestroy, whom he presented in his full stature as a powerful social satirist and linguistic genius. William Shakespeare was also a living force in Kraus's life, and between 1916 and 1936, the satirist recited his adaptations of thirteen Shakespearean plays, also publishing two collections of plays and the sonnets in his translation. Kraus's special relationship with Jacques Offenbach dated back to his boyhood; he adapted and performed, with a piano accompanist, many of Offenbach's operettas. He appreciated these in programmatic contrast to the Viennese operetta of his time, which he regarded as inane, meretricious, and unwholesome.

"Mir fällt zu Hitler nichts ein" ("I can't think of anything to say about Hitler") is the striking first sentence of Kraus's prose work *Die dritte Walpurgisnacht* (pb. 1952; the third Walpurgis Night). The title refers to both parts of Johann Wolfgang von Goethe's *Faust: Eine Tragödie* (pb. 1808, 1833; *The Tragedy of Faust*, 1823, 1838) as well as to the Third Reich. It was written in 1933 but not published in its entirety during Kraus's lifetime. That sentence, which lies at the heart of the misunderstandings and conflicts that marked and marred Kraus's last years, may have been indicative of resignation (though he could think of many things to say about Hitler and did indeed say them), but it was also a hyperbolic, heuristic device for depicting the Witches' Sabbath of the time. The satirist sadly realized the incommensurability of the human spirit with the unspeakably brutal and mindless power across the German border. Once again, language was in mortal danger, and the perpetrators of the new horrors obviously were not characters from an operetta.

In voicing genuine concern over Germany's pressure on his homeland, Kraus for once found himself in Austria's corner. Paradoxically, this led him to side with the clerico-fascist regime of Chancellor Engelbert Dollfuss, whose assassination in 1934 came as a severe shock to Kraus. Many of the satirist's erstwhile adherents expected him to join them in their struggle against Hitlerism, but they were disappointed at what they regarded as the equivocation of the essentially apolitical satirist. *Die Fackel* appeared at even more irregular intervals than before, and Kraus was content to reduce his readership to those who not only heard "the trumpets of the day" but also cared about Shakespeare, Nestroy, Offenbach, and German style, including Kraus's unique "comma problems." Preparing to "live in the safe sentence structure," Kraus strove pathetically and futilely to pit the word against the sword. His death of heart failure at the end of a long period of physical and spiritual exhaustion mercifully saved him from witnessing the Nazi takeover of Austria (to the cheers of most of its population), the destruction of his belongings, the deaths of close friends in concentration camps, and untold other horrors.

ANALYSIS

Karl Kraus's poetry was not fully appreciated in his lifetime, being decried as derivative and excessively cerebral. After his death, however, his poetry has come to be regarded as an integral and important part of his oeuvre, and critics such as Werner Kraft, Leopold Liegler, and Caroline Kohn have written perceptively about this aspect of Kraus's creativity. When one realizes that much of Kraus's prose is lyrical or poetic, it is easy to see his poetry as only a special coinage from the same mint.

Kraus began to write poetry relatively late in life; his first poems did not appear in *Die Fackel* until 1912 and 1913, but then nine volumes of poetry and rhymed epigrams were published between 1916 and 1930 under the modest collective title *Worte in Versen*. In his verse, Kraus admittedly was an epigone rather than an innovator, indebted to the Goethean and Shakespearean traditions. He was "unoriginal" in that he usually needed some occasion to trigger his art. The poems are seldom Romantic in the sense of being products of rapture or intoxication; rather, they spring from the inspirations of language and logic.

Some of Kraus's poems are versified glosses and polemics, lyric versions of prose texts, or satiric ideas given purified and aesthetically appealing forms; others represent autobiographical excursions. Their abstraction and concision often presuppose familiarity with Kraus's other works, his life, and his personality; in this sense, the poems add up to a lyrical roman à clef. "I do not write poetry and then work with dross," Kraus once wrote; "I turn the dross into poetry and organize rallies in support of poetry." To a certain extent, Kraus's poetry is *Gedankenlyrik* in Friedrich Schiller's sense—poetry with a cargo of thought, reflecting a tradition coming to an end and an effort to preserve that tradition. The satirical poems are really *Gebrauchslyrik*, pithy poetry with a purpose. However, Kraus's poetry also represents a kind of satirist's holiday in that the poet, so widely regarded as a hater, is here free to reveal himself fully and unabashedly in his love of humankind, the human spirit, nature, and animals. In this sense, it represents the "yea" of a great nay-sayer. Poetry to Kraus was like a freer, purer world, one harking back to the German classical tradition, in which the poet, freed from the goads of the satiric occasion and the burden of an ever-wakeful moral conscience, was able to reflect at leisure on love, nature, dreams, and wonderment.

THE ORIGIN AS THEME

The word *Ursprung* ("origin" or "source") figures prominently in Kraus's thought and poetry. In his orphic epigram "Zwei Läufer" ("Two Runners"), Kraus depicts two antithetical forces alive in the human spirit, one that he loves and one that he hates. The world is perceived as a circuitous route back to the *Ursprung*. Intellectuality may be the wrong road, but it does lead back to immediacy; satire is a roundabout way to poetry; and poetry, to Kraus, is a philosophical or linguistic detour on the way to a lost paradise. Kraus saw himself as being midway between *Ursprung* and *Untergang*, the "origin" or "source" of all things and the end of the world (or of the human spirit) as conjured up by his satiric vision, and he viewed language as the only means of going back to the origin—the origin that was forever the goal. This *Ursprung* represents a kind of naïve realism, a secular idea of Creation that is diametrically opposed to the tendency of speculative philosophy to make *homo cogitans*, cerebral man, the center of reality. In contrast to this, Kraus posits the unity of feeling and form from which all art, morality, and truth spring. This world of purity constitutes a timeless counterpoise to the world against which Kraus the satirist struggled, and such an inviolate nature stands in mute yet eloquent contrast to a contemporary world and society that Kraus, in a sardonic pun fully comprehensible only through an awareness of the subtleties of synonymous German prefixes, perceived not as a *Gegenwart* ("present time") but as a *Widerwart* ("repulsive age").

WORTE IN VERSEN

In his poetry, Kraus was guided by his conviction that the quality of a poem depended on the moral stature and ethical mission of the poet ("A poem is good until one knows by whom it is"). In his view, a satirist is only a deeply hurt lyricist, the artist wounded by the ugliness of the world. In *Worte in Versen*, rhyme and meaning are inseparably fused. Kraus's conception of rhyme is similar to that of the German Romantic critic Friedrich Schlegel, who described rhyme as the surprising reunion of friendly ideas after a long separation. Kraus's poem "Der Reim" ("The Rhyme"), for example, underscores this concept through the use of macaronic form: "Rhyme is the landing shore/ for two thoughts *en rapport*."

"NOCTURNAL HOUR" AND "THE DAY"

Two of Kraus's best-known poems make reference to his nocturnal working habits. "Nächtliche Stunde" ("Nocturnal Hour"), set to music by Eugen Auerbach

in 1929, is a profound and poignant expression of Kraus's situation, written with great visionary power and economy of syntax and symbolism. It is structurally notable for the recurring unrhymed first and last lines of each of its three stanzas and the reiteration of the theme of transitoriness in the opening line of each. There is an increasing sense of inwardness and depth until the final synthesis of night, winter, life, spring, and death. Kraus himself pointed out that three times the unrhymed last line belongs to "the bird's voice which accompanies the experience of work through the stages of night, winter, and life." Presumably, what the poet considers, weighs, and grades as he works is the possibility of changing this "language-forsaken" world through his efforts; a hero of creative work in Thomas Mann's sense, he continues to do his duty even as death approaches.

The beautiful poem "Der Tag" ("The Day"), set to music by Kraus's long-time piano accompanist, Franz Mittler, shares many of the motifs of "Nocturnal Hour." As the day breaks through the window, daring to disturb the claustrophobic intensity of the satirist's nocturnal labors, the bleary-eyed writer expresses surprise at the fact that the impure, desecrated day has the audacity to dawn after an apocalyptic night of struggle with the affairs of an ungodly, corrupt world—matters that the Zeitgeist keeps presenting in violation of an ideal, undefiled realm of pure humanity. The satirist has borne witness to the possibility of such humanity and has in mute, joyless toil erected an edifice of words in its support. The memento mori provided by a hearse outside, carrying some poor soul to his or her final resting place, gives the satirist an awareness of earthly evanescence and fills him with boundless sympathy with human suffering. His self-effacing, fanatical work in the service of the word, his ceaseless defense of language, and his search for eternal truths as a bulwark against the encroachments of the age have distinctly religious overtones: His prayer is for the poor soul outside as well as for himself but especially for a humankind gone astray and bound for perdition. It is properly understood, however, only in a larger context. Franz Kafka once described his obsessive writing as a form of prayer, and this was also Kraus's conception of his own work. One of his aphorisms is pertinent here: "When I take up my pen, nothing can happen to me. Fate, remember that!"

Ernst Krenek, who came under Kraus's spell at an early age, has included settings of both "Nocturnal Hour" and "The Day" in his song cycle *Durch die Nacht* (through the night), composed in 1930 and 1931, which also contains five other Kraus poems. "Schnellzug" ("Fast Train"), written in 1920 and set to music by Auerbach, has the evanescence and perceived meaninglessness of life as its theme and the dichotomy between inside and outside as its focus. The poet's staleness on a dirty, crowded train is contrasted with the fresh yet unspecific landscape outside, which tends to blur and blunt his perceptions. Though he is forced to stay aboard with the aimless multitude of his traveling companions, his disgust at his situation is a kind of rebellion. Being locked into his life of dedication and self-abnegation, he is fated to yearn for integration into the vanishing scenery.

TRIBUTE POEMS

A number of Kraus's poems are tributes to friends and other people he admired. Cases in point are "An einen alten Lehrer" (to an old teacher), a celebration of Heinrich Sedlmayer, his German and Latin teacher; "Die Schauspielerin" ("The Actress") and "Annie Kalmar," both in memory of the first of several women of uncommon physical and spiritual beauty in Kraus's life, a talented actress who died in 1901 at a tragically early age; "Peter Altenberg," a poetic obituary of one of the few contemporary writers whom Kraus befriended; and "An meinen Drucker" ("To My Printer"), a birthday tribute to Kraus's faithful printer, Georg Jahoda.

SATIRICAL POEMS

A number of satirical poems and songs form part of Kraus's plays. "Gebet" ("Prayer") is spoken by the Grumbler, the Kraus figure in *The Last Days of Mankind*, as is "Mit der Uhr in der Hand" ("With Stopwatch in Hand"), based on a 1916 news item about a submarine sinking a fully loaded troop transport in the Mediterranean in forty-three seconds. Also from that play is the trenchantly funny, self-exculpatory ditty sung by Emperor Franz Joseph in his sleep. "Die Psychoanalen" ("The Psychoanals"), from *Traumstück* (pb. 1923; dream play), is a long chorus of the killers of

dreams and blackeners of beauty, the exhibitors of inhibitions and purveyors of neuroses, people to whom even Goethe's poems are nothing but unsuccessful repressions. "Das Schoberlied" ("Schober's Song"), from *Die Unüberwindlichen*, is a mordant self-portrait of Vienna's police chief (and Austria's sometime chancellor), and "Das Lied von der Presse" ("The Song of the Press"), from the literary satire *Literatur: Oder, Man wird doch da sehen* (pr., pb. 1921; literature: or, we'll see about that), sums up Kraus's feelings about the press. Among Kraus's autobiographical poems are "Bunte Begbenheiten" ("Colorful Goings-On"), about the Salzburg Festival and its commercialization and vulgarization—for which Kraus blamed its prime movers, Hugo von Hofmannsthal and Max Reinhardt, as well as the Catholic Church—and "Nach dreissig Jahren" ("After Thirty Years"), which finds the satirist looking back on three decades of *Die Fackel* and taking stock of his achievements.

"SIDI" POEMS

Kraus evidently needed an idealized private sphere of wholeness, purity, and love to provide a counterpoint (and counterpoise) to the cacophony of corruption that he perceived all around him. Such a sphere was provided for him from 1913 to the end of his life by a Czech aristocrat, Baroness Sidonie Nádhérny von Borutin. Her family estate at Janovice, near Prague, became Kraus's *buen retiro*, a Garden of Eden six and a half hours from Vienna. A modern mythology about a Tristan and Isolde living through the last days of humankind is multifariously expressed in Kraus's letters to "Sidi" (long believed lost but rediscovered in 1969 and published five years later), in many of Kraus's poems addressed to her or inspired by shared experiences, and in the dedication of several volumes to the woman who, as Kraus once put it, had a true appreciation of only two books, "the railroad time-table and *Worte in Versen*."

Kraus proposed marriage to Sidonie on several occasions, but he was rejected and remained unmarried. Their relationship, however, survived Sidonie's engagements and marriages to other men. Among the approximately fifty "Sidi" poems are "Fernes Licht mit nahem Schein" ("Distant Light with Glow So Near") and "Wiese im Park" ("Lawn in the Park"), a poem with tragic undertones written on a sad Sunday in November, 1915. The poet wants to relieve the darkness of the times by recapturing the timeless past, in particular his childhood. His firm footing and reposeful communion with nature vanish, however, the spell is broken, and the present bleakly reasserts itself in the form of a "dead day."

USE OF SHAKESPEARE

Finally, mention must be made of Kraus's translations from William Shakespeare. Kraus, who knew little or no English (or any foreign language, for that matter), used existing German translations of Shakespeare as a basis for versions (*Nachdichtungen*, free re-creations in the spirit of the original rather than accurate translations) that, he felt, would capture Shakespeare's spirit more fully and would add his works to the treasure house of German letters more enduringly than other translations had done. In this effort, he was guided by his superior poetic sense and his unerring linguistic instinct. Commenting on Kraus's edition of Shakespeare's sonnets, Albert Bloch (Kraus's first translator into English) remarked that if Kraus had known English, his versions would not have been so beautiful. "Perhaps the result is not always immediately identifiable as Shakespeare," the reviewer admits; "certainly it is always undeniably Karl Kraus."

OTHER MAJOR WORKS

PLAYS: *Literatur: Oder, Man wird doch da sehn*, pr., pb. 1921; *Die letzen Tage der Menschheit*, pb. 1922 (*The Last Days of Mankind*, 1974); *Traumstück*, pb. 1923 (verse play); *Wolkenkuckucksheim*, pb. 1923 (verse play); *Traumtheater*, pb. 1924; *Die Unüberwindlichen*, pb. 1928; *Dramen*, pb. 1967.

NONFICTION: *Die demolirte Literatur*, 1897; *Eine Krone für Zion*, 1898; *Sittlichkeit und Kriminalität*, 1902, serial (1908, book); *Sprüche und Widersprüche*, 1909; *Die chinesische Mauer*, 1910; *Heine und die Folgen*, 1910; *Nestroy und die Nachwelt*, 1912; *Pro domo et mundo*, 1912; *Nachts*, 1918; *Weltgericht*, 1919, 1965 (2 volumes); *Literatur, oder Man wird doch da sehen*, 1921; *Untergang der Weltdurch schwarze Magie*, 1922, 1960; *Epigramme*, 1927; *Literatur und Lüge*, 1929, 1958; *Zeitstrophen*, 1931;

Die Sprache, 1937, 1954; *Die dritte Walpurgisnacht*, pb. 1952 (wr. 1933); *Widerschein der Fackel*, 1956; *Half-Truths and One-and-a-Half Truths: Selected Aphorisms*, 1976.

MISCELLANEOUS: *In These Great Times: A Karl Kraus Reader*, 1976; *No Compromise: Selected Writings of Karl Kraus*, 1977.

BIBLIOGRAPHY

Halliday, John D. *Karl Kraus, Franz Pfemfert, and the First World War: A Comparative Study of "Die Fackel" and "Die Aktion" Between 1911 and 1928*. Passau, Germany: Andreas-Haller, 1986. An examination of the political viewpoints of Kraus and Pfemfert as they were expressed in their periodical writings. Bibliography.

Howes, Geoffrey C. "Critical Observers of Their Time: Karl Kraus and Robert Menasse." In *Literature in Vienna at the Turn of the Centuries: Continuities and Discontinuities Around 1900 and 2000*. Rochester, N.Y.: Camden House, 2003. Howes examines the works of Kraus and Menasse and their worldviews. He examines the question of national identity and Kraus, and notes Kraus's conservatism.

Isava, Luis Miguel. *Wittgenstein, Kraus, and Valéry: A Paradigm for Poetic Rhyme and Reason*. New York: Peter Lang, 2002. Examines the poetry of Kraus, Ludwig Wittgenstein, and Paul Valéry from a phenomenological perspective.

Reitter, Paul. *The Anti-Journalist: Karl Kraus and Jewish Self-Fashioning in Fin-de-Siècle Europe*. Chicago: University of Chicago Press, 2008. Reitter argues that Kraus's criticism of Jewish journalists did not stem from anti-Semitism but rather was a constructive critique of assimilation strategies used by German Jews.

Theobald, John. *The Paper Ghetto: Karl Kraus and Anti-Semitism*. New York: Peter Lang, 1996. A study of Kraus's relationship with his Jewish heritage. Includes bibliographical references and index.

Timms, Edward. *Karl Kraus, Apocalyptic Satirist: Culture and Catastrophe in Habsburg Vienna*. New Haven, Conn.: Yale University Press, 1986. Kraus and his work in context, the first part of a biography.

_____. *Karl Kraus, Apocalyptic Satirist: The Post-*

War Crisis and the Rise of the Swastika. New Haven, Conn.: Yale University Press, 2005. Timms picks up the story in November, 1918, looking at the court cases Kraus pursued and his involvement in theatrical projects. He refutes the idea that Kraus responded with silence to the rise of Hitler.

Zohn, Harry. *Karl Kraus*. New York: Twayne, 1971. Intelligent introduction to Kraus's life and work.

_____. *Karl Kraus and the Critics*. Columbia, S.C.: Camden House, 1997. A history of the critical response to Kraus's work. Includes bibliographical references and index.

Harry Zohn

REINER KUNZE

Born: Oelsnitz, Germany; August 16, 1933

PRINCIPAL POETRY

Vögel über dem Tau, 1959
Aber die Nachtigall jubelt, 1963
Widmungen, 1963
Sensible Wege, 1969
Zimmerlautstärke, 1972 (*With the Volume Turned Down*, 1973)
Brief mit blauem Siegel, 1973
Auf eigene Hoffnung, 1981
Eines jeden einziges Leben, 1986
Nicht alle Grenzen bleiben, 1989
Am Krankenbett des Tierbildhauers, 1991
Ein Tag auf dieser Erde, 1998
Like Things Made of Clay, 2010

OTHER LITERARY FORMS

Although Reiner Kunze (KOON-sah) is known primarily as a lyric poet, he has also published two noteworthy volumes of prose and has distinguished himself as a prolific translator of modern Czech poetry. Kunze's first prose publication, *Der Löwe Leopold* (1970), was a collection of children's tales. Originally published in West Germany, the work subsequently appeared in a number of translations and was awarded the prestigious West German Youth Book Prize of 1971. It was never published in the German Democratic Republic (GDR). Kunze's second prose volume, *Die wunderbaren Jahre* (1976; *The Wonderful Years*, 1977), also appeared only in the West and consists of a series of short, critical vignettes describing various aspects of everyday life in the GDR. Kunze also worked closely with the producers of the film version of *The Wonderful Years* (1980).

ACHIEVEMENTS

Along with Günter Kunert, Volker Braun, Wolf Biermann, Sarah Kirsch, and Karl Mickel, to name only a few, Reiner Kunze belongs to the first generation of distinctively East German poets. These writers, who came of age in the late 1950's and early 1960's, took as their models poets from the preceding generation such as Peter Huchel and particularly Bertolt Brecht. Largely ignoring the prescribed canons of Socialist literary dogma, these poets lent an authentic voice to the experiences of their generation in the young GDR.

Kunze in particular helped to bring honor and credibility to East German literature, as attested by the numerous literary prizes he has won, including the aforementioned West German Youth Book Prize and the Literature Prize of the Bavarian Academy of Fine Arts. In the year 1977 alone, Kunze was awarded the Andreas Gryphius Prize, the Georg Trakl Prize, and perhaps the most prestigious of German literary prizes, the Georg Büchner Prize. He won the Eichendorff Literature Prize (1984), the Weilheimer Literature Prize (1997), the European Prize for Poetry, Serbia (1998), the Friedrich Hölderlin Literary Award (1999), the Christian-Ferber Honorary Prize of the German Schiller Foundation (2000), the Hans-Sahl Prize (2001), the Bavarian Maximilian Order for Science and the Arts (2001), the Jan-Smrek Prize (2003), the Thüringer Award for Lifetime Achievement (2008), and the Memminger Freedom Prize (2009). Because his poetic diction relies heavily on untranslatable wordplay, he is not as well known outside the German-speaking countries as he deserves to be, but few who find their way to him fail to be captivated by his sensitivity, quiet dignity, and courageous humanism.

BIOGRAPHY

Although Reiner Kunze was ultimately forbidden to publish in the GDR and even became a nonperson in the eyes of the cultural bureaucracy, it is also true that if he had not attained maturity and received his education there, he might never have taken up writing. Born to working-class parents in the region of Thuringia, Kunze was originally destined to become a shoemaker, and he was somewhat surprised to find himself in 1951 with a completed secondary school diploma, facing a choice between art studies at the Academy of Art in Dresden or studies in journalism in Leipzig. As the son of a father who had been trained as a plumber but spent most of his life as a miner and a mother who supplemented the family income by crocheting piecework in her home, Kunze was an unlikely candidate for a learned profession. In keeping with the policies of the new regime, however, Kunze's talents received active encouragement precisely because of his working-class background, and therefore, in spite of his father's strong reservations, he studied journalism, philosophy, and literature in Leipzig from 1951 to 1955. Kunze was young, idealistic, more than a little naïve, and extremely grateful to the new government that had granted him such unexpected opportunity. It is not surprising, then, that his earliest poetic works, written during this period, contain a great deal of uncritical praise of the state and of the Socialist Unity Party, which Kunze had joined in 1949. To a certain degree, he was simply repeating the clichés and formulas taught him by his teachers, but he also believed what he wrote. Although he later distanced himself from these early poems, which are now nearly inaccessible and justifiably forgotten, Kunze was sincere and cannot be charged with having consciously prostituted his art. At that time, he must have appeared to the authorities as everything they could wish for in the new generation of writers.

By 1959, however, Kunze's inability to reconcile Socialist theory with concrete experience led to severe political attacks on him. Disappointed and disillusioned, he was forced to suspend his doctoral studies and teaching activities in the journalism faculty at Leipzig. Later, Kunze came to regard the year 1959 as the absolute low point, the "zero hour," in his life. Ironically, the year 1959 also saw the publication of his first major collection of poems, *Vögel über dem Tau* (birds above the dew).

Following a period of work as a manual laborer in the heavy equipment industry and as a truck driver in Leipzig, Kunze lived in 1961 and 1962 in Czechoslovakia while recovering from a serious heart ailment and waiting for permission to marry a Czech citizen, Elisabeth Littnerová, an oral surgeon who had begun a voluminous correspondence with the poet after hearing one of the poems from *Vögel über dem Tau* read on the radio in 1959. It was during this period that Kunze established his close ties with contemporary Czech poets. By the time he returned to the GDR in 1962 and settled in Greiz as a freelance writer, he had published his second volume of poetry in the GDR, *Aber die Nachtigall jubelt* (but the nightingale rejoices), as well as the first of numerous volumes of translations of modern Czech poetry. It is difficult for a lyric poet to earn a living from his work, but Kunze's wife was able to establish a successful medical practice in Greiz, and in the years from 1962 to 1968, Kunze kept busy primarily with his translations and as a contributor to Czech literary journals. The year 1963 saw the first publication of Kunze's work in the West, *Widmungen* (dedications), a collection of poems mostly from the period of his residency in Czechoslovakia but also containing several earlier poems that he did not wish to disclaim. Kunze's poetry of this period did not fit the cookbook conception of Socialist Realism demanded by some cultural policymakers, but neither did most of the new poetry being produced by young writers in what must be seen as a lyric renaissance and one of the numerous "thaws" in the cultural history of the GDR, and Kunze was neither singled out nor repressed by the regime.

It was not until 1968 that a period of tension with the authorities began—tension that gradually came to dominate Kunze's life and work until his expulsion from the GDR in April, 1977. The proximate cause was the invasion of Czechoslovakia by Warsaw Pact troops in August, 1968, a development that triggered Kunze's immediate resignation from the SED, the East German Communist Party. This, in turn, resulted in an almost total blacklisting of the poet. Except for a volume of poetry selected from earlier collections that was published in 1973 under the title *Brief mit blauem Siegel* (letter with a blue seal), no work of Kunze's since appeared in the GDR. *Sensible Wege* (sensitive paths) and *With the Volume Turned Down* both appeared only in the West, and Kunze was fined in each instance under an East German law that prohibits authors from publishing material anywhere without first securing the permission of the Central Office for Copyrights.

As the East German repression of Kunze's works increased, so did the attention the poet received in the Western media. He was awarded numerous Western literary prizes but was often prevented from traveling to receive them. Some Western commentators were clearly more interested in Kunze as a political martyr than as a poet, and their attempts to stylize him into the "Solzhenitsyn of the GDR" served only to increase his difficulties. Matters came to a head following the publication of *The Wonderful Years*, when Kunze was first removed from the East German Writers' Union in October, 1976, an action tantamount to a total prohibition against practicing the profession of writing in any form, and then "invited" to leave the GDR, an invitation the poet could scarcely afford to decline in view of the campaign of vilification and intimidation launched against him and his family.

Kunze settled near Passau in Bavaria, saddened at having to leave the country he once said he "would choose over and over again" but happy to be able to write in relative peace. In spite of the fears of those who saw in Kunze only the beleaguered and eventually exiled political dissident and to the disappointment of those who wished to embrace him only as a Cold War propaganda tool, he has not allowed himself to voice a position of such bitter political opposition that he can no longer speak in the idiom of the poet. The first volume of poetry that Kunze produced after coming to the West, *Auf eigene Hoffnung* (of my own hope), indicated that he was able to give poetic expression to the full range of human experience, both political and private, with which he was confronted in the West.

Analysis

Although initially Reiner Kunze was in complete agreement with the ideals of humanistic Democratic Socialism, he is by nature a shy, sensitive, reflective man whose poetic interests have always tended toward the private sphere, and it is ironic that he first became known to a wider audience primarily as a political dissident. As is the case with any writer living in a system where literary questions are by definition also political issues, it is impossible to avoid the political dimension when discussing Kunze's work. His achievement as a poet, however, rests on the modest virtues of directness, honesty, and basic humanity, not on any polemical stance.

Kunze has always been a "popular" poet, both before and after his exile from the GDR to West Germany. His poetic images are concrete, drawn almost exclusively from everyday life, and easily accessible without being merely simpleminded or naïve. From Heinrich Heine, Kunze learned satire and wit, from Federico García Lorca a bold metaphoric vision, and from Brecht the knack of accommodating apparent opposites through dialectical thought; his chief claim to originality lies in his expansion of the possibilities of a lyric poetry of extreme brevity and concentration. His strength is the sudden, insightful aperçu, and some of his best work falls formally between epigram and graffiti. Kunze's playful, almost childlike view of the world, and of language in particular, allows him to exploit wordplay and create metaphors in ways that are both refreshingly original and genuinely insightful. He is capable of puckish good humor and wit, even when he has good reason for bitterness and despair. On the whole, his is a poetry of hope, however precarious. Kunze has said that he intends his poetry to reduce the distance and isolation between human beings, to make himself and his readers aware of their common humanity; at his best, he succeeds.

A fundamental characteristic of poetry can perhaps best be described as a tension between reason and emotion, between the demands of society and the needs of the private individual, between civilization and nature. In short, it is the clash of the Enlightenment with Romanticism. At different stages in his career, Kunze has resolved this tension now in one direction, now in the other, but his ultimate achievement lies in the dialectic reconciliation of opposites and the avoidance of false choices.

In Kunze's earliest poetry, contained in *Vögel über dem Tau, Aber die Nachtigall jubelt*, and, to a lesser extent, *Widmungen*, the Romantic elements clearly predominate. The first two volumes fulfill the promise of their titles, offering a great deal of nature imagery, with particular emphasis on birds and roses. The strophic forms as well as the rhymes of Kunze's early verse are simple, regular, and heavily indebted to folk poetry. Most of the poems of *Aber die Nachtigall jubelt* were intended to be set to music for use in East German puppet films for children, and Kunze has often said that he regards music as the queen of all the arts. The poet's preference for the realm of feeling is clearly apparent in the following lines from *Vögel über dem Tau*: "Love/ is a wild rose in us/ inaccessible to reason/ and not subjugated to it." Often the realm of nature and spontaneous feeling is defended against the demands or intrusions of a sterile, rational world of order and constraint, as in "The Song of the Strict Commander," whose troops are encouraged to break their close-order marching to pursue a pretty girl. Poetry itself is defended as a kind of refuge from an outside world that is often inimical to the spirit. Art and life become polarized, and there is no question what is to be preferred by the sensitive individual. In poems such as "Horizons" and "In the Thaya" (from *Widmungen*), the rose is regarded as being almost subversive of the prevailing order. The latter poem contains the lines: "do you see how a rose is blooming in his hands?/ Don't you see it? A rose!/ But we're not in favor of roses/ We are for order./ Whoever is for the rose/ is against order." To a great extent, Kunze was simply reacting against the excessive demands of the state for personal and poetic regimentation, as clearly suggested by these lines from *Aber die Nachtigall jubelt*: "Art—it flees commands./ Reason alone does not control it./ It wants the artist's soul." The predominance of Romantic characteristics in these early poems also reflects Kunze's poetic naïveté and the fact that his earliest literary models were drawn from that era.

Some of Kunze's early poetry is flawed by excessive pathos and sentimentality, and at times, he threatens to withdraw completely into a private realm of bird and flower metaphors. He was able to overcome that tendency by anchoring his poems in concrete, everyday experience. As he has matured, he has continued to portray landscapes, for example, but they have be-

come clearly identifiable geographical locations with specific historical and social coordinates. Similarly, Kunze has withdrawn from metaphysical speculation about universal truths, seeking rather to illuminate problems in their specific manifestation from his own experience. In this way, Kunze's poetry has become more clearly autobiographical and direct, and his understanding of its function has undergone an evolutionary change. Whereas the realm of feeling and poetry once offered an inward, private escape from or alternative to the sterile world of reason and society, Kunze now sees art and life less as irreconcilable opposites than as necessary complements. The realm of poetry is to be furiously defended not because it offers an escape from life but precisely because it offers a means of coming to terms with it.

DEFENSE OF POETRY

Kunze attributes his maturation as a poet primarily to his contact with modern Czech poetry and today regards *Widmungen* as his first significant work. In that volume and in the subsequent collections *Sensible Wege* and *With the Volume Turned Down*, it is clear that he has turned away from Romantic models, with the exception of the sharp wit and barbed irony of Heine. His defense of poetry becomes more sharply focused, and the threats to it are more clearly identified and engaged; a 1972 article by Manfred Jäger, one of the earliest studies of Kunze's poetry, is titled "Eine offensive Verteidigung der Poesie" (an aggressive defense of poetry). Kunze's chief weapon in the defense of poetry is a dialectical, epigrammatic style indebted particularly to the late poetry of Brecht. In his poems of this period, Kunze frequently adopts a satirical tone, and his diction, deflated of its pathos, could even be called reductionist. An entire poem may turn on a single metaphor or a bit of wordplay; grammatical markers fall away; and what is omitted is often more important than what is said. Sometimes, the polemical or didactic point of the poem lies in its title. All these features are evident in a poem titled "Gebildete Nation" (cultured nation): "Peter Huchel left the/ German Democratic Republic/ (report from France)/ He left/ The newspapers reported/ no loss." Kunze expresses dismay that a country that puts considerable emphasis on "storming the heights of culture" cannot feel or officially acknowledge the loss of a poetic talent of the magnitude of Peter Huchel. "Hymnus auf eine Frau beim verhör" (hymn to a woman being interrogated) illustrates Kunze's technique of setting the barb with a dialectical twist at the end: "Painful was/ the moment of/ undressing/ Then/ exposed to their glances she/ learned everything/ about them."

To be sure, the themes of Kunze's early lyrics do not altogether disappear, but they recede somewhat into the background; when they do appear, they share many of the stylistic features of the more overtly political poems. "Auf dich im blauen Mantel" (to you in a blue coat) is dedicated to the poet's wife: "Once more I read from the beginning/ the line of houses look for/ you the blue comma that/ makes sense of it." The fact that the poem itself desperately needs a comma between "houses" and "look" in order to make sense increases the poignancy of its thematic point. Kunze's ability to transform mundane experiences—such as the sight of his wife coming down the street—into a fresh poetic metaphor is one of his chief strengths. In *Widmungen* and subsequent collections, Kunze became a master of the short form, of the clever and penetrating but sometimes also moving aperçu. The previous romantic excesses gave way to a more balanced mixture of thought and feeling, and he emerged from an inward-turning lyricism to a poetry that engaged the world.

STRIVING TO COMMUNICATE

Indeed, the need for communication grew to occupy a central position in Kunze's life and art. One section of *Sensible Wege* is subtitled "Hunger nach der Welt" (hunger for the world), and the volume concludes with a cycle of twenty-one poems on the theme of the mail, a tenuous connection with the outside world for an increasingly critical East German poet whose standing with the authorities stood in inverse proportion to his growing reputation in both East and West. In one of these poems, Kunze refers to letters as "white lice in the pelt of the fatherland" awaiting the "comb" of the postal service.

Kunze fought all attempts at censorship and regimentation with the one weapon at his disposal, his poetry, which he could still publish in the West. The numerous literary prizes Kunze won in the West in the early 1970's afforded him a visibility that undoubtedly

helped to protect him from cruder forms of repression, and, together with another "thaw" in cultural policies, probably accounted for the surprising publication of *Brief mit blauem Siegel* in the East in 1973. Nevertheless, Kunze was increasingly caught up in a process of escalating politicization that threatened to destroy all balance between political and private concerns and overwhelm his ability to respond creatively to them. Particularly with the publication of *The Wonderful Years*, Kunze came to be regarded by many in both East and West as a purely political phenomenon. He was embraced in the Federal Republic by anti-GDR forces who hoped to use him only as a propaganda weapon, and he was vilified in the East as an "enemy of the state"; it appeared for a time that Kunze was not going to be allowed to be "merely" a poet, to continue to give poetic expression to the full range of human experience.

AUF EIGENE HOFFNUNG

Although some observers assumed, perhaps understandably, that Kunze was indeed primarily a political dissident who would probably fall silent after his exile to the West, the move was instead very beneficial to him as a poet. Freed from the bitterness of repression and the glare of sensational publicity, Kunze was gradually able to produce the poems contained in *Auf eigene Hoffnung*, published some nine years after *With the Volume Turned Down*.

If Kunze began his career retreating from the world into romantic excesses and was then prevented from maintaining a balance between private and public life by forces largely outside his control, then the poems of *Auf eigene Hoffnung* appear to represent an achievement of equilibrium. The first section of the book contains poems written between 1973 and 1975, before his expulsion from the GDR; his weariness and concern over the politicization of his work is apparent. The section is subtitled "Des Fahnenhissens bin ich müde, Freund" (I am tired of showing my colors, friend) a line from a poem based on a wordplay made possible by the dual meaning of the word *Fahne* ("flag" and "galley proof"). Ewald Osers, the British translator of *With the Volume Turned Down*, had written Kunze that he had just gotten the galley proofs (*Fahnen*) back from the printer and they were ready to be corrected, or "flown," depending on how one chose to understand the word. Kunze concludes his poem with the thought that the only *Fahne* to which he would care to swear an oath is one with a love poem on it. The same weariness with political themes is expressed in a poem titled "Tagebuchblatt 1980" (diary page 1980), obviously written during the West German election campaign: "The climbing roses are blossoming, as though the landscape were bleeding/ . . ./ Even the landscape, they will claim, may/ no longer simply exist, it too/ must be for or against." Nature's pure colors thus become stylized into campaign propaganda for the Social Democrats, just as Kunze had recently been used for political causes that were not his own.

It may be understood, however, that Kunze is not mourning here his own lost innocence, the time when landscapes and roses were a form of inward, private escape; rather, he desires the right (and the peace of mind) to produce landscape and love poetry. When he does so in this volume, the poems display the tautness of language and boldness of metaphoric vision characteristic of his best work. In "Your Head on My Breast," for example, the entire poem is constructed around a single metaphor or wordplay based on the word *Schlüsselbein* (which means "collarbone," but since a *Schlüssel* is a "key," the literal meaning is "key bone"). The abundance of landscape poems results in part, no doubt, from the poet's new freedom to travel. The latest volume even includes Kunze's impressions of America, gathered in 1980 when he held a guest professorship in the German Department at the University of Texas. Kunze's eye is open to natural beauty, but he also locates his landscapes within their concrete social context. The placing of natural settings within their human context is perfectly symbolized in the metaphor that Kunze chooses for the heading of the section of poems on America: "Amerika, der Autobaum" (America, the auto-tree).

Although Kunze by no means seeks to avoid political themes, he is concerned that they are sometimes unsuitable for poetic expression. He is very much aware of the apology in Brecht's well-known poem "An die Nachgeborenen" (to posterity), which acknowledges that even righteous indignation distorts the features, and as Kunze's poem "Credo on a Good Morning" sug-

gests, he would rather avoid certain painful areas: "When you are writing a poem, that is, going/ barefoot in your heart,/ avoid the places where/ something shattered in you/ The moss/ is no match for the fragments/ It exists, the/ poem without a wound." As suggested, however, this credo does not prevent Kunze from adopting a critical stance with respect to political aspects of West German society. One poem shows how neo-Nazi attitudes are revealed in everyday life, as when a young Bavarian watching an international soccer match in a neighborhood bar comments on a Dutch player who has just scored a goal: "Den ham's beim vagasn vagessn" ("they forgot to gas that one"). The man is obviously too young to remember the Nazi era, but the thoughtless remark reveals an appalling lack of sensitivity to Germany's past. Frequently, as in this poem, Kunze need only quote the target of his criticism directly to achieve a striking effect; the authorities in the GDR often made things easy for the poet in precisely this way.

THEMES BEYOND THE POLITICAL

Kunze has stated that he does not, in fact, choose his themes at all; rather, they choose him. In addition to its communicative intent, writing has for him also a personal, therapeutic function as a means of coming to terms with matters he can deal with in no other way. He vigorously rejects the thesis that he needs opposition in order to write and insists that he was never cut out for the role of political martyr. Kunze is relieved that the themes now choosing him—that is, the concerns impinging on his consciousness—are no longer almost all from the political sphere. Although he does not write prolifically, he has not fallen silent as many in the West feared he would, and the relative quiet that has grown around him has been productive, as expressed in the lines from a poem in *Auf eigene Hoffnung*: "Stillness gathers around me/ the soil for the poem/ In the spring we will/ have verses and birds."

EIN TAG AUF DIESER ERDE

Kunze has in fact not fallen silent, and he produced his first poetry collection in seven years in 1998. *Ein Tag auf dieser Erde* (a day on this earth) seems to indicate a diary approach to poetry. However, the scope and purpose of the work is discernibly larger than a series of journal entries. While the passing of time sets immediate and inexplicable barriers to confine the human condition, no such limits restrict Kunze's poetic imagination, which here elaborates on the tangible, not always comfortable, intimacy of the cosmic order. An elegant sparseness accommodates Kunze's method, and wide-spanning acumen guides him in his task. There are six sections, and the brevity and subdued diction of the verse throughout allow for subtle gradations to take hold. Section 1 hints at timeless, local precedents for universal myths. Inevitable realities in human aging are beautifully, seamlessly linked to nature in the poem "November." Section 2 expands to a tour of civilized history, with stops in a range of locales including Kyoto, for the cherry festival, and Namibia. The following two sections attend to events in recent German history and to the less-than-assuring ambivalence of ideal aspiration (two short poems in "Der himmel," the sky). The penultimate section, "Komm mit dem cello" (come with the cello), touches on the unqualified consolations of art.

The book ends with a coda that gives the collection its title, a meditation on mortality in fifteen sections. Fish, bird, and river are the vibrant signs of transcendent life here, and there is a one-sided confrontation with God. However, it is by a series of transformative, interwoven contrasts and reversals that the sequence becomes amazing, and so does the book as a whole, despite its emblematic familiarity. Without resorting to the readily available or conventional rhetoric of hope, *Ein Tag auf dieser Erde* builds to a quiet resolution, a calm right on the brink of a complete and devastating silence.

Other major works

NONFICTION: *Die wunderbaren Jahre*, 1976 (*The Wonderful Years*, 1977); *Das weisse Gedicht: Essays*, 1989; *Am Sonnenhang: Tagebuch eines Jahres*, 1993.

CHILDREN'S LITERATURE: *Der Löwe Leopold*, 1970.

Bibliography

Graves, Peter. "A Naked Individualist." Review of *Ein Tag Auf Dieser Erde. The Times Literary Supplement* (March 26, 1999): 26. Graves provides some biographical insights in his review of Kunze's work.

_____. "Reiner Kunze: Some Comments and a Conversation." *German Life and Letters* 41, no. 3 (1988): 312-322. A critical study of selected works by Kunze and an interview with the poet.

Hamburger, Michael. *After the Second Flood: Essays on Post-War German Literature.* New York: St. Martin's Press, 1986. A critical and historical study of several German poets including Kunze.

Kunze, Reiner, and Mireille Gansel. *"In Time of Need": A Conversation About Poetry, Resistance, and Exile.* Translated by Edmund Jephcott. London: Libris, 2006. Kunze and his French translator discuss poets under Nazism and Communism, including the German poet Peter Huchel.

Lasky, Melvin J. *Voices in a Revolution: The Collapse of East German Communism.* 1992. Reprint. New Brunswick, N.J.: Transaction, 2006. The chapter on Kunze describes his struggle to publish and the politicization of his writing.

Dennis McCormick
Updated by Sarah Hilbert

L

Jean de La Fontaine

Born: Château-Thierry, Champagne, France; July 8, 1621
Died: Paris, France; April 13, 1695

PRINCIPAL POETRY

Adonis, 1658 (English translation, 1957)
Le Songe de Vaux, 1659
Contes et nouvelles en vers, 1665 (*Tales and Short Stories in Verse*, 1735)
Deuxième partie des "Contes et nouvelles en vers," 1666 (*Part Two of "Tales and Short Stories in Verse,"* 1735)
Fables choisies, mises en vers, 1668-1694 (*Fables Written in Verse*, 1735)
Troisième partie des "Contes et nouvelles en vers," 1671 (*Part Three of "Tales and Short Stories in Verse,"* 1735)
Nouveaux Contes, 1674 (*New Tales*, 1735)
Poèmes et poésies diverses, 1697

OTHER LITERARY FORMS

The verse fable has attracted numerous writers over the centuries extending as far back as Aesop. The success of Jean de La Fontaine (lah fohn-TEHN) in the genre, however, surpassed them all. Though his verse novel *Les Amours de Psyché et Cupidon* (1669; *The Loves of Cupid and Psyche*, 1744) may be considered a major work and he wrote plays, librettos, translations, and letters, La Fontaine's name has become, for young and old, inseparably linked with the fable, a genre that he brought to its ultimate fruition.

ACHIEVEMENTS

Jean de La Fontaine is unquestionably one of France's most beloved poets. He is a classical writer in the true meaning of the word. For centuries, French schoolchildren have learned his fables by heart. He is so important in France that he has often been compared with Dante and William Shakespeare as a national literary monument. The poet's universal fame derives primarily from his verse fables; La Fontaine developed this literary genre to perfection, and there have been no great fabulists after him (with the possible exception of the Russian writer Ivan Krylov). The fables of La Fontaine culminated a long tradition in Western literature that began in antiquity with Aesop and Phaedrus. His works have been printed and reprinted in magnificent editions. They have been translated into many languages and have been illustrated by great artists down through the centuries: the *Fables* by Alphonse Oudry, Gustave Doré, and Marc Chagall; *Tales and Short Stories in Verse* by Charles-Dominique Joseph Eisen, Jean-Honoré Fragonard, and others.

La Fontaine unites the two major contrasting aesthetics found in the literature of seventeenth century France: artistic exuberance and classical restraint. Of the two, the former is best represented in poetry by the libertine poets, the so-called free spirits, such as Théophile de Viau and Marc-Antoine Saint-Amant. Temperamentally and in his general approach to life, La Fontaine belonged to this group of poets. His early works reveal a strain of playful sensuality and outspoken humor that are more representative of a hedonistic school of thought than one would normally expect from a renowned classical poet. Unlike other poets of his day, however, he was able to temper this natural tendency. One of La Fontaine's cardinal rules was that poetry should first of all give pleasure. He understood that pleasure is not an end in itself, that it must be deep and rich rather than facile or superficial. Wishing to please his readers, he hoped and believed that they would like what he himself liked.

Accordingly, he accepted the tenets of a classical doctrine that was very influential during this period. The influence of classical restraint is apparent in his mature works, especially the fables. In matters of style (he strove for simplicity, clarity, brevity), choice of language (a restrained vocabulary), versification, and the insertion of old materials among new, La Fontaine showed himself to be a genuine classical author. Moreover, the meter of classical French poetry, with the ubiquitous Alexandrine, was at times threatened with monotony and stiffness. Through his writings, La Fontaine managed to infuse new life in French versification. He achieved a melodic depth unsurpassed by his contemporaries and proved to be a superb craftsman. The quick movement of his verse, with those sudden short lines and that frequent suddenness of feminine rhyme that can create surprise, fun, or intimacy, has been emulated by generations of French poets. Above all, he had the gift of being sincere, personal, and completely natural in his finest poetry, at a time when it was not at all fashionable to be so.

BIOGRAPHY

Jean de La Fontaine was born in the province of Champagne at Château-Thierry in 1621. In spite of his name, he was not of noble birth. His father held a government post as an administrator of forest and water resources. It was in the lush, green countryside of Château-Thierry that the poet spent his first twenty years. He loved the surrounding neighborhood with its woods, waters, and meadows. He admired the natural world during a century when it went mostly unappreci-

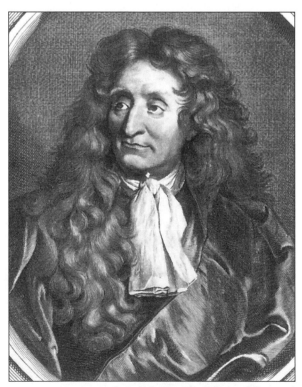

Jean de La Fontaine (Library of Congress)

ated; indeed, to most of his contemporaries the term "nature" meant primarily human nature. Thus, his early upbringing set him apart from the other great classical writers of France's Golden Age, and the influence of nature and of country people is apparent in many of his tales and fables.

It is well documented that as a boy, La Fontaine was dreamy and absent-minded. He was also cheerful and lively, possessing an amiable disposition that remained with him throughout his life. In 1641, at the age of twenty, La Fontaine decided to study for the priesthood at the Oratoire in Paris, but he abandoned this pursuit after eighteen months and turned to the study of law. In 1647, his father transferred his official post to La Fontaine and married him off to a girl from an affluent family. The match proved to be a disaster, and the couple formally separated after eleven years of marriage. During this period, La Fontaine lived the life of a dilettante. He showed a disinclination for steady work and was content to spend much of his time in idleness; he was a voracious reader. He eventually sold his father's post and took up permanent residence in Paris.

La Fontaine began writing comparatively late in life, in his middle thirties. Throughout his career as a man of letters, he relied on generous patrons for his support and well-being. His first patron was also his most important—the wealthy finance minister Nicolas Fouquet. La Fontaine became a pensioner of Fouquet in 1656 and wrote for him such early major works as *Adonis* and *Le Songe de Vaux* (the dream of Vaux). Unfortunately for La Fontaine, Fouquet soon fell into disgrace. His opulent lifestyle aroused the envy and anger of the young King Louis XIV. Fouquet was accused of appropriating state funds and spent the rest of his life in prison. During Fouquet's ordeal, La Fontaine exhibited that particular virtue that would always be characteristic of him as pensioner—a deep sense of loyalty. He did not abandon Fouquet as did so many others, and he even wrote poems, including the "Elégie aux nymphes de Vaux," begging the king to be lenient. For this display of allegiance, he incurred the king's lasting enmity. He thus never received a pension from the government, as did many other writers and artists, and his election to the prestigious French Academy was delayed on the king's order.

After Fouquet's downfall, La Fontaine was aided for a short time by the powerful Bouillon family and later by a royal patron, the dowager duchess of Orléans. He was by then forty years old, well into middle age for the times, and he was not a popular or well-known author. He realized that writing idyllic works such as *Adonis* would no longer be financially rewarding for him. Accordingly, he turned to more popular genres, such as tales and fables. He published *Tales and Short Stories in Verse* in 1665. They were written in the tradition of Giovanni Boccaccio and Ludovico Ariosto, among others, and they became an immediate success. A second collection appeared a year later, in 1666; a third collection was published in 1671; and the final collection appeared in 1674. At that time, La Fontaine also began to publish those works on which his fame rests—the *Fables Written in Verse*. The first collection appeared in 1668, when he was forty-seven years old; the second, ten years later; and the last collection, in 1694, one year before his death.

The success of the *Fables Written in Verse* placed La Fontaine at the forefront of French writers. In 1669, he published *The Loves of Cupid and Psyche*, taken from the tale of Cupid and Psyche in Lucius Apuleius's *The Golden Ass* (second century). La Fontaine continued writing many occasional verses of small importance for various patrons. In 1684, despite earlier opposition by the king, he was finally elected to the French Academy. In 1692, a serious illness occasioned a spiritual renewal, which, in turn, caused him to disavow publicly his earlier tales. In that same year, some of La Fontaine's fables were translated into English for the first time, by Sir Roger L'Estrange. In 1695, while attending a play, La Fontaine was struck ill and taken to the house of friends, the Haberts, where he died several days later. He is buried in the cemetery of the Saints-Innocents in Paris.

ANALYSIS

Jean de La Fontaine's poetic output mirrors the two major styles of seventeenth century French literature—that is to say, it lies between artistic exuberance, on one hand, and classical restraint, on the other. This has not always been apparent, however, since the fame of his *Fables Written in Verse* was such as to put his other po-

etic works in partial eclipse for a long period. Later scholarship has attempted to redress this imbalance. Such works as *Adonis*, *Le Songe de Vaux*, and *The Loves of Cupid and Psyche* reflect the grandiose splendor and fantasy characteristic of the Baroque style of the period. Conversely, the brevity, clarity, and logic of the *Fables Written in Verse* are more typical of the classical style associated with the authors of France's "grand siècle."

ADONIS

La Fontaine presented his first major poetic endeavor, *Adonis*, to his new patron, Fouquet, in June, 1658. It was a fine example of calligraphy by Nicolas Jarvey, with the title page illustrated by François Chauveau. The poem was a long pastoral work whose subject was borrowed from Ovid. It relates the legend of the goddess Venus's love for a youth, Adonis, and of his untimely death. La Fontaine's work is only half the length of William Shakespeare's better-known version, *Venus and Adonis* (1593). Furthermore, La Fontaine's Adonis is not a cold and reluctant character, as is Shakespeare's. Instead, La Fontaine chose to emphasize the theme of youth cut off in the flower of strength and beauty. For La Fontaine, Adonis symbolizes the agony of helpless strength, a paradoxical antithesis characteristic of the Baroque. The poet's vivid and enjoyable descriptions of nature create a self-contained poetic world. It is not the real world, yet La Fontaine, a true lover of nature, has managed to make the setting of his poem so directly appealing to the senses and simple instincts of his readers that the illusion is all but complete.

On the other hand, his amorous poetry is too artificial and conventional. He composed his idyll in the Alexandrines typical of French poetry: lines of twelve syllables, with four stresses to the line and rhyming in couplets. The stately Alexandrine was not well adapted to the subject matter of the poem. Even in the most tender passages, there is some monotony of cadence. A shorter verse line with its rapid movement would have smoothed the transitions between episodes in the narrative. Nevertheless, this first major poetic undertaking taught La Fontaine much about the writing of Alexandrines. For a long period unfairly neglected, *Adonis* deserves the recognition it has received during the past few decades. The poem contains verse worthy of La Fontaine at his best, and one can discern in it many of the traits that find fuller expression in his subsequent writings: skillful assimilation of source material, a refined musical style, close observation of human or animal life in a mythological setting, and, above all, an ability to infuse humor without compromising the decorous mood of the poem.

Le Songe de Vaux

Fouquet was pleased with *Adonis* and asked La Fontaine to undertake a new work in praise of Vaux, the magnificent white-stone palace that the finance minister was engaged in creating for himself with the help of the best architects, garden designers, and artists in France. La Fontaine accommodated his patron with *Le Songe de Vaux*, a work that, as a result of the disgrace of Fouquet, was never completed. Nine fragments have survived, written in a mixture of verse and prose. The poem fits marvelously into the parklike landscape of Vaux in which La Fontaine places it. It is enveloped in a world of fantasy. Artificial as it may be, there is enough imagination to give a touch of fairyland to the scene. Wishing to give posterity a picture of Vaux as it would appear in all the beauty of its maturity, the poet used his imagination in describing Fouquet's magnificent estate. He proposed to describe—in lyrical, allegorical, and mythological terms—what the Vaux gardens, newly planted and only shrub-high, would be like in years to come.

The plot of *Le Songe de Vaux* revolves around the discovery of some imagined buried treasure on the palace grounds. A mysterious inscription on a jewel case leads to a kind of beauty contest in which the four nymphs representing architecture, painting, gardening, and poetry contest the honor of being responsible for the chief beauties of Vaux. The poem evokes an ideal world from which all ugliness is banished. La Fontaine had the rare gift, unique in seventeenth century France, of communicating in poetry the sensations aroused by colors and forms. This is particularly apparent in *Le Songe de Vaux*, a work permeated with poetic feeling for beauty, peace, and sensual pleasure akin to one of Charles Le Brun's paintings, which it celebrates. The verse, more smooth and melodious than in *Adonis*, seems to have developed effortlessly. The limpid sim-

plicity of the shorter, octosyllabic lines assures a more flowing rhythm. The precious imagery and the choice of vocabulary help sustain the quiet enjoyment of varying moods.

The Loves of Cupid and Psyche

La Fontaine continued the practice of interweaving prose and poetry with *The Loves of Cupid and Psyche*, based on the classical tale of a jealous Venus who sends Cupid to make the beautiful maiden Psyche fall in love with an ugly creature, only to have Cupid fall in love with Psyche instead. This long novel-poem is set within the framework of a conversation in the park of Versailles among four friends—Polyphile, Acante, Ariste, and Gélaste. The gardens of Versailles and the surrounding area provide an atmosphere of fantasy similar in tone and style to the one depicted in *Le Songe de Vaux*. Indeed, La Fontaine transposed materials from the latter into this work. Once again, it is interesting to note the changes wrought by the poet on his source material—changes that enabled him to achieve effects unmatched by writers such as Vergil, Torquato Tasso, and Ariosto who had treated this myth before him. His Psyche is a much more complex character than any of her prototypes. She is sensual, tender, and open-minded, vain at times but always charming. Rather than portray her in bleak, isolated settings, as did his predecessors, La Fontaine shows her in beautiful surroundings. The joining of sensuous love and bucolic descriptions of nature bathe this work in an aura of voluptuous, Epicurean delight. *The Loves of Cupid and Psyche* is important as a transitional work in La Fontaine's oeuvre; it draws the curtain on the period of youthful ardor, of love and beauty, of preciosity and gallantry associated with the works of the Vaux period.

Tales and Short Stories in Verse

Second only to the *Fables Written in Verse* in their popularity, the *Tales and Short Stories in Verse* were first published in 1665. Three more collections of similar material appeared in 1666, 1671, and 1674. These tales belong to the Western literary tradition of stock ribald stories told and retold during the Middle Ages and the Renaissance by Boccaccio, Geoffrey Chaucer, Marguerite de Navarre, and many others. The predominant theme of these tales is illicit love: the frolicsome comedy of marital infidelity, the sexual prowess of men or lack of it, the frailty of women, the lustful desires of priests and nuns, and so forth. A total of thirty-five tales appeared over the years, of which "Joconde" and "Le Cocu battu et content" ("The Cudgelled and Contented Cuckold") are perhaps the most popular. In the later tales, the subjects include not only the illicit affairs of typically crafty women, paramours, and cuckolds but also the daily tribulations of ordinary people: a poor shoemaker, a cynical judge, a peasant and his master, among others. Like the fables, these tales first circulated in manuscript, soon winning favorable response from La Fontaine's friends. Licentious tales became extremely popular during the early reign of young Louis XIV; La Fontaine was aware of this trend and sought to cater to the salacious taste of the public. Nevertheless, the tales caused him enormous difficulties. Each collection was more licentious than its predecessors until the final published tales were ordered suppressed by the police. In his old age, La Fontaine publicly repudiated these tales, expressing regret at ever having written them; it should be noted, however, that this recantation was made during a period when strict moral severity prevailed at the court of Versailles.

NARRATIVE TECHNIQUE AND POETIC EXPRESSION

The fact that La Fontaine did not invent his plots—he borrowed freely from his precursors—enabled him to focus all his talents on details of narrative technique and poetic expression. It is in these two areas that he made his greatest contribution as a writer of tales. La Fontaine always had a flair for the dramatic, and in his tales he shows himself to be a master storyteller. His skill at creating action without impeding the progress of the plot (effected primarily by means of alteration in the rhythm of the poetry), his penchant for producing situations that shock or surprise, his ability to vary and freshen the treatment of old, banal themes—in brief, his talent for adroit handling of the strictly narrative aspects of the art—is his major appeal. Whatever plots he chose, his own special genius gave them new life.

In his tales, La Fontaine adopted a free-flowing conversational style. In fact, he seems to have gone to great lengths to ensure that the graceful, chatty style of these stories would appear as natural as possible to the reader. Toward that end, he employed an irregular and loose sort of verse, known as *vers libre* (not to be confused with modern free verse), consisting of lines in two or more meters without a fixed rhyme scheme. La Fontaine's two favorite verse forms were the eight-syllable line of the old French fabliaux and the ten-syllable line. These two verse lines, along with the lack of any clear-cut rhyme scheme, gave the tales a colloquial tone that one would normally expect to find only in prose. Such verse had greater flexibility than anything previously written in French. It allowed the poet to tell his stories in a familiar, relaxed style, addressing himself directly to the reader. Curiously enough, he frequently felt a need to justify his use of this form, declaring that it was the most suitable and that it had given him as much trouble as the writing of regular verse or prose. In truth, it must be said that La Fontaine employed *vers libre* with great restraint. He introduced other rhythmic patterns as well, but only on rare occasions. His poetic expertise was to be found elsewhere: in the subtle interplay of rhymes, in evocative combinations of sounds, in complex rhythmic gradations and contrasts, in the joining of heterogeneous stanza forms, in the interplay of thought patterns with metrical patterns—all the stylistic characteristics that became associated with his masterpiece, the *Fables Written in Verse*.

FABLES WRITTEN IN VERSE

In the *Fables Written in Verse*, as in his tales, La Fontaine was reviving a genre that had been popular throughout the Middle Ages and the Renaissance. The *Fables Written in Verse* is a work of maturity, nourished by wide reading and a long apprenticeship in poetic technique. They were published in three cycles spanning twenty-five years. The first cycle, containing 125 fables, appeared in 1668. Ten years later, La Fontaine added nearly one hundred more, and the 1694 edition—the last edition published during his lifetime—included two dozen new fables. Thus, he wrote nearly 250 fables in all. The early fables owe a great deal to classical sources, in particular Aesop and Phaedrus; the later ones find their inspiration in Asian stories.

These fables are the work of a man who had an intimate acquaintance with nature and an instinctive understanding of animals and country things. La Fontaine's *Fables Written in Verse* has always appealed to three distinct audiences: to children, because of the vividness and freshness of the stories; to literary students, because of their accomplished artistry; and to people of the world, because of their penetrating psychological observation of human behavior. Of these three disparate audiences, La Fontaine sought in particular the third category of readers, for he himself often said that his fables would be fully appreciated only by those who had had a long experience of life and people.

A comparison of La Fontaine's fables with others in the genre reveals the importance of his achievement. Traditional materials are handled with shades of feelings not to be found in earlier fables. In particular, his approach to the depiction of animals in the *Fables Written in Verse* is at variance with that of practically all the previous writers of fables who had found favor with the public. Like all fabulists, La Fontaine treats animals in anthropomorphic terms: They are used to depict certain human foibles. Moving beyond his predecessors artistically, La Fontaine's portrayals of the human as well as the animal aspects of his characters have not been surpassed by his followers and imitators. Strange, clumsy little creatures wander about, fiercely acting their parts to what is, at times, a merciless finish. These animals show the desires, appetites, and fears that are humankind's brutish inheritance. The dominant ones among them are forceful, secretive, cunning, and sharp-witted, and their ends are as elemental as their means are ingenious. Their victims are like those in the human world: muddleheaded, cringing before their masters, into whose maws they are ever ready to drop. The weak countenances of these victims remain plaintive, frightened, and pitiful—revealing the essential cruelty of existence.

What the *Fables Written in Verse* reveals, above all, is La Fontaine's conception of power (the first edition was dedicated to the future king of France). Animal hierarchies provided him with an opportunity to examine certain types of formal relations among control, resistance, and violence so that he could uncover, by implication, the same relationships in human society. In fact, the *Fables Written in Verse* constitute a survey of the struggle for power among men. La Fontaine views the political world as an arena in which the strong seek to defend and extend their powers and privileges. He posits a view of humankind that sees conflict as the only mode of action and insists that no moral considerations should be taken into account, the political aims justifying any means.

The prevalence of such motifs clearly indicates a substratum of belief that La Fontaine could not have derived from his learned sources alone. Themes such as these illustrate the extent to which he appropriated the idiom of the fable for his own wholly different ends. To study La Fontaine's fables is to investigate power *in extremis*. In the *Fables Written in Verse*, power must be exercised rather than merely possessed. It must be seized and maintained even at the cost of a progressive enslavement to its instinctive violence. The traditional concept of power as a societal mechanism that lays down the law for everyone alike no longer applies. Animals, men, and institutions are treated and studied mainly as objects of domination. There is no reason to doubt that La Fontaine's contemporaries understood perfectly the "message" of this important work—one that has become obfuscated down through the centuries by the rote memorizations of schoolchildren and the musty compilations of scholars. One can also understand better why Jean-Jacques Rousseau denounced the use of such texts to shape young sensibilities.

Each generation takes a different approach to La Fontaine's individual vision. Certain past generations saw him as a detached observer of the human comedy, while others have seen him as a dissatisfied man with a gift for caricature, as a poet of the picturesque in nature and in rural life, as a dilettante with dregs of smug morality, or merely as a pleasant storyteller. No subsequent writer of fables has sustained such an intense emotional vision of man and of the forces that dominate and shape the world in which he lives as did La Fontaine. Above all, his fables repay study because of their poetic beauty and simplicity; they are a deeply felt artistic manifestation of the human condition, derived mostly from the bitter truth of experience.

OTHER MAJOR WORKS

LONG FICTION: *Les Amours de Psyché et Cupidon*, 1669 (*The Loves of Cupid and Psyche*, 1744).

PLAYS: *L'Eunuque*, pb. 1654; *Clymène*, pb. 1671;

Daphné, pb. 1682 (libretto); *Galatée*, pb. 1682 (libretto); *L'Astrée*, pb. 1692 (libretto).

NONFICTION: *Relation d'un voyage en Limousin*, 1663; *Discours à Mme de La Sablière*, 1679; *Épître à Huet*, 1687.

MISCELLANEOUS: *Œuvres complètes*, 1933 (2 volumes); *Œuvres diverses*, 1942; *Œuvres, sources, et postérité d'Ésope à l'Oulipo*, 1995.

BIBLIOGRAPHY

Birberick, Anne L. *Reading Undercover: Audience and Authority in Jean de La Fontaine*. London: Associated University Presses, 1998. In her readings of La Fontaine's major poetic works, Birberick proposes the possibility of a "circular writing" resulting from the multiplicity of author/audience relationships in the poet's works, which allows La Fontaine room to criticize court patronage and tyranny, while nonetheless winning the necessary approbation of the Sun King.

_____. *Refiguring La Fontaine: Tercentenary Essays*. Charlottesville, Va.: Bookwood Press, 1996. In addition to Birberick's introductory summary of La Fontaine's critical reception since his death, this volume contains nine essays (three in French, six in English) that explore La Fontaine's adaptations of and challenges to literary structure, questions of discourse in the *Fables Written in Verse*, and new treatments of other, more neglected works by the poet. Of particular interest to an audience obliged to rely on translations from French is the last essay by David Lee Rubin, which examines three English translations of one fable in order to discuss how each translator's different approach informs, or distorts, the image of La Fontaine and his poetry.

Calder, Andrew. *The Fables of La Fontaine: Wisdom Brought Down to Earth*. Geneva: Droz, 2001. Arguing that it is essential to consider La Fontaine's *Fables Written in Verse* from a perspective both of utility and pleasure in some sixteen, self-contained chapters that look to the fables as lessons in life,

Calder's book is also of interest in that it explores La Fontaine's philosophical similarities with schools of thought in antiquity and with his Renaissance predecessors, such as Erasmus, François Rabelais, and Michel Eyquem de Montaigne.

Fumaroli, Marc. *The Poet and the King: Jean de La Fontaine and His Century*. Translated by Jane Marie Todd. Notre Dame, Ind.: University of Notre Dame Press, 2002. A biography of La Fontaine that details his relations with Louis XIV.

Guiton, Margaret. *La Fontaine: Poet and Counterpoet*. New Brunswick, N.J.: Rutgers University Press, 1961. Examines La Fontaine's competing visions of comedy and imaginative poetry. French passages translated. Contains chronological table of La Fontaine's life and works.

Lapp, John C. *The Esthetics of Negligence: La Fontaine's "Contes."* New York: Cambridge University Press, 1971. Refutes previous disparaging studies by demonstrating how La Fontaine's wit, eroticism, lyricism, and charm make the *Tales and Short Stories in Verse* superior to their sources.

Mackay, Agnes Ethel. *La Fontaine and His Friends: A Biography*. London: Garnstone Press, 1972. Examination of La Fontaine's relationship with intimate friends and influential patrons. French passages translated in chapter endnotes.

Sweetser, Marie-Odile. *La Fontaine*. Boston: Twayne, 1987. In this very approachable critical biography of La Fontaine, Sweetser organizes her chapters by the chronological appearance of each of the poet's major works. Her volume is also useful in that it makes available to a non-francophone readership a concise, well-documented synthesis of continental scholarship concerning La Fontaine.

Wadsworth, Philip A. *Young La Fontaine*. Evanston, Ill.: Northwestern University Press, 1952. A detailed study of La Fontaine's growth as a poet up to publication of his first fables in 1668. Good discussion of influences that shaped his early works.

Raymond LePage

JULES LAFORGUE

Born: Montevideo, Uruguay; August 16, 1860
Died: Paris, France; August 20, 1887

PRINCIPAL POETRY

Les Complaintes, 1885
L'Imitation de Notre-Dame la lune, 1886
Des fleurs de bonne volonté, 1888
Les Derniers Vers de Jules Laforgue, 1890
Poésies complètes, 1894, 1970
Œuvres complètes de Jules Laforgue, 1902-1903
    (4 volumes; 1922-1930, 6 volumes)
Poems, 1975
Selected Poems, 1998

OTHER LITERARY FORMS

In the short but prolific writing career of Jules Laforgue (lah-FAWRG), he produced more than two hundred poems and many works in other literary forms, only some of which have been rescued from the papers left at his death. His surviving verse dramas include "Tessa," written in 1877, existing in a manuscript only recently discovered; *Pierrot fumiste*, composed in 1882, first published in 1892; and *Le Concile féerique*, published in 1886, compiled from five poems originally written for *Des fleurs de bonne volonté* (poems that Laforgue composed between 1883 and 1886 and that first appeared in 1888). These three cabaret farces command the attention of scholars eager to explore Laforgue's developing themes and ironic dialogue; they are not major contributions to theatrical literature.

Masterpieces of an original genre are Laforgue's six fanciful prose tales, *Moralités légendaires* (1887; *Six Moral Tales from Jules Laforgue*, 1928), retelling myths in details both mundane and psychologically plausible. Among these, "Hamlet" and "Persée et Andromède" ("Perseus and Andromeda: Or, The Happiest One of the Triangle") have provoked considerable admiring commentary. The actor and mime Jean-Louis Barrault performed a memorable adaptation of "Hamlet" in 1939. Several works of fiction have apparently been lost, but there survive a short autobiographical novel, *Stéphane Vassiliew*, written in 1881, first pub-

lished in 1946, and a short autobiographical story, "Amours de la quinzième année," written about 1879, first published in 1887.

Laforgue's selected letters, especially those to his sister, created the legend of the poet as a self-conscious, sensitive, starving aesthete, but his letters to various other friends reveal his humor, his broad interests in philosophy, art, and music, and his acute observations of society. A fuller portrait of Laforgue's intellectual range emerges from his critical essays on Impressionist aesthetics, on the Symbolist poets Charles Baudelaire and Tristan Corbière, and on life in the German imperial court. Laforgue's translations of Walt Whitman's verse were published in 1886.

Among his other essays and drafts published posthumously are some provocative comments on the cultural definitions constricting the roles of women, including "La Femme—la légende féminine," among many others. Simone de Beauvoir, in *Le Deuxième Sexe* (1949; *The Second Sex*, 1953), and Léon Guichard, in his critical study of Laforgue, have evaluated these comments on feminine roles.

ACHIEVEMENTS

Jules Laforgue's poetry published in 1885 and 1886 earned for him praise from contemporary critics and established him as one of the leading innovators of poetic form at the time. The literary circle within which he moved made his classification as a Symbolist poet inevitable. His sudden death in 1887 gave his career a tragic plot, especially for literary historians eager to contribute to the mythology of doomed poets.

Laforgue's most significant contributions to the development of modern poetry are his rhymed free verse, his verbal playfulness, his juxtaposition of melancholy and gaiety in his ironic tone, and his psychologically complex monologues and dialogues, which give voice to the unconscious and to dream states, as well as to masks consciously assumed.

Although Laforgue has often been dismissed as a minor poet, his philosophical sophistication may deserve as much praise as his technical innovations. In his poetry, Laforgue explored the conflicts between the conscious and the unconscious, exposed the illusions of rational pessimism, and exploited the literary consequences of an idealist philosophy against those of determinism (as practiced by the naturalists), but he set all these metaphysical confrontations in the real, familiar world of trivial remarks and superficial gestures.

BIOGRAPHY

Born in Uruguay, Jules Laforgue was sent at the age of six to a boarding school in Tarbes, France, where he remained until he was fifteen. Laforgue felt isolated and persecuted at school; he left an account of his childhood and adolescence in the autobiographical novel *Stéphane Vassiliew*. His family returned from Uruguay in his sixteenth year, and the eleven children and two parents crowded into an apartment in Paris. That spring, his mother died after a twelfth pregnancy; she was thirty-seven. In "Avertissement," Laforgue wrote that he hardly knew his mother, but his awareness of her situation may be glimpsed in "Complainte du fœtus de poète," in which an unsympathetic and egotistic voice describes his birth, blithely unconcerned with any feelings but his own.

Laforgue attended the Lycée Fontanes (now Condorcet) but twice failed his oral examination for the *baccalauréat*. A paralyzing fear of failure afflicts many of Laforgue's poetic alter egos. After failing his examinations, Laforgue continued to study independently, reading omnivorously and attending lectures on the philosophy of art by the determinist Hippolyte Taine, whose assertions that art is completely determined by milieu, race, and historical moment Laforgue rejected.

In 1880, the twenty-year-old Laforgue met several influential men whose friendship helped launch his career. Gustave Kahn became a good friend, confidant, and literary editor. Kahn introduced Laforgue to the regular Tuesday readings by Stéphane Mallarmé and also to Charles Henry, an intellectual equally brilliant on scientific and literary topics. That same year, Laforgue also met the literary critic Paul Bourget, who generously criticized his writing and who arranged a job for Laforgue assisting the art critic Charles Ephrussi. He introduced Laforgue to the paintings of the Impressionists, and evidence from Laforgue's poems and essays indicates that the Impressionist aesthetic reflected his conviction that art aims at fusing a sensual and intellectual apprehension of life.

Late in 1881, Laforgue's father, who was dying from tuberculosis, moved the rest of the family to Tarbes, leaving Laforgue behind. Although he took a cheap room to remain in Paris, Laforgue was employed by Ephrussi, was writing poems, and was enjoying his literary life; ironically, a self-pitying letter written to his sister during this period, exaggerating his timidity and his loneliness and appealing for sympathy, later contributed to the legend of the starving poet.

That year, with the recommendations of Bourget and Ephrussi, Laforgue was appointed the French reader to the German Empress Augusta, a job that paid well, gave him leisure to write, introduced him to rich food and luxurious apartments, and required his residence in Germany. From November, 1881, through September, 1886, Laforgue lived with the peripatetic German imperial court for ten months of the year; he spent his long vacations of 1883, 1884, and 1885 in Paris, and his constant correspondence kept him in touch with contemporary literary developments in France.

Although he complained of his boredom in the German court, Laforgue worked steadily on his poems, and during the court's residence in Berlin, he enjoyed the company of musicians and artists (especially his friends the brothers Théophile and Eugène Ysaÿe, a pianist and a violinist) and amused himself at the aquarium, circuses, music halls, museums, the opera, the ballet, and orchestral concerts. His experience of Berlin's cultural life influenced the imagery of his poems, in which one finds clowns, harlequins, underwater creatures, sublime music, and playfully improper cabaret patter.

On New Year's Day, 1886, Laforgue, who identified his anguished self-consciousness with Hamlet's character, visited the castle of Elsinore; he later reworked his experience of Hamlet's haunt into his *Des fleurs de bonne volonté* and his prose fantasy about the indecisive Dane. Back in Berlin, late in January, Laforgue met an English woman, Leah Lee, who had chosen to live independently from her family and who was supporting herself by teaching English. As he fell in love with her, he was reaching his decision to leave the German court position. He spent three weeks in Paris in late June and early July, then returned to the German court, and by August, in the resort at

Schlagenbad, he was writing his first poems in free verse.

Laforgue returned to Berlin with the German court on September 1, 1886, Lee accepted his marriage proposal on September 6, and he left the employ of the Empress Augusta that month. By October, Laforgue was living in Paris, waiting for his own wedding, reworking and finishing his poems in free verse, completing his *Six Moral Tales from Jules Laforgue*, and discussing the movement newly named "Symbolist" with Édouard Dujardin and Teodor de Wyzewa (editors of *La Revue indépendante*) and his old friends Kahn (later editor of *La Vogue*) and Félix Fénéon (who edited and reshaped Laforgue's new poems in free verse). Laforgue's moral tales and his new poems were published in various issues of *La Vogue* and *La Revue indépendante*, so that by the autumn of 1886, Laforgue's star had burst onto the Parisian literary scene, with the publication of his tales, his free verse, *L'Imitation de Notre-Dame la lune*, and *Le Concile féerique*. Laforgue was being hailed as a leader in the avant-garde.

On the last day of that wonderful year, Laforgue and Leah married, in London (at St. Barnabas, where T. S. Eliot and Valerie Fletcher were married in 1957). Laforgue returned to Paris with a bad cough, which, as it developed, was a symptom of tuberculosis. For eight months, he was too ill to write much poetry, and he died on August 20, 1887.

ANALYSIS

Although the legend of his short, tragic life shaped the initial critical response to his work, Jules Laforgue is now recognized as one of the first modernist poets. Laforgue is notable for his technical innovations, for his ironic voices and psychologically complex personas, for his verbal and syntactic playfulness, and for his fusion of sublimely serious philosophical questions with the plainly vulgar language and concerns of ordinary life.

Laforgue developed the poetic form known as *vers libre*, or free verse, in which he used lines of varying length, subtle rhyming patterns, and diverse rhythms to correspond, flexibly, to shifts in mood and subject. Although Arthur Rimbaud also has been credited with inventing free verse (with his "Marine" and "Mouve-

ment," poems written earlier than *Les Derniers Vers de Jules Laforgue*), Laforgue's innovative verse forms were published in periodicals before Rimbaud's examples, and his *Les Derniers Vers de Jules Laforgue* more directly influenced the free verse of modernist poets.

Most English and American readers know Laforgue through his influence on Eliot, Ezra Pound, Hart Crane, and Wallace Stevens. In 1908, Eliot read about Laforgue in *The Symbolist Movement in Literature*, by Arthur Symons; in 1909, Eliot read Laforgue's poems and letters selected in *Œuvres complètes de Jules Laforgue*. Eliot's poems influenced by Laforgue's irony, dialogues, and verse forms include the 1909 "Nocturne," "Humouresque," and "Spleen," and the more famous "The Love Song of J. Alfred Prufrock," "Conversation Galante," "Portrait of a Lady," and "La Figlia che Piange," as well as sections of *The Waste Land* (1922). Pound and Crane both published translations of Laforgue's work, and Pound praised Laforgue's intellect dancing playfully among words. Laforguian irony and wordplay may be found in Pound's "Hugh Selwyn Mauberley" and in Crane's "Chaplinesque," among other poems. Stevens transformed Laforgue's Impressionist images and his verse forms extensively, but the French poet's diffused influence may be traced in such works of Stevens as "The Comedian as the Letter C," "Sea Surface Full of Clouds," "Peter Quince at the Clavier," and "Notes Toward a Supreme Fiction."

Laforgue anticipated the psychological narratives of both James Joyce and Marcel Proust in the interior monologue he developed in such poems as "Complainte de Lord Pierrot" and "Dimanches." He split his monologues and dialogues into multiple voices that are wittily self-aware and self-mocking. Although the contrapuntal dialogue of his "Complainte du soir des comices agricoles" was inspired by Gustave Flaubert (in a notorious scene in *Madame Bovary*, 1856, the overblown romantic language of a seduction is undercut by the vulgar realism of an animal auction at a country fair), Laforgue neither relied on simple antithesis nor assumed a superior moral stance; rather, his ironic conversations and monologues offer multiple perspectives that remain irreconcilable.

Pound and Joyce delighted in Laforgue's demolition and recombination of language. The amusing colloquialisms and revolutionary neologisms that appear in Laforgue's verse violated poetic etiquette but revealed the psychology of his speakers. They wittily or ignorantly combine two words from different realms to disclose an unexpected association. Examples include "sangsuelles," "éternullité," "voluptés," "spleenuosité," and "crucifige" (these neologisms are derived, respectively, from blood plus sensual, eternal plus nullity, violation or violence plus voluptuous, spleen plus sinuosity, and crucify plus to clot). Laforgue often fused common words, but he also correctly employed arcane, archaic, and slang words in lines of impeccably sublime diction. The shock of contrast, with the implied assertion of the validity and significance of these verbal intrusions, radically changes the poet's relationship to language.

In his images and subjects, Laforgue, like the Impressionists and the Symbolists in painting and literature, claimed for his art both a psychological and a physical definition of reality and envisioned correlations between the sublime and the ordinary, between the spiritual and the objective worlds. Eliot, in his celebrated definition of the "objective correlative," drew on Laforgue's example.

Laforgue's literary legacy also includes his black humor. In poems such as "Excuse macabre," "Guitare," and "Complainte des blackboulés" ("Lament of the Blackballs"), his ironic but not pompous stance treated the grim themes of death, frustration, self-doubt, boredom, melancholy, alienation, nihilism, and the failure of passion with a racy wit, slipping often into gaiety. In this, Samuel Beckett is one of Laforgue's heirs.

The bathetic, self-centered misery of the gloomy poems Laforgue wrote from 1880 to 1882, for *Le Sanglot de la terre* (first pb. in *Œuvres complètes de Jules Laforgue*), has provoked speculation about a period of depression he suffered, but these metrically conventional and sentimental verses, laboriously exploring correlations between an adolescent's passionate psyche and the world's turbulence, have a literary antecedent in the splenetic poems of Baudelaire, and they also betray the influence of the moral and metaphysical idealism of Arthur Schopenhauer. Recognizing the inadequacy of these early poems, Laforgue chose not to publish them.

From 1882 through 1884, Laforgue worked on a group of comic poems based on popular street ballads. In them, he experimented with unconventional metric forms and broken syntax, and introduced slang, puns, and vulgar words into poems that also played with liturgical images. In a letter, he described these poems as "psychology in the form of dream," and they contain free associations of words and sudden juxtapositions of sublime and tawdry images. These poems were written after Laforgue had immersed himself in the philosophy of Eduard von Hartmann, whose emphasis on the unconscious profoundly shaped the poet's definition of identity. The conflicting voices and shifting tones within Laforgue's poetry reflect his belief in the multiple selves that coexist in any personality. Consequently, his narrative verse seems to leap between dream states and waking; among past, present, and future experiences; and from unquestioning sympathy to biting mockery, while continuing to portray one persona. Publishing delays kept these poems from appearing until 1885, but, when *Les Complaintes* finally appeared, the volume was enthusiastically reviewed.

LES COMPLAINTES

Les Complaintes consists of two preliminary poems and fifty laments titled "Complainte de . . ." with the titles playing upon the subjective-objective ambiguity of the genitive. The ambiguous titles reflect the multiple voices speaking within these dramatic poems and also the poems' themes. For example, "Complainte de Lord Pierrot" is a divided interior monologue spoken by Pierrot, and his lament also defines his identity; "Complainte du soir des comices agricoles" is set during the night of the country fair and may also be heard as the lament of that night; "Complainte des pianos qu'on entend dans les quartiers aisés" is both a lament of a man walking in well-to-do neighborhoods, who hears and is aroused by the sounds of girls' piano practice, and an imaginary dialogue between the man and the pianos concerning the girls' inarticulate, romantic illusions, and their sexuality.

In "Complainte de Lord Pierrot," the individual is divided in time and in space, with Pierrot singing a self-mocking version of the ballad "Au clair de la lune," then commenting in rhymed couplets on his sexual timidity and inexperience, then in irregularly rhymed ten-syllable lines imagining himself under the influence of Venus, dressed as a swan, boldly coupling with Leda, then abruptly shifting to a mocking couplet, "—Tout cela vous honore,/ Lord Pierrot, mais encore?" ("All that pays you tribute,/ Lord Pierrot, but what next?"), which becomes a two-line refrain as it is repeated later in the poem. Similarly, in "Complainte des pianos qu'on entend dans les quartiers aisés," the lonely speaker meditates on desirable young girls who provoke his sexual longing, but a two-line refrain, echoing a popular song, seems to tease and mock him: "Tu t'en vas et tu nous quittes,/ Tu nous quitt's et tu t'en vas!" ("You depart and you leave us/ You leave us and you depart!"). As readers familiar with "The Love Song of J. Alfred Prufrock" will recognize, Eliot adopted Laforgue's device, the ironic couplet refrain, in his lines rhyming "come and go" with "Michelangelo."

Just as Pierrot's various moods are expressed in different verse forms, so the sexual longing, the self-doubting mockery, the erotic curiosity, and the contemptuous cynicism of a lonely man are represented in the shifting forms of "Complainte des pianos qu'on entend dans les quartiers aisés," in which the syllabic length of the lines changes with each stanza. The basic group of four verse forms, recurring five times in the same order, comprises a quatrain of irregular Alexandrines rhymed *abab*, followed by a rhymed couplet of seven-syllable lines, followed by a rhymed couplet of four-syllable lines, and concluded by a quatrain of seven-syllable lines rhymed *abab*, the first two lines being some version of the refrain, "Tu t'en vas et tu nous laisses,/ Tu nous laiss's et tu t'en vas." Although these shifts create the impression, on a first reading, of the free-flowing and disparate lines of thought within the lonely man's mind, the larger formal pattern is quite elaborate. The poem seems a patchwork of quatrains and couplets, in which the significant pattern of the whole shifts as one focuses on different combinations of the parts. Are the girls singing to the man? Is he imagining their mockery? The deliberate ambiguity reflects the psychological complexity of Laforgue's portrait and also the inevitability of change: from innocence to experience, from the sublimity of imaginary voyeurism to the vulgar reality of physical sexuality, from spiritual eroticism to the ordinary, routine materi-

alism of life—embodied in the ludicrous exclamations on the month, the underclothes, and the routine meal of the final line: "Ô mois, ô linges, ô repas!"

L'IMITATION DE NOTRE-DAME LA LUNE

The twenty-two poems for *L'Imitation de Notre-Dame la lune* were written at lightning speed, in six weeks of 1885, and dedicated to Laforgue's friend Kahn and to Salammbô, Flaubert's fictional pagan priestess. These litanies in praise of the moon ridicule the excessive zeal and overstated piety that characterize both Salammbô's behavior and most public professions of idolatrous worship. Utilizing the literary conventions associating the moon and the cultural archetype "woman," Laforgue mocks the lunatic lover who throws himself at the feet of the woman ("aux pieds de la femme," in the poem "Guitare"), and his obsessive myth defining woman as mysterious, cruel, changeable, and purely sensual is exposed in the allusions to Delilah, Eve, the Sphinx, and La Joconde (the Mona Lisa).

The eminent lunologist in *L'Imitation de Notre-Dame la lune* is Pierrot, whose ancestor is Pagliacco, of the commedia dell'arte, but who, in the French tradition, became fused with Harlequin. The Pierrot figure in Laforgue's poetry has contradictory characteristics: He is both a disappointed lover, melancholy and vulnerable, and a deceiving lover, frivolous and cynical. In either mode, Pierrot avoids the entangling responsibilities of love. This clown, in whiteface, with his long skinny neck, dilated eyes, reddened mouth, and black skullcap, both longs for a woman and fears passion. He closely resembles Eliot's Prufrock.

DES FLEURS DE BONNE VOLONTÉ

Des fleurs de bonne volonté is, in part, a response to Charles Baudelaire's *Les Fleurs du mal* (1857, 1861, 1868; *Flowers of Evil*, 1909). Written in 1886, these fifty-six poems reflect Laforgue's fascination with Hamlet's indecisiveness. Throughout these poems, he sprinkled epigraphs from Hamlet's and Ophelia's verbal duels, and his persona agonizes over his own inability to marry. Like Hamlet, this character cannot allow himself to trust a woman. Unlike Baudelaire, who treats the infidelity of woman as a cosmic truth, Laforgue focuses on the psychology of the lover whose fear of betrayal paralyzes him. Like Jaques in William

Shakespeare's *As You Like It* (pr. c. 1599-1600), this character's cynicism makes him miserable. His assertion in "Célibat, célibat, tout n'est que célibat" that human history is the history of one unmarried man at first seems ridiculous, a product of his obsession, but one may read the dramatic situation of these poems, the prolonged hesitation before risking a commitment, as an extended metaphor for human history.

Twelve different poems in this collection bear the title "Dimanches" (Sundays), and each portrays a profoundly melancholic state of mind; images of rain, gray skies, and the haunting refrain of a piano recur throughout. As Laforgue dissects ennui in these Impressionistic poems, it is self-generated and circles from dissatisfaction to longing for release, to fearing change, to resigning oneself to the misery of inaction.

"Dimanches" is representative. It consists of four stanzas, with the second and the fourth in parentheses. The first, invoking autumn, associates the fall of leaves with death and love's suffering; the second, replying parenthetically, pleads that the speaker can believe in himself only in moments when he is lost; the third raises the possibility of marriage; and the fourth replies with a hypothesis—what if he could believe in himself and then marry?—followed by a renunciation expressed in a self-wounding comparison: "C'est Galatée aveuglant Pygmalion!" (it is Galatea blinding Pygmalion!). Laforgue's use of myth here suggests that the artist, by dedicating himself to the abstract ideal of incorruptible beauty, comes to be transfixed by his own artifice; similarly, the woman, imprisoned in the statuesque role of perfect physical beauty, becomes a seductress as she embraces the one who created that role. The circular dialogue this speaker conducts with himself imprisons him in his own unhappiness.

When Laforgue decided to marry, he decided not to publish *Des fleurs de bonne volonté*, but he did rework several of the poems into his new poems in free verse. Laforgue's final poems develop his earlier themes with greater technical and psychological sophistication.

LES DERNIERS VERS DE JULES LAFORGUE

The twelve free-verse poems of *Les Derniers Vers de Jules Laforgue* cohere as twelve movements of one long symphony might; their interrelated themes and recapitulated forms reward close reading extended to the structure of the whole. Laforgue's extraordinary technical and thematic control reveals itself in the illusion of free-flowing lines, which, although irregular in length and grouped in no conventional stanzas, are linked by careful alliteration, internal harmonies, and end rhymes. The lines are grouped thematically, developing a mood, or symbol, or idea, in verse paragraphs, thus creating a verbal image of the memories, free associations, recurrent dreams, and self-conscious observations that compose an individual's interior universe.

Laforgue again treats the theme of an overly sensitive man, agonizing about the extent and the limits of his self-knowledge, who seeks release in a loving companion, but, associating sexuality with death, despairs of love. The personal tragedy, finally, is given broad cultural significance by Laforgue's allusions to historical events, to literary antecedents, to musical revolutions, to paintings, and to powerful myths. These poems, like Impressionist paintings, take into account the sensibility of the viewer and appeal to the imagination through associated sensual memories. Unlike Mallarmé, Laforgue does not invoke the poet as sole symbol for humankind; moreover, the ivory tower of abstract thought and artifice does not confine Laforgue's persona, whose feelings and sensual impressions reflect factory smoke as well as fog, spittle as well as the sun's blinding white disk, the pettiness of objects consumed daily as well as the tragic grandeur of human mortality glimpsed in a sunset or in the coming of winter.

"L'Hiver qui vient," the first poem of the collection, illustrates the broader references and more radical techniques. Laforgue breaks poetic convention with his first line: "Blocus sentimental! Messageries du Levant!" ("emotional blockade! Levantine carrier ships!"). The line nullifies syntax by exclamation and alludes by echo to the glory and grim cost of the Napoleonic War's Continental System (known as the "blocus continental") and the eastern packet ships running the blockade. Neither national history nor seasonal change is the subject; rather, both are employed as correlatives of the persona's mood, a complex mixture of self-indulgent pity, rage against frustration, and ironic mockery. Facing the coming of winter yet again, the persona recalls

associated feelings, images, and events: a child's loneliness at the *lycée*, the ennui of rainy Sundays, the end
of a love affair, the suffering of soldiers far from home,
the end of a foxhunt, each day's death of the sun, and
the misery of urban life. From the music of Richard
Wagner, Laforgue had learned to interweave distinctive themes representing complex passions. The weeping and sighing of autumnal rain and wind, the miserable coughing of a consumptive, the sad tones of hunting
horns (imitated in "Ton ton, ton taine, ton ton!") re-
sound in the poem, evoking compassion for the cor-
nered creature, nostalgia for a lost social order, and the
longing for an unattainable happiness. Laforgue's aim
in these musical, free-verse poems may be understood
in his last line of "L'Hiver qui vient": "J'essaierai en
choeur d'en donner la note" ("I will try, in this choir, to
give it its note").

Perceiving the human situation as essentially hopeless and feeling the tragic disparity between glorious
aspirations and sordid or merely ordinary lives, Laforgue nevertheless rejects the Romantic poet's uncon-
trolled sentimentalism, undercutting self-pity by vulgar language, tawdry details, and the wry commentary
of a rhymed couplet. His characteristic fusion of sensitivity and ironic distance, his representation of divided
psychological states, his masterful exploitation of free
verse to evoke shifting moods and associated ideas, his
consciously comic treatment of serious subjects, and
his playful re-creation of language mark Laforgue as
one of the first modernist poets.

OTHER MAJOR WORKS

LONG FICTION: *Stéphane Vassiliew*, 1946.

SHORT FICTION: *Moralités légendaires*, 1887 (*Six
Moral Tales from Jules Laforgue*, 1928).

PLAYS: *Le Concile féerique*, pb. 1886; *Pierrot
fumiste*, pb. 1892.

NONFICTION: *Berlin: La Cour et la ville*, 1922
(*Berlin: The City and the Court*, 1996); *Lettres à un
ami, 1880-1886*, 1941.

BIBLIOGRAPHY

Arkell, David. *Looking for Laforgue: An Informal Biography*. New York: Persea Books, 1979. A biographical study of Laforgue with a bibliography and index.

Dale, Peter, trans. Introduction to *Poems of Jules Laforgue*. London: Anvil Press Poetry, 2001. Dale's
twenty-page introduction provides a solid overview
of the poet, his body of work, and the history of the
texts. This bilingual English-French edition also offers notes on the text, a brief bibliography, and indexes of both French and English titles.

Franklin, Ursula. *Exiles and Ironists: Essays on the
Kinship of Heine and Laforgue*. New York: Peter
Lang, 1988. Critical analysis considering the influence of Heinrich Heine on Laforgue's work. Includes a bibliography.

Holmes, Anne. "'De Nouveaux Rhythmes': The Free
Verse of Laforgue's 'Solo de Lune.'" *French Studies* 62, no. 2 (April, 2008): 162. Holmes argues that
Larforgue's interest in music influenced the structure and detail of his free verse.

_____. *Jules LaForgue and Poetic Innovation*. New
York: Oxford University Press, 1993. A critical anal-
ysis focusing on Laforgue's innovations in technique.
Includes bibliographical references and index.

Howe, Elisabeth A. *Stages of Self: The Dramatic
Monologues of Laforgue, Valéry, and Mallarmé*.
Athens: Ohio University Press, 1990. A study of
the representations of the self in three nineteenth
century French poets. Includes bibliographic references and an index.

Ramsey, Warren, ed. *Jules Laforgue: Essays on a
Poet's Life and Work*. Carbondale: Southern Illinois
University Press, 1969. A collection of critical and
biographical essays with bibliographic references.

Watson, Lawrence J. *Jules Laforgue: Poet of His Age*.
Rev. ed. Mahwah, N.J.: Ramapo College of New
Jersey, 1980. A short introduction to Laforgue and
his work.

Judith L. Johnston

ALPHONSE DE LAMARTINE

Born: Mâcon, France; October 21, 1790
Died: Paris, France; February 28, 1869

PRINCIPAL POETRY

Méditations poétiques, 1820 (*Poetical Meditations*, 1839)
La Mort de Socrate, 1823 (*The Death of Socrates*, 1829)
Nouvelles méditations poétiques, 1823
Chant du sacre, 1825
Le Dernier Chant du pèleringe d'Harold, 1825 (*The Last Canto of Childe Harold's Pilgrimage*, 1827)
Harmonies poétiques et religieuses, 1830
Œuvres complètes, 1834
Jocelyn, 1836 (English translation, 1837)
La Chute d'un ange, 1838
Recueillements poétiques, 1839
Œuvres poétiques complètes, 1963

OTHER LITERARY FORMS

The attempts at drama of Alphonse de Lamartine (lah-mahr-TEEN) are poor, often embarrassing, imitations of the works of Jean Racine, Pierre Corneille, and Voltaire, as well as William Shakespeare. Lamartine was somewhat more successful in the realm of prose fiction. He wrote two semiautobiographical novels, *Graziella* (1849; English translation, 1871) and *Raphaël* (1849; English translation, 1849); the former was the more popular, while the latter is the better of the two. *Raphaël*, which is based on the poet's love affair with Julie Charles, has been criticized as a novel that was outmoded even in its time, as well as being excessively sentimental. Certainly, *Raphaël* bears the imprint of Jean-Jacques Rousseau's *La Nouvelle Héloïse* (1761; *Julia, or the New Eloisa*, 1773) but it is nevertheless an impressive treatment of Lamartine's favorite themes: religion, love, politics, and nature.

In the course of a long political career, Lamartine delivered some exceptionally eloquent and often politically perspicacious speeches before the French Chamber of Deputies. On the eve of the February Revolution of 1848, he published in eight volumes a fearless glorification of the French Revolution, *Histoire des Girondins* (1847; *History of the Girondists*, 1847-1848). While not a historian's history, it offers such a colorful and sweeping vision of a period that in many ways it is really a historical novel in the guise of nonfiction. Among many other works, Lamartine also wrote popular histories of the 1848 Revolution in France, the Restoration, Turkey, and Russia.

ACHIEVEMENTS

The critic Henri Peyre has observed that among the great French Romantics, Alphonse de Lamartine demonstrated "the keenest political insight." His work in politics was as important as the politics in his works, but his formal, aesthetic accomplishments in poetry were strong, too. He made his first and his most lasting mark in poetry with *Poetical Meditations*. This collection, which enjoyed tremendous success with the readers of its day, has been hailed as the first masterpiece of the Romantic movement in French poetry. Lamartine, seen by his contemporaries as an innovator, is often condemned by modern critics for his neoclassical diction, for his rhetorical flourishes, and for his sentimentalism. If one takes Lamartine's poetry on its own terms, however, and particularly if one appreciates its musical prosody, it will be clear why a handful of his poems have a permanent place in anthologies of French literature.

BIOGRAPHY

Alphonse de Lamartine's life can be schematized as a pattern that shifts among four points: political commitments, a sentimental intermixture of women and natural scenery, a personalized and heretical form of Catholicism, and a semiautobiographical approach to poetry. Each, either through circumstance or through the poet's whims, was allowed periodically to reach an ascendancy over the others and to dominate his time and energy. To give emphasis to one over the other is to understand none of them; all must be considered in due course. If one is to understand Lamartine's heavily autobiographical poetry, one must consider his politics, his religion, and his love of women and nature.

Given his family and the events of his early years, it

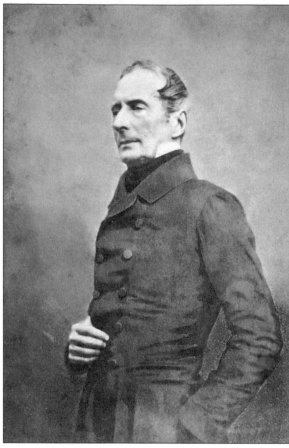

Alphonse de Lamartine (Hulton Archive/Getty Images)

is no surprise that the adult Lamartine was to demonstrate an active interest in politics—although the leftward direction of that interest could hardly have been predicted. On October 21, 1790, in the opening years of the French Revolution, Lamartine was born into a gentry family that was staunchly Royalist. His father was imprisoned for a long while during the Terror but was not executed. Lamartine's mother, a deeply religious woman who combined the ideas of Rousseau with Catholicism, gave Lamartine his early religious training and had a deep influence on him. At the Jesuit college at Belley, Lamartine again was exposed to liberal Catholic attitudes as well as to a broad range of world literature. It is a tribute to Lamartine's capacity for development that throughout his life he carried this liberalism in religion, as well as in politics, to points just short of radicalism, so much so that by old age he had evolved far beyond the paradigms of his youth.

An early and deep interest in nature and in love was to initiate Lamartine's metamorphosis. In 1811 and 1812, he visited Italy, which, as in the case of Johann Wolfgang von Goethe several decades before, proved a great impetus to Lamartine's development as a poet. An affair with an Italian cigar maker of loose morals named Antoniella (the probable model for Graziella) had the effect of loosening those of the poet. The scenery, particularly that of the Bay of Naples, left a strong impression on several of his lyrics.

The real turning point, however, came during the autumn of 1816. While convalescing at a fashionable bath in Savoy, Lamartine met Charles, who had all the requisite qualities for attracting the affections of a romantic poet: She was beautiful, consumptive, and married. They carried on an affair amid splendid alpine scenery, which helped to set the tone of pantheism in Lamartine's religious development. In spite of periodic separations, an amorous but perhaps unconsummated relationship continued until Charles finally died of tuberculosis in December, 1817. This affair left a permanent mark on Lamartine. Other affairs and even his marriage in 1820 to Marianne Birch, a wealthy Englishwoman, had no effect on his feelings for Charles and did not disperse the aura of melancholy that her death had imposed on him. Indeed, two further sorrows resulted from his marriage: the deaths of a son and a daughter.

Lamartine's career in the Chamber of Deputies, the elective legislative body of France during the first half of the nineteenth century and in the governments of the 1848 Revolution and the Second Republic is important historically and biographically. A consideration of this career is crucial to an understanding of Lamartine's political poetry. Charles-Maurice de Talleyrand-Périgord said of Lamartine that he had the acumen to penetrate to the heart of his country. He foresaw the dangers of military dictatorships—one of which was soon to materialize under Napoleon III. Lamartine also read an important message in the unsuccessful workers' riots in Lyons and in Paris (1831-1832). He foresaw the necessity for the political education of the working class, who he believed would initiate all future revolutions. (The events of 1848 and 1878 proved him, in great part, correct.)

Above all, Lamartine demonstrated an ability to adapt to a changing political climate—so much so that he was often a bit ahead of his time. Lamartine discovered to his sorrow that flexibility, no matter how logical, can be a fatal flaw in politics. What through twentieth century hindsight seems a sincere, if gradual, move from bourgeois liberalism to a moderately leftist stance seemed to his contemporaries to be inconsistency. Lamartine's sorrow was to have been a statesman in a time of political conservatives and opportunists, the worst and most formidable among whom was Napoleon III. Lamartine could easily have set himself up as a dictator, thereby gaining the support of the Right, but he decided instead to share his power as the head of the 1848 Provisional Government with the leader of the Left, A. A. Ledru-Rollin; this decision lost him the support of the wealthy ruling class.

Lamartine ran unsuccessfully for public office in 1848. Much of the remainder of his life was spent writing popular histories, biographies, and similar works to produce needed income. Lamartine's wife died in 1863; in 1867, the government of Napoleon III, acknowledging the relative poverty of the former statesman, granted Lamartine a substantial sum. Lamartine died in Paris on February 28, 1869.

ANALYSIS

Alphonse de Lamartine's poetry developed, as did everything in his life, by degrees, with no marked departures from the past. Rarely have life and art been so closely intertwined. All his passions became the stuff of his art, to be woven into complex patterns of alliteration and assonance. Perhaps he created only a handful of enduring works, but few poets can claim to have done more.

Lamartine's ability to accept and assimilate change as a Christian, a politician, and a poet demonstrates, more than any of his other qualities, his Romantic worldview. He did not merely accept nineteenth century historicism; he lived it. Change is the dominant theme of his poetry.

POETICAL MEDITATIONS

It is no surprise, then, that Lamartine's first collection of poems had a profound effect on the evolution of French poetry. Indeed, *Poetical Meditations* demon-

strates the same gradual development that characterized Lamartine the statesman. The work at the time seemed a radical departure from the neoclassical sensibility that continued to dominate French poetry under the directorate, the empire, and the early Restoration—indeed, it seemed so radical a departure that it was refused by the publisher to whom Lamartine first submitted it in 1817. What was acceptable in the prose of Vicomte François-René de Chateaubriand was, until 1820, not palatable in the more formalized realm of poetry. Lamartine took the first, appropriately cautious, step.

"THE LAKE"

The most famous and enduring work of this collection is "Le Lac" ("The Lake"); this lyric is also Lamartine's most frequently anthologized poem. The essential theme of the poem, mutability in the light of the permanence of nature, is introduced in the first stanza. Here, the natural world is treated metaphorically—"eternal night," "time's sea"—to suggest the uncertainty of human fate in the eternal flux. In short, the first stanza maintains a tradition that is at least as old as the first century Greek critic Longinus. Beginning with the second stanza, however, a new, albeit tentative, tone is struck. Natural objects, ceasing to be metaphors, have an existence all their own and are conveyed to the reader with a directness that had not been heard in French poetry for a long time. Although nature in Lamartine certainly lacks the concrete immediacy that it had already found in the poetry of William Wordsworth or Goethe, the lake, addressed as it is by the persona, is a natural object and not an imaginary shepherdess or an actual patron of the poet; thus, a new directness is gained. Stanzas 2 and 3 picture a time when the persona sat by an alpine lake with his beloved—a figure not individualized in the poem but based on Charles.

The fourth stanza deals with a third Wordsworthian "spot in time": The persona recalls a night when Charles and he were rowing on the lake. This complex layering of three events is characteristic of Lamartine's obsession with time. Stanza 5 introduces the motif of a nature sympathetically resonant with human relations. The persona's beloved begins to speak, causing the shore to be spellbound and drawing the attention of the waves. The beloved's reply in stanzas 6 through 9 is still in the eighteenth century tradition; personified time is now addressed far more conventionally than in the persona's earlier address to the lake. Stanza 9 is a twofold culmination of the beloved's address. First, it gives clear expression to the carpe diem theme to which it has all been leading: "So let us love, so let us love! let us hasten, let us enjoy the fleeting hour" ("Aimons donc, aimons donc! de l'heure fugitive,/ Hâtonsnous, jouissons!"). Second, the stanza returns to the opening image of the lyric, time as an expanse of water without a harbor: "Man has no harbor, time has no shore:/ It flows and we pass on."

In stanza 10, "jealous time" is addressed by the persona, who asks how time can take away the same "moments of intoxication" that it gives. In the last four stanzas, the persona addresses the "lake! mute rocks, grottos! dark forest!" asking them to keep alive the memory of the young couple's night on the lake. With measured rhythms, the poet appeals to all the different sounds of nature, "everything that is heard, seen, or breathed,/ Let all say: 'They loved!'" This musical voice of nature is a poetic credo that Lamartine repeats often in his poetry; the limpid rhythm and assonance that embody this natural music account for the great popularity of the poem.

"THE VALLEY"

A quick glance at another poem in the collection, "Le Vallon" ("The Valley"), indicates the unity of the *Poetical Meditations*. The theme and many of the motifs of "The Lake" are also found in "The Valley." Here, the persona again laments the brevity of life's pleasures, but the added motif of the anonymity of death sounds a new note. The waves and murmuring of the lake are replaced by those of two hidden streams, which meet to form one. The streams flow from their respective sources only to lose their individual identities by merging with each other. These natural images become metaphors for the persona's lost youth: "The source of my days like the streams has flowed away,/ It has passed without a sound, without a name, and without any hope of return."

In "The Valley," the poet employs one of his favorite metaphors: the capacity of sounds in nature to lull the senses and to heal hurts. These effects he sought, often with great success, in his lyrics: The persona says that, "Like an infant rocked by a simple chant,/ My soul is assuaged by the murmur of the waters" ("Comme un enfant bercé par un chant monotone,/ Mon âme s'assoupit au murmure des eaux"). The music of these lines, with their *n* and *m* sounds, creates precisely the soothing effect that they describe. The water of the brooks and other images taken from nature are used to symbolize the transience of human life; paradoxically, for the poet, nature has the ability to console humans because, although subject to change in its parts, it is permanent in its totality: "While everything changes for you, nature is the same." Behind nature is the quintessential permanence of God. For Lamartine, there is no consolation in change as manifested in natural phenomena such as water except in the thought that it is a part of some greater mystical whole.

NOUVELLES MÉDITATIONS POÉTIQUES

It is both the strength and the weakness of *Nouvelles méditations poétiques* that Lamartine continues to explore the themes of the *Poetical Meditations*. "Tristesse" (sorrow) is a poem that draws on Lamartine's experiences in Naples with Antoniella. As he often does in this volume, the poet draws on images found in the earlier collection. For example, the "laughing slopes" of "The Lake" appear again in "Tristesse." The lake is now a bay, but it is still an expanse of water that provides a place for lovers to listen "to the gentle noise of the waves or the murmuring wind" ("Au doux bruit de la vague ou du vent qui murmure"); indeed, any hasty glance at Lamartine's poetry will demonstrate the poet's predilection for the word *murmure*—whether it is the murmur of the waves, wind, or foliage. The persona of "Tristesse," as the title implies, suffers in a state of melancholy and nostalgia for a happy past that is lost, never to return. Life and death are joined, a final paradox in which the poet wishes "to die in the place where he has tasted life." There are, however, some new elements in "Tristesse": There is a growing specificity both in the poet's description of the locus of Vergil's tomb and as he conveys his youthful passion with images of "enflamed Vesuvius once again arising from the bosom of the waves."

HARMONIES POÉTIQUES ET RELIGIEUSES

Harmonies poétiques et religieuses reflects the concerns of Lamartine the political figure. Indeed, even the religious aspects of this work can best be understood in a political context, for the separation of church and state was a crucial issue in the politics of nineteenth century France. This relationship between politics and religion must be kept in mind if the reader of *Harmonies poétiques et religieuses* is to comprehend Lamartine's merging of Christianity with the secular historicism of eighteenth and nineteenth century France.

"Les Revolutions" (the revolutions) was first published in a review and later incorporated into *Harmonies poétiques et religieuses*. Inspired by the workers' uprisings in Paris and Lyon, which helped to provoke the turn left in Lamartine's politics, it demonstrates the concept of historical relativism that was to culminate in the works of Georg Wilhelm Friedrich Hegel, Charles Darwin, and Karl Marx. Lamartine shared a growing awareness that, in the evolution of social structures, whether religious or political, there are no absolute values. In this eloquent lyric, the poet expresses a genuine contempt for the backward-looking conservatism of the majority of his European contemporaries. He contrasts them metaphorically with the nomadic peoples of Arabia, who physically (if certainly not religiously or socially) packed up their belongings and passed on to new horizons. By contrast, the European conservatives are, as Lamartine tells them, "men petrified in [their] timid pride." Lamartine's preoccupation with change, previously applied to nature and to human relationships, is here applied to politics and religion; these human institutions are subject to the mutability that is part of a divine plan: "all things/ Change, fall, perish, flee, die, decompose" ("et toute chose/ Change, tombe, périt, fuit, meurt, se décompose") and all creation is subject to "divine evolutions."

Lamartine goes on, in a second section of "Les Revolutions," to say that the history of humankind is a course of changes, of rises and falls of empires: "All the course [of history] is marked out only/ By the debris of nations." The poet catalogs a variety of both religious and political forms that have been invented and discarded along the roadway of human history: "Thrones, altars, temples, porches, cultures, kingdoms, republics/ Are the powder covering the roadway." In this portion of the poem, Lamartine presents one of his comprehensive, universal visions of the history of Western civilization since ancient Egypt.

The final section of "Les Revolutions" gives perfect expression to Lamartine's conception of an evolutionary progression of human ethics and social structures—each valid only for a single day: "'Advance!' Humanity does not live by a single idea!/ Each night it extinguishes the candle that has guided it,/ it lights another from the eternal torch." Even religion evolves—even the sacred revelation of the Bible. Each generation reads its structures into the seemingly fixed text: "Page by page your epochs spell out the Gospel:/ Therein you have read but a single word, and you shall read a thousand;/ Therein your more venturesome children will read even more still!" God's revelation to humankind, for Lamartine, is not something fixed in time but is, rather, a dynamic, winged phenomenon: "In thunder and lightning your Word soars" ("Dans la foudre et l'éclair votre Verbe aussi vole"). Although many modern theologians share, in general outline at least, this notion of revelation, in Lamartine's day, it represented a clearly heretical conception of the relationship between humankind and God.

JOCELYN

According to Peyre, such a conception, which offers a new basis for Christianity, is also embodied in Lamartine's *Jocelyn*. The Church of Rome took such exception to the heretical nature of this work that it immediately placed it on the Index. *Jocelyn* is an epic work that was to be a part of an even larger, projected work, "The Epic of the Ages," never completed. A rather melodramatic narrative poem about a priest hiding in the Savoy Alps during the Terror, *Jocelyn* was nevertheless important in Lamartine's development, for in it he broke decisively with neoclassical norms of poetic diction, coloring his verse with real human speech.

LA CHUTE D'UN ANGE

Another work that was to form a part of "The Epic of the Ages," *La Chute d'un ange* (the fall of an angel) is little read today, but it contains an often anthologized passage, "Choeur des cèdres du Liban" (chorus of the Cedars of Lebanon), in which the poet reiterates his theme of the passage of time.

The ageless cedars are symbols for the continuity of nature and the transience of humanity: They have stood since before the Flood; they provided the wood for the

Ark; they have witnessed the passage of sacred and profane history in the Levantine. Holy men, philosophers, and poets come to do homage to these trees; Lamartine himself saw them on his voyage to the Orient. They are emblems of the creation, the making, the *poesis* that is nature itself—"the great vital chorus" ("le grand choeur végétal"). Nature is the inspiration for poetry: "And under our prophetic shadows/ They compose their most beautiful hymns out of the murmurs of our branches" ("Et sous nos ombres prophétiques/ Formeront leur plus beaux cantiques/ Des murmure de nos rameaux"). As Geoffrey Brereton has observed, this murmur of the cedars in the wind is an apt image for Lamartine's poetry, underlaid as it is with an all-important rhythm. The poet himself says that the trees roar "in glorious harmonies,/ Without articulated works, without precise language" ("en grandes harmonies/ Sans mots articulés, sans langues définies"). The emphasis on music over meaning that is found in Lamartine's most enduring lyrics foreshadows the verbal magic of Paul Verlaine and Stéphane Mallarmé.

OTHER MAJOR WORKS

LONG FICTION: *Graziella*, 1849 (English translation, 1871); *Raphaël*, 1849 (English translation, 1849); *Geneviève*, 1850 (English translation, 1850); *La Tailleur de pierres de Saint-Point*, 1851 (*The Stonesman of Saint-Point*, 1851).

PLAYS: *Toussaint Louverture*, pr., pb. 1850; *Saül*, pb. 1861; *Medée*, pb. 1873; *Zoraide*, pb. 1873.

NONFICTION: *Sur la politique rationelle*, 1831 (*The Polity of Reason*, 1848); *Voyage en Orient*, 1835 (*Travels in the East*, 1835); *Histoire des Girondins*, 1847 (*History of the Girondists*, 1847-1848); *Histoire de la révolution de 1848*, 1849 (*History of the French Revolution of 1848*, 1849); *Histoire de la Restauration*, 1851-1852 (*The History of the Restoration of Monarchy in France*, 1851-1853); *Histoire de la Turquie*, 1855; *Histoire des constituants*, 1855 (*History of the Constituent Assembly*, 1858); *Vie des grands hommes*, 1855-1856 (*Biographies and Portraits of Some Celebrated People*, 1866); *Correspondance inédite d'Alphonse de Lamartine*, 1994-1996 (2 volumes).

MISCELLANEOUS: *Œuvres complètes*, 1860-1866 (41 volumes).

BIBLIOGRAPHY

Barbin, Judith. "Liszt and Lamartine: Poetic and Religious Harmonies." *Comparatist: Journal of the Southern Comparative Literature Association* 16 (1992): 115-122. Compares religious elements and musicality in Lamartine's poems in his 1829 book with selected works by the great Polish Romantic composer Franz Liszt.

Betz, Dorothy M. "*Poetical Meditations*." In *Masterplots*, edited by Laurence W. Mazzeno. 4th ed. Pasadena, Calif.: Salem Press, 2011. A plot summary and an in-depth analysis of *Poetical Meditations*.

Birkett, Mary Ellen. *Lamartine and the Poetics of Landscape*. Lexington, Ky.: French Forum, 1982. Explores relationships between the representation of natural beauty in Romantic landscape painting and Lamartine's poetry. Examines the intimate connections between literature and the other arts that were so important during the Romantic period in France.

Bishop, Lloyd. "'Le Lac' as Exemplar of the Greater Romantic Lyric." *Romance Quarterly* 34, no. 4 (November, 1987): 403-413. This close reading of Lamartine's most famous poem explains how the poet's solitary meditation on the beauty of a lake reminds him of his deceased lover, with whom he often walked around the same lake. Argues that nature and death are important themes in Romantic lyric poetry.

Boutin, Aimeé. *Maternal Echoes: The Poetry of Marceline Desbordes-Valmore and Alphonse de Lamartine*. Newark: University of Delaware Press, 2001. Compares and contrasts the work of Desbordes-Valmore and Lamartine. Desbordes-Valmore published a similar work before Lamartine's *Poetical Meditations*, but her work did not receive the acclaim that Lamartine's did.

Fortescue, William. *Alphonse de Lamartine: A Political Biography*. New York: St. Martin's Press, 1983. Despite its title, this biography does not simply treat Lamartine's unsuccessful run for the French presidency and his opposition to the overthrow of the French Republic by Emperor Napoleon III in 1851. It also examines Lamartine's gradual evolution from a conservative Royalist to a fervent defender of democratic freedoms.

Lombard, Charles. *Lamartine*. New York: Twayne, 1973. Remains a clear introduction in English to Lamartine's lyric and epic poetry. Contains an annotated bibliography of important critical studies on the poetry.

Rodney Farnsworth

LUIS DE LEÓN

Born: Belmonte, Spain; 1527
Died: Madrigal de las Altas, Spain; August 23, 1591
Also known as: Fray Luis

PRINCIPAL POETRY

Poesías originales, 1637
*Poesías traducidas de autores clásicos y
    renacentistas*, 1637
Poesías traducidas de autores sagrados, 1637
*Poems from the Spanish of Fra. Luis Ponce de
    León*, 1883
Lyrics of Luis de León, 1928
*The Unknown Light: The Poems of Fray Luis de
    León*, 1979

OTHER LITERARY FORMS

Luis de León (LEW-ees duh lay-OHN) is considered the greatest Spanish prose writer of the sixteenth century as well as one of Spain's greatest poets. His prose masterpiece, *Los nombres de Cristo* (1583; *The Names of Christ*, 1926), is a treatise on the various names given to Christ in Scripture. *La perfecta casada* (1583; *The Perfect Wife*, 1943) is a commentary on Proverbs 31, with observations on marriage customs pertaining to medieval and sixteenth century women. His translations include the Song of Solomon, *El cantar de los cantares* (1561; *The Song of Songs*, 1936), and the Book of Job, *El libro de Job* (wr. c. 1585, pb. 1779).

ACHIEVEMENTS

Luis de León's life and work have come to symbolize for generations of Spaniards and Latin Americans

the struggle for truth within the intellectual tradition of the Spanish Golden Age (1492-1680), a tradition that valued faith above knowledge. During his career of forty-seven years at the University of Salamanca, in all his writings in Latin and Castilian, this Augustinian friar (frequently referred to as Fray Luis) fought valiantly to reconcile the Humanist tradition of the Renaissance with faith in the medieval Scholastic tradition based upon the authority of Aristotle and the church fathers.

In theology and exegesis, the two principal disciplines of the medieval university, the new learning implied for Fray Luis an uncompromising literalist position regarding sacred and classical texts. His insistence on an untranslatable spirit made concrete in language, his virulent criticism of his peers' imperfect understanding of texts, and the occasional unorthodox position that was a consequence of his understanding of Hebrew and Greek resulted in five years of prison while the Inquisition investigated his work for signs of heresy. Legend, unfounded in fact, has it that after his exoneration, he resumed his university lectures in the usual manner with the words, "As we were saying yesterday . . ." Fray Luis has grown to represent the quality of forgiveness of those who misunderstood his passionate dedication to the pursuit of knowledge.

Fray Luis's translations from Greek, Latin, and Italian into Spanish, which constitute two thirds of his poetic production, attest eloquently his knowledge of the nature of language and the art of translation. His work within the Augustinian Order and his prose writings reveal his belief in the perfectibility of humans and human institutions as well as the strength of his faith. Most important, however, Fray Luis's original verse established the Salamancan school of Spanish poetry, which rejected the full aesthetic force of the language in favor of a simplicity of style and profundity of thought that would lay bare the poet's struggle to reconcile modern concerns with awesome traditions.

BIOGRAPHY

One of six children, Luis de León was born Luis de León y Varela, the son of Lope de León and Inés Varela, in 1527 in the town of Belmonte. His family on both sides was extremely successful and included a professor of theology, a royal treasurer, a lawyer at the royal court, the secretary to the duke of Maqueda, and the general Cristóbal de Alarcón, who had won fame and wealth in the Italian campaigns of Charles V. Lope de León himself was a successful lawyer in Madrid and Valladolid and was able to give his sons an outstanding classical education. When Luis was fourteen years old, he began to follow his father's and uncles' footsteps in the Faculty of Law at the University of Salamanca.

Perhaps because of the international reputation of the Salamancan theologians, perhaps because of a strong religious vocation, at age seventeen Luis de León professed in the Order of Saint Augustine and, instead of studying law, began to study in the Faculty of Sacred Letters. His first public speech before the order reveals his determination that no kind of intimidation would force him to swerve from the truth as he perceived it. In that speech, Fray Luis claimed that, having given his life to Christ rather than to personal ambition, neither hypocrisy nor deception could constrain him to obedience. Within six years, he had begun the career that he would continue until his death, that of professor of theology at Salamanca.

Fray Luis was faced with winning and then every four years defending his position in public debates until he won a *cátedra*, or lifetime appointment to a chair with a fixed salary. These appointments became the source of fierce rivalry and heated debates between Augustinian and Dominican friars, and Fray Luis used every legal means available to guarantee his post until he had won a chair. Even then, to improve his position, he continued to challenge other professors for better-paying chairs as death provided opportunities. In one such opposition, he brought to trial Fray Bartolomé de Medina, a Dominican, for irregularities in Medina's appointment. The Salamanca conference decided in Medina's favor because of the latter's popularity among his students and colleagues. Fray Luis took the case to the royal council of Philip II, which decided in Fray Luis's favor by virtue of his seniority. This process and similar cases soon incurred his colleagues' disfavor and mistrust.

Fray Luis remained undefeated at Salamanca until he opposed León de Castro. Fray Luis denounced the latter's *Comentarios sobre Isaias* (1570) to the In-

quisition and succeeded in having it suppressed. The *Comentarios sobre Isaias* contained a thinly veiled assault on the dangers of the Humanists' approach to Scripture because of their reliance upon Greek and Hebrew. León de Castro preferred the traditional Scholastic method of syllogistic deduction to the literalist method of translation, claiming that the literalist approach, particularly in the work of Martínez de Cantalpiedra and Gaspar de Grajal, represented a threat to the authority of the Vulgate (vulgar Latin) Bible. On a personal level, León de Castro attacked Martínez and Grajal and, by association, Fray Luis, as heretics.

In March of 1572, the seeds of dissension bore fruit. An accusation against Fathers Grajal and Martínez implicating Fray Luis was filed with the Inquisition in Valladolid, calling for an investigation into their orthodoxy. Fray Diego González initiated the process, declaring that he had learned from León de Castro that, like Grajal and Martínez, Fray Luis taught that the rabbinical interpretation of Scripture was as valid as that of the saints, that the prophets' words are meaningful to Christian and Jews alike, that there was no promise of eternal life in the Old Testament, and that the Vatablo and Pagninus Bibles were superior to the Vulgate. All three men, Diego González claimed, were *conversos* (converted Jews) who desired to observe the faith and law of their Jewish ancestors.

It is well known that Fray Luis, like Teresa de Jesús and much of the Spanish nobility, had Jewish forebears, that Fray Luis's maternal grandmother and great aunt had renounced Christianity and had been put to death in an *auto-da-fé*. During the Counter-Reformation in Spain, as during the plague-ridden fourteenth century, Spanish popular concern with *limpieza de la sangre* (purity of blood) reached fanatical proportions. On March 30, 1572, Fray Luis was arrested in Valladolid, where he would remain until 1577.

While in prison, Fray Luis finished *The Names of Christ*. The record of the trial reveals that Fray Luis valiantly refused to confess or to acknowledge his accusers' interpretations of the texts in question. While his judges declared that they felt Fray Luis was a dissembler and a deceiver, they refused to submit him to torture because of his delicate health. He was declared innocent of the charges only after the principal

Augustinian professor of theology at Salamanca, Fray Domingo Báñez, turned the trial around by giving a Catholic meaning to Fray Luis's more ambiguous theological proposals. Báñez afterward advised Fray Luis that regarding scriptural studies, one might think with the minority but must speak with the majority. He was released with the threat of excommunication should he discuss the trial with anyone or try to seek out his accusers.

Fray Luis returned to Salamanca in triumph, but not to his original chair; he was given a lectureship in theology instead. On another occasion, he was denounced again to the Inquisition for opposing the teachings of Saint Thomas Aquinas and Saint Augustine regarding the nature of grace and predestination. Fray Luis held that grace was not a free gift of God but determined in part by people's actions or merit. This time the Inquisition refused to try the case.

Fray Luis left Salamanca in 1585 to represent the interests of the University in Madrid, specifically to defend the Colegio del Arzobispo against charges of irregularities in the granting of degrees. He was never to return, in spite of the efforts of Salamanca to have him back. Instead, he remained in Madrid, finished his commentary on the Book of Job, and became a close friend of Madre Ana de Jesús, a follower of Saint Teresa of Ávila in the establishment of Reformed Carmelite convents.

Fray Luis's friendship with Madre Ana de Jesús and his sympathy with the Carmelite reforms were to become the strongest concerns of the last years of his life. When an opportunity arose in Salamanca to act upon the very issue for which he had been imprisoned by the Inquisition—the opportunity to correct the Vulgate in the light of Hebrew and Greek texts—he turned it down. He stated that such an undertaking was interminable and impossible since what was requested was not a literal translation but a re-creation of the spirit of the original texts, with the inevitable result that each revision would be worse than the last. Instead, in 1588, he visited Philip II at El Escorial Palace to speak with the king's confessor about the establishment of cloistered monasteries for Augustinian friars. The request was granted.

Later, Fray Luis aided Madre Ana de Jesús's efforts,

as did Saint John of the Cross, to establish autonomy for the Reformed Carmelite nuns from the ambitious rule of Jesús María Doria. Fray Luis and Teresa de Jesús's favorite, Father Gracián, wrote Pope Sixtus V and received permission to provide a separate council for the nuns. Doria reacted by appealing to Philip II, and the king, in turn, ordered Fray Luis to desist in his support for the nuns. Fray Luis reacted by calling a general council to act immediately upon the directive of Pope Sixtus V. Doria appealed to the king, who sent an order to the meeting forbidding any innovations until the opinion of the new pope, Gregory XIV, could be assessed.

Reportedly, Fray Luis left the meeting saying that none of his Holiness's orders could be carried out in Spain. This comment was overheard and reported to Philip II, who retaliated by temporarily blocking Fray Luis's appointment to provincial of his order. Pope Gregory XIV eventually revoked the brief of Sixtus V, and Fray Luis died soon after in Madrigal de las Altas, having finally been appointed provincial.

ANALYSIS

The poetry of Luis de León presents the pursuit of knowledge as a form of spiritual exultation. For him, the intellectual's contemplation of creation constitutes a joy approaching mystic rapture. In almost all his original poems, he holds Neoplatonic philosophy and medieval Christianity in a tenuously balanced, unstable harmony that creates tremendous aesthetic tension. During his early years, his poems circulated in random manuscript form until he collected them at the request of his friend Don Pedro Portoarrero as a defense against misinterpretation. He divided his work into three books: original poems; translations from Horace, Vergil, Pindar, and Pietro Bembo; and translations of Holy Scripture.

In 1631, a similarly spirited poet, Francisco Gómez de Quevedo y Villegas, published all of Fray Luis's poetry. Quevedo recognized Fray Luis's depth and clarity, qualities that contrasted strongly with the elaborate Baroque preciosity of the style that was to become known as *Gongorismo*. Quevedo likewise recognized that Fray Luis's translations were in keeping with the classical orientation that informed his theory of language in *The Names of Christ* and that had led him to conclusions often dangerously at variance with those of his colleagues. In *The Names of Christ*, Fray Luis asserts that language when used by true and sound minds will reflect reality accurately without distortion; the triple complexity of words—in thought, speech, and writing—can obtain absolute truth. This absolute, shared by many minds, leads to a harmonious world. Within this essentially Neoplatonic framework, Fray Luis includes the tradition of the Kabbala and attributes to words an unconscious depth of meaning, realized through secret references and arbitrary associations.

RELIGIOUS POETRY

In Fray Luis's religious poetry, there is an intimacy of feeling and an occasional self-doubt that appear nowhere else in his work. The poem "En la fiesta de todos los santos" ("On the Holiday of All Saints' Day") illustrates the characteristic antithetical organization of his verse. The greatness of the remote past contrasts so strongly with the inadequacies of the present that the devotion to the early Christian saints continues to increase with each generation. A sense of being abandoned imbues his poem "En la ascensión" ("On the Ascension"), in which the poet asks Christ where his sheep will turn now that he has left them.

In one of his songs dedicated to the Virgin, "A Nuestra Señora" ("To Our Lady"), Fray Luis, in the depths of his despair at the persecution he has suffered, calls upon the Virgin Mary and, protesting his innocence and declaring his unworthiness, beseeches her to intercede for him against the hatred of his enemies and against their deceptions. He asks her to free him from the prison in which their misunderstanding has cast him. In this poem, Fray Luis expresses self-doubt, saying that if indeed he has succumbed to evil unknowingly, the Virgin's virtue will shine more brightly in forgiving a darker sin.

"TO CHRIST CRUCIFIED"

The song "A Cristo crucificado" ("To Christ Crucified"), by virtue of the brutal realism of the imagery and the poet's legalist perspective, reveals Fray Luis's faith in the law. While (for Fray Luis) the Virgin is the summa of the Divine Essence, Christ's humanity and suffering make him humble in Fray Luis's eyes and, therefore, accessible. The poem elaborates the theme of

Christ the advocate fulfilling the law by granting pardon to all who call on him. He cannot flee because his feet are nailed. His heart is revealed through his gaping wounds, and two words from a thief are sufficient to steal it. He dictates his will and New Testament before dying and, from the Cross, can deny no one's wish. His head drops upon his chest, and Fray Luis calls upon witnesses to affirm the gesture as a sign that the poet's request for pardon has been granted. Finally, since no testament is legally valid until the testator is dead, Christ fulfills the law to the letter and dies. While concluding the poem with the lines that Heaven, Earth, and Sun mourn Christ's death, the poet, because of his intellectual and legalistic perspective on the Crucifixion, demands—rather than seeks—justice.

"TO SANTIAGO"

The same intensity found in "To Christ Crucified" characterizes Fray Luis's *liras* dedicated to Saint James the Apostle and Moor Slayer, "A Santiago" ("To Santiago"). The poet portrays Saint James as the disciple who, after bringing Spain to Christ and returning to the East to suffer martyrdom, reappears during the Wars of Reconquest (780-1492) to avenge Spanish blood spilled by the Infidels. The poem exalts the theocratic dynamics of Spain's imperial expansion: the Spaniard's thirst for vengeance against the Moor, the Isabeline politics of African expansion, and the taste for awesome power, wealth, and fame acquired by the valiant conqueror who wages war for Christ. In this poem, Fray Luis proves that his range includes the grandiloquence associated with his contemporary Fernando de Herrera, founder of the Sevillian school.

THE PERFECT WIFE

Fray Luis's book *The Perfect Wife* still enjoys popularity in the Spanish-speaking world. Through a commentary on the last chapter of Proverbs, Fray Luis acknowledges that love between husband and wife is the strongest of all human bonds. It is forged by nature and enhanced by grace, being the only institution in existence before the Fall of Adam and Eve. It is reinforced by social custom and tied by intricate mutual obligations. Fray Luis writes that the role of wife is more difficult than that of the average husband because, aside from the chastity that is universally assumed, she is duty bound to profit her husband by managing his household economically, rearing his children wisely, and bringing him comfort and joy. Fray Luis contrasts the ideal wife with vain women who are incapable of physical work because they spend their days with cosmetics and jewelry, who scold servants to prove their authority, or who destroy their neighbors' reputations with frivolous gossip. Because of her role as wife and mother, Fray Luis insists, a virtuous woman is the most powerful agent in society, providing she speak wisely and gently. He writes that, since reason cannot deceive and love does not wish to deceive, a loving and reasonable woman can bring her husband to perfection.

PEACE THROUGH SERVICE

For Fray Luis, in *The Names of Christ* and *The Perfect Wife*, perfection consists simply of fulfilling well one's station in life. In his own life, as a friar and scholar, service to the Church was of paramount importance. The poem "A la vida religiosa" (on the religious life) reveals through a dream the nature of Fray Luis's vocation. In the pastoral setting he so often prefers, he is called to exchange the glory of Earth for the glory of Heaven by renouncing present contentment, comfort, and wealth. Rather than follow the career of his father and uncles, the rewards of which he believes are feigned, he chooses the monk's bare cell, plain frock, hair shirt, and flagellation in order to free himself of vice, the world, the Devil, and the flesh. Thus freed, Fray Luis believes he will have everything the secular person strives for simply by serving God.

For Fray Luis, the ascetic life does not lead, as it did for Saint John of the Cross, to mystic union with God. Rather, it frees him to engage in intellectual pursuits unencumbered by personal concerns. Through acquired rather than infused knowledge, he hopes to envision, enjoy, and realize in a social context his ideal of peace. His most famous and successful poems present this theme of peace through knowledge. This peace is obtained by achieving the Neoplatonic ideal of harmony, first within the soul, next between the individual and nature, and, finally, between the individual and a well-ordered society. Thus, in his poem "Morada del cielo" ("Dwelling Place in Heaven"), Fray Luis harmonizes the Renaissance idea of utopia with the Christian concept of Heaven through the conventions of the pastoral tradition. The Good Shepherd leads his flock to fields where knowledge becomes aesthetic delight, obliterating the sorrow, pain, and injustice of an imperfect temporal world.

This vision of peace stands in marked contrast to Fray Luis's combative life, yet in spite of his fierce competitiveness, in spite of his tendency to win through litigation what he could not win through friendship and approval, there are in his poems moments of that wholeness he so desperately desired. In "Dwelling Place in Heaven," Fray Luis reveals the height of his spiritual ambition, to hear the divine, silent music of the spheres played by God himself, the music that will transport him from his prison of imperfection to the eternal companionship of those who live free from error.

Fray Luis reveals his empirical certainty that such a paradise exists in his three most famous poems, "Vida retirada" ("The Secluded Life"), "A Salinas" ("To Francisco Salinas"), and "Noche serena" ("Serene Night"). Whenever he perceives the concert of number and harmony of disparities as he does in these poems—whether it be in the pastoral vision of nature, in the aesthetic pleasure of polyphonic music, in observing the heavens within a mythic Copernican perspective, or in the language of Humanistic dialogue and Renaissance verse forms—Fray Luis reaffirms his ideal of perfection and his belief in the perfectibility of humanity and its institutions. Because of the intensity of his struggle to harmonize the new learning of the Renaissance with the medieval traditions of Post-Tridentine Spain (after the Council of Trent, 1545-1563) and because of the valor of his struggle for intellectual integrity against his contemporaries' lack of understanding and his own self-doubts, Fray Luis has a permanent place in the history of Spanish culture.

OTHER MAJOR WORKS

NONFICTION: *La perfecta casada*, 1583 (*The Perfect Wife*, 1943); *Los nombres de Cristo*, 1583 (*The Names of Christ*, 1926).

TRANSLATIONS: *El cantar de los cantares*, 1561 (*The Song of Songs*, 1936); *El libro de Job*, 1779 (wr. c. 1585).

BIBLIOGRAPHY

Bell, Aubrey. *Luis de León*. Oxford, England: Clarendon Press, 1925. A biographical study in the context of the Spanish Renaissance.

Durán, Manuel. *Luis de Léon*. New York: Twayne, 1971. An introductory biography and critical study of selected works by Fray Luis. Includes bibliographic references.

Fitzmaurice-Kelly, James. *Fray Luis de León: A Biographical Fragment*. Oxford, England: Oxford University Press, 1921. A brief biography issued by the Hispanic Society of America.

Gaylord, Mary Malcolm, and Francisco Márquez Villanueva, eds. *San Juan de la Cruz and Fray Luis de León: A Commemorative International Symposium*. Newark, Del.: Juan de la Cuesta, 1996. This collection of works from a symposium examines mysticism in literature, focusing on John of the Cross and Fray Luis. Includes index.

Hildner, David Jonathan. *Poetry and Truth in the Spanish Works of Fray Luis de León*. Rochester, N.Y.: Boydell & Brewer, 1992. A critical analysis of selected works by Fray Luis. Includes bibliographical references.

Nowak, William J. "Virgin Rhetoric: Fray Luis de León and Marian Piety in 'Virgen, que el sol más pura.'" *Hispanic Review* 72, no. 4 (Autumn, 2005): 491-510. Nowak examines Fray Luis's poem "Virgen, que el sol más pura" and argues that it is not simply an expression of the poet's Marian piety.

Thompson, Colin P. *The Strife of Tongues: Fray Luis de León and the Golden Age of Spain*. 1988. Reprint. New York: Cambridge University Press, 2009. A critical study of Fray Luis's works with an introduction to the history of Spain in the sixteenth century.

Vossler, Karl. *Fray Luis de León*. Buenos Aires: Espasa-Calpa Argentina, 1946. A short biography of Fray Luis.

Kenneth A. Stackhouse

LEONIDAS OF TARENTUM

Born: Tarentum (now Taranto, Italy); fl. early third century B.C.E.
Died: Place and date unknown

PRINCIPAL POETRY

Epigrams, third century B.C.E.

OTHER LITERARY FORMS

Leonidas of Tarentum (lee-AHN-ihd-uhs uhv tuh-REHN-tuhm) is not known to have written anything but epigrams.

ACHIEVEMENTS

Although a poet of the second rank in a period of scant literary achievement, Leonidas of Tarentum is notable for his attention to classes of people who had been ignored before the Hellenistic era. He was greatly admired by later epigrammatists, as is shown by scores of imitations produced in subsequent generations. More than any other Hellenistic writer, Leonidas can be credited with the expansion of poetry's vision to include the poor, the farmers, hunters, fishermen, tradesmen, merchant seamen, prostitutes, weavers, and others whose lives, although in no way remarkable, bore the common stamp of humanity in their labors. Although he did not limit his scope to the working world, Leonidas made proletarian life his special preserve, much as Theocritus made singing shepherds his poetic domain. Judging by the number of his immediate imitators, in fact, it would appear that Leonidas had a greater influence in his own time than the more celebrated Theocritus. When Vergil revived the pastoral, Theocritus had inspired barely two imitators (Bion and Moschus), whereas Leonidas's followers, both before and after Vergil's time, were legion.

The great paradox of Leonidas's achievement is his remarkable affinity for elaborate language to describe simple people. His poetry is full of ornamental adjectives and novel compounds and is characterized by a vocabulary that appears nowhere else in ancient Greek. His style is commonly characterized as baroque, exuberant in its highly calculated arrangement of words and ideas. Leonidas is an excellent Hellenistic example of the phenomenon of a writer vastly popular and influential in his own time but virtually unread today. Modern estimations vary widely: Gilbert Highet has called him "the greatest Greek epigrammatist of the Alexandrian era," but C. R. Beye finds him "heavy-handed, pedantic, and [overly] detailed"; Marcello Gigante sees him as the high-minded prophet of a new egalitarian society, and A. S. F. Gow as "a competent versifier, [but] hardly ever more than that." Whatever his merits as a poet, Leonidas deserves a careful reading by anyone who wishes to understand the dynamics of the age that gave classical Humanism its definitive shape.

BIOGRAPHY

Leonidas of Tarentum's biography, like that of most Hellenistic poets, is strictly conjectural and, in the absence of contemporary references to him, is completely dependent on the evidence of his epigrams, in which he says very little about his own life. Most authorities place him in the first or second generation of Hellenistic poets, either early in the third century B.C.E., with Asclepiades, Callimachus, and Theocritus, or nearer the middle of the century, closer to such poets as Dioscorides and Antipater, whose epigrams echo his style. An epigram purporting to be his own epitaph (epigram 715 in book 7 AP. or Leonidas 93 G. P.) represents him as a wanderer who died far from his native Tarentum, itself a plausible claim, because his one hundred-odd surviving epigrams represent people and places scattered all over the Greek-speaking world, the eastern Mediterranean littoral loosely referred to as the *oikoumenē*.

Though a native of Italy, Leonidas (like the Sicilian Theocritus) was in every sense of the word a member of the Greek world. His city (the modern Taranto) was colonized at the end of the eighth century B.C.E. by Spartans, and from the middle of the fifth century B.C.E. it was the leading Greek city of southern Italy. By the end of the next century, however, Tarentum came under pressure from Italian tribes to the north and depended on various mercenary leaders for protection. The last of these was Rome's famous adversary Pyrrhus, who left Tarentum to the Romans in 275. From about

that time until the Hannibalic wars at the end of the century, the city regained stability and prosperity under Roman rule. Leonidas's supposed departure from Tarentum has been linked to the period of insecurity early in the third century, though, like other literary and intellectual figures from the Greek west, he would have been naturally attracted to such Greek capitals as Athens and Alexandria. His epigrams do not, however, suggest residence in any particular place, but rather an itinerant existence and a life shared mainly with the rural poor. Would-be biographers have leapt to the conclusion that Leonidas was in fact a destitute wanderer by choice who wrote about people with whom he shared his meager existence. This speculation is strengthened by occasional suggestions in Leonidas's epigrams that he was an admirer of the Cynic philosopher Diogenes and shared Cynic beliefs concerning poverty, simplicity, and the frailty of human life. It is possible that he followed in the footsteps of the popular Cynic philosopher Crates, adopting poverty as a way of life and traveling about the *oikoumenē* spreading a gospel of voluntary poverty and independence and consoling the victims of hardship, perhaps by celebrating their simple lives in his epigrams. Crates himself is said to have written poetry as a vehicle of his teaching, and some students of Leonidas see him as playing a similar prophetic role in his poetry.

Such speculation is difficult to reconcile with the highly sophisticated style of Leonidas's actual poems, which are seldom as austere or simple as the people he liked to write about. There is also the cosmopolitan range of his subjects, which include the most celebrated artistic, literary, and intellectual events of his time and, indeed, of previous generations. Wherever he spent his time, Leonidas did not isolate himself from the tastes or the events and concerns of his age. The public for whom he wrote was urban and well educated, with a sophisticated nostalgia for the simple lives of peasants and rural tradespeople. Like Theocritus's shepherds, Leonidas's working folk are as much a product of imagination as of observation, and there is no need to speculate that he spent most of his life among them. In short, no solid facts can be drawn from the epigrams to illuminate the mystery of Leonidas's life.

ANALYSIS

It is not known in what form Leonidas of Tarentum published his epigrams. A large number were published after his death in the *Garland* of Meleager, an anthology of epigrams put together early in the first century B.C.E., but it is probable that Meleager himself depended on earlier collections. Meleager's *Garland* is lost, although large parts of it were included when Constantine Cephalas, a church official in the palace at Constantinople in the late ninth century C.E., made a larger anthology of Greek epigrams. Within a century, Cephalas's collection (itself also lost) became a source of a still much larger anthology of Greek epigrams from the Byzantine, Roman, and earlier Greek eras, now known as the *Greek Anthology* or the *Palatine Anthology*. Cephalas's collection was also the source of an independent selection of epigrams put together in 1301 by the Byzantine monk Maximus Planudes. Eight or nine epigrams by Leonidas are extant only in the *Planudean Anthology*. The *Palatine Anthology* is so called because of its rediscovery in the Count Palatine's library at Heidelberg in 1606; modern editions are based on that tenth century codex as supplemented by the later Planudean collection. The numbering system used for references is either that of the *Palatine Anthology* (AP.) or that of the standard edition, *The Greek Anthology: Hellenistic Epigrams* (1965), edited by A. S. F. Gow and D. L. Page (G.-P.).

THE EPIGRAM FORM

Historically and etymologically, an epigram is an inscription on something, usually a tomb, a statue, or a dedicatory plaque. At an early stage, epigrams were sometimes set to verse, and in time it was customary to write them in elegiac couplets consisting of a dactylic hexameter followed by a shorter pentameter line. The conciseness required of an inscription on metal or stone was a special challenge to the first epigrammatists, and from these circumstances evolved a miniature literary form that became extremely popular in the Hellenistic age, whose reading public was tired of rambling heroic poetry and prized concise workmanship.

One effect of this development was that by Hellenistic times, the epigram had become more or less independent of its origins as an inscription, not being intended for actual writing on anything more substantial than a piece of paper; still, it sometimes retained vestiges of its origins by masquerading in the form of an inscribed dedication or epitaph.

New types were also invented: The epideictic, or display, epigram is a versified comment about a statue, poem, or any other object, such as a fig tree or a carved piece of incense. The love epigram is a short poem about love, often not even ostensibly inscriptional or memorial in character. The protreptic, hortatory, or admonitory epigram is likewise not formally associated with an object; it is simply a versified bit of wisdom— "what oft was said but ne'er so well expressed"— usually in Hellenistic times a commonplace of popular Stoic, Cynic, or Epicurean philosophy. The tone as well as the type could vary, from somber to declamatory, playful, or mocking.

GREEK ANTHOLOGY

Leonidas of Tarentum's epigrams are arguably all epideictic, although most of them take the form of an epitaph or a dedication. If any of them were actually inscribed, however, it was probably after the fact and beyond the intentions of the author. The *Greek Anthology* preserves them, scattered among epigrams by other authors, under three main categories: Book 7, devoted to epitaphs or sepulchral epigrams, includes the largest number; book 6, containing dedicatory epigrams, has nearly as many; fifteen are preserved as epideictic epigrams in book 9. These three books of the *Greek Anthology* account for nearly all of Leonidas's epigrams, with a dozen others distributed elsewhere, chiefly in Planudes' collection. The assignment of categories in the *Greek Anthology* is often careless, however, and is useful only as the most general guide to the kind of poems that Leonidas wrote.

RURAL THEMES

Too much attention to Leonidas's special interest in peasants, artisans, and the poor can obscure the fact that these subjects account for scarcely more than one-third of his epigrams. He can be credited with the "discovery" of simple folk as a subject of epigram, and he made himself their poet laureate, so to speak, but he did not limit himself to that subject any more than Theocritus limited himself to the poetic shepherds that made him famous. As has already been noted, Leonidas's complex style seems made for purposes other than the depiction of simple folk.

A survey of Leonidas's poems reveals, more than anything else, a love of complexity and variety. His work is a miscellany of people, places, and events that would seem novel to his city readers: They enjoyed reading about subjects outside their usual cosmopolitan ambit in Tarentum, Syracuse, Athens, or Alexandria. Hence the prominence of rural artisans, seamen, and the countryside and the significant absence of urban scenes and subjects. Hellenistic life was concentrated as never before in the cities, but taste was for anything but the here and now. Hence, also, the love of paradoxes, novelties, and curiosity items in Leonidas. He had no special loyalty to the class of people he put in his epigrams, no political posture, and no philosophical ideology with which to indoctrinate his readers. Everything was subordinated to writing an epigram that his audience might find interesting, clever, and unconventional.

TIMELESSNESS

For these reasons, Johannes Geffcken's attempts to read historical allusions into Leonidas and Gigante's discovery of revolutionary protosocialist sentiment in the epigrams has had a cool reception among students of Hellenistic poetry. Leonidas is anything but topical; his epigrams, although often ostensibly tied to specific events, such as a fisherman's death or the dedication to Bacchus of some casks of wine, are almost always timeless or look back to an event in the distant past.

A small number of epigrams may be exceptional in this regard, such as a pair of quatrains dedicating spoils taken from Tarentum's ancient enemies, the Lucanians (epigrams 129 and 131 in book 6 AP. and Leonidas 34 and 35 G.-P.), but Leonidas's language is not specific enough to permit a definite dating within his probable lifetime; the epigrams may well be epideictic and patriotic rather than specific to a certain battle. An epigram on the occasion of Antigonus Gonatas's defeat by Pyrrhus in 273 B.C.E. (epigram 130 in book 6 AP. or Leonidas 95 G.-P.) is a much better candidate for specific contemporary dating, if the ascription to Leonidas is correct.

Of the poets and artists celebrated in some eleven epigrams, only one belongs to Leonidas's own century: Aratus, the author of a poem on astronomy, the *Phainomena*, written shortly after 277 B.C.E. In his tendency to avoid the contemporary, Leonidas is like other poets of the third century: They preferred to write about the timeless or the mythical, and they tended to find only the poets and artists of earlier generations to be fit subjects for their praise.

ESCAPISM

This affinity with things set apart from the poet and his audience was not entirely new to Greek poetry; Homer wrote about events that took place nearly five centuries before his own time, and the Greek tragedians used even older myths for their plots. However, the comedies of Aristophanes were unabashedly topical at the end of the fifth century B.C.E., and in the fourth century, Menander's comedies were also set in contemporary times (although they were not as politically topical). A certain escapism distinguishes Hellenistic poetry from that of earlier periods. Although some of their classical predecessors had used remote settings and characters only as a background for the presentation of their own immediate concerns and controversies, the Hellenistic poets—Leonidas, Callimachus, Apollonius Rhodius, and Theocritus—used similarly removed situations as a means of turning away from their own milieu, which held little interest for them, to worlds more to their liking.

POETRY AS CRAFT

As a corollary of this impulse, art was cultivated for art's sake rather than for the traditional purposes of education and inspiration. When it inspired, it inspired disengagement rather than the heroic commitment that was typical, say, of Sophoclean tragedy. Poetry came to be viewed more as a craft than as a vehicle for great ideas. The many epigrams that Leonidas and his contemporaries composed in praise of ancient poets and artists suggest something like a cult of the artist whose art transcends rather than reflects. At the same time, they felt inferior to the geniuses of the past, and, rather than try to compete with them in epic or tragic poetry, the better poets sought uncharted territory for themselves, new kinds of poetry in which they would not be in the shadow of the grand masters of the past. With something of a pioneering spirit, every poet of talent sought to bring his readers something new and distinctive. In this way, Hellenistic poetry was a means of escaping the past as well as the present.

SUBJECT MATTER

Leonidas's novel attention to common people attracted many imitators—and, one must assume, a large audience. Some of what he provided his readers is now found in "human interest" journalism: "Man Half-Eaten by Sea Monster Buried Today" (epigram 506 in book 7 AP. or Leonidas 65 G.-P.), "Lion Takes Refuge with Herdsmen" (epigram 221 in book 6 AP. or Leonidas 53 G.-P.), "Four Sisters Die in Childbirth" (epigram 463 in book 7 AP. or Leonidas 69 G.-P.). Others are less sensational curiosities, such as a die carved on a gambler's tombstone (epigram 422 in book 7 AP. or Leonidas 22 G.-P.) or a fisherman who dies a natural death after a lifetime in a perilous trade (epigram 295 in book 7 AP. or Leonidas 20 G.-P.).

Most of Leonidas's subjects are bland in themselves: Three sisters dedicate their spinning and weaving implements to Athena on retiring from their labors (epigram 289 in book 6 AP. or Leonidas 42 G.-P.); a gardener prays to the nymphs to see that his garden is well watered (epigram 320 in book 9 AP. or Leonidas 6 G.-P.). The tone of such imaginary epitaphs and dedications is predictably calm; rarely does Leonidas inject the emotion expressed in epigram 466 in book 7 AP. or Leonidas 71 G.-P., where a father grieves for his son, dead at eighteen. More often, there is a humorous note of mockery, as in the imaginary epitaph of a lady who drank too much and has a cup on her tomb: Her only regret in death is that the cup is empty (epigram 455 in book 7 AP. or Leonidas 68 G.-P.). There are other joke epigrams, such as epigrams 236 and 261 in book 1 AP. or Leonidas 83 and 84 G.-P., in which a statue of the tutelary god Priapus threatens to abuse troublemakers with his overgrown phallus.

Sometimes an epigram will be built around a paradox: a cult statue of Aphrodite bearing warlike gear (epigram 320 in book 9 AP. or Leonidas 24 G.-P.); a figure of Eros carved in frankincense that will be burned, although not with the fires of love (epigram 179 in book 9 AP. or Leonidas 28 G.-P.). For the most part, Leonidas avoids erotic topics, although they were a favorite preoccupation in nearly all Hellenistic art and literature. He shows a greater interest in the com-monplaces of Cynic philosophy; his longest poem is a sepulchral elegy of sixteen lines made up of Cynic sentiments on the frailty of life (epigram 472 in book 7 AP. or Leonidas 77 G.-P.). Leonidas is not always consistent in his Cynic views, however, especially on the subject of poverty. Sometimes he praises it in good Cynic fashion because it implies independence and self-sufficiency, but in a rare autobiographical moment he prays that Aphrodite will save him from his "hateful poverty" (epigram 300 in book 6 AP. or Leonidas 36 G.-P.). Moreover, he is as ready to make fun of a ragged Cynic guru (Sochares in epigrams 293 and 298 in book 6 AP. or Leonidas 54 to 55 G.-P.) as he is to mock a man who goes to his grave without ever drinking too much (Eubulus or "Wiseman," in epigram 452 in book 7 AP. or Leonidas 67 G.-P.). Less a philosopher than a poet, Leonidas shifts his point of view to suit his subject.

CHALLENGES OF TRANSLATION

Without reading Leonidas's epigrams in the original Greek, one is not likely to understand why they were read, copied, and imitated, even by generations whose tastes were not those of the modern world, because so much of Leonidas's art is invested in his use of language itself. The literary qualities most admired by Hellenistic readers and authors were highly formal, with relatively little emphasis being placed on the substance of a piece of writing. What mattered was not so much what one said, but how well one said it.

In translation, most of Leonidas's poetry will seem intolerably bland—as it will even in Greek, so long as one reads for propositional content. To read Leonidas as his admirers did, one must read through Hellenistic eyes focused on felicity of phrasing, effective manipulation of word order (which is much more flexible in Greek than in English), freshness of diction, and creative management of the reader's expectations to stimulate curiosity, evoke surprise, and elicit humor. In his subordination of content to form, Leonidas (like many of his contemporaries) can be called a poet's poet. Christopher Dawson has shown by close analysis of several epigrams how successfully Leonidas exploited his material for maximum effect and, in particular, how he arranged his epigrams for a climactic focus at the end. His creation of poems leading up to a play of wit at the end took the epigram a step closer to the modern form first fully realized by the Roman poet Martial.

BIBLIOGRAPHY

Bing, Peter, and Jon Bruss, eds. *Brill's Companion to Hellenistic Epigram*. Boston: Brill, 2007. Part of the Brill's Companions in Classical Studies series, this work brings together many experts to create an introduction to all aspects of the epigram. Provides context and touches on Leonidas.

Clack, Jerry. *Asclepiades of Samos and Leonidas of Tarentum: The Poems*. Wauconda, Ill.: Bolchazy, 1999. A collection and translation of the complete extant works of these two Greek epigrammatists, who set the course for this particular genre of poetry. As the book points out, for Leonidas the poetic form of the epigram went beyond the purely personal feelings of the author and allowed for social commentary, often alluding to the suffering and miseries of the poor, the infirm, and the aged.

Fowler, Barbara Hughes. *The Hellenistic Aesthetic*. Madison: University of Wisconsin Press, 1989. A general survey of the artistic thought and movements of the period that produced Leonidas. Although slight in its treatment of the poet and his individual poems, it is valuable for placing him and his work into an overall context.

Gutzwiller, Katheryn. *Poetic Garlands: Hellenistic Epigrams in Context*. Berkeley: University of California Press, 1998. A full-length study of the later, more literary Greek epigrams written by professional poets such as Leonidas. Gutzwiller traces the themes in Leonidas's work, including death, eroticism, and morality, and comments particularly on his epigram for the sponge-fisher Tharsys, attacked and half-eaten by a shark and so buried on both land and sea.

White, Heather. *New Essays in Hellenistic Poetry*. Amsterdam: Gieben, 1985. A good study of Leonidas and his contemporaries. The essay on Leonidas's work is useful, although somewhat technical in its examinations of the poetic and linguistic devices of the works of Leonidas. This is the sort of resource best used in conjunction with other more general studies of the poet and his writing.

Daniel H. Garrison

GIACOMO LEOPARDI

Born: Recanati, Papal States (now in Italy); June 29, 1798
Died: Naples (now in Italy); June 14, 1837

PRINCIPAL POETRY
Versi, 1826
Canti, 1831, 1835 (includes expanded version of *Versi*; English translation, 1962)
I paralipomeni della batracomiomachia, 1842 (*The War of the Mice and the Crabs*, 1976)
The Poems of Leopardi, 1923, 1973
Poems, 1963
Selected Poems of Giacomo Leopardi, 1995

OTHER LITERARY FORMS

Giacomo Leopardi (lay-oh-POR-dee) was a child prodigy who began exercising both his talents and his erudition at the age of eleven. While as a poet he is best known for the *Canti* (literally, "songs") and to some extent for the political satire *The War of the Mice and the Crabs* and other lyrical poems not included in the *Canti*, he did leave a great number of shorter poetic pieces or fragments, including translations, together with a similar number of brief prose pieces that in the aggregate round out an active literary personality. His philosophical "Imitazione," on Antoine Vincent Arnaut's "La Feuille," is possibly of 1818, or of 1828, the year of his polemical poem on style, "Scherzo." Four or five years before, he had freely translated a fragment of Simonides and followed it with another translation of the same author. As early as 1809, inspired by Homer's *Iliad* (c. 750 B.C.E.; English translation, 1611), Leopardi produced his first poem, "La morte di Ettore," and in 1812, he wrote *Pompeo in Egitto*, a tragedy denouncing tyranny. A number of extant poetic fragments cannot be dated accurately. In 1819, Leopardi wrote the pastoral tragedy *Telesilla*. In addition, he created many prose works, such as the remarkably erudite *Storia dell'astronomia* (1813; *History of Astronomy*, 1882), ranging from the beginning of the science to the comet of 1811, and the long *Saggio sopra gli errori popolari degli antichi* (1815; *Essay on the*

Popular Superstitions of the Ancients, 1882), which revealed, among other things, the budding philologist. This philological dedication was to produce a number of projects in translation, vulgarization, and editing throughout his life, albeit more frequently in his earlier than in his later years because of his failing eyesight and health. As examples, one might mention his translations from the poetry of Moschus in 1815; the *Discorso sopra la vita e le opere de M. Cornelio Frontone*, the essay *Il salterio Ebraico*, and various vulgarizations of Homer and Vergil, all of 1816; and the *Crestomazia* (1827-1828) of Italian literature in two volumes, as well as editions of Cicero and Petrarch, and an *Enciclopedia delle cognizioni utili e delle cose che non si sanno* during the 1820's, many volumes of which he never completed. A fundamental work is his 4,526-page notebook titled *Zibaldone*, which he began in 1817 and which represents an encyclopedic medley of thoughts and analyses, observations and recollections—philosophical, philological, critical, and personal—that occupied his mind until the end of 1832. It was published from 1898 to 1900. From this notebook, in large part, he compiled a collection of thoughts titled *Cento undici pensieri* that was also published posthumously, in 1845 (*Pensieri*, 1981). To be noted, too, is his essay *Discorso di un Italiano intorno alla poesia romantica* (*Discourse of an Italian Concerning Romantic Poetry*) of 1818. Next to the *Canti*, Leopardi's most important work remains the collection of twenty-four short masterpieces of satirical prose known as the *Operette morali* (*Essays and Dialogues*, 1882), published and augmented three times during his lifetime: 1827, 1834, and 1836. Finally, an indispensable companion to Leopardi studies is his published correspondence, *Epistolario* (its nucleus was published in 1849), not only for its wealth of biographical indications but also, often in the manner of the *Zibaldone*, for its innumerable intellectual premises.

ACHIEVEMENTS

Giacomo Leopardi left an indelible mark on Italian poetry, in which category he is considered second only to Dante, and while Leopardi's influence on European letters does not match that of a number of transalpine contemporaries (Lord Byron, Victor Hugo, and Ludwig Tieck, for example), he is surely a greater poet than most of them and closer to the modern psyche—indeed, one of the truly significant poets of the nineteenth century. Leopardi was not only a consummate philologist in the classical sense, with all the linguistic and historical erudition that that term implies, but also one of those rare poets who, like Dante and Johann Wolfgang von Goethe, have been deemed worthy of consideration as a philosopher. Lyrical expression and philosophical reflection maintain a harmonious balance in his poetry at all times. Some critics see Leopardi chiefly as a scholar of broad humanistic and historical dimensions; others, as one of the sacred voices inspiring the movement for Italian unification; still others, as a pessimistic philosopher, a precursor of twentieth century Existentialism. Even in *Essays and Dialogues*, however, Leopardi was above all a poet—which is perhaps the most appropriately encompassing term available for him.

BIOGRAPHY

Count Giacomo Talegardo Francesco di Sales Saverio Pietro Leopardi was born in Recanati, in the province of the Marches, of a wealthy and noble family with a long tradition of service to the Church. His father, Count Monaldo, prided himself on his intellectual accomplishments, among which he included reactionary and scholarly writings and the building of an extensive and erudite family library in which the young Leopardi spent most of his formative years. Monaldo's sense of infallibility did not help him manage his inherited fortune, a responsibility undertaken by his wife, Marquise Adelaide Antici, an austere, bigoted, and despotic woman, whose harshness toward the sensitive Giacomo contrasted with her husband's affectionate paternal disposition. The priest who tutored Giacomo until he was thirteen declared at that time that there was nothing more he could teach the boy, who read and studied daily until very late. Leopardi's interests—theology, mathematics, history, rhetoric, Greek, Latin, Spanish, French, Hebrew, English, German, the philosophers, the Enlightenment, the Italian classics, the commentators, and astronomy—encompassed an encyclopedic range of intellectual activities, as described in *Zibaldone*, a "mad and most desperate [regime of] study," which inevitably and irreparably damaged his naturally frail constitution. His eyesight, his bones (rachitis), his back (he became a humpback), and other ailments (such as a cerebrospinal disease) were to plague him painfully for more than half of his brief life.

At first, Leopardi's consuming ambition was the acquisition of fame, "a very great and perhaps immoderate desire," but as the years passed, he realized that he had sacrificed his youth in pursuit of his ambition. Youth, "dearer than fame and laurels, than the pure light of day," lost "without a pleasure, uselessly," became a recurrent theme in his poetry. Frequently, he sat depressed in the library, or, during an afternoon stroll around the countryside, waves of melancholy overcame him, "an obstinate, black, horrible, barbarous melancholy," which convinced him that life could produce only misery.

Pietro Giordani, an Italian writer and patriot, befriended Leopardi, and for a while his spirits lifted. The subdued tones of earlier poems such as "Le rimembranze," "Appressamento della morte," "Primo amore" ("First Love"), and "Memorie del primo amore" were replaced by the more energetic tones of patriotic songs such as "All'Italia" ("To Italy") and "Sopra il monumento di Dante che si preparava a Firenze" ("On the Monument to Dante"). He tried to leave his "native savage town" of Recanati, but his parents discovered and frustrated the attempt, in the wake of which they imposed a close surveillance of his actions, complete with censorship of his correspondence. This situation produced meditations of deep melancholia, out of which grew a philosophy of sorrow, which for him constituted the necessary condition of the universe, in which beauty, love, glory, and virtue emerge as illusions that deceive wickedly and promote universal unhappiness. However, illusion provided the only refuge from devastation occasioned by reason and reality, and the need for it made repeated claims on his soul and his worldview. During this period, from around 1819 to around 1822, many fine idylls came to light, such as "Il sogno," "L'infinito" ("The Infinite"), "La vita solitaria" ("The Solitary Life"), "La sera del dì

di festa" ("Sunday Evening"), "Alla luna" ("To the Moon"), as well as the philosophical canzones "Ad Angelo Mai" ("To Angelo Mai"), "Nelle nozze della sorella Paolina," "A un vincitore nel pallone," "Bruto Minore" ("The Younger Brutus"), "Alla primavera, o delle favole antiche" ("To Spring: Or, Concerning the Ancient Myths"), "Inno ai patriarchi" ("Hymn to the Patriarchs"), and "Ultimo canto di Saffo" ("Sappho's Last Song").

Finally, in 1822, Leopardi received permission to journey to Rome—an experience that he anticipated with great enthusiasm, only to find in a short time disappointment and disillusionment. The capital, once the classical city of Caesar and Brutus, now the pontifical abode of Pius VII, academically still unemancipated from the corruption and veneered pomp of the eighteenth century Arcadia, appeared like everything else: It partook of the vanity of all things.

In 1823, the Milanese editor Antonio Stella offered Leopardi, by then returned to Recanati, the job of pub-

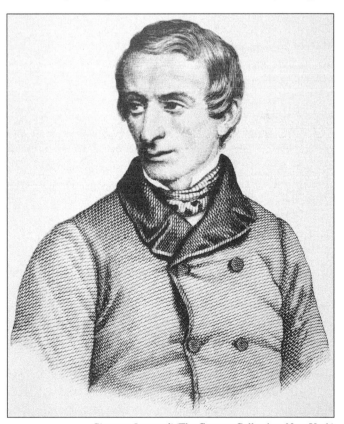

Giacomo Leopardi (The Granger Collection, New York)

lishing the complete works of Cicero, a venture that saw the poet leave "the sepulcher of the living" for the Lombard capital in 1825. Completed by this time were the philosophical poem "Alla sua donna" ("To His Lady") and his famous prose work, *Essays and Dialogues*, his acid reflections on an undependable world. In Milan, he also worked on a commentary on Petrarch's poetry and on a double anthology of Italian verse and prose. Another poem, also in the philosophical vein, "Al Conte Carlo Pepoli" ("To Count Carlo Pepoli"), appeared. His reputation spread beyond Italy, so that offers of chairs reached him from the universities of Bonn and Berlin, but fear of the intemperate northern winters prompted him to refuse.

After a lapse of several years, Leopardi returned to his creative writing: "A Silvia" ("To Sylvia"), "Il risorgimento" ("The Revival"), "Il passero solitario" ("The Solitary Thrush"), "Le ricordanze" ("Memories"), "La quiete dopo la tempesta" ("The Calm After the Storm"), and "Il sabato del villaggio" ("Saturday Evening in the Village") are poems of sorrow and illusion, of simple joys and lost youth, of evil and the pain of living. One of his greatest poems, "Canto notturno di un pastore errante dell'Asia" ("Night Song of a Nomadic Shepherd in Asia"), is dated 1829. Financial difficulties, aggravated by his parents' characteristic insensitivity, dented his pride when, in 1830, he accepted a sum of money raised by charitable friends headed by the historian Pietro Colletta. "I have lost all; I am a trunk which feels and suffers." In 1832, Leopardi was forced to ask his family for a modest allowance, an improbably small sum that, together with the previous year's Florentine printing of the augmented *Canti* (the idylls had appeared in Bologna in 1826 as *Versi*, and the broader and final collection appeared again in Naples in 1835), provided some economic respite.

Life continued to disillusion Leopardi, especially in his experience of unrequited and disappointing love. First, there had been a distant cousin, Gertrude Cassi, a lovely young lady of twenty-six who had come to Recanati for a brief visit that had filled the somber family mansion with some cheer, but had left the shy youth disenchanted ("First Love," written in 1817); then came Countess Carniani-Malvezzi of Bologna, a poet herself, with whom he established a comfortable

intellectual relationship until his own emotions, growing warmer, forced a reluctant break in 1826; finally, between 1830 and 1833, having fallen in love with the wife of a Florentine professor, Fanny Targioni-Tozzetti, Leopardi discovered that she had merely been flattered by the attentions of a great man and had given him insincere encouragement. She became his "ultimate deception," the wounding return to reality from his illusions, echoes of which are heard in "Il pensiero dominante" ("The Ascendant Thought"), "Aspasia," "Amore e morte" ("Love and Death"), and "Consalvo," as well as in his most bitter poem, "A stesso" ("To Himself").

Leopardi knew many of the important figures of his day, and many others yearned to know him. Still, his circle of friends remained limited. Toward the end of his life, he became close companions with a young Neapolitan exile, Antonio Ranieri, first in Florence and then, after Ranieri was pardoned by King Ferdinand II, in Naples. Leopardi's health, already strained, declined rapidly, despite the more salubrious climate of Torre del Greco in the neighborhood of Mount Vesuvius; the loving attention of Ranieri and his sister Paolina, as well as the doctors, could do nothing for Leopardi. By this time, he had written "Sopra un basso rilievo antico sepolcrale" ("On the Ancient Sepulchral Bas-Relief"), "Sopra il ritratto di una bella donna" ("On the Portrait of a Beautiful Lady"), and "Palinodia al marchese Gino Capponi," as well as his monumental poem "La ginestra, o il fiori del deserto" ("The Broom: Or, The Flower of the Desert"). On his deathbed, just before he died, he dictated to Ranieri the end of his last poem, "Il tramonto della luna" ("The Setting of the Moon"). Death, which he had so often invoked as a liberation from the anguish of having been born, overtook him on June 14, 1837. He was buried in the small church of San Vitale in Fuorigrotta. Giordani provided the epitaph, in the course of which one reads: "philologist admired outside of Italy, consummate writer of philosophy and poetry, to be compared with the Greeks. . . ."

ANALYSIS

Giacomo Leopardi's prominence as a poet stems from the lyrical greatness of the *Canti*, but as *Essays and Dialogues* demonstrates, there was in him a talent for biting sarcasm and sardonic humor that *The War of the Mice and the Crabs* brings forth in no uncertain terms. He thought about this work from 1830, when he conceived it in Florence, to the end of his life, in Naples, where he completed it. An ironic fantasy, ringing with sociopolitical overtones, it was published abroad (by Baudry, in Paris), posthumously, in 1842, thanks to the faithful guardianship of Ranieri. The work, whose full original title means "things left out of the [pseudo-Homeric] War of the Frogs [also Crabs] and the Mice," is in eight cantos of eight-line stanzas (Leopardi had translated the original *Batrachomyomachia*, a work originally attributed to Homer, three times), and takes to task any optimism based on the notion of social progress, liberals who claim to have the solution for national problems, the antimaterialistic postures of early nineteenth century philosophers, and political absolutism. Mixing together many elements, including the grotesque (the hell of the mice), the lyrical (a nocturne), and the polemical (statements against nature), Leopardi alludes to many Italian and European political realities of the first third of his century, without leaving too much room to doubt the identities of some of his characters, such as Camminatorto (Prince Clemens von Metternich), Senzacapo (Francis I of Austria), Mangiaprosciutti (the Bourbon Ferdinand I), Rubatocchi (Joachim Murat, the "Dandy King" of Naples and Napoléon's ally), and so on. To regard the poem strictly as a political allegory of contemporary events, however, does not do it justice, for beyond the satirical and grotesque presentation in all its varied fantasy is a panoramic view of human society conceived in broad, historical terms.

CANTI

The poetry of the *Canti* is elegant in its classical simplicity, its unpretentious yet effective imagery, its meditative philosophical tone, and its profoundly human tenderness. It reveals an overabundant inner life characterized by endless searching and by intellectual sincerity, a sincerity that found no compromise with reality. In the long run, Leopardi explained nothing (the mystery of life, after all, defies explanation), but he said everything. The "beautiful and mortal thing passes and lasts not"; all is vanity to which humans fall prey, and those things they think they can turn to and rely on—

such as love, beauty, and nature—deceive them cruelly, for each person is a microcosm in a macrocosm, subject to the universal destiny of sorrow existing in a world of ultimate nothingness. However, as often as Leopardi proclaims universal disillusionment, the poet continues to nourish illusions of love, goodness, beauty, and human fraternity. The paradox harbors one implied refuge: art, that shaper of benign illusions. This is why he was a poet.

The *Canti* as read today follow the arrangement of the poems, approved by the poet, in the posthumous Florentine edition of 1845, faithfully executed by Ranieri. The form is free, usually in blank verse in lines of varying length but with sparse rhyme and above all a sophisticated use of assonance. For Leopardi, the lyric represented the summit of literary expression. With a truly classical regard for the importance of the word, he aimed at Homeric clarity—eschewing complexity and the pathological somberness of many of his northern contemporaries—no matter how pessimistic the thought. Suppleness and the cleanly contoured line had to coexist to maintain the tone of serenity that made for a feeling of beauty and a sense of music. In addition, the free style of the canzones allowed a more relaxed incorporation of philosophical reflection than would have been possible in a more rigid versification. At no time, however, did the poet lapse into discursiveness or pedantry. Meditations, like emotions, were subject to the simplicity and directness of Leopardi's style.

PATRIOTIC CANZONES

The first poems in the *Canti*, the patriotic canzones "To Italy" and "On the Monument to Dante," do not fit the ideological profile of a person who stood, ultimately, like his contemporary Alessandro Manzoni, above the political fray. Indeed, in later years, liberals who expected more utterances in this vein from Leopardi were disappointed. His conversations with Pietro Giordani undoubtedly underlie the nationalistic, youthful fervor reflected in these early poems, though as the years went by, his philosophical nature could not yield to political pragmatism, and he adopted more and more a metaphysical view of life's vicissitudes.

Of the two patriotic canzones, "To Italy" has enjoyed somewhat greater acclaim. It contains seven strophes of twenty lines each. The poet portrays a prostrate and reviled Italy, once so glorious yet today subject to foreign masters; its sons die fighting on alien ground, unlike the handful of noble Greeks, victors over the Persians at Thermopylae, who died for their own land. The poet Simonides could sing of that deed to posterity and thereby commingle his own fame with that of the Hellenic heroes. Tainted by occasional tones of "high-sounding oratory," in the opinion of Gian Carlo D'Adamo, the poem betrays the idealistic background of Petrarch and Ugo Foscolo, yet more personally it also rings with sincere concern and reveals that at twenty years of age, Leopardi was already an accomplished poet.

IDYLLS

Unlike the classical, Theocritan idylls that resembled verbal vignettes, Leopardi's idylls bear an autobiographical imprint. He defined them as "experiments, situations, feelings, historical adventures of my soul." Five poems in hendecasyllabic blank verse, the "small" idylls "The Infinite," "Sunday Evening," "To the Moon," "Il sogno," and "The Solitary Life," constitute the first significant phase in Leopardi's poetic development.

"The Infinite" is a mere fifteen-line idyll, yet it is a work of extraordinary depth. The poet is near Recanati, atop a hill that has always been dear to him. A hedge blocks his view of the horizon, but he imagines the silence of boundless space beyond it. The factor of time intrudes through the sound of the wind in the leaves, reminding him of eternity, of history, and of the present. "And so," he concludes, "in this immensity my thought is drowned: and in this sea is foundering sweet to me." The meditation strikes the reader because of the absence of concrete details; its indeterminateness is made vital by the evocative power of the words, the pauses, the enjambments, the oxymoronic arrangement of "foundering" and "sweet"—indeed, a whole rhythm of inner contemplation that halts on the threshold of fear before nothingness and reverts to losing itself completely in the immensity of being. A miniature drama played out in the mind, the poem has been considered Leopardi's masterpiece.

"Sunday Evening" recounts in forty-six lines how the poet cannot, like his beloved, indulge in pleasant fantasies during the calm evening after the holiday; na-

ture allows him only tears. He compares the experience to the artisan's song that vanishes in the night's silence; on a grander scale, to the fall of the Roman Empire; and finally, to the anxiously awaited holiday that deceived him as a youth and choked his heart. The private theme of deception following in the wake of expectation is treated more objectively in "Saturday Evening in the Village." The effectiveness of this "holiday" poem derives from the moonlit setting, the sad, sentimental recollection, the dimmed semblance of a loved one, and the harshness of nature that favors others in preference to the poet.

"The Solitary Life" anticipates "The Solitary Thrush" with its theme of yearned-for solitude. A whole day is traced in its four unequal stanzas comprising 107 lines, from the morning patter of raindrops and the hen's fluttering wings, through the poet's lazy meditation by a quiet lake at noontime, where he remembers—despite the moving song he hears sung by a working girl from a nearby house—a disillusionment in love, to his greeting of the moon, which, unlike a thief or an adulterer, he wholly welcomes, as it sees him "wander through the woods and by the verdant banks, mute and solitary, or sit upon the grass, content enough, if only heart and breath be left for me to sigh." The movement of thought here surrenders to the motionlessness of silence.

PHILOSOPHICAL CANZONES

The next group of poems in the *Canti* is distinguished by a loftier language, and by a shift in subject matter from private to public concerns. These philosophical canzones number seven in all: "To Angelo Mai," "Nelle nozze della sorella Paolina," "Hymn to the Patriarchs," "A un vincitore nel pallone," "The Younger Brutus," "To Spring," and "Sappho's Last Song." This group of the early 1820's is usually expanded to include two poems composed slightly later, "To His Lady" and "To Count Carlo Pepoli," which share similar motifs.

In "To Angelo Mai," written in twelve fifteen-line strophes, Leopardi takes his Italian contemporaries to task because of their neglect of their illustrious past. To his "dead century" he opposes the philological discoveries of the erudite philologist and head librarian of the Ambrosiana and Vatican library, Angelo Mai, who had resurrected many significant texts. Philology is transfigured here to serve as a metaphor for civic regeneration. Though the poet feels decimated by sorrow and by lack of faith in the future, he evokes those "heroes" who lived and wrote before nature lifted the veil of comforting illusions from reality, before too much knowledge of the truth diminished humanity's imagination, before the sole certainty of existence—sorrow—had been fully disclosed, and before common opinion's notion of the sciences had pushed poetry into the background. Dante, Petrarch, Christopher Columbus, Ludovico Ariosto, Torquato Tasso, and Conte Vittorio Alfieri—all (except Ariosto) experienced deep sorrow, to which Leopardi relates his own experience in a manner that adumbrates the dominant pessimism of his subsequent poetry.

"The Younger Brutus," in eight fifteen-line stanzas, recalls the Roman hero after the Battle of Philippi ridiculing the concept of virtue. The gods, he opines, are not moved by the fate of humans, who accept death with resignation. The hero claims a limited victory over such a destiny through suicide, which the gods are incapable of understanding. Why the divine injunction against suicide? Animals are not ruled by it, only the sons of Prometheus. Beasts and birds are ignorant of the world's destiny, and the stars are indifferent (adumbrations of the coming song of the Asian shepherd). On the threshold of death, Brutus will not invoke the gods or the stars or posterity; his greatness will not enjoy understanding among men, so let his name and memory be lost. The poem stresses the hero's isolation; virtue, bitterly denounced at the outset, is exalted at the end. Leopardi's "agonism," as it has been called, consists of an active, if finally resigned, acceptance of fate, together with an eloquent protest against the laws of nature.

"Sappho's Last Song" portrays, in four sixteen-line stanzas, a legendary rather than historical Sappho: in Leopardi's words, "the unhappiness of a delicate, tender, sensitive, noble, and warm soul located in an ugly and young body," and, like Brutus, near suicide. The serene night and setting moon disclose a natural spectacle that once had brought comfort, but now, because of an adverse destiny, brings only misery. Why? No one can understand the lot of humankind; all is suffering, all

is externality—the music and poetry of the deformed find no appreciation. Sappho will die; with illusions and youth gone, she will descend into the infernal black night. The poem mixes with great lyrical fantasy some of Leopardi's favorite themes, particularly the ironic contrast between the beauty of the world and the bleakness of human infelicity.

GREAT IDYLLS OF 1828-1830

As distinguished from the "small" idylls of 1819 to 1821—a term that many critics hesitate to accept (there is certainly nothing "small" about "The Infinite")—the "great" idylls of 1828 to 1830, perhaps better identified simply as further *canti*, treat Leopardi's familiar themes with more complex meditation and richer inspiration. They number seven: "The Revival," "To Sylvia," "The Solitary Thrush," "Memories," "The Calm After the Storm," "Saturday Evening in the Village," and "Night Song of a Nomadic Shepherd in Asia." Most of them are canzones in free form; they marked Leopardi's return to writing poetry after a lapse of several years.

"To Sylvia" underscores the theme of lost youth and the insensitive deception of nature. In its sixty-three lines in six uneven, free-form stanzas, the poem recalls the daughter of a coachman in Recanati, whose "happy and elusive" eyes and "constant song" he remembers. His life then was bright with hopes in a lovely landscape of gardens outlined in the distance by mountains and sea, but all those hopes died, as Sylvia died, the victim of nature's cruelty, of a "strange disease" that preempted even her first acquaintance with words of love and praise for her beauty: "And with your hand you pointed from afar at chilling death and at a naked tomb." The poet, living on, can only lament the shattered illusions of youth, yet he does so without bitterness, with exquisite melancholy and refined sorrow that find relief in the re-creating power of the word.

"The Solitary Thrush," its three stanzas comprising fifty-nine lines, is a melancholy elegy evoking a festive spring day in the village, stressing, along with the theme of lost youth, the notion of isolation. The reasoning poet compares himself to the instinct-guided thrush that sings alone all day long while the other birds frolic in the sky. As the poet walks away from the celebrants in the village, the thrush leaves behind the joys of love and youth. It is an ending, in a way, and the sunset symbolizes it; while the bird will not mourn its losses, the poet will "many times look back at them, but quite disconsolate." Leopardi always revered solitude as a balm for the spirit and the imagination, but at the same time he recognized that it precludes communion with other people, and he saw in his penchant for solitude a dangerous inability to cope with life.

Written in seven free-style stanzas comprising 173 hendecasyllables, "Memories" recalls a train of images that had left their imprint on Leopardi's mind during his earlier years in Recanati. Returning to Recanati, the poet remembers how the "bright stars of the Bear" used to kindle dreams at night, and how by daytime the mountains suggested happiness beyond them. At that time, he did not know the malevolent crassness of his townsmen, nor did he expect a life without love. The pealing of the bell on city hall used to comfort his midnight fears, even as the "old halls" and the "frescoed walls" stirred his imagination then—when life held some promise. There was, too, the fountain in whose waters he had "thought of ending . . . my dreams." He remembers all this with tenderness and regret, all these "dulcet illusions," now that he has seen life in all its squalid reality. No one can ever forget the lovely illusions of youth, like those associated with young Nerina, who was stripped of life when it seemed most promising. She has remained for him the lamented image of all that has departed. The poem is characteristic of Leopardi's more mature style in its blend of the lyrical with the reflective.

To the double tone of the lyrical and the reflective, "The Calm After the Storm" adds a third, the descriptive. It contains fifty-four lines in three free-style stanzas. After the storm, the town's rhythm resumes: the song of birds and the "refrain" of the hen, the artisan's tune, the women hustling after rainwater, and the screeching cart on the highway. Life truly seems welcome, as when one has escaped death. This is "bounteous" nature's sole gift: the avoidance of sorrow; pleasure is "relief from pain." The human race is "blest only when death relieves you from all sorrow." The original idyll becomes—not untypically for Leopardi—an ironic meditation.

"Saturday Evening in the Village," in four very un-

even stanzas comprising fifty-one lines, again presents a series of images, all of villagers eager to complete their chores before the next day's holiday: the young lady with a bouquet of roses and violets, the old lady spinning at the wheel and recalling her youth, the children playing in the square, the farmer returning from the fields, the carpenter working until dawn. However, the festive expectation will yield only ennui and the sad thought of the continuing drudgery of tomorrow. Youth is like Saturday—one should not be so eager to leave it behind. Echoes of Vergil and Tasso give this poem an archaic flavor, as do the moralizing hints at the end. Leopardi's idea is clear: Happiness is a factor of the imagination that anticipates, and to which one should cling, for it inevitably surpasses realization. The charm of the poem, however, resides in the gentleness with which it treats a potentially sermonic subject matter.

Generally acclaimed as one of Leopardi's finest poems, "Night Song of a Nomadic Shepherd in Asia," consisting of six stanzas comprising 143 lines, drew its inspiration from an item in the September, 1826, issue of *Journal des savants* concerning the Kirkis, a north-central Asian nomadic tribe, some of whom "spend the night seated on a rock and looking at the moon, and improvising rather sad words on equally sad airs." The idea, however, had occupied Leopardi's mind for some time before 1826. The shepherd watches the "eternal pilgrim," the moon, as it crosses the sky and in turn watches the land. He does the same from dawn until evening, but what is the sense of the eternal movement of the stars and humanity's brief sojourn on Earth? Such is life: an old man who finally reaches his goal and disappears. Birth is difficult to begin with; then the parents must comfort the child "for being born"—so why struggle to live out the misery? Maybe the moon knows the why of things. The shepherd asks, but the question remains unanswered. Happy is the flock that knows nothing of destiny, though perhaps the lot of animals is equally unenviable, since "the day of birth is black to anything that's born." A surrogate for the poet, the shepherd in his primitive state knows as little about existence as the poet in his advanced modern age. Humans has always asked themselves the ultimate question, long before they started organizing their thoughts in writing; the shepherd always sensed that life is but an arduous journey toward death. All whys remain unanswered, and the moon, like the one Brutus saw, shines cold. Here again, because of the themes of pain, solitude, destiny, and universal mystery, the term "idyll" seems less suited than the term "elegy." In either case, however, the poem's supple rhythms give it a haunting, dirge-like quality.

THE ASPASIA CYCLE

The Aspasia cycle consists of "The Ascendant Thought," "Love and Death," "Consalvo," "To Himself," and "Aspasia," the last being a fictional name given by Leopardi to a woman he loved—unhappily: Pericles' beautiful and cultured courtesan represents the poet's Fanny Targioni-Tozzetti. All the poems in the cycle are in blank verse, and with the exception of "Consalvo" and "Aspasia," which are in hendecasyllables, the style is free.

"The Ascendant Thought," in fourteen stanzas comprising 147 lines, refers to the effects of love, to the way in which the poet's mind is dominated by the thought of love "like a tower gigantic and alone in a solitary field." To him it seems impossible that he has tolerated unhappiness without turning to love, which thwarts death and gives life meaning. Love allows one to withdraw from reality as in a dream. What more can the poet ask than to look into the eyes of his beloved? The Platonic ideal of Leopardi's earlier "To His Lady" here modulates into a moving passion, sustained from beginning to end not with dreamy tones, but with energetic emphasis. Here, Leopardi willingly throws himself into the arms of illusion.

On the other hand, "Love and Death," a slightly shorter poem of four stanzas comprising 124 lines, opposes death to the pleasures of love. The first effect of love is a languorous desire for death: While one needs love to escape the aridity of life, one knows also its "furious desire." Often, a lover in the heat of passion invokes death, and young lovers who kill themselves do so under the indifferent eyes of the crowd (for whom the poet ironically wishes emotionally barren longevity). As Benedetto Croce suggested, Leopardi addresses here the ravaging power of the senses: love as a "sweet and tremendous, elementary force of nature."

"To Himself" is Leopardi's most despairing utterance on the delusion of love, all the more powerful for its compression into a mere seventeen lines. The poet's heart will rest forever after the latest deception of love: "Bitter and dull is life, nothing more ever; and the world is mire." The only certainty is death; for himself, he has scorn, as he has also for nature, "and the infinite vanity of all things." Leopardi's style is as tense as his message; it is full of aesthetic silences that conjure up a wasteland of emotions, yet vibrant with the energy of disillusionment.

"Aspasia," consisting of 112 lines in four stanzas, concerns the mythologizing of woman. The poet sees Aspasia as a mother of incomparable beauty, elegance, and maternal femininity, a "ray divine." When he discovers that his image of her is largely fantasy, he blames her unjustly; in turn, she is unaware of the noble feelings that feed his delusion. The enchantment broken, the poet thinks of Aspasia in his tedium, "for a life bereft of sweet illusions and of love is like a starless night," but he finds comfort in lying on the grass to smile at "mortal destiny." The poem confesses Leopardi's humiliation for having been a slave in the throes of love, then rises to smile at the vanity of all things.

THE SEPULCHRAL CANZONES

The sepulchral canzones are only two in number: "On the Ancient Sepulchral Bas-Relief" and "On the Portrait of a Beautiful Lady." Both are written in free style, in lines of uneven length.

In the 109 lines of "On the Ancient Sepulchral Bas-Relief," the poet hesitates to call the dead young lady fortunate or unfortunate; perhaps she is happy, but her destiny inspires pity, since she passed away in the flower of her beauty. How could nature bring this on an innocent person? If death, a "most beautiful young maiden," is good, why lament it? Nature engenders illusions and struggles, so why should death appear frightening? If nature were not indifferent to humans, it would not "tear a friend from friendly arms . . . and killing the one, the other keep alive." Sadly, Leopardi meditates, questioning the finality of things human; humankind's lot leaves not even death as the ultimate comforter. Against this despair, the poem adumbrates the theme of human solidarity, "brother [for] brother, child [for] parent, beloved [for] lover," that informs his last great poem, "The Broom."

"THE BROOM"

"The Broom," the poem that concludes the *Canti*, is Leopardi's most profoundly philosophical canzone. Its seven uneven stanzas comprise 317 lines. The setting is the sloping wastes of Mount Vesuvius, where solitary broom plants grow. Under the lava once flourished famous cities; now there is only the plant's consoling scent. If one believes in humanity's "magnificent progressive destinies," one might come here to take note of nature's destructive powers and of humanity's impotence before nature. The poet's "proud and mindless age" only thinks it progresses; its intellectuals praise the supposed accomplishments of the age, but the poet, who will be forgotten because of the bitter truths he utters, knows better. A humble, sick, yet generous man has nothing to hide about himself, but the one who foolishly ignores the misery of the human condition keeps making glorious promises to those who can be wiped out by natural disasters. On the other hand, those who admit humankind's frailty are noble—he who realizes that nature is the enemy and urges self-defensive brotherhood and the renunciation of wars. Under the starry sky where the poet sits, one cannot reconcile such immensity with the self-centered importance that humanity, "a mere dot," gives its members: "Laughter or pity, I know not which prevails." Nature treats humankind as the apple that falls from the tree and crushes the ant colony. After nearly two thousand years, the husbandman tending the vineyards still watches the crater closely and with constant apprehension. Tourists visit the unearthed Pompeii while the volcano keeps smoking, and nature does not heed human affairs. The broom plant, too, will succumb to the lava, but, free of "overweening pride," it is "far wiser and so much less infirm than humans," who believe in their immortality.

As a compendium of the *Canti*, "The Broom" reveals most of the best in Leopardi, although it does not achieve the melodic magic of "To Sylvia" or "Night Song of a Nomadic Shepherd in Asia." In the course of the collection, Leopardi establishes for himself a position of marked individuality in the poetic traditions of love, beauty, death, and nature, often by virtue of his melancholy cosmic view, emotionally powered by a deep sense of wonder. Narrowing his vision to a few common and familiar objects that serve as his points of departure, he opens them up, as it were, drawing himself away into the "infinite spaces" where his thought likes to roam freely. From this vantage, serenity dominates, rather than a pathological concentration on the ego. Although Leopardi is always at the base of his poetry, he stands there as an example, not as a display, of the human condition.

In the background of this seminal poem lie some of Leopardi's basic philosophical beliefs. "Against a reborn Catholic spiritualism and the idealistic currents," explains D'Adamo, "Leopardi places his unchanged faith in materialistic and sensationalistic doctrines . . . ; he regrets that this body of thought that, after originating in Renaissance philosophy and developing successively during seventeenth century rationalism, freed us from medieval superstition and error, should be abandoned by the intellectuals of his day . . . in favor of new spiritualistic positions"—which included Catholic liberalism. Also in the background was the accusation of misanthropy leveled at Leopardi for his antiprogressivism, as well as the cruel charge that his pessimism was merely a consequence of his unfortunate physical condition.

As a symbol of humanity's helplessness, the broom plant encourages the poet in his message of brotherhood, which, after all, dates back to the origins of human life on Earth, and which bespeaks an innate moral sense in humanity. Leopardi appeals to humankind's reason; he wanted to end the *Canti* in this vein. The lyrical and the philosophical remain intertwined in this poetic discourse, though, as the composition unfolds, the two modes develop separately from each other in a brilliant interplay of reason and emotion.

OTHER MAJOR WORKS

PLAYS: *Pompeo in Egitto*, wr. 1812; *Telesilla*, wr. 1819.

NONFICTION: *Storia dell'astronomia*, 1813 (*History of Astronomy*, 1882); *Saggio sopra gli errori popolari degli antichi*, 1815 (*Essay on the Popular Superstitions of the Ancients*, 1882); *Discorso sopra la vita e le opere de M. Cornelio Frontone*, 1816; *Il salterio Ebraico*, 1816; *Discorso di un Italiano intorno alla poesia ro-*

mantica, 1818 (*Discourse of an Italian Concerning Romantic Poetry*, 1882); *Operette morali*, 1827, 1834, 1836 (*Essays and Dialogues*, 1882); *Crestomazia*, 1827-1828 (2 volumes); *Cento undici pensieri*, 1845 (*Pensieri*, 1981); *Epistolario*, 1849; *Zibaldone*, 1898-1900; *The Letters of Giacomo Leopardi, 1817-1837*, 1998.

BIBLIOGRAPHY

Barricelli, Jean Pierre. *Giacomo Leopardi*. Boston: Twayne, 1986. A basic biography of Leopardi, examining his life and works.

Broggi, Francesca. *The Rise of the Italian Canto: Macpherson, Cesarotti and Leopardi—From the Ossianic Poems to the "Canti."* Ravenna, Italy: Longo, 2009. Examines the works of Leopardi, James Macpherson, and Melchiorre Cesarotti and traces the development of the Italian canto.

Carsaniga, Giovanni. *Giacomo Leopardi: The Unheeded Voice*. Edinburgh, Scotland: Edinburgh University Press, 1977. A critical introduction to Leopardi's works with bibliographic references and index.

Chambers, Ross. "On Inventing Unknownness: The Poetry of Disenchanted Reenchantment (Leopardi, Baudelaire, Rimbaud, Justice)." *French Forum* 33, no. 1/2 (Winter, 2008): 15-35. Examines the poetry of Leopardi, Charles Baudelaire, Arthur Rimbaud, and Donald Justice for what he terms "invented unknownness." He argues that poems do not discover the unknown but rather create it. Leopardi's "The Infinite" is analyzed.

Nisbet, Delia Fabbroni-Giannotti. *Heinrich Heine and Giacomo Leopardi: The Rhetoric of Midrash*. New York: Peter Lang, 2000. Provides a critical analysis of similarities between the rhetorical strategies of Heine's *Ludwig Börne: Eine Denkschrift von H. Heine* (1840; *Ludwig Börne: Recollections of a Revolutionist*, 1881) and Leopardi's "Il Cantico del Gallo Silvestre" and the Midrashic process. Heine and Leopardi refer to biblical and historical events in their narratives and relate them to a contemporary situation to present their interpretation of an existential experience.

Press, Lynne, and Pamela Williams. *Women and Feminine Images in Giacomo Leopardi, 1798-1837.* Studies in Italian Literature 7. Lewiston, N.Y.: Edwin Mellen Press, 2000. A study of female images and man-woman relationships in Leopardi's works. Includes bibliographical references and index.

Rennie, Nicholas. *Speculating on the Moment: The Poetics of Time and Recurrence in Goethe, Leopardi, and Nietzsche*. Göttingen, Germany: Wallstein, 2005. Examines the themes of time and recurrence in the poetry of Leopardi, Johann Wolfgang von Goethe, and Friedrich Nietzsche. An entire section is devoted to Leopardi, although much of the discussion concerns *Zibaldone*.

Veronese, Cosetta. *The Reception of Giacomo Leopardi in the Nineteenth Century: Italy's Greatest Poet After Dante?* Lewiston, N.Y.: Edwin Mellen Press, 2009. Examines Leopardi's reception in Italy and other countries. Looks at early critical analysis of Leopardi.

Jean-Pierre Barricelli

ELIAS LÖNNROT

Born: Sammatti (now Lohja), Nyland, Swedish Finland; April 9, 1802
Died: Sammatti (now Lohja), Nyland, Russian Finland; March 19, 1884

PRINCIPAL POETRY

Kalevala, 1835 (enlarged 1849 as *Uusi Kalevala*; English translation, 1888)
Kalevalan esityöt, 1891-1895 (3 volumes)
Alku-Kalevala, 1928 (*The Proto-Kalevala*, published in *The Old Kalevala, and Certain Antecedents*, 1969)

OTHER LITERARY FORMS

Although the international fame of Elias Lönnrot (LUHN-rawt) rests primarily on the compilation of *Kalevala* and his extensive contributions to collecting, editing, and popularizing Finnish folklore, he is also recognized as a prominent linguist and literary scholar who helped secure for the Finnish language and oral culture the status of a national language and culture. Lönnrot assembled a massive Finnish-Swedish dictionary. His contributions to the Finnish hymnal are equally copious. Interest in his field trips to eastern Finland and Russian Karelia and Ingria triggered numerous posthumous publications of his travel accounts, diaries, and letters.

Achievements

Since its publication in 1835, Elias Lönnrot's *Kalevala* has continuously provided both national and international validation for Finland's cultural heritage. Widely acclaimed for having laid the foundations of Finnish as a literary and national language, *Kalevala* has been translated into forty-seven languages. It has inspired works in literature, the fine and performing arts, design, and architecture, both in Finland and abroad. In Finland, writers, playwrights, and poets Aleksis Kivi, Zacharias Topelius, Lauri Haarla, Juhana Erkko, Eino Leino, Veikko Koskenniemi, and Paavo Haavikko; composers Johan Filip von Schantz and Jean Sibelius; painter-sculptor Akseli Gallen-Kallela; and photojournalist Into Inha all found fruitful source material in *Kalevala*. Abroad, the work inspired American poet Henry Wadsworth Longfellow, Swedish painter Johan Blackstadius, and Swedish sculptor Carl Sjöstrand, among others. Finland celebrates February 28 as Kalevala Day, thereby granting Lönnrot's epic formal recognition as a national symbol.

Biography

Elias Lönnrot, the fourth of seven children, was born in Sammatti, a Finnish-speaking area in Swedish Finland, to a poor tailor and his wife. Financial difficulties and the need to learn Swedish, the country's official language until 1863, prevented Lönnrot from attending college until he was twenty years old. In 1822, he enrolled at the University of Turku, where he studied classical and modern languages and literatures (Greek, Latin, Hebrew, Swedish, and Russian), history, philosophy, and the natural sciences. A major influence on him was the Romantic nationalism of Finnish historian Henrik Gabriel Porthan and Turku professor of Finnish Reinhold von Becker, both of whom advocated the col-

lection, study, and popularization of folklore and the vernacular as depositories of Finnish national and cultural identity. Encouraged by von Becker, in 1827, Lönnrot defended a thesis on the Finnish epic and cultural hero Väinämöinen. Later that year, because of a fire in Turku, Lönnrot transferred to Helsinki, where he obtained a degree in medicine in 1832. His thesis, "On the Magical Medicine of the Finns," again reflected a strong intellectual investment in Finland's indigenous traditions. Medical degree in hand, Lönnrot became a district physician in Kajaani, northeastern Finland.

Part of Lönnrot's duties in Kajaani involved making health inspection trips, which created rich opportunities to further his study of the Finnish language and folklore. The leaves of absence he took between 1828 and 1844 allowed Lönnrot to embark on eleven field trips to northeastern Finland, Karelia, and Ingria, areas associated with the mythological lands of Kalevala and Pohjola. The fifth trip, in April, 1834, proved especially fruitful: Within two weeks, Lönnrot had collected more than thirteen thousand lines of poetry. In 1835, the Finnish Literary Society published Lönnrot's *Kalevala*, which he later expanded and published as *Uusi Kalevala*. Lönnrot's conscious effort to disclose the ethnographic authenticity of the folk material integrated into his epic is reflected in his editing and publishing several volumes of lyric and epic songs, ballads, tales, charms, proverbs, and riddles between 1829 and 1840.

In the 1840's, Lönnrot took a longer leave of absence to begin to compile a Finnish-Swedish dictionary that contained more than 200,000 words and took more than thirty-five years to complete. Lönnrot was appointed professor of Finnish language and literature at the University of Helsinki in 1853, a position he held until 1862, when he retired to his native Sammatti. He continued working on the dictionary, the first volume of which appeared in 1867. As chairman of the Finnish Hymnal Committee, Lönnrot was the hymnal's most prolific contributor, compiling three hymn collections between 1867 and 1870. During his lifetime, Lönnrot founded, edited, or published several language and literary periodicals: Kajaani's *The Bee*, *Finnish Review*, a Swedish-language literary periodical, and *Oulu Weekly*. He died in Sammatti at the age of eighty-one.

ANALYSIS

Elias Lönnrot attempted to revive a sense of Finnish nationality by using its oral tradition to actively reconstruct a culture unified by a common language, historical continuity, and an indigenous artistic tradition. Lönnrot's efforts are evident in *Kalevala*'s composition, dominant themes, and reception. Having been a Swedish province for seven hundred years, Finland had developed deep sociocultural divisions: The Swedish-speaking urban elites had little in common with the Finnish-speaking lower classes, whose cultural self-awareness remained rooted in the country's rural and oral customs and traditions. In 1809, when Finland was incorporated into the Russian Empire as an autonomous grand duchy, it faced an identity crisis: The Romantic nationalists who sought to create a Finland independent from Sweden's cultural legacy also needed to take into account fears of being assimilated by the Russians.

Lönnrot's *Kalevala* responded to this identity crisis by providing Finns with a national symbol that gave them direct access to Finland's mythical heritage and historical past, the feats of its epic and cultural heroes, and its indigenous pre-Christian rituals, customs, and beliefs. These are embedded in *Kalevala*'s main cycles, which center on the exploits of four ancient heroes, Väinämöinen (the shaman or "eternal sage"), Ilmarinen (the primeval smith), Lemminkäinen (the adventurer), and Kullervo (the tragic hero), who protect Kalevala's order and prosperity, which are threatened by its northern neighbor Pohjola. Lönnrot's adaptation of folklore produces several levels of epic allegory: While the Kalevala-Pohjola conflicts reflect an archetypal struggle between the forces of light and darkness, they also mirror Finland's struggle for cultural and national self-definition against two powerful neighbors, Sweden and Russia. Framed by Väinämöinen's birth and departure from Kalevala, the epic's narrative adds a historical dimension to the mythological world: It recounts the rise and fall of Finnish paganism, its downfall sealed by the arrival of Christianity.

In the interest of creating a historical time line and safeguarding the mythological characteristics of the epic narrative and characters, Lönnrot eliminated the Christian and modern elements in the folk songs and discarded those that posed narrative or stylistic contradictions. He preserved the metric characteristics of the folk poetry: The Kalevala meter contains eight-syllable trochaic lines, with alternating long (stressed) and short (unstressed) syllables. *Kalevala* makes frequent use of alliteration and is consistent in its reliance on parallelism. Every other line of verse presents a paraphrased repetition of the idea or image introduced in the first line.

THE SAMPO CYCLE

Kalevala's main plot line encompasses the world's creation, Väinämöinen's birth, and the events leading to the forging, retrieval, and loss of the Sampo, a miraculous object associated with spiritual and material prosperity. The narrative incorporates epic songs, mythic in nature, that reveal the female origins of creation; Väinämöinen's role in ordering Kalevala's natural, agricultural, and moral spheres; and his prestigious position as an "eternal sage," whose singing (poetic insight) manifests both his unmatched magical powers and ability to communicate with the otherworld. In canto 3, when Joukahainen, envious of the bard's fame, challenges Väinämöinen to a singing contest and is defeated, the epic songs transform into shaman songs, giving rise to a dominant theme: Spells and magic occupy a more powerful position in *Kalevala* than physical violence. This theme also underlies the relationship between Väinämöinen and Ilmarinen, the sky's forger. In cantos 7-8, for example, Väinämöinen looks for a wife in Pohjola. As the land's mistress, Louhi promises her daughter to the man who can create the Sampo. Väinämöinen's spells transport the reluctant Ilmarinen to Pohjola, where he has no other choice but to forge the Sampo (canto 10). Väinämöinen also resorts to magic in cantos 16-17 when he travels to Tuonela, the land of the dead, in search for the spell that would allow him to accomplish an impossible feat and win Louhi's daughter, who had refused to marry Ilmarinen. In the epic's closing cantos, Väinämöinen resorts to violence only after his magic has failed to stop Louhi's revenge on Kalevala for the theft of the Sampo. As Väinämöinen and other characters often resort to incantations as a way of curing disease or injuries and securing help from the otherworldly, scholars have often classified *Kalevala* as a shamanistic epic.

THE WOMEN

In addition to the epic poetry and ritual/healing incantations typical of the repertoire of male folksingers in Karelia, Lönnrot integrates into *Kalevala* elaborate examples of lyric poetry, wedding songs, and lamentations, which are traditionally associated with female singers. Such lyric passages create a nuanced literary language, well-suited to articulating the psychological subtleties of a national culture and also to magnifying the emotional intensity of both character motivation and setting, prompting critics to describe *Kalevala* as both folk epic (with clearly identifiable folklore sources) and literary epic (an individual creation). The sorrowful stories of Aino (cantos 4-5) and of Louhi's younger daughter (canto 38), neither of whom is willing to marry Väinämöinen or Ilmarinen, reveal that the female characters' wishes are clearly subordinate to the needs and desires of the male characters, thus emphasizing thematic and narrative continuities between wooing and war in the epic. A woman can escape an unwanted marriage only by merging (or being forced to merge) her identity with nature: Aino drowns in a lake and gets transformed into a mermaid, while Ilmarinen, unable to endure the sorrowful lamentations of his unwilling bride, "sings" her into a seagull.

OTHER MAJOR WORKS

NONFICTION: *Om det Nord-Tschudiska språket*, 1853; *Finsk-svenskt lexikon*, 1874, 1880 (2 volumes); *Elias Lönnrotin matkat*, 1902 (2 volumes); *Elias Lönnrots svenska skrifter*, 1908, 1911 (2 volumes).

EDITED TEXTS: *Kantele*, 1829-1831 (4 volumes); *Kanteletar*, 1840 (3 volumes; *The Kanteletar: Lyrics and Ballads After Oral Tradition*, 1992); *Suomen kansan sananlaskuja*, 1842; *Suomen kansan arvoituksia*, 1844; *Vanhoja ja uusia virsiä*, 1865; *Viisikymmentä virttä*, 1869; *Suomalainen virsikirja valiaikaiseksi tarpeeksi*, 1870; *Alku-Kanteletar*, 1929.

BIBLIOGRAPHY

DuBois, Thomas A. *Finnish Folk Poetry and the "Kalevala."* New York: Garland, 1995. Offers comparative readings of select folk poems from *The Kanteletar* and excerpts from both *Kalevala* editions, tracing Lönnrot's formal and aesthetic transformations of folklore into literature. Especially valuable are the contrasts between communal aesthetics reflected in Karelian and Ingrian folksingers' repertories and the subsequent suppression of female experience and point of view in Lönnrot's epic.

Honko, Lauri, ed. *The "Kalevala" and the World's Traditional Epics*. Helsinki: Finnish Literature Society, 2002. A collection of studies on *Kalevala* and other epics.

_____. *Religion, Myth, and Folklore in the World's Epic: The "Kalevala" and Its Predecessors*. New York: Mouton de Gruyter, 1990. Wide-ranging and accessible studies of *Kalevela*'s epic models (Homeric, Roman, Old Norse, Germanic, and Celtic) and the processes of its conception; also contains insightful comparisons between Finland's epic tradition and those of Europe, Africa, and Asia.

Kolehmainen, John I. *Epic of the North: The Story of Finland's "Kalevala."* New York Mills, Minn.: Northwestern, 1973. An extensive study of the mythological, folklore, intellectual, cultural, and literary origins of *Kalevala*, with special attention given to its influence on Finnish national and cultural self-awareness, establishing Finnish as a literary language, popularizing Finnish-language schools, and inspiring new Finnish literature, fine and performing arts, and films.

Lönnrot, Elias. *The Kalevala: An Epic Poem After Oral Tradition by Elias Lönnrot*. Translated by Keith Bosley. New York: Oxford University Press, 2009. A translation of the great Finnish epic by a prize-winning translator and English poet. Bosley has provided a lengthy and informative introduction.

Mazzeno, Laurence W., ed. *Masterplots*. 4th ed. Pasadena, Calif.: Salem Press, 2011. Contains a plot summary and a detailed critical analysis of *Kalevala*.

Oinas, Felix J. *Studies in Finnic Folklore: Homage to the "Kalevala."* Helsinki: Suomalaisen Kirjallisuuden Seura, 1985. Situates the Finnish lyric and epic folklore tradition underlying *Kalevala* in the larger folklore context of Russian Karelia and Ingria and the Estonian epic *Kalevipoeg*; focuses on parallel and divergent narrative elements; prominent songs, rituals, and divinities; and epic and cultural heroes.

Pentikäinen, Juha Y. *"Kalevala" Mythology*. Bloomington: Indiana University Press, 1989. A seminal study of *Kalevala*'s major characters, conflicts, and mythic-cultural symbols. Especially valuable are the critical explorations of *Kalevala* as a shamanistic epic, the allegorical stories of creation and cultural origins, and the mythical and historical aspects of time, life, and death.

Miglena Ivanova

LUCAN

Born: Corduba, Roman Province of Spain (now Córdoba, Spain); November 3, 39 C.E.
Died: Rome (now in Italy); April 15, 65 C.E.
Also known as: Marcus Annaeus Lucanus

PRINCIPAL POETRY
Bellum civile, 60-65 C.E. (*Pharsalia*, 1614)

OTHER LITERARY FORMS
Thirteen of the lost works of Lucan (LEW-kuhn) were known to Vacca, one of his major biographers, living in the sixth century. Vacca implied that these works were still extant; and several of them were confirmed by Suetonius, another biographer. Vacca is clear that the thirteen are minor works compared with the epic on the civil war, *Pharsalia*, but feels that some, at least, are valuable. The items on Vacca's list include the *Iliacon* from the Trojan cycle; the *Laudes Neronis*; the *Orpheus; De incendio urbis*, a description of the great fire that nearly destroyed Rome; *Saturnalia*, on the gaities of December; ten books of miscellaneous *Silvae*; the unfinished tragedy of *Medea*; a series of letters called *Epistulae ex Campania* (which, if they had survived, would surely have proved to be a fascinating addition to our specimens of ancient letter writing); as well as speeches for and against Octavius Sagitta. The latter suggest that (in 58 C.E.) Lucan, perhaps acting on the detective instinct, seized upon one of the most exciting murder trials of the day as material for two clever rhetorical showpieces.

ACHIEVEMENTS
Lucan's poetry covered a great variety of genres, although only his incomplete epic, the *Pharsalia*, is extant. Based on the titles, the subjects of a number of lost works range from tragedy to satire to occasional verse. The bulk of Lucan's poetry, including the ten books of the *Pharsalia*, was probably produced in about five years, beginning in 60 C.E. In the light of this information, his production can only be described as prodigious. The output is all the more remarkable when one considers that Lucan composed much of his poetry while he was involved in a political career. Most poets of antiquity who were also politicians postponed their poetic endeavors until they had withdrawn or retired from state business.

Lucan, then, enjoyed neither the leisure time of the retired senator nor the professional poet's singleness of purpose. Vergil was able to spend eleven years of his mature creative life working almost exclusively on the *Aeneid* (c. 29-19 B.C.E.; English translation, 1553), and the *Thebais* (c. 90 C.E.; *Thebiad*, 1767) occupied Statius for twelve years, but Lucan, still in his early twenties, worked on the *Pharsalia* for no more than five years and possibly less than three. While he worked, he held an augurate and a quaestorship and joined a conspiracy to kill the emperor Nero.

BIOGRAPHY
Marcus Annaeus Lucanus was born in Corduba on November 3, 39 C.E. The determining factors in his career were his descent from two prominent Spanish families and his rhetorical education. His father, Marcus Annaeus Mela, was the brother of Seneca the Younger (the philosopher, poet, and statesman) and the son of Seneca the Elder. Lucan's mother was the daughter of Acilius Lucanus, a Corduban speaker of note. Thus, by birthright Lucan belonged to one of Spain's most distinguished families, whose talents had been widely recognized and who had obtained considerable wealth. Lucan was brought to Rome at an early age, where he enjoyed all the wealth and prestige that the Annaei could provide, particularly after 49 C.E., when Seneca was recalled from exile to become the tutor to Nero, the heir apparent to the throne. After formal training at the school of a grammarian, Lucan became the pupil of the

Stoic philosopher Annaeus Cornutus, whose name suggests that he may have been a freedman of Lucan's own family.

Considering Seneca's position in Roman public affairs, which grew even stronger between 49 C.E. and 60 C.E., it is not surprising that Lucan was quickly drawn into the very heart of Roman social and political life. While this introduction to court life proved to be an incentive to Lucan, it ultimately caused his ruin. Lucan probably spent considerable time with Nero himself. After all, Lucan and Nero were only two years apart in age and both had a keen interest in literature. When Lucan left Rome for Athens to pursue his education, Nero recalled him to join his entourage, the *cohors amicorum*. Soon, honors were being conferred upon Lucan, such as the quaestorship before the regular age of twenty-five and an augural priesthood. In 60 C.E., then twenty-one years old, he achieved his first public literary triumph with his *Laudes Neronis* at the festival of the Neronia, a newly established celebration in honor of the emperor.

At that time, Nero and his young admirer were on the best of terms; Lucan's position, however, became less secure as Nero's dislike for his tutor Seneca increased. Lucan, perhaps foolishly, entered a competition against Nero and so incurred the enmity of the emperor, who was clever, conceited, and egotistical. Suetonius, a biographer of Lucan, implies that the break between Lucan and Nero arose partly from Lucan's imagining that Nero's attitude toward his works was deliberately insulting and partly from Lucan's unbecoming mockery of the emperor's verses. Vacca attributes the quarrel to Nero's jealousy of Lucan's genius. In any case, Lucan was forbidden to engage in further poetic production or the pleading of law cases. The only avenue left open to the poet was covert satire, and he was prompted by Nero's persecution to join the Pisonian conspiracy. When the intrigue was discovered, Lucan was condemned to death. To avoid execution, after a sumptuous feast, he had his veins opened. His last moments were spent reciting a piece of his own about a soldier similarly bleeding to death. When the emperor cut short Lucan's career, his epic was incomplete and published only in part.

ANALYSIS

Lucan was an audacious author. In touch with an imperial court, he dared to write his long poem *Pharsalia* glorifying the opposition to the founder of imperial power in Rome. Lucan must have been sufficiently aware of the arbitrary tyranny of Nero to recognize that in writing such an epic he played a game involving the highest of stakes. Conscious of his genius, independent in spirit, and impetuous in his youth, he was perhaps fascinated by a hazard with double danger. It was dangerous enough to challenge Nero in literary competition, but it was even more perilous to celebrate the defenders of the ancient Republican system. Theirs had been a lost cause, yet Lucan makes idols of Pompey and Cato and so implicitly challenges Caesarism. There were several justifications for this anti-Caesarism. Corduba, the Spanish seat of his family, acknowledged a traditional allegiance to Pompey, and Lucan's own youthful imagination dreamed up rosy visions of a Republican past. His readings of Livy, the great propagandist for the Republic, confirmed his attitude. Nero's unfairness in trying to silence him drove him to detest the Caesarean dynasty.

Lucan's independent spirit affected not only the subject of his epic but also its composition. He broke away from epic tradition by resolutely rejecting mythology. Lucan's originality lay not so much in the choice of a Roman historical theme—there had been many epics, renowned and unrenowned, on national history—but in the treatment of his theme without the conventional introduction of the gods. The way in which Lucan introduced mythology as an appendix to geography served only to measure his contempt for it. When he described a region that had a legend, he told the legend with the proviso that it was not true. For Lucan, the strongest motive for relating a legend was that it was an incredible explanation of facts for which no credible explanation was forthcoming. Aware of the intrinsic greatness of the figures in a colossal struggle, Lucan relied for his effects more on history than on romance. In his theme, therefore, he broke away from Vergilian precedent and for legendary glamour substituted interest in a human conflict of a comparatively recent time.

PHARSALIA

Pharsalia is the only work by Lucan extant, and only ten books survive. This epic treats the war between Caesar and Pompey that erupted in 49 B.C.E. The title *Pharsalia* is borrowed from book 9, verse 985 of the poem. It consists of more than eight thousand hexameters but still does not complete the poet's design; the tenth book, about 150 lines shorter than the next shortest, ends abruptly, leaving Caesar at war in Egypt.

Modern critics have tended to condemn Lucan as tasteless and uninspired, and his *Pharsalia* is frequently (as has been said about John Milton's *Paradise Lost* of 1667, 1674) more talked about than read. In the Middle Ages, however, few classical authors were more widely read or praised than Lucan. In eighteenth century England, the *Pharsalia* not only was popular but also was considered to be the work of a poet even greater than Vergil. Lucan must be given credit for picturesque and striking language, but above all for his attempt to reinfuse a somewhat wilted Roman literature with the spirit of life. As Vergil had correctly seen, historical themes were not well suited to epic treatment. Nevertheless, Lucan was right in perceiving that Roman literature could not go on forever dealing with mythological fantasy, with ancient never-never lands and legendary history. If literature was to have any real meaning, it had to bring itself back to reality.

Lucan's attempt to make philosophy and science serve as the divine and mythological machinery had once served, however, is less than successful. The philosophical portions of the poem seem pompous, forced, and insincere, and require entirely too much argument. The scientific and pseudoscientific episodes are too long and detailed and clog the narrative. Lucan also failed to notice that if he was to write about real people and real history, he must write about them in "real" language and not in the high-flown, artificial style of the rhetorical schools.

The conflict between character and circumstance, each always victorious on its own ground, is the subject that gives interest and dignity to the *Pharsalia*. The poem opens with a delay of the action as Lucan describes the emperor Nero as a god and addresses him as sufficient inspiration for a poet. Lucan anticipates Nero's apotheosis and acknowledges that civil war was

not a heavy price to pay for the blessings of Nero's reign. This opening probably owes something to Seneca, and certainly the poet is not at first so violently opposed to Caesar as he later becomes. Lucan is able to recognize that the war was a result of Pompey's inability to endure an equal and Caesar's inability to endure a master. It is a solitary gleam of insight. Referring to Pompey's lack of recent battle experience, Lucan unduly stresses his advanced age. In his fifty-seventh year, he was only four years older than his opponent, and, as Lucan more than once reminds his readers, had become Caesar's son-in-law by marrying Julia, whose death made the breach between them more probable. The poet, although sincerely embracing Pompey's cause, perceives him as a man overconfident because of previous battles and too trusting in the power of his name. The contrasting figure of Caesar is drawn forcefully although not sympathetically. He is a character who relies much on the sword and who enjoys creating havoc.

The strict narrative begins with Caesar's passage across the Alps, bringing his big plans to the small river Rubicon. (The adjectival antithesis is Lucan's.) Caesar is confronted with the majestic image of his native country protesting against further advance. The Rubicon is crossed; Arminium is taken; Caesar is met by his supporters. A summons for troops from Gaul presents an opportunity for digressions on Gallic tribes, tides, and Druids; then, a description of panic in Rome at Caesar's approach leads to the introduction of omens and expiatory rites. The book ends gloomily amid presages of disaster. Lucan, while he removes from his historical epic the conventional gods of epic poetry, puts in their place the supernatural, represented here by the symbolic figure of Roma, by portents, and by the prophecy of both an astrologer and a clairvoyant matron who has a vision of Pompey already lying dead.

Philosophy hesitantly opens book 2. The philosophical foundation of the *Pharsalia* is popular Stoicism, and the Stoics were perpetually confronted with the problem of reconciling belief in fate with divination. Why, asks Lucan, is humanity allowed to know future unhappiness through omens? He ends his philosophical discussion with a prayer that there might be hope amid fear and that the human mind be unaware of the coming doom. Mourning falls on Rome, and men pray for a foreign attack in preference to civil war. The passage is rhetorical in its earlier portion and argumentative at its close. The chief incidents of the book are: first, the remarriage of Cato to his former wife Marcia; second, the resistance to Caesar offered by Domitius, pointedly introduced because he was an ancestor of Nero; and, finally, the retreat of Pompey to Brundisium and overseas. Padding consists of digressions on the civil wars between Marius and Sulla and on the rivers of Italy. The introduction of Cato here is significant for book 9, where he plays a commanding part. For Lucan, Cato is the incarnation of virtue, never before guilty of shedding his country's blood, but now drawn by force into the struggle. Full of admiration for Cato's ascetic ordering of his life, the poet proudly describes his Stoic ability to combine self-sufficing virtue with altruistic claims.

Book 3, mainly concerned with Caesar's activities on his return to Rome and his siege of Massilia, is ruined by a wearisome list of Pompey's eastern allies and the account of an interminable series of ingeniously horrible deaths that befall the soldiers. Among the compensating passages, however, are descriptions of Pompey's farewell to Italy and the eerie forest near Massilia. The former opens the book with a note of poetry and pathos, and the latter, describing the grave of the Druids, is a somber study touched with the spirit of Celtic romance. The reader is placed in a haunted wood at twilight, a place polluted by inhuman rites, shunned by birds, beasts, and forest deities. The leaves of the trees quiver, although there is no wind, and the whole forest is awesome with decay and nameless terrors.

Three episodes constitute most of the action of book 4: Caesar's Spanish operations, the failure of one of three Caesarean rafts to escape the Pompeian blockade in Illyria, and the arrival of a Caesarean general, Curio, in Africa, where he is defeated by Iuba and meets his death. The thirst suffered by the Pompeians in Spain prompts one of Lucan's denunciations of luxury, while the advice of the Caesarean commander to his men trapped on the raft to commit "mutual" suicide rather than surrender is argued in the strained style of a course in rhetoric. When the crew carries out their mutual slaughter, characteristic realism is employed to de-

scribe the crawling, bleeding, writhing agony of the lacerated men. This mass suicide closes with a reflection that consoled many of Nero's subjects as well as Lucan: Death is a ready way to elude tyranny. It is the Stoic speaking, recognizing the theoretical obligation of suicide and admitting that it was in certain circumstances defensible.

Book 5 opens with the assembly of the Senate friendly to Pompey and closes with his decision to send his wife, Cornelia, to Lesbos for safety. Nevertheless, Caesar is the dominant figure, especially when he cows the mutineers and crosses the Adriatic in a small boat on a stormy night to bring Antony. Caesar's willpower is dramatized in his defiant braving of the storm despite a fisherman's warning. He is content to have Fortune as his sole attendant in crossing the sea, but the storm is irresistibly tempting for Lucan. He exhausts his use of contending winds and then turns to hyperbole; mountains, having struggled in vain, crumble into the sea, as the waves roll portentously. Still full of hyperbole, but much more human, is the concluding episode, in which Pompey, deeply affected, can scarcely bring himself to tell his wife that for her safety they must part.

Overloaded with digressions, details of Caesar's scheme to enclose his enemy at Dyrrachum, and hyperbolical praise of the repulse of Pompey, book 6 is not on the whole successful. The action concentrates on one outstanding Caesarean who offers the resistance of an African elephant, tearing out and stamping on his own eyeball along with the arrow that pierced it. This and much more is neither poetry nor common sense. The rest mainly concerns the temporary setback of Caesar, who retreats to Thessaly and is followed there by Pompey. The mention of Thessaly offers the opportunity for digressions on geography and magic. There is a catalog of Thessalian spells for love, weather, rivers, mountains, and laws of the universe. The witches of Thessaly are more convincing in the work of Apuleius; yet Lucan does achieve a gruesome effect through Sextus Pompey's morbid longing to learn the future, not from oracles but from necromancy. He makes his way to the sorceress Erichtho and holds a midnight séance with her. Agreeing to his request, she selects a dead warrior, who is brought back to life by loathsome ingredients in order to foretell the future. The revelation is that the shades of the dead await both Sextus's father and his house. With that ominous response, Sextus returns to his father's camp before daybreak.

Although book 7 is not free from extravagance, it is the greatest book of the poem. It describes the feelings of both rivals before Pharsalus, as well as their fortunes in the battle. Pompey's men shout for battle and criticize their leader's caution. In a historically inaccurate scene, Cicero, who was not actually present, is introduced as urging Pompey to give battle. Pompey consents under protest. His men have their way, but many presage death in their pale coloring. The harangues to each side by the respective commanders are vigorous, full of bravado, and very readable. Despite Pompey's claim that his is the better cause, tyranny—in Lucan's view—is triumphant at Pharsalus. Lucan contrasts the fugitive Pompey, looking back upon lost greatness, with Caesar, whose adversary from this point on is not Pompey but freedom and who, to discerning eyes, might be an object of pity: It was worse to win. The picture of the conqueror is not flattering. According to Lucan, Caesar encouraged his men to plunder, was the leader of the guilty side, callously surveyed the dead, withheld rotting corpses from cremation, and was hunted, Orestes-like, by avenging Furies.

The main interest of book 8 lies in Pompey's flight to Egypt and his murder as he is about to land. It is broken by reflections and apostrophes on both Egypt and Pompey. A prey to nervous fears, the defeated warrior escapes in a small boat to Lesbos, where he tries to console his grief-stricken wife. He sets sail with her in anxiety great enough to make unnatural his conversation with the pilot about astronomy. He holds a council of his supporters on his destination, suggesting they land in Parthia. His advisers consider this action dishonorable and persuade him to try Egypt, whose king, Ptolemy, owes his throne indirectly to Pompey. Thus does Pompey sail to meet death. Overmastering fate arranges that Pompey is enticed into a small boat where, in view of his wife and son, he is stabbed by a traitor. Pompey's head is cut off and carried to the boy-king Ptolemy. Having noted the majesty of Pompey's looks as preserved in death, Lucan yields to his obstructive passion for realism and spoils the pathos of the scene. Instead of Vergil's dignity in the face of sorrow, or

beauty of simile, there are repulsive details of the still-gasping mouth and the drooping neck laid crosswise to be hacked through; there are sinews and veins to be cut; there are bones to break. Such realism is rendered unnecessary by the moving description of Pompey that follows. The headless body is retrieved from the sea by one of Pompey's Roman attendants and, after an incomplete cremation, is hastily buried. The book ends with imprecations and wild rhetoric on Egypt.

Pompey's apotheosis begins book 9. The lamentations of Cornelia, the threats of vengeance by Pompey's son, and Cato's dignified praise of the dead leader are preliminaries to the central theme of the book: the heroism of Cato. He marches with his men to Africa and gives many demonstrations of his endurance and courage. Cato's inspiring bravery is, however, almost smothered by a mass of irrelevant details about the origin of serpents in Africa and by catalogs of various species of serpents and various sorts of deaths from snakebite.

Book 10, on Caesar in Egypt, would fit better into an epic on mighty Julius than into the *Pharsalia*, yet it has energy in spite of a digression on Alexander the Great. The principal events are Caesar's visit to Alexander's tomb, his affair with Cleopatra, her magnificent banquet after a reconciliation with Ptolemy, and the plot to kill Caesar. The tenth book is incomplete, and there are many indications of an unfinished scheme. There is, for example, a reference to the postponement of a fated penalty, which implies that the poem was designed to continue up to Caesar's assassination in 44 B.C.E.

LEGACY

When it is remembered that the aim in academic rhetoric was to appear clever and striking at all costs, the central characteristic of Lucan's epic is at once grasped. The dominant note is one of display. The object is not to be natural but above all to be piquant and impressive. The parade of erudition that leads to catalogs and digressions employs Lucan's rhetorical training. The realistic detail is calculated to cause a shudder, the subtlety of argument makes a debating speech cogent, the hyperbole arrests attention, and points, epigrams, and antitheses produce memorable phrases.

Realism in Lucan is morbid and grotesque. Too often it is paired with the desire to terrify the audience by dwelling on the horrible. Hence he enjoys describing tortures, the agonies of the wounded, the repulsive ghoulishness of a witch, and the revolting aspects of cremation. When realism is strained to the breaking point, it becomes unreal.

Despite such overemphasis on gory realism and hyperbole, Lucan's rhetoric is often brilliant, expressing his thought in brief, pointed form, often assisted by antithesis. These economical lines and phrases epigrammatically summarize a character, a situation, or—in the older meaning of *sententia*—a general truth.

Lucan's mannerisms and willful faults can blind his audience to his merits. It is true that he is rhetorical and sensational, yet when all his inaccuracies, distortions, and digressions have been held against him, his great passages prove that in spite of artificiality he can be fiery and irresistible.

BIBLIOGRAPHY

Bartsch, Shadi. *Ideology in Cold Blood: A Reading of Lucan's "Civil War."* Cambridge, Mass.: Harvard University Press, 1997. Bartsch approaches Lucan's *Pharsalia* as a paradoxical work, a combination of poetry and history in which the historical "facts" are less important than the underlying "meanings" that Lucan imposes on them.

Braund, S. H. Introduction to *Civil War*, by Lucan. 1992. Reprint. New York: Oxford University Press, 2008. Braud's solid, meticulous translation of *Bellum civile* is put into literary and historical context through his introduction, which reviews both the subject matter and style of the work and its altering reputation over the centuries.

D'Alessandro Behr, Francesca. *Feeling History: Lucan, Stoicism, and the Poetics of Passion.* Columbus: Ohio State University Press, 2007. This study examines Lucan's poem, especially his use of apostrophes (figures of speech in which an absent or dead person is addressed as if present or alive).

Henderson, John. *Fighting for Rome: Poets and Caesars, History and Civil War.* New York: Cambridge University Press, 1998. Henderson looks at Lucan's *Pharsalia* as an attempt to rewrite history in terms of explaining its meaning if not changing its course. An interesting approach to what Lucan was attempting to do with his poetry and how successful he was in the task.

Johnson, W. R. *Momentary Monsters: Lucan and His Heroes.* Ithaca, N.Y.: Cornell University Press, 1987. Studies the flaws in Lucan's "heroes"—Caesar, Cato, and Pompey—which cause them to become "momentary monsters" at crucial periods during the action of the poem. The question, which Lucan never resolves, is whether these flaws are prompted by events or are themselves the cause of those events.

Joyce, Jane Wilson. Introduction to *Pharsalia*, by Lucan. Ithaca, N.Y.: Cornell University Press, 1993. Wilson prefaces her lively and intelligent translation of Lucan with an introduction that places the poem in historical and literary context. While accepting much of the traditional scholarship that addresses the "poetry vs. history" puzzle the poem raises, she goes further to point out the underlying qualities that link the poem to other epics of the ancient world.

Masters, Jamie. *Poetry and Civil War in Lucan's "Bellum Civile."* New York: Cambridge University Press, 1992. Lucan's *Bellum civile* not only is about civil war, Masters explains, but also manages to mimic the conflict in its structure, style, and characters. The tensions of the poem thus help re-create the struggle of the civil war itself, making form and contents merge.

Matthews, Monica. *Caesar and the Storm: A Commentary on Lucan "De bello civili," Book 5, Lines 476-721.* New York: Peter Lang, 2008. This work closely examines a section of the fifth book of *Pharsalia*.

Sklenář, R. *The Taste for Nothingness: A Study of Virtus and Related Themes in Lucan's "Bellum Civile."* Ann Arbor: University of Michigan Press, 2003. This work looks at the concept of *virtus*, Latin for heroism on the battlefield and rectitude in the conduct of life, and how Lucan did or did not use it in his writing.

Shelley P. Haley

LUCRETIUS

Born: Probably Rome (now in Italy); c. 98 B.C.E.
Died: Rome (now in Italy); October 15, 55 B.C.E.

PRINCIPAL POETRY

De rerum natura, c. 60 B.C.E. (*On the Nature of Things*, 1682)

OTHER LITERARY FORMS

Lucretius (lew-KREE-shuhs) is remembered only for *On the Nature of Things*.

ACHIEVEMENTS

Lucretius wrote a single poem, not intended for public performance. The poem, *On the Nature of Things*, consists of the exposition of a philosophical system in exalted and ornate language and of an exhortation to follow that system and attain happiness.

BIOGRAPHY

Little is known about the life of Titus Lucretius Carus. Apart from the date of his birth, his literary activity, a curious statement concerning the publication of his poem, a possibly spurious anecdote of his intermittent insanity and possible suicide, and the date of his death, little else has survived. Modern scholars have argued against Lucretius's insanity by appealing to the intellectual stability and range, the subtlety, complexity, and orderliness of *On the Nature of Things*. The poem, while it does not solve the problem of Lucretius's insanity, does give some valuable insights into the history and personality of its author. *On the Nature of Things* shows that Lucretius was a scholar, and his knowledge of works such as the *Odyssey* (c. 725 B.C.E.; English translation, 1614) glows throughout his poem. He uses the story of Iphigenia to make the central point of his poem, which is the elimination of dangerous superstition. Lucretius was familiar with ancient science, Thucydides, Epicurus, and Empedocles, as well as early Roman authors. There are echoes of Quintus Ennius, the one Roman poet whom Lucretius praises by name, as a kindred rationalist in religion.

Lucretius's poem reveals his extensive knowledge, which in turn indicates his aristocratic, moneyed, and cultured background. Like many other Roman youths in the same financial circumstances, he probably journeyed to Athens and so was introduced to science. Although the poem holds clues concerning Lucretius's library, as well as his literary habits, education, and social status, these assumptions can never be taken at face value.

In keeping with the allegation of insanity, Lucretius is said to have died by his own hand. According to another legend, followed by Alfred, Lord Tennyson, in his *Lucretius* (1868), Lucretius's wife killed him with a love potion. This notion has nothing to support it, and there is no evidence that Lucretius even had a wife.

ANALYSIS

Any discussion of the *On the Nature of Things* inevitably involves an explanation of the philosophical system that is its topic. The system is Epicurean, and Lucretius is, in fact, the chief authority of that system. Epicurus followed the atomistic theory, proposed by Leucippus. The philosopher Democritus worked out

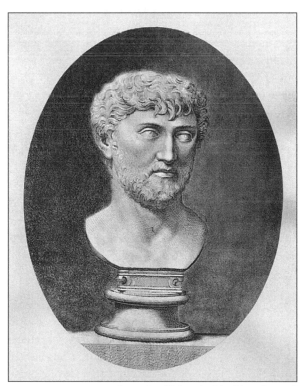

Lucretius (Hulton Archive/Getty Images)

the theory, and through Epicurus, it reached Lucretius. Like Epicurus, Lucretius cared for physical speculations only insofar as they might help people live happy lives. Democritus made it his main goal to seek causes; he would prefer, he said, to discover a true cause than to possess the kingdom of Persia. Epicurus and Lucretius were satisfied if they were convinced that something was the result of a number of possible causes, so long as these would not interfere with the happy life.

Epicurus held that both this and innumerable other universes, which he supposed to exist, are the result of chance conglomerations of atoms. These atoms are of all shapes but are very minute and fall eternally through space. As they fall, they swerve in an erratic way, making their motions unpredictable. Nothing is immaterial, although some things such as the soul are the result of the combinations of comparatively few and very fine, mobile atoms. As all things are, therefore, accidental compounds, all things are capable of dissolution. The two exceptions to this are the atoms themselves, which are too small to be broken into anything smaller, and the void, which, being nothing, cannot be injured. Man, therefore, has nothing to fear from death, which is mere dissolution followed by complete absence of consciousness. Humans' one good is pleasure, yet this is not to be found in overindulgence of physical desires, which results in a surplus of pain, not of pleasure. The right course is to satisfy the physical needs in the simplest ways (hunger for example, by a reasonable amount of plain food) and to concentrate on gratifying and pleasing the mind. There is no need to disturb the mind with ambition, desire, or fear of death. The good Epicurean will live a quiet life and withhold himself from public employment and from all that would mar his tranquillity. He should devote much time to philosophic reflection and study. Such is the Epicurean system, which Lucretius set forth with much eloquence.

ON THE NATURE OF THINGS

On the Nature of Things is divided into six books. After a hauntingly beautiful address to Venus, Lucretius gives as his aim the release of humans from fear by means of a philosophy that delivers humankind from the impieties of superstition. After laying down the fundamental principle that nothing can come from

nothing or pass into nothing, book 1 then proceeds to state the atomic theory of matter as understood by the Epicureans.

After an introduction in praise of philosophy, book 2 continues the subject and states the doctrine of "swerve." Book 3, which begins with praise of Epicurus, explains the nature of the soul. There are two parts of humans: the *animus* or *mens*, which is situated in the chest, and with which humans think and feel, and the *anima* or soul, which is dispersed throughout the body. Both the *animus* and the *anima* are composed of several sorts of minute atoms and both are mortal, passing out of the body and dispersing at death. Death, therefore, is not to be dreaded. The legendary tortures of the other world are nothing more than allegories of the woes that beset the foolish in this life.

The fact that book 4 has no introduction is one of many indications that the work never received final revision. It explains the Epicurean theory of perception, and from this, it passes to a discussion of sexual passion, explained as the effect of external stimuli acting on a system already suffering from an internal disturbance. Recognition of the purely physical nature of sexual passion and of the nonsupernatural causes of such conditions as barrenness will guard against the miseries of extravagant lovers and of the superstitious. Book 5, again having for its prologue an eloquent praise of Epicurus, is one of the most interesting of the poem. It gives the Epicurean theory of the history of the universe and of humanity. The universe is neither perfect, everlasting, nor divinely governed, and it will have an end as surely as it had a beginning. All its phenomena, such as sunrise and sunset, have perfectly natural explanations. Book 6, clearly the least finished of all, progresses, after another tribute to Epicurus, to a somewhat miscellaneous series of discussions—first of celestial and meteoric phenomena, then of the curiosities on the surface of the earth (Mount Etna, the flooding of the Nile, and so on). Finally, the book moves on to the causes of disease, which are said to be largely the result of unwholesome or even unfamiliar air that is driven from one part of the surface of the earth to another. The poem concludes with Lucretius's rendering in verse of Thucydides' account of the plague at Athens.

STYLE AND LANGUAGE

Stylistically, Lucretius, the most Roman in character (honest, fearless, austere, and orderly) of the Roman poets except perhaps for Ennius, is as an artist the most Greek. He has many traits associated with Hellenism. His science is Hellenistic and his didactic poems, full of learned lore, were much the fashion from Alexandrian times forward.

The excellence of *On the Nature of Things* is principally of two sorts: first, in the command of the language, and second, in the eloquence of the passages of moral reflection and the descriptions of nature. Lucretius lived at a time when the Latin speech with which he was most familiar was the idiom of the Ciceronian Age. It was a clean and straight medium, more refined than the earlier language of Cato the Censor, but still natural and direct, retaining many expressions drawn from the law, the market, and the political arena.

It was during the Ciceronian Age that the literary force known as Alexandrianism made itself strongly felt in Roman poetry. Lucretius, however, was not attracted to Alexandrianism. At any rate, he did not imitate its wearying niceties of phrase and its emphasis on form. His deep although latent patriotism may have made him averse to a style so clearly foreign. Perhaps his own energetic nature craved a more energetic mode of expression. Because he was a devoted pupil of Epicurus, Lucretius may have believed that an intense preoccupation with the minutiae of style was unworthy of a poet who sought to free people from the haunting terror of death. Whatever the reason, Lucretius turned, rather, to the past, and there found a congenial model. He followed in the footsteps of Ennius; consequently, archaism is the most notable mark of Lucretius's style and diction.

By virtue of its dignity and energy, the older Latin speech seemed to be an appropriate medium through which Lucretius could proclaim Epicurus. Lucretius did not, however, imitate without discretion and taste, nor did he attempt to recapture the style and diction of a century before. For the most part, Lucretius avoided the extreme characteristics of Ennius's language: its uncouthness and grotesqueness. Lucretius's position in the history of Latin poetic style and diction is intermediate and transitional. Adopting the best that the past

offered, he impressed upon Latin style his own energy and directness and passed it on to his younger colleague Vergil, who developed its qualities of gravity and flexibility still further.

Lucretius borrows many words and phrases directly from Ennius, but his archaism is not confined to such borrowings. In his fondness for the past, and in his desire to integrate his own poem with the traditions of older Roman literature, Lucretius often employs old words, old spellings of familiar words, and old idioms. The first of these categories strikes the attention of even the most casual reader (in Latin, of course, and not in translation). The reader is also at first surprised by a variety of old verbal forms.

Despite his conscious archaism, Lucretius was in no way a thoroughgoing and consistent antiquarian. He made no attempt to resurrect in its entirety the speech of Ennius and other early Latin poets and to write solely in their dying idiom. Had he done so, he probably would have ceased to be a poet and would have become simply a technician of words, devoid of energy and authenticity.

Another striking element of Lucretius's style is the fluidity and variety of his language. Like any other great poet, Lucretius used the literary sources at his disposal, but from them he developed a style that was uniquely his own; in so doing, he unified the several elements from which his style was drawn. One goal that Lucretius strove for was clarity. He hated obscure and pretentious language because it was objectionable in itself, but still more because of its exploitation by philosophers. Clarity of language may have been Lucretius's first aim, but it was, perhaps, also his greatest problem.

Epicurus had behind him a long tradition of philosophical writing in Greek. Lucretius was a pioneer in Latin in this field. His public was relatively unfamiliar with philosophical concepts and presumably with Greek philosophical terms. Lucretius found Latin equivalents for these terms but took care to insert them in contexts that help clarify their meaning. Paradoxically, Lucretius had to be clearer than his master had been, and yet, as a poet who wished to write true poetry according to well-understood traditions, he was denied the full freedom of prosaic explanation and endured the tyrannies imposed by the hexameter. He did the best he could by employing different forms of words, adopting contracted forms, and borrowing or creating linguistic oddities. These practices account for the fluid nature of *On the Nature of Things*.

One of the conditions imposed by the need for clarity was a greater acceptance of repetition than was considered elegant by most contemporary poets, together with a comparative neglect of the conventional virtue of variety. Lucretius was disinclined to seek variations, although he did not exclude them, because he was not willing to sacrifice precision and clarity. What repetition Lucretius does use is sometimes rhetorical; he will repeat unusual or idiosyncratic words or phrases, thus attracting added attention to them. The repetition is deliberate and is used more as an artistic than as a didactic tool. Its object is to enliven expression, emphasize a point, or express the poet's feelings, which may be, in Lucretius's case, feelings of didactic earnestness.

Lucretius wrote his didactic poem in the epic medium, following the example of Empedocles, but he adapted the form to his own purposes. The ornamental epic simile (characteristic of Homer, Vergil, and John Milton) held little attraction for Lucretius. His similes, picturesque though they may sometimes be, are predominantly functional. The most famous Lucretian simile of all, about physicians administering wormwood to children (book 1, lines 936ff.), looks more like a conventional simile than most of his. It is, in fact, a severely practical personal statement of his own position as a philosopher-poet, and its language is strictly linked with the reality it is designed to illustrate. When Lucretius's similes are longer than usual, there is no extension of the simile as a picture in its own right, but as an additional illustration or further analogy. In fact, the longer similes often contain a series of analogies designed for the fullest possible clarification.

The functional character of the similes is closely connected with the Epicurean insistence on the validity of sense evidence. The normal function of these similes is to explain or illustrate, by an appeal to familiar experience, concepts or theories about invisible things (such as the atoms) or things remote in space (such as the movement of heavenly bodies) or in time (such as the infancy of the earth and the life of primitive man). The comparison is most commonly with man (his body or his actions), with living creatures familiar to man (such as dogs and cattle), or with the events of his life (such as a shipwreck) and things visible in his daily experience (such as smoke, flowing water, or sunrise). Since the similes are not conventional embellishments, they are not usually heralded by conventional introductory phrases, such as *ac veluti* (and just as), which distinguish a simile from its context and direct special attention to it. They slip in simply and naturally, remaining closely integrated with the context, but are dismissed as soon as their task is done. They prove to be illustrations, comparisons, or analogies rather than similes in the conventional sense; however, they are, in fact, another example of Lucretius's individualistic and serious-minded use of an element from the epic medium that he had adopted.

IMAGERY

Lucretius excels in another important feature of the poetic tradition: imagery. It has been said of Lucretius that he had that acute sensory awareness essential to all great poets. He was physically aware of textures, colors, and patterns of every kind. Imagery is an integral part of Lucretius's method, not at all in the conventional and superficial way in which it was to appear in the imperial poets.

Probably no poet of the Latin language, not even Vergil, exhibits so vast a range of imagery, so universal a vision of the world and its poetic possibilities as does Lucretius. The feel of a pebble in a shoe; the touch of the feet of an insect or of a strand of cobweb brushing across the face; the acrid smell of a just-extinguished wick; the taste of bitter medicine; the various parts of the human body—eyes, nose, hands, ears, internal organs, nerve fibers, and even teeth and their agonizing ache; the dead body tumescent and full of worms; a pig's-bladder balloon exploding; the hiss of a hot iron dashed into water; sparks flying from stone struck against stone or steel; the crash of a falling tree; clothes that grow damp when laid out near a body of water and then grow dry again when hung in the sun; the rumbling of carts over the paving stones of a Roman street; the wobbling of a vase when the water within it is disturbed; sheep on a mountainside; armies clashing on the plain; the foot of a bronze statue worn smooth and shiny where passersby have touched it; the light of the sun shining through varicolored awnings stretched over a theater; the springtime gaiety of birds and animals and even of fish; the curious snakelike majesty of the elephant and his trunk; and the sloppy contentment of pigs in the mud: These are only some of the many aspects of life that Lucretius uses for poetic and argumentative purposes. Although he is not often thought of in this respect, he was, in fact, one of the most brilliant word painters of life in the ancient world. His poem offers a wide panorama of the Mediterranean in the first century B.C.E. Lucretius saw that ideas are to be found only in things and that nothing proves a point quite so neatly as an appropriate series of pictures from life.

Consistently, Lucretius's images, down to the smallest detail, are functional, and their function is to clarify and enforce the argument of the poem. The raison d'être of Lucretius's poetry is that it sweetens the seemingly bitter but life-giving dose of Epicureanism. The raison d'être of the images is the rigorous logical work they are set to do in their contexts. This is one of the things that gives such intensity to the poetry of Lucretius, and it is a quality often lost in translation.

Lucretius expounds a materialist philosophy that explains the whole of the world and of experience in terms of the movements of invisible material particles. Therefore, repeatedly, he must infer the behavior of these particles from the behavior of visible phenomena—rivers, wind and sea, fire, light, and all the rest. The philosophical subject matter of this poem is not an impediment to the poetry, but rather the stimulus for the impassioned observation and contemplation of the material world that contributes so much to the poetic intensity of the work.

GREEK MYTHS AND ALLEGORY

Another aspect of Lucretius's art is the use of Greek mythology for the purpose of allegory. Normally, Lucretius brushes aside myth as totally misleading, particularly the stock representations of Hell or the personalities of the Olympian gods. He does use the names of the gods as appropriate paraphrases, provided that nothing further is intended. Quite different is the opening of the first book, with its extended address to Venus and Mars, a fully developed allegory. There can be no doubt that Lucretius enjoys this sort of symbolism for

its own sake. That is confirmed in his elaborate version of the sacrifice of Iphigenia in book 1, which is related with great force and pathos to demonstrate the moral of the evils of superstition.

The story of the Trojan War in book 1 is purely decorative. It is related in true epic style, simply as an example of an event that could not have happened had not the universe contained space as well as matter. The story of Phaëthon in book 5 is given as an illustration of the domination of the four elements over the others. Lucretius, however, dismisses it immediately as hopelessly naïve and unscientific. The poet takes delight in relating both myths, and they serve the purpose of adding a personal interest to passages in which the human content is small.

In his imagery, sublime or lowly, Lucretius appears as a man who observes natural phenomena with a keen eye and expresses their essential significance in simple but effective language. If Lucretius is still worth reading, it is not only because of the brilliance of his descriptions or the power of his poetry, but also because he has something to say.

BIBLIOGRAPHY

Dalzell, Alexander. *The Criticism of Didactic Poetry: Essays on Lucretius, Virgil, and Ovid.* Toronto, Ont.: University of Toronto Press, 1997. Explores how Lucretius used poetic forms to express his philosophical views.

Fowler, Don, and Peta Fowler. Introduction to *Lucretius on the Nature of the Universe*. 1997. Reprint. New York: Oxford University Press, 2008. Places Lucretius's philosophical and scientific poem within the contexts of Latin literature, Epicurean philosophy, and classical science. A good overview of the work and its contents that grounds it for the modern reader in terms of a vigorous translation.

Gale, Monika. *Myth and Poetry in Lucretius.* New York: Cambridge University Press, 1994. Lucretius's distinctive use of poetic imagery is analyzed in a study that sheds light on his methods and metaphysics.

_____. *Virgil on the Nature of Things: The "Georgics," Lucretius, and the Didactic Tradition.* New York: Cambridge University Press, 2000. Good for helping the modern reader understand how a hand-book on agriculture and a scientific treatise could be written in disciplined Latin verse.

_____, ed. *Lucretius*. New York: Oxford University Press, 2007. This collection of essays discusses many topics, including the source of Lucretius's inspiration, his interpretation of the plague, his use of analogy, and his Epicureanism.

Gillespie, Stuart, and Philip Hardie, eds. *The Cambridge Companion to Lucretius*. New York: Cambridge University Press, 2007. Experts in the history of literature, philosophy, and science examine Lucretius's poem from its ancient context and its legacy.

Hardie, Philip. *Lucretian Receptions: History, the Sublime, Knowledge*. New York: Cambridge University Press, 2009. Discusses the influence of Lucretius on Vergil and Horace.

Johnson, W. R. *Lucretius and the Modern World*. London: Duckworth, 2000. In this description of Lucretius's influential poem, Johnson surveys major texts from the eighteenth and nineteenth centuries in the works of John Dryden, Voltaire, Alfred, Lord Tennyson, and others. Emphasizes Lucretius's version of materialism and his attempt to devise an ethical system appropriate to the universe.

Marković, Daniel. *The Rhetoric of Explanation in Lucretius' "De rerum natura."* Boston: Brill, 2008. The author examines rhetoric in the writings of Lucretius. Also discusses Epicureanism.

Sedley, D. N. *Lucretius and the Transformation of Greek Wisdom*. New York: Cambridge University Press, 1998. Shows how Lucretius built on and departed from Greek traditions that informed the context in which he worked.

Shelley P. Haley

M

ANTONIO MACHADO

Born: Seville, Spain; July 26, 1875
Died: Collioure, France; February 22, 1939

PRINCIPAL POETRY

Soledades, 1902 (dated 1903)
Soledades, galerías, y otros poemas, 1907
    (*Solitudes, Galleries, and Other Poems*, 1987)
Campos de Castilla, 1912 (*The Castilian Camp*,
    1982)
Poesías completas, 1917
Nuevas canciones, 1924
De un cancionero apócrifo, 1926
Obras, 1940
Eighty Poems of Antonio Machado, 1959
Antonio Machado, 1973
Selected Poems of Antonio Machado, 1978
Selected Poems, 1982
Times Alone: Selected Poems of Antonio Machado,
    1983
*Roads Dreamed Clear Afternoons: An Anthology of
    the Poetry of Antonio Machado*, 1994
*Lands of Castile / Campos de Castilla, and Other
    Poems*, 2002 (bilingual)
*Border of a Dream: Selected Poems of Antonio
    Machado*, 2004

OTHER LITERARY FORMS

Although the majority of the published work of Antonio Machado (mah-CHAH-doh) is poetry, he collaborated with his brother, Manuel, on a number of plays for the Madrid stage. These began in 1926 with adaptations of Spanish dramas of the Golden Age and culminated in 1929 with the very successful *La Lola se va a los puertos* (the *Lola* goes off to sea). The last of their plays to be staged in Madrid was *El hombre que murió en la guerra* (the man who died in the war), in 1941. Several series of prose commentaries on a variety of sub-jects, principally literary and philosophical, originally appeared in periodicals and were eventually collected and published in 1936 in the somewhat amorphous yet interesting *Juan de Mairena* (English translation, 1963).

ACHIEVEMENTS

Antonio Machado was one of the two great lyric poets of Spain's Generation of '98, the other being Juan Ramón Jiménez. In 1927, Machado was elected to the Royal Spanish Academy.

BIOGRAPHY

Antonio Cipriano José María y Francisco de Santa Ana Machado was born into an interesting family of relatively successful professionals. His paternal grandfather had been to the New World, studied medicine in Paris, and practiced for a time in Seville, where he published a philosophical and scientific journal and became governor of the province. Machado's father studied but never practiced law, devoting himself to the study of Spanish folklore, especially flamenco song and poetry, and publishing four important collections. His mother was a vivacious woman who dedicated herself to her family and four sons, most particularly to Antonio, who was attached to her throughout life and whose death preceded hers by only a few days. Machado's memory of the home where he was born and for eight years led a peaceful existence in charming surroundings never left him.

When Machado's grandfather received a professorship in Madrid, the family accompanied him there. Life in the capital was turbulent and somewhat more hazardous than in Seville. Machado and two of his brothers were enrolled in the Free Institute, a private school founded by Francisco Giner de los Ríos, a friend of the Machado family, and dominated by the principles of *Krausismo*, named after an obscure German philosopher Karl Christian Friedrich Krause (1781-1832), whose system of philosophy, which attempted to combine pantheism and theism, was promoted in Spain by Julián Sanz del Río in an effort to establish a new, liberal educational system. Although Machado completed his secondary education in Catholic institutions, he was to remain faithful to the tenets of *Krausismo* and anticlerical to the end. When Machado concluded this first phase of his education, his family was undergoing a reversal of fortune, and in 1892 and 1895, respectively, his father and grandfather died.

Although Machado became "the man of the family," he did not assume any responsibilities. Rather, he led a somewhat Bohemian life, as before, and began a literary career by writing satirical sketches for *La caricatura* under the pseudonym of "Cabellera" ("Long Hair")—his brother Manuel wrote as "Polilla" ("Moth")—meanwhile thinking of entering the theater. In 1899, Antonio and Manuel at last obtained paid positions as translators and editors for Garnier Brothers in Paris. What they accomplished at Garnier Brothers is not clear, but they did frequent the literary circles of Paris and became acquainted with many of the celebrities of the day, such as Jean Moréas and Rubén Darío. At the same time that the Machados were exploring new interests, they were reading, discussing, and beginning to write poetry.

Little is known of Antonio's first efforts in France and Spain, but the small volume *Soledades* appeared in 1902 (although it was dated 1903) and soon began to enjoy some success in Madrid. Dissatisfied with the *Modernista* aestheticism of these early poems, however, Machado immediately started work on an expanded *Soledades*, in which the spiritual and the ethical would dominate and from which a number of the earlier poems would be excluded. During this period of rapid growth and maturation, the great influence on the poet was that of Miguel de Unamuno y Jugo, who, in an open letter of 1904 in *Helios*, had urged Machado to abandon the principle of art for art's sake. In an article of 1905 on Unamuno's *La vida de Don Quijote y Sancho* (1905; *Life of Don Quijote and Sancho*, 1927), Machado admires his mentor's re-creation of Miguel de Cervantes' hero, in which spirit and feeling transform ideas into poetry.

As a result of his contact with Unamuno, Machado abandoned his semi-Bohemian life and, during 1906 and 1907, prepared for a serious profession. Considering himself too old to attend a university, he studied French and Spanish language and literature at home and passed the arduous examinations to become a professor. He was appointed to a post at the Institute in Soria, in the heart of Old Castile, where he spent five years. Soria was not what it had been in ancient and medieval times, and the Institute ran pedagogically and politically in ways far removed from the principles of *Krausismo*. Patient and unassuming, Machado adjusted to the school's dull atmosphere, accepting old-fashioned patterns of unenthusiastic teaching and rote learning and ignoring local politics. His salvation lay in a few friendships with men of strong cultural interests and in the setting, steeped in the history and traditions of Spain.

Although an attractive man, Machado was timid and unaggressive with women, as was characteristic of the generally unromantic Generation of '98, who placed the blame on old Spanish customs regarding courtship. In late 1907, however, when he was past thirty, Machado met Leonor Izquierdo, the daughter of the family in whose boardinghouse he lived. The girl was only thirteen at the time, and Machado had to wait until she was fourteen to court her; they were married in 1909. A simple, provincial girl of limited education, augmented only by short stays in Madrid and Paris, Leonor nevertheless pleased her husband, and his love for her endured well beyond the grave. While they were in Paris in 1911, where Machado had been awarded a fellowship, she fell seriously ill with tuberculosis. She died in 1912, some time after their return to Soria.

After his wife's death, Machado secured a transfer to Baeza in Jaén. His native Andalusia did not comfort him, however, and he sank into a depression that brought him close to suicide. His mother joined him for a time, which must have helped, and the success of *The Castilian Camp* made Machado aware that he possessed a useful talent that he did not have the right to destroy. His faith in life was restored above all by a serious study of philosophy, including not only the work of modern philosophers, especially Henri Bergson, but also that of the ancients and the languages to read them in the original. Unable to emulate Unamuno in his mastery of Greek, Machado nevertheless managed during several summers in Madrid to pass the necessary examinations to acquire his doctorate in 1918, at the age of forty-three.

In Baeza, Machado, older, heavier, and careless of his appearance, resumed his old way of life. He was a seemingly aimless, somewhat lame, but indefatigable walker, usually alone. He sought the company of a few friends in a *tertulia*, at the Institute, or in the local pharmacy. Sometimes there would be an organized excursion to visit a point of interest; other times he would participate in the literary homages that are a part of Spanish culture, as when he read his "Desde mi rincón" (from my corner) in Aranjuez to honor José Martínez Ruiz (Azorín) and Castile. In 1915, Federico García Lorca, also an Andalusian, came to meet Machado at a cultural gathering in Baeza. Machado continued his work as a critic of Spanish society, concentrating on that of Baeza as most typical of the nation, except for Madrid. In his correspondence with Unamuno, he decried the state of religion in Baeza, dominated as it was by women. Both Machado and Unamuno were evolving from the Cain-Abel theme applied to Spain to a reaffirmation of Jesus's principle of Christian charity, yet Machado was not yet prepared to be an open activist.

Resigned but not satisfied in Baeza, and his inspiration grown thin, Machado obtained a post in Segovia in 1919. Segovia possessed everything that Soria had offered the poet and more, and Madrid was near. He would toil during the week in Segovia, pursuing other interests, especially in the theater, on his weekends in Madrid. Machado's scant poetic production during this time is varied in nature and high in quality. Outwardly he revealed little of his thoughts and feelings, but his mind was teeming with ideas and projects. One project that Machado eagerly worked to realize was the Segovian activists' Popular University. To it he contributed, with all its political overtones, his philosophy of an active Christian brotherhood outside the hierarchy of the Church. Further, he delivered a lecture on Russian literature in which he declared the Revolution a failure because of a lack of philosophical tradition, but praised Russian literature for its universality, founded on Christian brotherhood.

In the mid-1920's, Machado began to feel discontented with his image as a somewhat eccentric widower and schoolteacher and as an isolated poet exploiting a few memories. Furthermore, the poets of the Generation of '98 were being displaced by those of the Generation of '27. It was time to do something new. During this period, Machado began to collaborate with his brother on a series of plays. His desire for rejuvenation

also led him henceforth to use pseudonyms and to seek and find a new love. As Machado's passion was at first for an imaginary lady, it was long thought that his "Guiomar" did not exist, but he met Pilar Valderrama in 1926 and soon was in the grip of a schoolboy's infatuation for the mediocre poetess, who was also a married woman and a mother of three. It was an infatuation that, despite her coolness, he maintained for many years, deriving from it a metaphysical system for all consolation.

Except for the theater, Machado's significant production after 1925 consisted of two open-ended, interrelated works. In 1926, he published a brief, intensely concentrated book in prose and verse, *De un cancionero apócrifo* (apocryphal songbook), in which his first important persona, Abel Martín, expresses Machado's persistent belief that the poet is constantly torn between philosophy and poetry. All great poets must be backed by an implied metaphysics, so that, like Plato and perhaps Machado, poet and philosopher are one. The prose parts explain Machado's ideas, each of which is illustrated by a poem. The idea of love is expressed, for example, in "Canciones a Guiomar" ("Songs to Guiomar"). *Juan de Mairena*, published as a series in the *Diario de Madrid* and as a book in 1936, was entirely in prose, with increased emphasis by Mairena-Machado on political themes, for the Spanish Civil War was then in progress.

In 1927, Machado was elected to the Royal Spanish Academy, normally the greatest of honors for a man of letters in Spain, but his increasingly revolutionary political ideas made him less sympathetic toward the conservative academy, and he never completed his acceptance speech. In 1931, under the Republic created after the abdication of Alfonso XIII, Machado was appointed professor of Spanish literature at the Instituto Calderón de la Barca in Madrid, but his hope for the future of Spain could not keep him from putting all his creative energy into *Juan de Mairena*, and he continued to be a dry, dull professor.

In the tradition of civil wars, the Spanish Civil War set the Machado brothers against each other, Manuel producing propaganda for the Nationalists in Burgos, Antonio performing the same service for the Republicans, first in Madrid, then in Valencia, and finally in

Barcelona. In January, 1939, as that city was about to fall to the Nationalists, Antonio, his mother, and others of the family fled to France. Both mother and son were gravely ill, and Antonio died in Collioure of pneumonia on February 22; his mother died three days later. After the war, Machado's work continued to be honored, and today the poet is widely recognized as one of the greatest of the Hispanic world.

Analysis

The two great lyric poets of the Generation of '98, Jiménez and Antonio Machado, were both Andalusians. The latter is equally representative of Castile, however, in his preference for intellectual, philosophical, and classical solutions to existential problems. At first influenced by the *Modernismo* of Darío, who characterized him as profound, Machado soon abandoned that style as superficial in its constant striving for effect. For him, true lyricism consisted of deep spirituality, of an animated exchange between the soul and the world.

Machado's output was not large, and his themes were few in number. His *Soledades* (solitudes) stressed recollections of his youth and the dreams of a young man in an Andalusian setting. In *The Castilian Camp*, the landscape with which Machado communes is that of the province that historically and culturally came to epitomize Spain, and that after many years of residence, he adopted as a second native region. In this collection as in *Nuevas canciones* (new songs), there are also memories of Leonor Izquierdo, the young woman whom Machado met, married, and soon lost to death in Soria; wishes for the renaissance of Spain, shared with the other intellectuals of the Generation of '98; and meditations on the passage of time, life, death, and the search for God. Discarding early in his career the influences of Impressionism, French Symbolism, and Hispano-American *Modernismo*, Machado forged a personal yet traditional style. His restrained, highly concentrated verse provided a valuable alternative to the aestheticism of his great contemporary, Jiménez.

Soledades

The editions of Machado's *Soledades* dating from 1917 remained substantially unchanged and represent the mature poet. Despite successive modifications and excisions, the collection continues to reflect important influences of earlier poets. Gustavo Adolfo Bécquer, a Sevillian post-Romantic who wrote intimate lyrics in opposition to the realistic or bombastic poetry of his day, persisted in Machado's literary affections. Bécquer's idea of poetry as high perfection, impossible to attain, is symbolized by a disdainful virgin or a fleeing doe (poem 42 in *Soledades*), or, as life became sadder and more disappointing, illusion turned to chimera (poems 36 and 43). Like Bécquer, Machado became the poet of reverie par excellence, creating brief, intimate lyrics of traditional octosyllabic lines and subtle assonance.

Inevitably, he was somewhat influenced also by Darío's work, especially the brilliant and erotic *Prosas profanas* (1896; *Prosas Profanas, and Other Poems*, 1922). Although Machado, like the others of his grave generation, eschewed the sensual, he fell under the spell of Darío's "Era un aire suave" ("The Air Was Soft") when he composed "Fantasía de una noche de abril" (fantasy of an April night) in elegant *arte mayor*, musical twelve-syllable lines of balanced hemistichs. Although Machado relegated the poem to a minor section of *Soledades*, he did not reject it. In the poem, the poet ardently seeks love one night in Moorish Seville, but lacking confidence and considering himself an "anachronism," his hopes disintegrate with the elaborate form of the poem.

Another strong though brief influence on Machado's work was that of Paul Verlaine, particularly the Symbolist's use of nature, as in the garden with a fountain, to express the poet's feelings at a given moment, as well as the Edgar Allan Poe-like theme of fatality discovered through the French poet. Although by 1907 he had rejected most of his poems in the manner of Verlaine, Machado became a poet who, like Marcel Proust in his poetic novels, developed memory as a powerful instrument to reveal his inner self.

The poetic renovation accomplished by Machado's *Soledades*, a traditional title well suited to his purpose, progressively and rigorously excluded frank confession and the anecdotal as well as the stylistic excesses of Luis de Góngora y Argote. Here, Machado is preoccupied with time, and as he reworks a few symbols, such as the gallery, the road, the fountain, and the river, he seeks constantly to re-create the past and meditates on a possibly better future. Many lines in these simple poems strike deep and lasting chords in the reader responsive to the same existential problems.

THE CASTILIAN CAMP AND NUEVAS CANCIONES

Although somewhat late in joining Unamuno, Azorín, and Pío Baroja in their celebration of Castile, with *The Castilian Camp*, Machado earned membership in the Generation of '98, the only poet to do so, for Jiménez chose not to write on the Spanish theme. Influenced above all by Unamuno and Azorín, considerable portions of *Nuevas canciones* exploited the theme further. Machado dealt with the problems and destiny of Castile and Spain, centered on Soria as typical of the region and nation. Along the same lines, another group of poems praised those who advanced the culture of Spain. A third group gave the history of Machado's love for his wife, the shock of her death, and the continuing sense of loss, all in the same setting of Soria.

In the long run, however, the outer view was not the one with which Machado felt most comfortable. Toward the end of *The Castilian Camp*, in a poem unique in tone, "Poema de un día" or "Meditaciones rurales" ("Poem for a Day" or "Rural Meditations"), he offhandedly details his extreme loneliness and expresses his intention to withdraw once more into philosophy. The form is a rather complex variation of Jorge Manrique's medieval elegy; in his solitude, the poet is intensely conscious of his surroundings—the changing winter weather outside, the constant ticking of the clock inside. The latter causes him to think about the meaning of time, and the former leads him mentally to follow the raindrops to the fountain, then to the river, and finally to the sea, which symbolically evokes the anguish of the agnostic. Machado's only consolation lies in his books, particularly those of Unamuno, whose latest work, probably *Del sentimento trágico de la vida en los hombres y en los pueblos* (1913; *The Tragic Sense of Life*, 1921), he possesses. As for his old master, Bergson, Machado ironically accepts the author's conclusion in *Essai sur les données immédiates de la conscience* (1888; *Time and Free Will*, 1910) that time and being according to his definitions made free will inescapable. After a walk amid the banalities of Baeza and its provincials to clear his head, the poet returns to

his study, again ready to face solitude and his own efforts to cope with the human condition.

Despite the inclusion of many different kinds of poems, *The Castilian Camp* presents a relatively unified picture of Machado in his effort to reach out to the reality of Spain—its landscape, its problems, its important cultural figures—and to create a meaningful personal life. Moreover, there is a strong continuity from *Soledades* to *The Castilian Camp*, for many of the symbols of the former became realities in Soria, and the poet's obsession with time found a firm basis in the strong sense of history in the typical Castilian town. When his wife's death forced him back into himself, Soria became more vivid as he sought to re-create time and life in memory. It is interesting to note in passing that what the Andalusian Machado did for Castile, his contemporary, Robert Frost, did for his adopted New England.

PROVERBIOS Y CANCIONES

The third and most complex body of poems by Machado is that in which he strove hardest to reconcile his metaphysical and aesthetic concerns. First in *The Castilian Camp*, then in *Nuevas canciones*, one finds long series of "Proverbios y canciones" (proverbs and songs), poems of one stanza presenting a bit of philosophy in highly concentrated form. They culminated in the major poems with prose commentaries, somewhat in the tradition of Saint John of the Cross, of the two parts of the *De un cancionero apócrifo* in *Obras completas de Manuel y Antonio Machado* (1946). This collection clearly reflects the poet's need to renew his inspiration and his desire to find love again.

DE UN CANCIONERO APÓCRIFO

As his protagonists represent Machado in his dramas, so do a series of related personas in the *De un cancionero apócrifo*. Lacking systematic training in philosophy, the poet hesitated to express himself directly. Moreover, the use of spokesmen permitted him a degree of objectivity in dealing philosophically with the great themes of love, God, and death, which were either disturbing personally or shocking to a Catholic readership. Noteworthy, too, is the mask of ironic humor that the poet wears throughout to conceal his anguish.

It is clear that Machado thought of poetry as the expression of intimate, personal experience. When, in the second part of the prose discussions in the *De un cancionero apócrifo*, he attacks Spanish Baroque poetry of the seventeenth century as too conceptual and artificial and insufficiently intuitive, he is attacking also the poetry of his day and of all the vanguard to the present. More important, Machado, through another of his spokesmen, Jorge Meneses, satirizes the mechanistic, materialistic society of the contemporary world, which has rendered individual sentiment unnecessary and ineffectual for poetry. Meneses has invented a kind of protocomputer into which are fed the terms significant in the kind of poetry desired; the machine thus produces a poem for the masses. When, with the words "man" and "woman," the computer is programmed to create a love poem, however, the result merely proves that love and the heightened existence that it is supposed to provide are illusory. As before, then, Machado acknowledges defeat for lyric poetry and for himself as a poet, a defeat brought about by excessive intellectualization. However accurate his predictions for the future of lyric poetry, Machado's poetic work nevertheless lives on, as fresh and human as when he conceived it.

OTHER MAJOR WORKS

PLAYS (with Manuel Machado): *Desdichas de la fortuna, o Julianillo Valcárcel*, pr., pb. 1926; *Juan de Mañara*, pr., pb. 1927; *Las adelfas*, pr., pb. 1928; *El hombre que murió en la guerra*, pr. 1941 (wr. 1928); *La Lola se va a los puertos*, pr., pb. 1929; *La prima Fernanda*, pr., pb. 1931; *La duquesa de Benamejí*, pr., pb. 1932.

NONFICTION: *Juan de Mairena*, 1936 (English translation, 1963).

MISCELLANEOUS: *Obras completas de Manuel y Antonio Machado*, 1946 (includes *De un cancionero apócrifo*).

BIBLIOGRAPHY

Cobb, Carl W. *Antonio Machado*. New York: Twayne, 1971. An introductory biography and critical study of Machado by an expert in Spanish poets and the translation of Spanish poetry into English. Includes a bibliography of Machado's work.

Hutman, Norma Louise. *Machado: A Dialogue with Time—Nature as an Expression of Temporality in the Poetry of Antonio Machado*. Albuquerque: University of New Mexico Press, 1969. A critical analysis of selected poems by Machado. Includes a bibliography of Machado's poetry.

Johnston, Philip G. *The Power of Paradox in the Work of Spanish Poet Antonio Machado (1875-1939)*. Lewiston, N.Y.: Edwin Mellen Press, 2002. In this study of paradox in Machado's writing, chapters 2 and 4 examine the poetry.

Krogh, Kevin. *The Landscape Poetry of Antonio Machado: A Dialogical Study of "Campos de Castilla."* Lewiston, N.Y.: Edwin Mellen Press, 2001. Krogh analyzes Machado's description of the countryside of Castile. Includes bibliographical references and indexes.

Ribbans, Geoffrey. *Antonio Machado, 1875-1939: Poetry and Integrity*. London: Hispanic and Luso Brazilian Council, 1975. A transcription of a lecture dealing with Machado's life and poetry. Ribbans has written extensively on various figures in Spanish literature and has edited collections of Machado's poetry.

Round, Nicholas Grenville. *Poetry and Otherness in Hardy and Machado*. London: Queen Mary and Westfield College, 1993. A critical study comparing the poetic works of Thomas Hardy and Machado. Includes bibliographical references.

Walters, D. Gareth. *Estelas en el mar: Essays on the Poetry of Antonio Machado*. London: Grant and Cutler, 1992. This collection of essays from the Glasgow Colloquium focuses on technical aspects of specific poems. Studies such as "Questioning the Rules: Concepts of Deviance and Conformism in *Campos de Castilla*," by Robin Warner, reevaluate the works' meanings in their historical contexts. Other studies analyzing neomysticism, the nostalgic vision of Canciones a Guiomar, and the poetry of cultural memory offer fresh approaches to contemporary classics.

Whiston, James. *Antonio Machado's Writings and the Spanish Civil War*. Liverpool, England: Liverpool University Press, 1996. A study of the influence on Machado's writing of Spanish Civil War propaganda and the resulting schism between the poet and his brother.

Richard A. Mazzara

FRANÇOIS DE MALHERBE

Born: Caen, France; 1555
Died: Paris, France; October 16, 1628

PRINCIPAL POETRY

Les Larmes de Saint Pierre, 1587
À la reine, sur sa bienvenue en France, 1600
Consolation à Monsieur Du Périer sur la mort de sa fille, c. 1600
Prière pour le roi Henri le Grand, 1605
Prière pour le roi allant en Limousin, 1607
Ballet de Madame, 1615
Poésies, 1626

OTHER LITERARY FORMS

Friendship with the Stoic Guillaume Du Vair brought François Malherbe (mah-LEHRB) in contact with the writings of Livy and Seneca, some of which he began to translate as early as the turn of the seventeenth century. The first of these efforts was published in 1617, and most of the rest posthumously. These translations are of little if any interest to the modern reader. Of greater import are his numerous letters to many of the major literary figures of his time; some of these were anthologized as early as 1625, although most of them did not see print until 1645; of particular interest to students of the history of ideas are his letters to Nicolas Fabri de Peiresc, perhaps the most universally learned man of the era. His commentaries on contemporary poems and plays—marginalia published posthumously—are essential to an understanding of the poet's doctrine, but they must be taken with a grain of salt: Sallies of a very temperamental man, they are always excessive, and perhaps were intended more to draw attention to the ambitious Malherbe than to detract from the work of his colleagues (although unpublished, these commentaries were widely circulated).

ACHIEVEMENTS

"At last, [François] Malherbe came," said Nicolas Boileau-Despréaux in 1674, giving credit to him for having brought order and reason to poetry. "Everyone followed his rules [of prosody]," continued Boileau, al-

though some twenty years later, in a letter to François de Maucroix, he was to admit that "in truth, nature had not made [Malherbe] a great poet; but he made up for that . . . with work, for no one worked harder than he over his poems." This composite has misled many generations of students and critics who insisted on overstating François Malherbe's influence and teachings while belittling or disregarding his genuine achievements as a poet. Thanks to the efforts of scholars such as René Fromilhague, David Lee Rubin, and Philip A. Wadsworth, that error has been largely rectified. It should further be stated that it is precisely in that area of poetics in which Malherbe's influence was most categorically posited—prosody—that close analysis shows it to be minimal. In matters of prosody, Malherbe had little or no effect on the poets of his century, not even on "pupils" such as François Maynard and Honorat de Racan. It would be dangerous, however, to limit one's vision to prosodic matters, for to do so would be to allow the mechanics of the genre to obscure its essence. In his pronouncements, Malherbe concentrated on (indeed, limited himself to) the former; in his own poetry, particularly in his "grandes odes," he most definitely strove for that "higher, hidden order" in which the latter resides.

Unlike the posturing and opportunistic theoretician, Malherbe the poet arranged syllables and words not because such intellectual games had intrinsic value, but because he saw that clarity and harmony were essential to the aura of grandeur and majesty with which he wished to imbue his official poetry. His labors over finding the one right word or expression were the butt of many jokes, but they yielded sensible, rational images, striking in their accuracy and psychological truth. These images are never mere ornaments, as they tend to be in Mannerist poetry, but integral parts of the symbolic and metaphoric structures from which the poems derive their profound unity. Through them, commonplaces are given life and raised to new evocative powers.

One has but to read one of Malherbe's odes aloud to realize that this "arranger of syllables," as he called himself, thoroughly understood what most of his contemporaries did not—that lyric poetry, by definition and by nature, is a musical art. His balanced phrases and carefully chosen words not only give strength to his lines but also are pleasing to the ear; their all-pervasive harmony makes the auditor forget about the labors detected by the punctilious critic. It then becomes evident that all of Malherbe's prosodic strictures were born of his concern for order and harmony.

In Malherbe's poetic world, intricate (hidden) structural patterns are made to reinforce poetic abstractions representing the material, historic reality. Few poets, if any, followed Malherbe's specific prosodic rules; many saw that such strictures were motivated by the profound conviction that craftsmanship was necessary if the poet were ever to imbue his work with any semblance of metaphoric coherence and with any degree of lyricism. These loftier considerations behind the specific rules and practices were understood by poets such as Tristan L'Hermite and Jean de La Fontaine, and in that broader understanding of poetry, they, and not the likes of Maynard and Racan, are perhaps to be considered the true "students" of Malherbe.

BIOGRAPHY

François Malherbe received his early education in his native Caen. When he was sixteen, he was sent by his father, newly converted to Protestantism, to study in Germany for two years. In 1577, Malherbe became the secretary of Henri d'Angoulême, illegitimate son of Henry II, and glad to get away from his father's extreme Protestantism, which he loathed, he followed his new master to Provence, where the young prince was to assume the role of governor. A devoted political servant, Malherbe was to remain with his master in the south of France for nearly ten years. There, he married the daughter of a local *président* and, except for a preliminary piece written for a colleague's poem, gave little indication of having literary aspirations. In 1586, Malherbe and his wife were back in Caen when his master was assassinated in Aix. The following year, Malherbe was in Paris, where he presented his first major poem, *Les Larmes de Saint Pierre* (the tears of Saint Peter), to King Henry III; he was given a sizable financial reward, but not the pension or post he had sought. In 1594, he was elected alderman of Caen, but this duty did not keep him from spending more of the next ten years in his wife's native province—particularly in its

dazzling capital, Aix—than in his native Normandy. He was in Aix in 1600 when the new queen, Marie de Médicis, on her way to meet Henry IV, whom she had married by proxy, stopped in that city. A member of the welcoming party, Malherbe presented her with his first official ode, the 230-line *À la reine, sur sa bienvenue en France*.

In 1605, Malherbe went to Paris and was presented to Henry IV, who requested a poem of him. The resulting *Prière pour le Roi allant en Limousin* so pleased the king that he granted the poet a pension and a job with his master of the horse, Bellegarde. It was to be the beginning of a lifelong association with the court: Malherbe became the official poet of the Crown until his death in 1628. Astute, careful, fawning, Malherbe survived the unsettled regency of Marie de Médicis, singing her praises as he had sung those of her husband and as he was to sing those of the ambitious Cardinal de Richelieu when he early perceived his rising star.

Fundamentally—and admittedly—lazy, Malherbe was a great lover of law and order. He was sincere in his

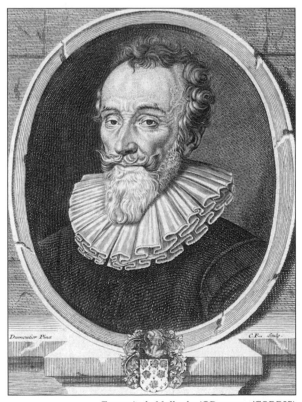

François de Malherbe (©Bettmann/CORBIS)

vehement defense of Crown and Church and lavishly praised the martial inclinations of a king if aimed at quelling anarchy. His orthodoxy, in short, political or theological, was more a question of desire for peace than one of philosophic cogitation and decision. Antoine Adam is quite right when he suggests that in London, Amsterdam, or Zurich, Malherbe would have been a good Protestant. The bitterness so prevalent in his later poems, and so diametrically opposed to the quiet Stoicism he professed and demonstrated in earlier works, is undoubtedly due to the sorrows (such as the death of his son in a duel) and travails (such as the endless pains to which he had to go to collect his various pensions) that banished peace and contentment from the last years of his life. Marie de Médicis had appreciated the sallies of his wit and the pomp of his pen; her son, Louis XIII, did not share her sensitivity. Although Malherbe never lost his position at court, he readily sensed and deeply resented his diminished presence. When he died in 1628, it was not simply because his health had been broken; his spirit too seemed to have given up.

ANALYSIS

François Malherbe's poetic production is far from extensive; it is, nevertheless, considerably varied and of uneven merit. Much of his success at court was due to the ballet libretti that he wrote; these are of interest to court historians, but their literary value is negligible at best. His epigrams today seem derivative and forced. Of primary interest are his great odes and other solemn occasional poems such as the *Prière pour le Roi allant en Limousin*. Also of interest are his religious poems and, to a lesser degree, his erotic ones.

"RÉCIT D'UN BERGER"

Nearly everything that Malherbe wrote for public consumption was a political statement. That is the case even for seemingly innocuous poems such as the "Récit d'un berger" of the *Ballet de Madame* of 1615, a lavish court festivity celebrating the marriage of Elizabeth, sister of Louis XIII, to the future Philip IV of Spain. The "ballet" was really a revue of court notables in sumptuous costumes parading through equally sumptuous settings activated by what were then astonishing machines. Malherbe's "Récit d'un berger" allowed its

speaker to praise the efforts of the young king and of the Queen Mother on behalf of peace, and to vaunt the advantages of what was a far from popular alliance of royal families. Malherbe's lines had been commissioned by the Queen Mother, and in addition to the usual flattery, they faithfully reflected her policy and desires. It is almost impossible to divorce Malherbe the poet from Malherbe the political animal. In 1617, with the rise to power of D'Albert de Luynes, Malherbe lost his privileged status at court; the need to write disappeared, and he seriously thought of "abandoning the Muses." In fact, until 1623—by which date de Luynes had died and Richelieu was quickly rising in power, welcoming Malherbe back into the official fold— Malherbe concentrated his literary efforts on his letters and translations; the poet was silent.

Under the circumstances, it is no wonder that these poems are so hyperbolic in their flattery and allusions as to defy credibility—an ingredient no one expected anyway—and to verge on sycophancy. The most indecisive military encounter could, with such a pen, be transformed into a momentous and stupendous triumph. Today, the reader of such excesses may be tempted to smile, but it must be kept in mind that for an official court poet, as for the painters of the *portraits d'apparat*, the presentation of the royal apotheosis was a very serious matter.

Asked why he did not write any elegies, Malherbe is said to have answered, "Because I write odes," referring to the form he considered to be the ultimate endeavor in lyric poetry. He used the term only for long poems dealing with great matters of state, and he called "stances" those poems dealing with less lofty subjects—or, as in the case of his famous *Prière pour le Roi allant en Limousin*, briefer treatments of lofty themes—a distinction his successors were not to maintain. It is these odes that are today considered the omphalos of Malherbe's official poetry.

For generations, the guardians of academic truths steadfastly maintained that Malherbe's odes were characterized by rigorous composition, striking articulation, and, above all, a strictly logical discourse from which all digressions were ruthlessly banished. Recently, however, Wadsworth, by closely analyzing the great odes, has shown that "a forceful argument . . . is not necessarily a logical one," and that these poems, using a certain fragmentary, accumulative process, do in fact violate the rules of deductive logic more often than not. For all that, Wadsworth does not suggest that Malherbe's official poems lack structure. Rather, he points to the age-old theory of the ode as an inspired creation, one "in which elevation of style mattered much more than obedience to rules of composition." He hints that beyond that apparent "beautiful disorder," there might be found a higher, hidden order. It is precisely this more subtle order that Rubin has analyzed. Looking closely at the six completed odes, he concludes that they contain both literal and figurative structural elements; that the literal ones include successions of facts "from whose less-than-rigorous presentation stems the surface disorder noted by Professor Wadsworth"; that the figurative ones, however, contain "the techniques by means of which Malherbe integrated the fragmentary literal elements into a [higher, hidden order]." It is at this level that the poet established—through intricate, yet coherent, systems of figures—series of correlations yielding a not-too-obvious but profound metaphorical unity.

"ALLANT CHÂTIER LA REBELLION DES ROCHELOIS"

In his prosody, Malherbe avoided the unusual, achieving striking variety within the framework of conventional forms. Five of the six completed odes are in isometric (octo- and heptasyllabic) *dizains*, the variety deriving from the diverse rhyme scheme and syntactic breaks. Much the same can be said of the poet's manipulation of metaphors, which are relatively few and conventional. The allusions are set up early in the poem so that all comparisons may be derived therefrom. Thus, in the opening stanza of the ode to the king "Allant châtier la rebellion des Rochelois," the first line contains a reference to the (Herculean) labors of the king; the second line deifies Louis by references to Jupiter's thunderbolt and to the Lion of Judah; the third and fourth lines represent the rebellious enclaves as so many Hydra's heads, of which this godlike Hercules will now strike off the last.

It is noteworthy that in the last stanza of this ode, Malherbe explicitly demonstrates what he has only implied earlier, that the king and his bard enjoy a symbiotic relationship. He enters into his poetic tableau much as a medieval painter introduced himself into a lordly fresco. The king's glory is made eternal precisely because Malherbe's poetry, a verbal temple, will last forever, unlike the bronze or marble of monuments. In this temple, both the icon (Louis) and the high priest (Malherbe) are simultaneously of this world and transcend it, but for the king to be assured of eternity, he must rely on his poet's pen, which alone can make a god of him. Malherbe would be nothing without his monarch's generosity and would be mute were it not for Louis's deeds, which furnish him with suitable subject matter; but without these odes, Louis would also be unable to fulfill his destiny. As Rubin concludes, "thus the poet establishes himself as the king's greatest—that is, most powerful and efficacious—subject and, paradoxically, his most generous patron."

CATHOLICISM AND MALHERBE

It would be difficult to ascribe with certainty any sort of deep religious feelings to Malherbe, in view of his private behavior and admissions to friends. Most critics agree that to him, religion was a matter of political orthodoxy and social compliance; he was a Catholic in much the same way that he was a royalist. However, it is impossible to read the best of his religious poems without admiration: A thorough professional, he took modes of expression—such as the paraphrase of Psalms, *stances spirituelles*, and consolations—and avoided the prevalent excessive ejaculations of facile penitence and humility to produce poems of pure religious expression that were to serve as models for generations to come. There is no exaltation to be found here but, as in the occasional poetry, an aura of grandeur and solemnity.

Malherbe's Catholicism, as expressed in these poems, is one strongly affected by his preoccupation with Seneca, but that Stoicism never interferes with the expression of a most orthodox dogma. It adds to a primordial aura of pomp and majesty one of resignation and melancholy. It should not be thought, however, that Malherbe advocated an ascetic or contemplative faith; rather, he saw the Monarchy and the Church as inextricably conjoined, the former being the temporal arm of the latter, and several of his works dealing with this relationship cannot be categorized as either exclusively spiritual or exclusively temporal. Such is obviously the case with *Prière pour le Roi allant en Limousin*, but there are others—less self-evident, perhaps, yet revealing the close relationship that Malherbe espoused.

Such a poem is the paraphrase of Psalm 128, written for the Queen Mother in 1614. In that year, a league of princes had rebelled against the regency of Marie de Médicis, who bribed them into submission. It is this purchase of peace that Malherbe treats by having the young king praise God for saving him and his realm from evil and turmoil. The praise of God is intertwined with castigation of the perfidious rebels whose snares the youthful Louis escaped only because of the powers watching over him. It is here that a deliberate ambiguity is introduced. God is the watchful Father protecting his royal son. God has turned the tide, but it is the Queen Mother who has implemented his wish. Not only is the benevolent paternity shared by God and the queen, their roles and attributes so closely intertwined as to make distinctions impossible, but also the king is depicted as that offspring of a noble race who, now that he is delivered from the hands of his foes, will bring happiness to his once-oppressed people. His role in establishing a peaceful realm on Earth is nothing short of messianic. This is not blasphemy: A monarch by divine right, Louis could be expected to do no less, at least in theory.

It can readily be seen that such a poem, although inspired by the Bible, is entirely Gallic in tone. The references are French, as are the expressions. Even the short biblical formulations yield to more sophisticated compound sentences, and the artistic expression is delicately enhanced by qualifiers rare or absent in the Psalms. By definition, a "paraphrase" suggests that the author has been struck by a thought he wishes now to comment on and amplify. In Malherbe's case, the impetus is not biblical—spiritual or historic—but official or personal. It is intended as an exposition of a rational and coherent concept or attitude. There is lyricism; even more, there is drama; above all, there is persuasive reason. Dramatic beginnings in these poems—such as those of the paraphrase of Psalm 145 or of the famous *Consolation à Monsieur Du Périer sur la mort de sa fille*, the latter's striking exordium sustained by tightly knit and sustained images—are part and parcel of a unified structure for which the word "theatrical" would not be out of place. After such an initial exhortation, there are always reiterations of imperatives (as in the paraphrase of Psalm 145) and energetic rhythms to sustain the initial impact. To people in the twenty-first century, drama and theology may seem like ill-suited partners; such was not the case in a century in which the stage and the pulpit were the centers of attention and of admiration. When, in 1715, before the crowned heads of Europe and their representatives, Jean-Baptiste Massillon, of humblest origins, began the funeral oration of Louis the Great with "God alone is great, my brothers," he was electrifying his audience in much the same way that Malherbe had startled his readers a full century earlier.

Malherbe's production in the realm of spiritual poetry is even less voluminous than in the official, occasional arena. Quality cannot be assessed on the basis of volume, nor can influence. Racan, Pierre Corneille, Antoine Godeau especially—all the successful writers of spiritual verses—show the undeniable imprint of Malherbe's daring and forceful creation.

OTHER MAJOR WORKS

NONFICTION: *Commentaire sur Desportes*, 1605-1606 (literary criticism); *Lettres à Peiresc*, 1628; *Les Lettres de Monsieur de Malherbe*, 1630.

TRANSLATIONS: *Le XXXIIIe livre de Tite Live*, 1616 (of Livy's history *Ab urbi condita libri*); *Traité des bienfaits de Seneque*, 1630 (of Seneca's treatise *De beneficiis*).

MISCELLANEOUS: *Œuvres complètes*, 1862-1869 (5 volumes).

BIBLIOGRAPHY

Abraham, Claude K. *Enfin Malherbe: The Influence of Malherbe on French Lyric Prosody, 1605-1674*. 1971. Reprint. Lexington: University Press of Kentucky, 1982. A good discussion of Malherbe doctrine, giving insight into the importance of Malherbe and the role he played in the development of literature in France.

Campion, Edmund J. "Poetic Theory in Théophile de Viau's 'Élégie à une dame.'" *Concerning Poetry* 20 (1987): 1-9. Describes why Malherbe's contemporary Théophile de Viau rejected Malherbe's attempt to impose one standard on all poets. Unlike Malherbe, Viau believed that a truly original poet must develop his or her unique style and voice.

Chesters, G. "Malherbe, Ponge, and Revolutionary Classicism." In *The Classical Tradition in French Literature*. London: Grant and Cutler, 1977. Describes well the arguments in Francis Ponge's 1965 book *Pour un Malherbe* in which this eminent twentieth century French poet attempted rather successfully to rehabilitate Malherbe's poetry but not his poetics.

Conway, Megan, ed. *Sixteenth-Century French Writers*. Vol. 327 in *Dictionary of Literary Biography*. Detroit: Thomson Gale, 2006. Contains a short biography of Malherbe and some analysis of his poetry.

Gershuny, Walter. "Seventeenth-Century Commemorative Verse." *Cahiers du dix-septième* 3, no. 1 (Spring, 1989): 279-289. Explains very clearly formal poems that the court poet Malherbe wrote to honor the French kings Henry IV and Louis XIII.

Gosse, Edmond. *Malherbe and the Classical Reaction in the Seventeenth Century*. 1920. Reprint. Philadelphia: R. West, 1977. This classic study deals specifically with Malherbe's importance to the creation of French classical literature.

Rubin, David Lee. *Higher, Hidden Order: Design and Meanings in the Odes of Malherbe*. Chapel Hill: University of North Carolina Press, 1972. A book-length study on the rhetoric of praise and blame in the numerous odes that Malherbe wrote during the late sixteenth and early seventeenth centuries. Rubin argues that Malherbe was a more successful and effective poet than traditional criticism indicates.

Winegarter, Rene. *French Lyric Poetry in the Age of Malherbe*. Manchester, England: Manchester University Press, 1954. A useful consideration of Malherbe's work in the light of that of his contemporaries.

Claude Abraham

STÉPHANE MALLARMÉ

Born: Paris, France; March 18, 1842
Died: Valvins, France; September 9, 1898

PRINCIPAL POETRY

L'Après-midi d'un faune, 1876 (*The Afternoon of a Faun*, 1936)
Les Poésies de Stéphane Mallarmé, 1887
Un Coup de dés jamais n'abolira le hasard, 1897 (*A Dice-Throw*, 1958; also as *Dice Thrown Never Will Annul Chance*, 1965)
Igitur, 1925 (English translation, 1974)
Poems by Mallarmé, 1936 (Roger Fry, translator)
Herodias, 1940 (Clark Mills, translator)
Selected Poems, 1957
Les Noces d'Hérodiade, 1959
Pour un "Tombeau d'Anatole," 1961 (*A Tomb for Anatole*, 1983)
Poésies, 1970 (*The Poems*, 1977)
Collected Poems, 1994

OTHER LITERARY FORMS

Stéphane Mallarmé (mah-lahr-MAY) is known chiefly for his poetry. A selection from his numerous critical essays and reviews, including some important theoretical statements, was published in *Divagations* (1897; English translation, 2007). Following the example of Charles Baudelaire, Mallarmé translated Edgar Allan Poe. He also published an idiosyncratic introduction to English philology, *Petite Philologie à l'usage des classes et du monde: Les Mots anglais* (1878; little philology for classroom use and for society: English words). It should be noted that Mallarmé wrote a number of prose poems, treated by some critics as prose works. The best edition of Mallarmé's poetry and essays is the Pléiade *Œuvres complètes de Stéphane Mallarmé* (1945), prepared by Henri Mondor and G. Jean-Aubry, although it is not a complete collection.

ACHIEVEMENTS

Stéphane Mallarmé's work is both the culmination of French Romanticism and the harbinger of the more hermetic poetry of the twentieth century. His vision of poetry as a sacred art, created with considerable sacrifice by an elite, derives from the Romantic image of the poet as prophet, typical of Victor Hugo. Mallarmé's "pure poetry," without reference to history or to social reality and characterized by a dense and elliptical style, however, deliberately abandons the attempt of many Romantics to bring poetry closer to life and to make it a social force. Very early in his career, Mallarmé said that it was heresy to try to make poetry understandable to a large audience. He sought instead to give expression to a higher form of intellectual experience in a language that is suggestive and indirect. Mallarmé's disciples, notably Paul Valéry, used the term "symbolism" to describe the new poetry. Mallarmé exerted a great personal influence on the theories developed in modernist artistic circles through his Tuesday receptions in his apartment on the rue de Rome in Paris.

BIOGRAPHY

Stéphane Mallarmé was born Etienne Mallarmé into a middle-class Parisian family of government administrators. His mother died when he was five. He was taken in by his maternal grandparents, who placed him in a series of boarding schools from the time he was ten. This forcible separation from a family environment was particularly painful because it deprived him of the company of his only sibling, his sister, Maria, who was younger by two years. He continued to write to her until her death at the age of thirteen. This disappearance of mother and sister, both idealized figures strongly linked in Mallarmé's mind to the religious life, seems to have caused Mallarmé to abandon conventional religious beliefs and to seek in his adolescent poetry a way of preserving the memory of these beloved presences. At the same time, Mallarmé's active sexual life seems to have left him disappointed and perhaps guilty about physical pleasure.

In 1860, Mallarmé took a position with the French administration, then went to London in 1862 with a young German woman, Maria Gerhard, whom he married in 1863. At the end of that year, he took his first position as a teacher of English. His entire professional career consisted of a series of appointments in secondary schools, first in the provinces and then, after 1871, in Paris. He retired in 1894. During the 1870's, Mal-

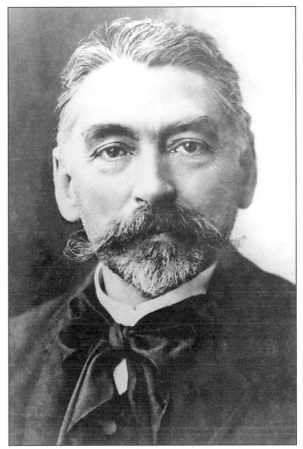

Stéphane Mallarmé (Hulton Archive/Getty Images)

larmé published translations, textbooks, a women's fashion magazine, and his own poetry.

His period of great celebrity began around 1884, when Paul Verlaine and Joris-Karl Huysmans acclaimed him in their own works. During the last fifteen years of his life, Mallarmé exercised enormous influence on the younger poets, who hailed him as the prophetic exemplar of Symbolism. Mallarmé himself did not seek honor or public attention. He left the publication of manifestos to his followers and preferred to devote his time to research for his oeuvre, his great "work," which he never finished. His poetic works, considerable as they are, did not live up to his ambition, although his manuscripts give evidence of intense labor.

ANALYSIS

"Everything in the world exists to end up in a book," wrote Stéphane Mallarmé in 1895. It is this attitude toward reality and toward the importance of the book that makes Mallarmé the preeminent Symbolist poet. For him, reality exists only in the symbol, which, in poetry, is constructed out of language. This position, apparently influenced by Hegelian idealism, does not mean that poetry is necessarily about language—although a number of Mallarmé's poems are about language and poetry themselves—but rather that language provides the only systematic and rational framework, the only escape from randomness, in a world in which there is no sign of a personal God. Mallarmé's poetry is a kind of metaphysical poetry, in that it aspires to go beyond the physical reality of everyday life to uncover the mysterious world of a pure ideal that can exist nowhere except in the mind and in language.

Even though many of Mallarmé's poems seem at first to be completely obscure, in most cases careful reading will reveal that a kernel drawn from everyday life has been transformed into a spare, unsentimental, timeless formal variation (in the way that a composer makes a variation on a musical theme). The effect is neither an enshrinement of a particular moment, place, or picturesque character nor an appeal to emotional sympathy. It is still less a moral or political message. Instead, such poems invite the reader to experience the power of the mind and of language.

For Mallarmé, the most important experience is the experience of the poem itself, and if such a statement seems commonplace and even trite, it is because Mallarmé's influence has been so pervasive. For him, however, the experience of the poem was particularly concrete and precise, and he frequently wrote about acts and objects connected with writing and reading with a kind of religious awe. The word *livre* (book) and such kindred terms as *grimoire* (book of magic incantations) and *bouquin* (old book) have in his vocabulary an importance rarely found in other bodies of poetry except in religious texts, where "the book" is the sacred scripture explaining and justifying the world. Mallarmé attempted during his life to create a nonreligious scripture.

Most of his poems, however, are playful occasional pieces such as "Eventail de Madame Mallarmé" ("Madam Mallarmé's Fan"); brief poems written in honor of other artists, such as the "Hommage" to Richard Wagner and "Le Tombeau d'Edgar Poe" ("The Tomb of Edgar Poe"); erotic poetry based on elliptical sexual fantasy, such as *The Afternoon of a Faun* and "Victorieusement fui le suicide beau" ("The Beautiful Suicide Victoriously Escaped"); or the long series of poems lamenting the difficulty of escaping from the base material world and of writing the higher kind of poetry. The last category includes the well-known "L'Azur," sometimes called the "Swan Sonnet," "Les Fenêtres" ("The Windows"), and "Le Pître châtié" ("The Clown's Punishment"). Only the three longer poems, *Herodias, Igitur* (read to friends in unfinished form and published posthumously), and *Dice Thrown Never Will Annul Chance* (published in the magazine *Cosmopolis* in May, 1897, but not published in book form until 1914) give some idea of the form of Mallarmé's more ambitious projects.

There is nevertheless a stylistic and thematic coherence in Mallarmé's work, which proceeds by a kind of condensation and subtraction. The extremely difficult but logical grammar absorbs the reader in the enigmatic possibilities of meaning, thus fixing attention on the poem's language. Objects and persons named in the poems are described as absent or "abolished."

"ALL THE SOUL INDRAWN . . ."

A good way to begin with Mallarmé's poetry is to look at his brief poem "Toute l'âme résumée . . ." ("All the Soul Indrawn . . ."), which is a witty response to a survey on free verse. Mallarmé compares making poetry to smoking a cigar. The successive rings of smoke are "abolished" by those that follow, and the ash keeps falling away from the "bright kiss of fire." Poetry is not what is left behind, Mallarmé implies; it is rather the process itself, momentary but renewed. Because the word *âme* can mean both "soul" and, with some etymological delving, "breath," and *résumée* means both "summed up" and "drawn in," Mallarmé has put into play a metaphor for the content of poetry that eludes the traditional distinction between form and content, vehicle and tenor. The breath is what permits the cigar to keep burning; it is also the proof that one is alive. Yet this thing, which is so essential to smoking and to life, is empty. Similarly, the burning tip of the cigar, the thing showing that the cigar is "alive," is the fire that can survive only by emptying itself of the ash. Like smoking,

Mallarmé suggests, poetry should be regarded as pure activity, without product and without connection with any external reality. After making this comparison explicit in the third quatrain, which advises writers to exclude vile reality, Mallarmé concludes with a distich that pointedly inverts the usual literary and rhetorical values of his day: "A too precise meaning scratches out/ Your vague literature." The more definite and specific the reference a poem makes to reality, the less it can be considered precisely literary.

"MY OLD BOOKS CLOSED AT THE NAME OF PAPHOS"

Another celebrated poem centered on the powers of literature, considered this time from the point of view of the reader, is "Mes bouquins refermés sur le nom de Paphos" ("My Old Books Closed at the Name of Paphos"). The speaker of the poem tells of closing his book and looking out on a snowy landscape where he imagines a Mediterranean scene. There is a parallel between the foam of the sea splashing against a ruin in the first quatrain and the white snow presented as part of the reader's material reality in the second quatrain. The speaker makes clear, however, that he will not wail a funereal lament (*nénie*) if the snowy reality does not coincide with his imagined seascape. The tercets make clear why the speaker so calmly accepts the divorce of dream from reality. The absence of things, which one notices because literature draws one's attention to such lacunae, is presented as a superior value. Mallarmé's negative approach, his preference for hollowing out a dream world by "abolishing" elements of the everyday world, appears in the speaker's claim: "My hunger, which is satisfied here by no fruits/ Finds in their learned lack an equal savor." To be satisfied by "no fruits" is not the same as being unsatisfied. It is a state in which the learned vision imposes a preference for the dream.

The second tercet goes even further, recalling that absence is not merely in the speaker's present world but in the scene imagined as well. Apparently addressing a lover, he confesses: "I think longer, perhaps desperately,/ Of the other, with the seared breast of an ancient Amazon." The scene is not only absent but also organized around an absence, the missing breast of one of the legendary warrior-women who founded the city of Paphos. Even these two absences are not all one can find here. The adverb translated as "desperately" or "distractedly" to describe the speaker's preoccupation with the Amazon is *éperdument*, which contains the word *perdu* (lost). The speaker, as reader, is thus also in some way lost to the everyday world and to ordinary love.

"HER PURE FINGERNAILS ON HIGH OFFERING THEIR ONYX"

The procedure of creating a scene by "abolishing" is taken closer to Mallarmé's project of a great magical work in the sonnet "Ses purs ongles trés haut dédiant leur onyx" ("Her Pure Fingernails on High Offering Their Onyx"), known as the "Sonnet in yx" because of its unusual rhymes. This sonnet apparently describes a deserted parlor belonging to a magician, the "Master," who has gone to get tears in the underworld from the river Styx. The vessel the Master will use is a *ptyx*. This is a word that has a meaning in Greek but none in French. Mallarmé may have meant it to remain meaningless, for the *ptyx* is called "this unique object of which Nothingness is proud." Furthermore, the *ptyx* is designated in the poem only as an absence: "in the empty parlor: no ptyx,/ Abolished trinket of sonorous inanity."

Scholars have studied the problem of the *ptyx* at length with reference to its ancient meanings, ranging from "book" to "seashell." As one scholar has noted, however, the more meanings that are proposed for the word, the less it actually signifies. It has become an empty form that traps the reader into deep and repeated investigations of semantic, phonetic, and etymological networks in the sonnet in the hope of finding some meaning. This sonnet certainly follows the precepts of "All the Soul Indrawn . . ." in avoiding a "too precise sense." It also exemplifies the kind of dream to which Mallarmé wanted to lead his readers. Although psychoanalytic readings of Mallarmé have been among the most interesting, Mallarmé himself did not use the word *rêve* (dream) to designate a person's unconscious. For Mallarmé, "dream" suggested both the aspiration to a world of pure thought without material limitation (this is particularly clear in "The Windows") and the realm in which language unfolds in all its ambiguity. The Master's absence from this parlor could be interpreted as the author's desire to absent himself from the scene within which the reader can experience the possibilities of language, including the possibility that the most important words exist anagrammatically within the evident ones.

HERODIAS

Of Mallarmé's longer poems, those that seem to be part of his "great work," only *Herodias* and *Dice Thrown Never Will Annul Chance* gave the public some idea of the synthesis of poetic research of which he often spoke. Those works and the posthumous publications are all extremely difficult to interpret, but they seem to have at their core a struggle between the magic of the poetic symbol and the Nothingness (*le Néant*) that, for Mallarmé, constituted the universe. Because he rejected the physically present world for an ideal one and yet did not believe in religious spirituality, the magic of the great work would be to create a place where the ideal could exist. The language of the great work would have to be a special one, not the "unrefined and immediate" but the "essential" word free from the "chance" of usage, as he wrote in a preface to a work by René Ghil.

Herodias, a verse drama with little of the apparatus of a theater script, unites the themes of incantation, abolition, cerebral eroticism, and the preservation of the memory of the beloved dead. In most editions of Mallarmé, *Herodias* is divided into an "overture," in which the nurse of Princess Herodias describes the imaginary setting; a "scene," consisting of a dialogue between Herodias and her nurse; and a "canticle," in which the voice of John the Baptist sings at the moment of his decapitation. In the overture, the palace is evoked as empty and abandoned, like the parlor of the "Sonnet in yx." The king is long absent, the basin deserted by its swan, the sun rising red for the last time.

Even if one could create such a setting on the stage, the words of the overture make it clear that the real stage for these words is in the mind. The nurse, for example, speaks of a voice that evokes the past and then asks, "Is it my voice ready for the incantation?" If the speaker responsible for the exposition is not sure whether she has spoken, this suggests that she has merely thought the words. Moreover, the words that her voice may be ready to pronounce are an evocation of the past. Future and past thus join to create a situation in which imminent doom, nostalgia, and uncertainty about time coexist in a paradoxical equilibrium. The abstract quality of this setting is further emphasized by such metaphors as "the bed with pages of velum." The princess's bed is thus characterized as entirely chaste, while the whole drama takes on the aura of something entirely within a book.

In "Scene," the nurse tries to persuade Herodias to satisfy her awakening sexuality, while the princess insists that she loves the "horror" of being a virgin and that she cannot tolerate any touch. In place of touch, sight becomes the only sense through which Herodias can open herself to sexuality or even to consciousness. The scene is full of mirrors, described as cold and distant like "water frozen from boredom." All the mirrors serve to reflect the princess's image, excluding the menacing outside world. In the last lines, Herodias, at the departure of the nurse, announces that she is waiting for an unknown thing and that she has lied to her nurse about her voluntary solitude.

The connection between "Scene" and "Canticle," which follows it, is not clear, although the fragments edited by Gardner Davies in *Les Noces d'Hérodiade* permit some conjectures. Several critics have advanced the idea that John the Baptist has seen Heriodas, who then feels that only his death can restore her sense of intactness. The saint is what the fragment calls the "somber pretext" for the princess's full achievement of self-consciousness. His crime is to be different from a mirror, which offers a neutral image without judgment. According to "Canticle," there is a tension between the ideal and the physical in John as well, and this tension is released by the decapitation, in which the saint sees salvation. Mallarmé, however, avoids religious statement by concluding with the word *salut*, which can mean both "salvation" and "salute." The word describes both the movement of the head as it follows its trajectory up and then down and the hope expressed by baptism. In the unfinished version of this drama, Herodias seems to have captured the dying glance of John and to consider herself united to the prophet in a wedding that is both sexual and ideal. She addresses the head, saying "I reason for you, head, not about you."

Herodias's hope to snatch consciousness from death

was apparently the long-term result of Mallarmé's adolescent poetic meditations on death. It is also a hope that appears in the fragmentary *A Tomb for Anatole* (edited by Jean-Pierre Richard), in which the poet tried to recreate the life of his dead son through imagination. In a passage similar to that in which Herodias declares that she will think for John, Mallarmé tells his dead son that the poet will *be* the son hereafter. The question of the apparent futility of such a project is addressed by two other long poems by Mallarmé, *Igitur* and *Dice Thrown Never Will Annul Chance*.

IGITUR

Igitur, a prose poem written between 1867 and 1870 and left unfinished at Mallarmé's death, was edited by the scholar Edmond Bonniot, the poet's son-in-law, who discovered the manuscript in 1900. The poem relates the adventures of Igitur, a prince haunted by a supreme "Idea" and by the destiny imposed by his race, which has somehow projected Igitur outside time. The next-to-last section is titled "A Roll of Dice" and takes place in the family tomb. There, Igitur confronts the problem of the relationship among personal action, necessity, and chance. Understanding that action is absurd except as a return to infinity, which is a form of the pure absolute, he throws the dice before laying himself on the ashes of his ancestors. This metaphysical hero, described by critics as a Hamlet stripped of psychology, confronts the problems of individual time-bound existence (versus a timeless ideal) and of the tradition of a nation or race. This can be considered as Mallarmé's own problem, for the poet is both haunted by the literary and scriptural tradition and faced with the apparent randomness of his own efforts. Mallarmé's flight from a psychological and emotional poetry toward an intellectual and apparently impersonal one corresponds to the desire to escape from chance into a pure rationality in which everything would be determined and necessary, although not foreseeable to the human mind.

DICE THROWN NEVER WILL ANNUL CHANCE

Dice Thrown Never Will Annul Chance follows from *Igitur* and seems to be the work that most closely approaches Mallarmé's ambition for "pure poetry." This work has had a wide influence on such twentieth

century movements as Dada, Surrealism, and Lettrism, not because of its theme but because of its innovative typographical form. Mallarmé had the text set in type of various sizes and specified the exact location of each word on the double-page layouts. Some pages have as few as four words, while others have nearly a hundred. The poet can control more than the verbal aspect of the poem by dealing directly with the visual domain usually left to the printer. Mallarmé here manifests his obsessive concern for the concrete aspects of the book, for the obliteration of the distinction between form and content, and for the reduction of chance in the production of a literary work. The title of the poem runs in the largest type through the poem in such a way that the last word, "Chance," appears only on the ninth double-page unit (out of a total of eleven). Interrupting the title sentence are qualifications expressed in subordinate clauses and in various forms of apposition in various smaller type sizes. The effect is one of suspense, like that which attends a throw of the dice. The last small line of the poem reveals an application of the metaphor of the dice: "Every thought makes a roll of the dice."

Even though Mallarmé eschewed appeals to a broad public, and despite the fact that, aside from a half-dozen shorter poems frequently taught in *lycées* and colleges, his work does not have a wide readership, he has had an enormous influence on twentieth century poets, artists, and critics.

OTHER MAJOR WORKS

NONFICTION: *Petite Philologie à l'usage des classes et du monde: Les Mots anglais*, 1878; *Les Dieux antiques*, 1880; *Divagations*, 1897 (English translation, 2007); *Correspondance*, 1959-1984 (10 volumes); *Documents Mallarmé*, 1968-1971 (3 volumes); *Mallarmé in Prose*, 2001 (Mary Ann Caws, editor).

TRANSLATION: *Les Poémes d'Edgar Poe*, 1888.

MISCELLANEOUS: *Album de vers et de prose*, 1887; *Pages*, 1891; *Vers et prose*, 1893; *Œuvres complètes de Stéphane Mallarmé*, 1945; *Selected Prose Poems, Essays, and Letters*, 1956; *Mallarmé*, 1965; *Selected Poetry and Prose*, 1982; *Divagations: The Author's 1897 Arrangement, Together with "Autobiography" and "Music and Letters,"* 2007.

BIBLIOGRAPHY

Cohn, Robert Greer, ed. *Mallarmé in the Twentieth Century*. London: Associated University Presses, 1998. A collection of essays by many of the most eminent figures in the study of Mallarmé, including Julia Kristeva, Mary Ann Caws, Albert Cook, Anna Balakian, and Robert Cohn. An important summary of the state of scholarship on the poet.

Lloyd, Rosemary. *Mallarmé: The Poet and His Circle*. Ithaca, N.Y.: Cornell University Press, 1999. A literary biography of the poet and his period. Mallarmé hosted gatherings attended by writers, artists, thinkers, and musicians in France, England, and Belgium. Through these gatherings and voluminous correspondence Mallarmé developed and recorded his friendships with Paul Valéry, André Gide, Berthe Morisot, and many others. Includes bibliographical references and index.

Millan, Gordan. *A Throw of the Dice: The Life of Stéphane Mallarmé*. New York: Farrar, Straus and Giroux, 1994. This biography of Mallarmé, who has a reputation for difficulty and obscurity, proves equally valuable to students and specialists. The narrative is aimed at the general reader while the ample footnotes provide material for the specialist. The text draws on previously unpublished correspondence and new documentation and includes bibliographical references and an index.

Pearson, Roger. *Unfolding Mallarmé: The Development of a Poetic Art*. New York: Oxford University Press, 1996. An account of the development of Mallarmé's poetry from his earliest verse to his final masterpiece. Close readings demonstrate the intricate linguistic and formal play to be found in many of his major poems.

Sartre, Jean Paul. *Mallarmé: Or, The Poet of Nothingness*. Translated by Ernest Sturm. University Park: State University of Pennsylvania Press, 1988. A leading existentialist's view of Mallarmé.

Sugano, Marian Zwerling. *The Poetics of the Occasion: Mallarmé and the Poetry of Circumstance*. Stanford, Calif.: Stanford University Press, 1992. Focuses on Mallarmé's occasional poems.

Takeda, Noriko. *The Modernist Human: The Configuration of Humanness in Stéphane Mallarmé's "Hérodiade," T. S. Eliot's "Cats," and Modernist Lyrical Poetry*. New York: Peter Lang, 2008. Takeda examines modernist humanity as evidence in the poetry of Mallarmé and Eliot. Contains a general discussion of Mallarmé's poetry.

Temple, Michael. *The Name of the Poet: Onomastics and Anonymity in the Works of Stéphane Mallarmé*. Exeter, England: University of Exeter Press, 1995. Study of the use of place-names versus personal anonymity in Mallarmé's work.

_____, ed. *Meetings with Mallarmé*. Exeter, England: University of Exeter Press, 1998. Critical interpretation of Mallarmé's major works. Includes bibliographical references and index.

John D. Lyons

ITZIK MANGER

Born: Czernowitz, Bukovina, Austro-Hungarian Empire (now Chernivtsi, Ukraine); May 28, 1901
Died: Gadera, Israel; February 20, 1969

PRINCIPAL POETRY

Shtern oifn Dakh, 1929
Lamtern in Vint, 1933
Khumish Lider, 1935
Demerung in Shpigl, 1937
Volkens ibern Dakh, 1942
Der Shnyder-gezeln Nota Manger Zingt, 1948
Medresh Itzik, 1951, 1969, 1984 (reprintings of the *Khumish Lider* with later additions)
Lid un Balade, 1952
Shtern in Shtoib, 1967

OTHER LITERARY FORMS

In 1938, Itzik Manger (MAYNG-ur) published in the Warsaw Yiddish press his *Noente Geshtaltn* (intimate figures), a newspaper series of bittersweet, fictionalized portraits of twenty forerunners of Yiddish poetry: troubadours, rhyming wedding jesters, itinerant actors, and writers of the nineteenth century and earlier. These popular artists expressed themselves in

Yiddish when it was considered, even by its speakers, a language fit not for literature but for low-class entertainment. They were Manger's first heroes; from their earthy folk style, he learned the art of simplicity.

Manger's only novel, *Dos Bukh fun Gan-Eden* (1939; *The Book of Paradise*, 1965), is a fantasy set in Paradise—a humorous vision of the afterlife in which familiar human weaknesses and pains persist. In *The Book of Paradise*, fantasy is the everyday norm, and the wrinkles are provided by earthly reality: the reality of human nature and the folkways of the Eastern European Jewish community. In Manger's novel, Yiddish culture—its folklore, faith, parochialism, and beauty—is celebrated, satirized, and memorialized. *The Book of Paradise* was published in Warsaw in August, 1939, and nearly the entire edition was destroyed at the printer's a month later by the invading German army. Only a handful of review copies mailed to the United States survived.

Although Manger's poetry places him in the line of the English and German Romantics and the French Symbolists, the cultural movement in which he was personally active was the Yiddish theater. Seeing himself as the modern heir of the itinerant Yiddish entertainers of older times, Manger was drawn to the musical theater as a medium for direct contact with his audience. His unusual popularity as a poet brought him the opportunity to write for several Yiddish theater productions in the 1930's. *Hotzmakh Shpiel*, Manger's adaptation of Abraham Goldfaden's operetta, *Di Kishufmakherin* (the sorceress), was performed in Warsaw in 1936. (Goldfaden founded the Yiddish theater in the 1870's in Romania, producing his first musicals in wine cellars and barns. His troupes played throughout Eastern Europe and in England in the 1880's and 1890's. In Manger's gallery of portraits in *Noente Geshtaltn*, Goldfaden appears on his deathbed, hallucinating scenes.)

Sometime in the 1930's, Manger wrote the lyrics for the Warsaw musical production of Sholom Aleichem's novel, *Blondzne Shtern*, 1912 (*Wandering Star*, 1952), a romance based on the lives of early Romanian Yiddish actors. In 1935, he wrote the lyrics for the first Yiddish musical film, *Yidl mitn Fidl* (released 1936; *Yiddle with His Fiddle*).

Manger's best-known work for the theater is the tragicomic operetta *Megillah Lider*, published in 1936 but not staged until thirty years later, when it was set to music by Dov Seltzer and performed in Israel and on Broadway as *The Megillah of Itzik Manger*. The first production of Manger's operetta played from 1965 to 1969. It stirred much interest in Manger among the Yiddish-scorning youth of Israel and led to the Hebrew-speaking public's discovery of Manger's more serious poetry. It began to appear in translation in newspapers and magazines, and belatedly, Manger became the first Yiddish writer since Sholom Aleichem to win a wide readership in Israel.

ACHIEVEMENTS

Itzik Manger's place in the cultural history of the Jews was officially recognized in 1969 with the first annual awarding of the Manger Prize for Yiddish Literature. Among the twelve founding members of the Manger Prize Committee were the Hebrew writer S. Y. Agnon (corecipient of the 1966 Nobel Prize in Literature); two prime ministers of Israel, Levi Eshkol and Golda Meir; the then-president of Israel, himself a poet, Zalman Shazar; and the committee's chairman, Shalom Rosenfeld, editor in chief of the Tel Aviv daily, *Maariv*.

The committee made public what had been the private sentiment of many readers. Both for the older generation who knew the poet from prewar years in Europe and for the younger generation who had just discovered him, Manger was an intimate figure, a teacher, muse, and friend. For people whose beliefs in various opposing movements of Judaism and European humanism had failed, Manger's gentle yet hardheaded, sensuous poetry was a spiritual renewal. His poems had the power to evoke feelings and discoveries of religious intensity, but with a light touch, a lighthearted, cheerful acceptance of the evanescence of all meaning. This acceptance made possible, or necessary, Manger's anarchistic eclecticism. His poems assimilated and refined diverse sensibilities and philosophies, from Hasidism to nihilism, from Saint Francis to Friedrich Nietzsche and Sigmund Freud. Manger gleaned from these sources all that answered a human yearning; that which was abstract and therefore susceptible to rigidity and mystification, he sloughed off.

Manger's poetry readings in the 1930's drew audiences of thousands in the major cities of Poland. Local musicians played the tunes they had composed for his words. Not since the days of Aleichem's public reading tours a generation back had the flowering Yiddish cultural scene experienced such festivity. Within a decade of the publication of Manger's first book, his works were in the curriculum of every grade in the secular Jewish school system of Poland, from kindergarten through secondary school.

Manger's artful mixture of innocence, irony, deviltry, and tenderness charmed away his culture's old, argumentative obsessions with justice and truth, offering instead less instructive but more deeply satisfying ideals: love, beauty, and wisdom. Among poets, these preferences are not new; what is unusual is how far Manger's love strove to outgrow itself, to reconcile the reckless thirst for meaning and beauty with the sober, responsible cultivation of wisdom. His works offered a way to live between beauty and wisdom—between the beauty of sensation, illusion, and faith and the wisdom of memory and detachment.

BIOGRAPHY

Itzik Manger was born in 1901 to Hillel Manger and Khava Voliner Manger, the first of three children close in age. His birthplace was the ethnically Romanian and Jewish city Czernowitz (now Chernivtsi, Ukraine), capital of Bukovina, a province of the Austrian Empire. The city was situated at the intersection of Bukovina, the Russian-ruled Ukraine, and the independent state of Romania; its official language was German. When the Russian army invaded Bukovina in 1914, the Manger family fled to Jassy, capital of the Romanian province of Moldavia, and settled there. The Mangers moved often, going from one single-room apartment or basement to another when the rent was due. Their home served also as the family's tailor shop. "A roof I didn't inherit from my parents," Manger wrote, "but stars—plenty." They were a happy family. The mother was pious and barely literate, but she knew thousands of Yiddish folk songs.

The future poet, together with his brother and their younger sister, spent childhood summers in the country, in their paternal grandparents' home. Riding through the countryside with his grandfather, Zaida Avremel the wagon driver, revealed wonders of nature and perspective to the boy from the slums. The misty Carpathian Mountains, where the spirit of the Baal Shem Tov, the founder of the Hasidic movement, had roamed seven generations before, haunted Manger, and over the years he returned again and again to this setting in his poetry.

After finishing the traditional Jewish school for boys, Manger was enrolled in a state secondary school in Czernowitz but was expelled in the second semester. This left him time to frequent cafés and wine cellars where Gypsy fiddlers played and to volunteer as a stagehand in the Yiddish theaters of Czernowitz and later Jassy, where he absorbed the folklore of his nineteenth century forerunners.

In Czernowitz, an apprentice-tailor working for Manger's father introduced the boy to the works of Johann Wolfgang von Goethe, Friedrich Schiller, and Heinrich Heine. At thirteen, Manger began writing poetry in German. His teens were an exhilarating time for him and his brother, Nota; together they discovered Rainer Maria Rilke, Friedrich Nietzsche, Paul Verlaine, and "Saint" Baudelaire. (Manger gave that title to only two others: Homer and the Baal Shem Tov.)

Before the late nineteenth century, Yiddish had no tradition of poetry other than primitive folk writings and inspirational polemics. During Manger's childhood and youth, the stories of I. L. Peretz and Aleichem created a body of modern Yiddish literature. Their example attracted the young writer of German poetry to his mother tongue and its speakers. At fifteen, Manger started to write in Yiddish, wondering whether modern poetry could be written in the language of wagon drivers, Hasidism, peddlers, and uneducated women. His doubts were banished when, in his late teens, he encountered the work of two immigrant Yiddish poets who were writing in New York. The gutsy and delicate lyricism of Moishe Leib Halpern and Mani Leib gave new power to Yiddish and set Manger on his course: He would refine the spirits of his ancient and modern fathers in the language of his mother's lullabies.

During his twenties, Manger was based in Bucharest, where he was active in the Yiddish avant-garde grouped around Eliezer Steinbarg. The group's influences were Russian, French, and German literature mixed with Slavic, Gypsy, and Jewish folklore. The spirit of the group reflected that of the times: Europe was in ferment and the Jews were in turmoil. World War I, the Bolshevik Revolution, and the Russian Civil War broke up what was left, after the mass migration to the United States, of the old Eastern European Jewish communities. In 1923, the immigration quotas set by the United States Congress closed the "Golden Door," and Jews came in increasing numbers to the large cities of Eastern and Central Europe.

Throughout the nineteenth century and into the twentieth, the religious faith of the Jews had been eroded by contact with the outside world and its liberal ideas. A minority clung zealously to fundamentalism; for the rest, the intensity of the lost faith became converted into various new drives: assimilation, economic and professional ambition, public service, leftist radicalism, political and cultural nationalism, intellectual activity, and art. In the popular Gentile mind, the traditionally despised Jews became the symbol of all the changes that were hitting Europe too fast: inflation, labor conflict, sexual revolution, and radical "modern" ideas of all kinds. Anti-Semitic parties and economic boycotts proliferated in Poland, Romania, Lithuania, and Germany. For the newly "emancipated" Jews, the world seemed to totter between salvation and ruin.

Amid the welter of mass movements promising the Jews a brighter future, Manger, after an adolescent leftist period, raised the unlikely banner of the renewal of Yiddish folk song. "Our wounds need balm," he wrote in a manifesto in his twenties. "All roads lead to Rome and all roads lead to the kingdom of Beauty." Some of the roads taken by Yiddish poets in the 1920's came under his attack. He criticized the radical modernists who were influenced by trends in Germany and the Soviet Union for breaking away from their Jewish roots and experimenting with deliberately unmusical verse. With his brother's meager earnings as a tailor and the occasional support of culture patrons, he traveled throughout the Jewish centers of Romania, Poland, and Lithuania, addressing crowds in outdoor markets, political meetinghouses, and wine cellars, reading poetry and lecturing on Yiddish folklore and Aleichem's sad humor. For a people whose religion was built on preserving strict dichotomies, Manger dissolved such rigid

categories as old-fashioned or modern, popular or classical, secular or sacred. Manger's effect on his audience was described by a poet who grew up in Poland in the 1920's, Avraham Sutzkever, in the autumn, 1958, issue of *Di goldene Keit*, the Israeli Yiddish literary journal that he edited: It was "like a child with a mirror throwing a drop of sun on an old man."

In 1928, Manger moved to Warsaw, the main center of Yiddish life and culture. When his first book, *Shtern oifn Dakh* (stars on the roof), was published in 1929, he instantly became a folk hero, known throughout Eastern Europe. Nourished by an enthusiastic public in Warsaw, he wrote more than half of his lifework there and nearly all his best. Nevertheless, tired of writers' feuds and of the scandals caused by his penchant for wine, women, and what rabbis called Decadent poetry, Manger left Warsaw in 1938, traveling to Paris, where there was a colony of expatriate Eastern European Jewish artists and intellectuals. Not much is known of his two years in France. It was there that he wrote his fantasy novel, *The Book of Paradise*, a wistful, gently mocking love letter to the world he had left behind.

As the German army approached Paris in 1940, Manger fled to Algiers, where thousands of legally stateless refugees scrambled for the limited opportunities of transport to safer destinations. The glint in Manger's eye caught the interest of a boat captain and won Manger a space on a boat to Liverpool in late 1940. During the war, Manger managed the German section of a London bookstore owned by Margaret Waterhouse, a great-granddaughter of the poet Percy Bysshe Shelley; she was Manger's companion and nurse for most of his ten years in England. The two months that he spent in a Liverpool hospital upon his arrival from Algiers did not completely cure him of the effects of the hunger and exhaustion he had suffered while fleeing the Nazis, and his poor health was aggravated by his increased drinking in England.

While his people were being massacred in Europe, Manger immersed himself in English and Scottish folklore: "From Herrick to Burns" was his title for an unpublished anthology of English poetry that he did not finish translating into Yiddish. In 1942, Manger's brother, Nota, died on a Soviet collective farm from hunger, exposure, and battle wounds. He had joined the Army of the Red Star as a believer in Socialism.

During his years in England, Manger waited for a U.S. visa. He considered the Yiddish-speaking immigrant community of New York as the closest thing to a home and as the only audience that could support him. In 1951, he left England for Montreal, whose Jewish community had invited him to give a series of readings and lectures during the last months of his wait for a U.S. visa. The enthusiasm with which he was received both in Montreal and, later that year, during a tour making public appearances in American cities, attended by crowds in the thousands, helped to restore his spirits. In 1951, he met and married Genya Nadir, the widow of the Yiddish writer Moishe Nadir. They lived in Brooklyn for the next fifteen years.

New York was a disappointment. It was clear that its Yiddish cultural scene had little future beyond the generation then growing old. Finding a society more open and tolerant than they or their ancestors had ever had, the Jews of America were rushing to assimilate. For most of those who clung to their ethnic roots, the compelling myths and visions were those of a Hebrew future (Zionism) or past (traditional Judaism). Yiddish was the language of the ghetto, whose history Jews wanted to forget. The humanistic renewal of Jewish culture that had been carried on in Yiddish squandered much of its idealism and prestige in leftist ideological squabbling that seemed anachronistic, at best, to most of the generation that grew up after the Great Depression.

After the passing excitement of his arrival in the United States, Manger fell into the mood that his poetry had taught others to transcend: bitterness. The little poetry that he wrote in New York had a tired feeling. He managed to antagonize and alienate most of his friends. In the midst of the largest, freest, and richest Jewish community in history, he and his works were neglected. The remnants of the thriving Yiddish cultural scene of prewar Europe had become concentrated in a few neighborhoods of New York, with each writer coveting a share of a shrunken audience. In Israel, the bitterness of the Holocaust survivors was sublimated by the positive determination to build a country. In New York, the bitterness of the non-Zionist Yiddishists spilled out on the only people with whom they had

much contact: one another. Manger complained in his letters that he was being boycotted by the Yiddish journals of New York, whose literary editors and their friends were his rivals for the title of the "Last Great Yiddish Poet." As if to belittle his stature as the most popular poet by far in the history of Yiddish, critics in New York referred to him as a mere "balladeer" or "satirist."

Manger, however, lived to see the redemption of the years he had spent facing oblivion. Ironically, it came to him in Israel, the country that had struggled to do away with the history of the Jewish Diaspora—the Diaspora whose language, ethos, and *schleppers* he had celebrated, liberated, enlightened, and exalted. As he lay in Israeli hospitals for the last two and a half years of his life, totally crippled and speechless from a nervous disease but still able to show something of a smile, he heard the news of the nation's rediscovery of his works. On the radio, he heard pop stars and schoolchildren singing his poems, in Hebrew translation, to their old tunes and to new ones as well. He read of the Manger festivals presented by the nation's cultural elite. Three weeks after the return of his power of speech, he died.

ANALYSIS

Using the verse patterns and simple language of traditional Yiddish folk songs, Itzik Manger created a style that brought modern poetic sensibilities to an ordinary audience. In style and theme, his poems transform the commonplace into something subtle, wondrous, and beautiful. His subjects are sad—loneliness, disappointment, death, confusion, frustration—but his poems usually evoke smiles.

Manger's voice changes not only from poem to poem but also often within the same poem. With seeming indiscriminateness, he mixes nursery rhymes, gangster jargon, regional Yiddish dialects, classical mythology, traditional prayers, and burlesque theater with the poetic traditions of Europe. His anachronisms have their own integrity, and the same can be said of his irrationalities and contradictory traits in general. Their coming together feels perfectly natural to a reader, like an intuitive click or a rhyme. In the same moment that one of Manger's paradoxes hits the reader, it also resolves itself; it is as if the reader has secretly sensed it already, so that all that is left to do is smile at a crumbled convention.

The poetic clichés that Manger enjoyed using would make a novice blush. He loved the moon and brings it in dozens of times: as a big loaf of bread for a hungry family, a crescent twinkling in Hagar's hair, an earring for Rachel, but usually just as the moon. He went out of his way to use it in rhymes. Equally unoriginal is the form in which he almost always wrote, rhymed quatrains: He meant for his poems to be sung. A list of the poets and other sources he both plagiarized and collaborated with would run as long as the Jewish exile.

BALLADS

Of the many kinds of poems that Manger wrote—ballad, lyric odes, mystical fancies, still lifes, prayers, confessions, ditties, love poems, elegies, children's songs, lullabies, mood reflections, satires, autobiographies, scenes of local color—it is the ballads that have most interested literary critics.

In his essay "The Ballad: The Vision of Blood," published in 1929, Manger acknowledged that he was influenced by the traditional British ballad of the supernatural. This influence was already apparent in "Ballad of a Streetwalker," his first published poem, which appeared in 1921 in the Bucharest Yiddish journal, *Kultur,* edited by the fabulist-poet Eliezer Steinbarg. The poem anticipates Manger's mature verse, with its emphasis on the primacy of the moment, provocative understatement and paradox, plain speech, twilight blurring of the natural and the supernatural, psychological realism, compassion for characters on the fringe of society, distant, detached perspectives, and word music. Indeed, of his essential traits, only lightheartedness and folk traditionalism were missing.

In "The Ballad of the Bridal Veil," published in Manger's first collection, a maiden is spinning thread for her bridal veil. At midnight, when the thread runs out, seven aged women enter, and with the white thread of their hair they weave her a veil. At dawn, they depart, and the maiden turns to the mirror. Her face has turned white.

In the ballads Manger wrote after his twenties, there is a lighter touch, as if he had been released from a spell. While he continued to explore the irrational and to develop his ghostly, grotesque symbolism, he filled his later ballads with incongruous turns of phrase and rhythm, nuances of bittersweet irony, a homey Jewish warmth, and a respect for mundane exigencies as an escape from spiritual tension. He became more resigned to chaos, alienation, cruelty, and perplexity.

"The Ballad of Hanna'leh the Orphan" exemplifies this later style. An orphan girl is visited by her mother's grave. The tears she sheds on the grave, on her mother's instruction, sprout a wonderful husband. With scissors, the daughter snips him apart from the grave, and after she brushes off the worm dangling from his nose, they introduce themselves. As soon as they meet, they go to get married, and the mother's grave waits outside the officiating rabbi's house. On her mother's instruction, the daughter cries again—this time for a baby girl—and one sprouts from the grave. The groom then dismisses his dead mother-in-law, as "we no longer need you." The young family goes off, carrying a thin thread tied to the grave. With unsentimental compassion and delicately eccentric charm, the poet exposes the powerful secret fears and the twisted longings and loves of his heroes. With a folksy Yiddish playfulness that belies the tension latent in the ballad, he makes a dance of the strange collisions and collusions of instinct.

"THE BENT TREE"

A tragic sense pervades Manger's work, yet none of his works is tragedy. In "The Bent Tree," a child looks outside and sees birds flying away for the winter. He decides that he must become a bird. His mother warns him of the dangers, but he insists. Just as he is about to take flight, she rushes to bundle him up against the weather, from head to toe. He lifts his wings, about to fly, but he is now too heavy. All he can do is sing, "I look sadly in my Mama's/ Eyes, without a word./ It was her love that didn't let/ Me become a bird." What in real life is a bitterly tragic conflict is ameliorated in the poem by the enchantingly grotesque and comic action, by the fact that it is the frustrated child who expresses the generously tragic perspective of the final sentence, and by the poet's setting of the lyrics to a lullaby tune, so that they are sung (confessed?) by parents to their children.

RELIGIOUS INFLUENCES

Manger's folkloristic approach to family situations was in the tradition begun in the Book of Genesis, the collection of prose poems about sibling rivalries, marriage problems, and intergenerational relations that is the foundation of Jewish civilization. For adult Jewish men, the traditional course of study has been the interpretation and argumentation of the Talmud, the body of law that developed as an attempt to fix a detailed code of behavior based on the teachings of the Torah (the books of Moses, the first five books of the Old Testament). For Jewish women and children, the path along which the tradition developed has been the study of the Old Testament stories themselves and of the *Midrashim*, legends included in the Talmud, which embellish the original biblical texts. In Manger's religious education, the key influence was his mother, a woman who could read only haltingly and could not write at all. Her knowledge of the Bible came from the *Tsena Urena*, a sixteenth century Yiddish version of the Bible, adapted for women. The book is a rambling narrative of retellings of the original stories according to the *Midrashim*, interwoven with fairy tales, exhortations to piety, household advice, and anecdotes about modern-day heroes (such as Jewish tailors) and villains (such as Christian gentry). The characters in the *Tsena Urena* are portrayed with the quaint reverence of the rabbinic tradition, but with an intimacy and historical naïveté that presents them as if they were members of the reader's family several generations removed.

KHUMISH LIDER

With an imagination whose first literary influence was the *Tsena Urena*, Manger wrote his own *Midrashim*, his *Khumish Lider*, transporting the patriarchs to a nineteenth century Eastern European Jewish setting. With his wagon driver, Eliezer, Abraham rides with Isaac to the sacrifice:

> "Where are we riding to, Daddy?"
> "To Lashkev, to the Fair."
> "What are you going to buy me, Daddy,
> In Lashkev, at the Fair?"
> "A porcelain toy soldier,
> A trumpet and a drum,
> And some satin for a dress
> For Mama back at home. . . ."

Fully a third of the *Khumish Lider* is about women caught in a man's world: Abishag the Shunamite (five

ballads), Bathsheba, Ruth (eight ballads), Dinah, Jephthah's Daughter, and Hagar (three ballads). In one of the last-named ballads, Abraham dismisses his concubine, Hagar, the mother of his son Ishmael, at the instigation of his wife, Sarah. As Hagar packs her things to leave, she pauses to look at a straw summer hat, a silk apron, and some beads that Abraham gave her in better days. She sighs, "This must be what was meant for us;/ Ishmaelik'l, don't be scared . . . Such were the ways of the Patriarchs/ With their long and pious beards. . . ."

One month after its publication in 1935, the *Khumish Lider* was banned by Agudas Yisroel, the rabbinical council of Poland, as "poison for Jewish children" and "blasphemy against the People, Torah and God of Israel." From another perspective, Manger's accomplishment was to infuse the sacred stories with a sensitivity developed by a people's long and varied experience of living with them—a gift back to its source.

THE HOLOCAUST

For a Yiddish poet, and one who was so intimately attuned to the yearnings of his people, Manger wrote surprisingly little about the Holocaust. He told an interviewer in 1958 that much time would have to pass before hatred of the Germans and their helpers faded enough for artistic objectivity. In his few poetic attempts to face the destruction of his people and culture, he took two approaches: involving Jewish folk motifs and legendary figures in the reality and its aftermath, and bringing the horror down to the small scale of a personal and subjective view. The sad streak that had always run through his poetry grew more pronounced in the 1940's; the tone of some of his poems recalls the pessimism of Ecclesiastes, though Manger is more gentle. In his poetry, visionary experience prevails over sorrow. In poems that only obliquely show signs of struggle or historical awareness, he ekes enchanting meaning and music out of the quotidian. In the survey of Yiddish literature that appears in *The Jewish People: Past and Present* (an English-language reference work published between 1952 and 1955), Shmuel Niger, the preeminent Yiddish critic, referred to Manger as "a hopeless romantic"—an apt judgment, if taken as an affectionate tribute to the poet's childlike capacity for wonder.

OTHER MAJOR WORKS

LONG FICTION: *Dos Bukh fun Gan-Eden*, 1939 (*The Book of Paradise*, 1965).

PLAYS: *Hotzmakh Shpiel*, pr. 1936; *Megillah Lider*, 1936 (libretto; *The Megillah of Itzik Manger*, pr. 1965).

NONFICTION: *Noente Geshtaltn*, 1938.

MISCELLANEOUS: *Gezamlte Shriftn*, 1961; *Shriftn in Proze*, 1980; *The World According to Itzik: Selected Poetry and Prose*, 2002.

BIBLIOGRAPHY

Davin, Dan. *Closing Times*. New York: Oxford University Press, 1975. A collection of correspondence and reminiscences by several authors, including Manger.

Kahn, Yitzhok. *Portraits of Yiddish Writers*. Translated by Joseph Leftwich. New York: Vantage Press, 1979. A collection of biographical essays on Yiddish writers, including Manger.

Manger, Itzik. *The World According to Itzik. Selected Poetry and Prose*. Translated and edited by Leonard Wolf. Introduction by David G. Roskies and Leonard Wolf. New Haven, Conn.: Yale University Press, 2002. This selected collection of Manger's prose and poetry begins with an introduction by two experts on Manger that provides history, biography, and literary criticism.

Roskies, David G. "The Last of the Purim Players: Itzik Manger." *Prooftexts: A Journal of Jewish Literary History* 13, no. 3 (September, 1993): 211-235. A biographical and critical overview of Manger's life and work.

Sherman, Joseph, ed. *Writers in Yiddish*. Vol. 333 in *Dictionary of Literary Biography*. Detroit: Thomson Gale, 2007. Contains an essay on Manger, discussing his life and works.

David Maisel

JORGE MANRIQUE

Born: Paredes de Nava, Palencia, Castile (now in Spain); c. 1440
Died: Castle of Garci-Muñoz, Cuenca, Spain; 1479

PRINCIPAL POETRY

Coplas por la muerte de su padre, 1492 (wr. 1476; *Coplas on the Death of His Father*, 1833)

OTHER LITERARY FORMS

Jorge Manrique (mon-REE-kay) is known only for his poetry.

ACHIEVEMENTS

Jorge Manrique was a major Spanish poet. His *Coplas on the Death of His Father* is celebrated as a philosophical and theological reflection on the brevity and fragility of life. It is perhaps the most famous elegy written in Spanish and is still read in the twenty-first century.

BIOGRAPHY

It is generally believed that Jorge Manrique de Lara y Figueroa was born in the town of Paredes de Nava in about 1440; however, some scholars conjecture that Manrique's birthplace was Segura de la Sierra. Manrique's father, Rodrigo Manrique, was the count (*conde*) of Paredes de Nava, constable (*condestable*) of Castile, grand master (*maestre*) of the Order of Santiago, and one of the principal figures of the Kingdom of Castile in the fifteenth century. Manrique followed a great line of forebears who had distinguished themselves in their literary virtuosity. He was the great-nephew of Iñigo López de Mendoza (the marqués of Santillana); nephew of Gómez Manrique, the famous soldier and poet; and a descendent of Pero López de Ayala, the famed author of the *Libro Rimado de Palacio* (c. 1378-1403). Manrique's mother died while he was still a child, and the boy was raised largely by his father in the courtly tradition of humanism and the arts of war. Like his forebears, the young Manrique became a soldier, a courtier, and a literary figure.

Politically, the Manrique family allied itself with the Infante Alfonso, brother to King Henry IV and a pretender to the throne of Castile. In 1470, Manrique married Guiomar, one of his stepmother's younger sisters. Upon Alfonso's death, the Manriques took up the cause of Isabella, Henry's half-sister, and denied their support to Henry's daughter, Juana ("La Beltraneja"). Manrique fought at his father's side in support of Isabella in numerous clashes with Henry's supporters, such as those at Montizón, where in 1474, he distinguished himself for his bravery; Calatrava; Uclés; and at the castle of Garci-Muñoz, where, according to the historian Hernando del Pulgar, he was killed in battle in 1479. Some scholars, such as Jerónimo Zurita, believe that Manrique survived the battle only to die several days later in Santa María del Campo de Rus. It is believed that both Manrique and his father, Rodrigo, are buried in the cathedral of Uclés, in the province of Cuenca, although this has not been scientifically verified.

Analysis

Jorge Manrique's secular verse, which mostly treats of love, is typical of fourteenth and fifteenth century courtly poetry. Modeled in large measure after Ovid's *Ars amatoria* (c. 2 B.C.E.; *Art of Love*, 1612) and following the great tradition of Spanish adaptations of this work, most notably Juan Ruiz's *Libro de buen amor* (c. 1330; *The Book of Good Love*, 1933), Manrique's work was published in *cancioneros*—collections of poetry—with verse by other poets. Most of his poems are located in Hernando del Castillo's celebrated *Cancionero general* (1511). No autograph manuscript of Manrique's work is known to exist. Manrique's love poetry was not published separately until the latter half of the sixteenth century and not in its entirety. Even in the sixteenth century, critics recognized that Manrique's greatest contribution to Spanish literary history lay in his *Coplas on the Death of His Father*. Manrique's love poetry is typical of late-medieval and early-Renaissance works in its return to classical allusions and its pagan outlook on life, especially in questions of love. It was strongly influenced by the Provençal poets of southern France, whose work had become popular among nobles and in courtly circles in northern Spain during the late twelfth and thirteenth centuries. Manrique was a man of his day and, as such, embodied the great tradition of the courtier—the man of arms and letters, of war and of liberal arts.

Love poetry

Manrique's love poetry was published in *cancioneros*, or collections of poems by various writers. His composition, "De Don Jorge Manrique quexándose del dios del amor, y cómo razona el uno con el otro" (of Jorge Manrique complaining to the god of love, and how the one reasons with the other") is reminiscent of Ruiz's rendition of the dispute between the Arcipreste and don Amor in the *Libro de buen amor*. Manrique's composition shows no particular innovation, in that he follows the late-medieval and Renaissance convention of a return to a classical vision of love that depends on the actions of don Amor (Sir Love). In Manrique's case, the "debate" shows a curious mixture of the pagan and the Christian, which is also typical of fifteenth century Spanish love poetry. The poetic voice, who seeks love but does not find it, complains to don Amor that he has promised much and given nothing. In each instance, don Amor responds to the accusations leveled against him, urging that the "plaintiff" appeal his case to a "higher God" who can judge them both. The "plaintiff" doubts that God will help him:

> That high God without equal
> well do I know that he is the mightiest
> but, with my erring,
> I have made Him very upset

Other poems are directed to Fortune ("A la Fortuna"; this may also be understood as fate), a blind force that annihilates the hopes and dreams of lovers and soldiers alike, bringing all to a bitter end.

Coplas on the Death of His Father

Manrique's father, Rodrigo, died in Ocaña in 1476 after a protracted struggle with facial cancer, sending the young poet into a state of psychological and spiritual distress. Manrique's creative response to this disaster is the celebrated *Coplas on the Death of His Father*, his greatest work, and one of the most famous works of the entire Hispanic literary canon. The coplas are composed of forty strophes of *pie quebrado* verse (two eight-syllable lines followed by a four-syllable line, repeated four times per strophe) that follow *rima perfecta* (full rhyme) of *abc-abc-def-def*. The forty strophes can be divided into four thematic sections. The theme of the first section, strophes 1-15, is a general consideration of the shortness and purpose of life on Earth (in Latin, the *topos*, or literary commonplace, is called *tempus fugit*). The second, strophes 16-24, deals with the question of where all the great and powerful people of the past have gone (in Latin, this *topos* is called *ubi sunt*). The third section, strophes 25-37, is a panegyric to Rodrigo Manrique. The fourth section, strophes 38-40, deals with Rodrigo's acceptance of death and his prayer to Jesus, as well as a description of Rodrigo as an example to others. The first strophe of *Coplas on the Death of His Father* is one of the most famous in all of Spanish literature:

> Recuerde el alma dormida,
> abiue el seso e despierte
> contemplando
> cómo se passa la vida
> cómo se viene la muerte
> tan callando,
> quánd presto se va el plazer,
> cómo, después de acordado,
> da dolor;
> como, a nuestro parescer,
> qualquiere tiempo passado
> fue mejor.

> Let the sleepy soul remember,
> let the mind come to life and awaken
> contemplating
> how life passes by,
> how death comes
> creeping up so silently,
> how quickly pleasure fades,
> how, after being remembered,
> it brings us pain
> how, in our eyes,
> any time in the past
> was better.

This strophe sets the theme for the entire poem, namely, that time and life slip away before one knows it, and thus, every minute is to be savored and used wisely. While Manrique adduces two great topoi of classical and medieval Western literature, *tempus fugit*

and *ubi sunt*, he locates them squarely in the realm of Roman Catholic theology. Manrique uses the Spanish of his day, which differs significantly from contemporary Spanish. Note the use of "u" for "v" in "abiue," the double consonant in "passa," the "z" for "c" in "placer," the "sc" for "c" in "parescer," and the use of "q" with "uá" in "quánd"; unusual also is the phrase "cómo se viene la muerte/ tan callando" and the use of the medieval form "seso" for "mind."

Manrique employs a simple, yet beautiful, metaphor to speak of the endless movement of time and of people's lives toward death: "Nuestras vidas son los ríos/ que van a dar en la mar" ("Our lives are rivers/ that will empty into the sea"). This evocation of nature is at once filled with the beauty of creation, the inexorableness of the "flow" of time, and a recognition that human beings are merely a small part of a much bigger world. It is interesting to note that Manrique uses the feminine form, *la mar* (the sea), rather than the more common masculine form, *el mar*, a convention often employed by native speakers to show tenderness and affection for the ocean. The metaphor is particularly moving in that Manrique applies this form of endearment to the sea that is "el morir" (death) in the following line. Indeed, as the poet explains, this sea (death) is the great leveler that erases all differences between the great and the small, the rich and the poor.

In the fifth copla, Manrique presents the metaphor of life as a road that leads to everlasting life, the kingdom of heaven, where there are no worries and where people will find rest. The poet urges people to hurry along the road of their present lives, so as to reach the goal of their eternal reward without delay:

> Este mundo es el camino
> para el otro, qu'es morada
> sin pesar;
> mas cumple tener buen tino
> para andar esta jornada
> sin errar;
> partimos quand nascemos,
> andamos mientra viuimos,
> y llegamos
> al tiempo que fenecemos:
> assí que quando morimos
> descansamos.

This world is a road
to the other, that is a dwelling place
without worry;
it is well to move quickly
in making this journey
without erring;
we leave when we are born,
we travel while we live,
and we arrive
at the time when we die:
such that when we die
we rest.

The *Coplas on the Death of His Father* are celebrated for their lyrical beauty, their vivid images and examples from history, their directly stated message, and their clear affirmation of the Roman Catholic understanding of the present life as a time of preparation for the eternal life to come. Manrique's praise of his father as a model Catholic courtier is heartfelt, endearing, and a singularly powerful confession of faith in an age of great religious and intellectual confusion in Spain.

BIBLIOGRAPHY

Darst, David. "Poetry and Poetics in Jorge Manrique's *Coplas por la muerte de su padre*." *Medievalia et Humanistica* 13 (1985): 197-206. A brief but valuable study of the medieval attitudes and poetic theories at work in Manrique's work.

Domínguez, Frank. "Body and Soul: Jorge Manrique's *Coplas por la muerte de su padre*." *Hispania* 84, no. 1 (2001): 1-10. A brief review of the theological question of the relationship between the body and the soul, as this is presented in the Manrique's work.

_____. "Jorge Manrique (circa 1440-21 April 1479)." In *Castilian Writers, 1400-1500*, edited by Frank Domínguez and George Greenia. Detroit: Gale, 2004. A general study of the life and works of Manrique, written by one of the best authorities to publish in English on the subject.

_____. *Love and Remembrance: The Poetry of Jorge Manrique*. Lexington: University of Kentucky Press, 1988. This study of Manrique's works is thorough and carefully researched and is among the most important studies of the subject in English.

Grossman, Edith, trans. *The Golden Age: Poems of the Spanish Renaissance*. New York: W. W. Norton, 2006. This anthology contains a translation of Manrique's most famous work, along with information about the poet. An introduction by Grossman and one by poet Billy Collins provide context for understanding Monrique.

Kennedy, Kristin. "Fame, Memory, and Literary Legacy: Jorge Manrique and the *Coplas por la muerte de su padre*." In *Negotiating Heritage: Memories of the Middle Ages*, edited by Mette B. Bruun and Stephanie Glaser. Turnhout, Belgium: Brépols, 2008. This article is helpful in understanding the complex relationship between the medieval topoi (commonplaces) of fame and memory as these are expressed through the cultural patrimony of Christian literature.

Krause, Anna. *Jorge Manrique and the Cult of Death in the Cuatrocientos*. Berkeley: University of California Press, 1937. One of the earliest full-length studies in English of Manrique's major work, situating the coplas in the literary and theological context of fifteenth century Spain.

Montgomery, Thomas. "Jorge Manrique and the Dynamics of Grieving." *Hispania* 18, no. 3 (1995): 483-490. This brief study seeks to go beyond the study of theological aspects of Manrique's work so as to understand it as an expression of Manrique's grief at the loss of his father.

Mark DeStephano
(including original translations)

ALESSANDRO MANZONI

Born: Milan, Lombardy, Austria (now in Italy);
    March 7, 1785
Died: Milan, Italy; May 22, 1873

PRINCIPAL POETRY
"Il trionfo della libertà," 1801
Sermoni, 1801-1804
"A Francesco Lomonaco," 1802
"Ode," 1802-1803

"L'Adda," 1803

"In morte di Carlo Imbonati," 1805-1806

"Urania," 1808-1809

Inni sacri, 1812-1815 (*The Sacred Hymns*, 1904)

"Il cinque maggio," 1821 ("The Napoleonic Ode," 1904)

"Marzo 1821," 1821, 1848

OTHER LITERARY FORMS

Alessandro Manzoni (mond-ZOH-nee) is remembered chiefly for a single work, *I promessi sposi* (1827, 1840-1842; *The Betrothed*, 1828, 1951)—his only novel. He was, however, a prolific writer of astonishing range and intellectual depth. Manzoni was a historian, the author of such works as the *Discorso sopra alcuni punti della storia longobardica in Italia* (1822), the *Lettre à Alphonse de Lamartine* (1848), and *La storia della colonna infame* (1842; *The Column of Infamy*, 1964), which accompanied the 1842 edition of *The Betrothed*. He was also a writer of religious and philosophical works, including *Lettre à Victor Cousin* (1829), *Dell'invenzione* (1850), and *Osservazioni sulla morale cattolica* (1819), and a philologist, author of *Sulla lingua italiana* (1850) and *Dell'unità della lingua e dei mezzi di diffonderla* (1868). His bibliography includes many more works, among them volumes of literary criticism such as *Lettera sul romanticismo* (1846) and *Del romanzo storico* (1845), and two historical tragedies, much admired by Johann Wolfgang von Goethe and Charles-Augustin de Sainte-Beuve, *Il conte di Carmagnola* (pb. 1820; *Count of Carmagnola*, 2002) and *Adelchi* (pr., pb. 1822; English translation, 2002). Finally, his published correspondence, *Epistolario* (1882), makes fascinating reading.

ACHIEVEMENTS

Alessandro Manzoni emerged as a dominant figure during his long and extraordinarily productive life, particularly on the Italian peninsula. His novel, *The Betrothed*, remains one of the greatest novels of the Western world, not merely of the 1800's but of all time. It is a compendium of various novelistic styles and genres, including the historical, in which context the narrative unfolds from a humble beginning concerning two peasants to epic dimensions involving a whole world in moral and physical turmoil. With his tragedy *Adelchi*, which recalls William Shakespeare's *Hamlet, Prince of Denmark* (pr. c. 1600-1601) and *Henry IV* (*Part I*, pr. c. 1597-1598; *Part II*, pr. 1598), Manzoni reached the apogee of Christian fatalism in the theater. *The Column of Infamy* is an uncategorizable work that offers psychological insights into the evil of torture; its seventeenth century characterizations reveal a novelist's skill. Finally, as a poet, his fame rests primarily on his religious poetry, *The Sacred Hymns*, an occasional political piece such as "Marzo 1821" (March, 1821) and the "historical" ode on Napoleon, "The Napoleonic Ode."

BIOGRAPHY

Alessandro Francesco Tommaso Antonio Manzoni belongs to Lombardy, in whose capital he was born on March 7, 1785. His putative father, Count Pietro, and his mother, Giulia—the daughter of the distinguished jurist and political economist Cesare Beccaria—were incompatible and were legally separated seven years after Manzoni's birth. Though as a child he studied in various religious schools in and around his native region, and though as a youth he suffered from excessive shyness, he developed strong sympathies with the libertarian ideas of the French Revolution, as the Jacobin flavor of his 1801 poem, "Il trionfo della libertà," clearly indicates. His mother had run off to Paris in 1795 with her new lover, Carlo Imbonati, and the young Manzoni accepted an invitation, ten years later, to join them there. He had traveled in the meantime, but Paris seemed like a shiny goal. While there, he came in contact with many liberal philosophers and politicians, a number of whom (including the historian Claude Fauriel, with whom he formed a lifetime friendship) contributed significantly to his intellectual development and to his experience of the world. He wrote some poetry during these years—"L'Adda," *Sermoni*, and "Urania" (on the civilizing virtues of the arts)—which revealed his lingering classical leanings; he also wrote an elegy in which he began to come into his own as a poet, "In morte di Carlo Imbonati," for his mother's lover, who had died when Manzoni arrived in Paris, and had left him a goodly inheritance.

In 1808, Manzoni married Henriette Blondel, the lovely sixteen-year-old daughter of a Genevese banker,

Calvinist by faith. Always attracted to matters of the spirit, Manzoni found Henriette's strong sense of religious devotion a stimulus to regain acquaintance with his original Catholic faith, and it was not long before he underwent a conversion in which several Jansenist clerics played an important role. His wife switched to Catholicism as well, and his mother returned to it after many years. From this point on, back in Lombardy, Manzoni led a long life of semiretirement between Milan and his country retreat in Brusuglio, where he performed a number of agricultural experiments. His conversion inspired him to write a series of religious poems, among them, in 1812-1813, *The Sacred Hymns*: "La resurrezione" ("The Resurrection"); "Il nome di Maria" ("The Name of Mary"); and "Il natale" ("The Nativity") followed in 1815 by "La passione" ("The Passion") and in 1822 by "La pentecoste" ("The Pentecost"). He began *The Betrothed* in 1821, and composed "The Napoleonic Code" and "Marzo 1821," his two finest compositions in verse apart from the exceptionally beautiful choruses in *Adelchi*.

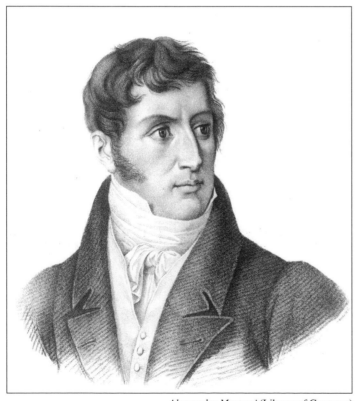

Alessandro Manzoni (Library of Congress)

With these works, Manzoni's significant poetic period came to an end. What followed was a long list of intellectual works—historical, philosophical, and linguistic—in each of which his scholarly gift for documentation and analysis, to say nothing of his perpetually gentle, serene way of arguing his subjects, made a profound impression on his readers. His novel occupied a good part of his time as well, from 1823, when its first version was published under the title of *Fermo e Lucia*, to 1827, when its next version appeared as *Gli sposi promessi*, and finally to 1842, when the final version, polished in the pure Tuscan idiom and titled *The Betrothed*, came off the presses. *The Column of Infamy* accompanied this publication.

Such an apparently serene, productive life was not shielded from sorrow. One of the harshest blows came in 1833 with the death of Manzoni's beloved wife; eight years later, his mother died (his father had died before). Manzoni remarried, in 1837, but his second wife, Teresa Borri, died in 1861. Of his eleven children, he was survived by only two; even his son-in-law, the well-known author Massimo D'Azeglio, died before him, as did the celebrated theological philosopher Antonio Rosmini, who had been one of the most important intellectual mentors of Manzoni's later years.

Many honors were accorded to Manzoni, though in general he shunned them—indeed, refused them in many instances. Maximilian of Austria, John Henry Newman, and William Ewart Gladstone wanted to be counted among his acquaintances. He turned down the French Legion of Honor, the grand duke of Tuscany's Order of Merit, and a deputyship in the Piedmontese Chamber, but he did accept a lifetime pension from King Victor Emanuel II, senatorship in the newly founded kingdom, and the honorific Roman citizenship. Italians up and down the peninsula looked to him as a national conscience, as he lent his name to several important political actions of his day, and withdrew it symbolically from others: For example, he refused to consider Eugène de Beauharnais for king of Italy (1814), rejected Austrian honors, and withdrew from participation in Milan's celebrations for the Bourbon Ferdinand I (1838). In 1848, he signed a petition to induce Carlo Alberto to intervene in the north, and in 1860, his vote helped to effect the transfer of the national capital from Florence to Rome.

Little wonder that when he died in Milan on May 22, 1873, of cerebral meningitis, Manzoni was honored by a state funeral and was mourned by all Italy. The occasion inspired Giuseppe Verdi to resume work on his *Messa da requiem*, which was performed, dedicated to Manzoni, one year later to the day. The musical remembrance represents a just tribute.

ANALYSIS

The product of a classical culture, Alessandro Manzoni held the written word in high regard: the fitting expression, the eloquent turn of phrase, the correct vocabulary. Poetry, which emphasized all these things, was seen as the most fitting genre for artistic utterance. More than this, however, poetry was to be concerned with moral and civic problems rather than indulging itself in languid lyricism and autobiography. Hence, Manzoni's early verses contained barbs against the Church, tyrants, poetasters, the decadent rich, unworthy teachers, and dissolute women. In part, the impetus for this manner came from idealistic pronouncements made during the Napoleonic era (concerning justice, reason, human rights, artistic value, and civic duty) that were never translated into practice, a double standard that easily aroused the indignation of a youthfully vigorous poet.

Although in the background of Manzoni's poetry, besides a list of French authors headed by Voltaire, one finds Alfonso Varano, Giuseppe Parini, Vittorio Alfieri, Ugo Foscolo, and the early revolutionary Vincenzo Monti, the spirit of imitation never guided Manzoni's pen. Conscious of this, in the 1802 sonnet "Alla musa," he bids the deity to show him "new paths."

Manzoni's best poetry exudes a Christian ethos. Hence Goethe's praise, which went beyond Manzoni's "new" poetic manner and his "simplicity of feeling"; Goethe extolled the poet's "boldness of genius, metaphors, transitions," Manzoni's way of being "Christian without fanaticism, Roman Catholic without sanctimo-

niousness, zealous without hardness." Put otherwise, Manzoni's art was an inspired function of his humanitarianism.

"IL TRIONFO DELLA LIBERTÀ"

Manzoni's first significant piece was his still somewhat classical "Il trionfo della libertà," written after the peace of Lunéville (1801), in four cantos and hendecasyllabic tercets, heavy with references to ancient heroes and myths. Typically pessimistic in approach, the poem at one point considers the figure of the French General Louis-Charles Desaix, who died fighting for the independence of an indifferent land, where he lay a "barbarian . . . foreign corpse." Liberty's "triumph" is limited by the extent of the crimes committed in her name. A similar lament echoes in "A Francesco Lomonaco," a political sonnet chastising Italy for not extolling the heroic martyr for liberty—who, to make matters worse, was even exiled from his native Naples. The true sense of liberty, therefore, cannot be imposed from without; it must grow from within.

Perhaps beauty, instead of liberty, may emerge as the noblest ideal—beauty in a woman of moral and spiritual perfection, "whose sweet mouth conceals a pure smile wherein speaks the soul." This is found in Manzoni's Vergilian "Ode," though late in the poem, he turns incongruously to thoughts of bloodstained Italy. He found it hard to relinquish his youthful pessimism, which also colors a group of four sarcastic poems gathered under the title of *Sermoni*: the Horatian "A Giovan Battista Pagani," the Petronian satire on the enriched plebeian "Panegirico di Trimalcione," the invective against poetasters "Della poesia," and the pungently bitter "love" poem "A Delia." Manzoni blames individuals rather than institutions for a corrupt society in which women become playthings of lust, parlor games mask eroticism, inept poets recite "hard verses," and lovers chase after "incautious virgins"—a society symbolized by rich Trimalchio's vulgar ostentation. A brief attempt to break out of the pessimistic mold, when in 1803 he wrote an idyll on his beloved Lombard river, "L'Adda," found Manzoni this time erring in the direction of stiltedness, bound as he was to classical formulas in composing elegiac verses. The same rigidity appears in his mythologico-philosophical poem of 1808-1809, "Urania," a disquisition on the moral and utilitarian value of poetry, which is so oratorical that he himself later described it to Fauriel as "hateful."

"In morte di Carlo Imbonati"

Manzoni had, however, gone to Paris in 1805, and his best poem of that time, "In morte di Carlo Imbonati," reveals greater detachment and intellectual depth, avoiding the polemical and aggressive manner of his other pieces of the time. The young poet, very devoted to his mother, justifies on the grounds of pure love her cohabitation with Imbonati, defends it against the petty gossip of Milanese society, and places her consort in a paternal role, delivering a Polonius-like counsel to Manzoni, who must be guided by feeling and meditation:

> with little
> be content; never bend your eyes
> from your goal; with things human
> experiment only so much as you need
> to care not for them; never become slave;
> with the base never make peace; never betray
> the holy Truth; nor proffer ever a word
> that applauds vice, or virtue derides.

This poem, along with "A parteneide," was the last of Manzoni's early lyrics; it gave evidence that his invocation to the Muse to find "new ways" was about to be realized. He put aside indignant resentments, violent satire, and rhetorical formulas, and his postconversion poetry bears the imprint of an artist who has gained control both of himself and of his medium. To a friend, Manzoni wrote: "[Verse is] a form which above all likes to express what each one of us can find inside himself, but something no one yet has thought of saying, and which is capable only of rendering those thoughts that develop along with it, and mold themselves on it, as it were, as they are born. . . ."

The Sacred Hymns

Manzoni's new mastery is evident in the religious poems gathered under the title *The Sacred Hymns*. Though the collection is uneven, it is informed by a genuine and compelling poetic voice, and its concerns prefigure those of Manzoni's great novel. The civic and moral concerns that animated his early poems are elevated to universal ethical views on society. As Francesco De Sanctis has commented, *The Sacred Hymns* offer an evangelized version of the triad of liberty, equality, and fraternity. Because of their pervasively biblical tone, they may sound more didactic than intended, for in his mature years Manzoni avoided the hortatory manner; he placed revelation above inculcation, and in this he differed from those such as Parini, Alfieri, Foscolo, and Victor Hugo, who believed in the sacerdotal function of the poet.

Fittingly, the first of the *The Sacred Hymns* is called "The Resurrection," six octosyllabic lines capped by a final heptasyllabic line, giving each stanza a liturgical gait, consistent with Christ's victory over sin and death: "Like a strong man exhilarated/ The Lord was reawakened." Occasional faulty imagery and brusque changes of pace, coupled with an inconsistently dramatic representation, mar the genuine sense of *gaudeamus* that the messenger-poet wishes to convey. "The Name of Mary," the second hymn, is, by comparison, musically fluent. Three hendecasyllables and one heptasyllable per stanza in alternate rhyme make for compelling sweetness (despite a rather incongruous final image) and comfort in the eternal mother: "In the fears of his dark waking/ The child names You. . . ." In typical fashion, Manzoni is always alive to human miseries, fears, and needs. This spirit underlies the next poem, "The Nativity," which responds to the query of what would have happened if Christ had not come:

> . . . the people
> Know not the child who's been born;
> But . . .
> in that humble repose,
> . . . inside that dust inclosed,
> They'll recognize their King.

Manzoni's worldview centers on the key word "humble," and through it the angels rending the night to sing of the holy Nativity acquire inspiring visibility. This final setting of gladsome song contrasts successfully with the opening metaphor of a boulder plunging into a valley. Here again, the poet changes the metrical scheme—seven lines of eight, seven, eight, seven, seven, seven, and six syllables respectively with rhymes of lines 2 with 4, line 5 with 6, and line 7 of one stanza with line 7 of the next—as he does, too, in the subsequent hymn, "The Passion"—octaves composed of two groups of four lines in a syllabic pattern of ten, ten, ten, and nine, rhyming *abacbddc*. More sermonic and therefore less engaging than the rest, the hymn still gathers noticeable power when a choral prayer invokes God's forgiveness for those who trespassed against Jesus:

> Cease now your tremendous anger;
> And . . . may that Blood descend all over them;
> May it be but a rain of mild bathing;
> We all erred . . .

"THE PENTECOST"

These hymns, however, fade before the beauty of "The Pentecost," which was begun in 1817, completed in 1822, and revised in March, 1855. Perhaps because it took him so long to arrive at a final version of this hymn, Manzoni never completed the projected series of twelve. As with the poetry of Saint John of the Cross, the distinction between literature and theology disappears when feeling and meditation blend and when concept translates into image with lyrical intensity:

> Oh Spirit! in supplication
> Before your solemn altars;
> Alone through inauspicious woods;
> Wandering o'er desert seas;
> From Andes chilled to Lebanon,
> From Eire to bristling Haiti;
> Scattered over every shore,
> Through You, singlehearted,
> We implore you
>
> . . . . . .
>
> Breathe inside the ineffable
> Smiling lips of our children.

The eight- and seven-syllable octaves with a rhyme scheme similar to that of "The Nativity" release Italian poetry (with a helping hand from Giacomo Leopardi) from the traditional manner of versification established by Petrarch, Torquato Tasso, and the Arcadians. At the same time, Manzoni strikes a very influential personal note with his unobtrusive pessimism, his reasoned resignation.

"MARZO 1821"

Resignation is a component of Manzonian serenity, his most attractive quality, apparent even in his great political poems, in which it is clear that all nations and all individuals share in the common experience of suffering. "Marzo 1821," consisting of thirteen eight-line stanzas with a rhyme scheme of *abbcdeec*, was written when the Piedmontese crossed the Ticino River and rushed to the aid of the Lombards, whose insurrection was aimed at Austrian oppression; the poem was dedicated to Theodor Koerner, the German poet-martyr for freedom from Napoleon who had died in the Battle of Gadebusch (1813). The ode appeals not only to Italians but also to all civilized nations to rise for freedom. Even so, the oppressor is not challenged with hatred or invective; justice dons the cloak of universal love, as in *Le mie prigioni* (1832; *My Prisons*, 1836), by Manzoni's contemporary Silvio Pellico, who found the same transcending answer to the horrors of the Spielberg dungeons where he had been thrown.

"THE NAPOLEONIC ODE"

Manzoni's finest poem is the historical ode "The Napoleonic Ode," marking the day Napoleon died on St. Helena. These eighteen stanzas of six lines each (with rhymes on lines 2 and 4 and a pattern involving the last line of each stanza) elicited the admiration of Goethe, always a great promoter of Manzoni's poetry, and publication in the periodical *Über Kunst und Althertum*. The poem stands above all other European expressions of celebration or criticism of the emperor because the poet is determined not to pass moral judgment, preferring to let history do the judging on the basis of a central question: "Was his true glory?" Napoleon's life embraced triumph, peril, flight, victory, sovereignty, exile, "Twice low in the dust,/ Twice high on the altar," straddling two centuries and two eras. The warring despot turns into the sorrowing prisoner who remembers in a series of images all his exhilarations: "A heap of memories!" In the light of such ephemerality, temporal glories appear hollow, and the imposing emperor has reached the brink of despair, while a superior force looks on, symbolized by the crucifix that "On the deserted bedding/ He placed next to himself." In a string of moving, lyrical, and reflective passages, the historical view modulates into poetic vision, a unique contribution to the literature on Napoleon.

OTHER MAJOR WORKS

LONG FICTION: *I promessi sposi*, 1827, 1840-1842 (*The Betrothed*, 1828, 1951).

PLAYS: *Il conte di Carmagnola*, pb. 1820 (*Count of Carmagnola*, 2002); *Adelchi*, pr., pb. 1822 (English translation, 2002); *Alessando Manzoni: Two Plays*, 2002 (includes *Count of Carmagnola* and *Adelchi*).

NONFICTION: *Osservazioni sulla morale cattolica*, 1819; *Discorso sopra alcuni punti della storia longobardica in Italia*, 1822; *Lettre à M. C*** sur l'unité de temps et de lieu dans la tragédie*, 1823; *Lettre à Victor Cousin*, 1829; *La storia della colonna infame*, 1842 (*The Column of Infamy*, 1964); *Del romanzo storico*, 1845; *Lettera sul romanticismo*, 1846; *Lettre à Alphonse de Lamartine*, 1848; *Dell'invenzione*, 1850; *Sulla lingua italiana*, 1850; *Dell'unità della lingua e dei mezzi di diffonderla*, 1868; *Lettera intorno al vocabolario*, 1868; *Epistolario*, 1882; *Saggio comparativo su la rivoluzione francese del 1789 e la rivoluzione italiana del 1859*, 1889; *Sentir Messa*, 1923.

BIBLIOGRAPHY

Barricelli, Gian Piero. *Alessandro Manzoni*. Boston: Twayne, 1976. An introductory biography and critical study of selected works by Manzoni. Includes bibliographic references and an index.

Colquhoun, Archibald. *Manzoni and His Times: A Biography of the Author of "The Betrothed" ("I promessi sposi")*. 1954. Reprint. Westport, Conn.: Hyperion Press, 1979. One of the basic resources in English, this biography is by one of the best-known scholars of Italian literature. Illustrated.

Ferlito, Susanna F. *Topographies of Desire: Manzoni, Cultural Practices, and Colonial Scars*. New York: Peter Lang, 2000. Drawing on a wide range of current disciplinary debates in the fields of comparative politics, anthropology, cultural studies, and comparative literature, this book examines how Manzoni's French and Italian writing produced differences between cultural discourses in a nineteenth century Europe that was not yet thought of as "naturally" divided between nation-states. Bibliography and index.

Ginzburg, Natalia. *The Manzoni Family*. Translated by Marie Evans. New York: Arcade, 1989. An especially good background study of the tradition and the history out of which Manzoni's work was created. Ginzburg includes a family tree, a list of characters, and a map of Italy in the Risorgimento.

Matteo, Sante, and Larry H. Peer, eds. *The Reasonable Romantic: Essays on Alessandro Manzoni*. New York: Peter Lang, 1986. An anthology of seventeen original essays (a few using deconstruction techniques) written by new and established Manzoni scholars to introduce Manzoni. The first section is a general introduction, followed by sections on the poet and Romanticism, language, history, and religion.

Pallotta, Augustus. *Alessandro Manzoni: A Critical Bibliography—1950-2000*. Pisa, Italy: F. Serra, 2007. A bibliography of Manzoni's works and works about him. Contains a section on Manzoni's reception outside Italy.

Wall, Bernard. *Alessandro Manzoni*. New Haven, Conn.: Yale University Press, 1954. Chapters on the life and times, the poet and dramatist, *The Betrothed* and its place in literature, and controversial issues: Manzoni's religion, the problem of language, and Romanticism. Provides biographical and bibliographical notes.

Jean-Pierre Barricelli

MARIE DE FRANCE

Born: Île de France; c. 1150
Died: England(?); c. 1215

PRINCIPAL POETRY

Lais, c. 1167 (*Lays of Marie de France*, 1911; better known as *The Lais of Marie de France*, 1978)

Ysopet, after 1170 (*Medieval Fables*, 1983; also known as *Fables*)

La Vie seinte Audrée, after 1179 (*The Life of Saint Audrey*, 2006)

Espurgatoire Saint Patriz, 1208-1215 (translation of *Tractatus de purgatorio Sancti Patricii*, attributed to Henry of Saltrey)

OTHER LITERARY FORMS

In addition to two collections of short narrative poems, *The Lais of Marie de France* and *Fables*, Marie de France (mah-REE duh FRAHNS) translated a long poem, the *Espurgatoire Saint Patriz* (purgatory of Saint Patrick). The Latin original, *Tractatus de purgatorio Sancti Patricii* (1208), has been attributed to Henry of Saltrey. Although the particular version Marie translated is no longer extant, virtually all its lines are to be found in surviving manuscripts. The translation is a faithful one, to which a brief prologue and epilogue (and only a few "asides" or editorial comments) have been added. Because it is a translation and not an original work, its chief interest—if it is properly attributed to Marie de France—is in the testimony it bears to the poet's thorough knowledge of Latin and to her concern, expressed in the epilogue, that the treatise be accessible to the layperson. The narrative also bears some resemblance in form to the genre of the *roman* (romance), which was becoming increasingly popular in this period. Saint Patrick's "purgatory" is a cave on an island in Lough Derg, Donegal, which to this day still draws pilgrims; it was said to have been revealed to Saint Patrick in answer to a prayer, and those who enter it hope to witness or experience the sufferings of the souls in purgatory. The treatise translated by Marie describes the adventures of a particular knight, Owein, who entered the cave and was tempted by demons but was saved by invoking the name of Christ. One motif is of particular interest to students of medieval romance: To cross the river of Hell, Owein must resort to a high and dangerously narrow bridge, which widens as soon as he has the courage to start across. Lancelot, the hero of Chrétien de Troyes's romance *Lancelot: Ou, Le Chevalier à la charrette* (c. 1168; *Lancelot: Or, The Knight of the Cart*, 1913), must cross a similarly narrow bridge in order to rescue the abducted Queen Guinevere; once he has crossed it, the lions who seemed to be guarding the farther end have disappeared. In contrast to most romances, however (and in contrast to Marie's own *The Lais of Marie de France*), the *Espurgatoire Saint Patriz* involves no profane love story; its inspiration is purely religious.

Other works have been attributed to Marie de France. The current scholarly consensus, however, is that none of them is hers, with the possible exception of another translation, *The Life of Saint Audrey*, which would confirm her interest in religious themes.

ACHIEVEMENTS

Marie de France was probably not the first woman to write poetry in the French vernacular. She is, however, the earliest whose name has been recorded. In fact, she is one of the few twelfth century poets, male or female, whose names are known. This is partly because she wished to be remembered; thus, she "signed" her works by naming herself in their opening or closing lines. It is almost certain that she is also the Marie mentioned by a contemporary, Denis Piramus; if so, she was already well known and "much praised" in the aristocratic circles of her day, where her lays were often read aloud. (Piramus's further observation that her stories were "not at all true" may even indicate some jealousy of her popularity.)

Marie's originality is harder to gauge, for although she claims to retell "Breton lays," there are no direct parallels to her tales in extant Celtic literature. She gives Celtic names to most characters and places and uses recognizable Celtic motifs (such as the fairy lover, the magic boat, and the hunt for a white animal), but her plots hinge on affairs of the heart, and her characters bear a closer resemblance to those of twelfth century romances than to the heroes and heroines of Celtic folk literature. One critic, Lucien Foulet, has gone so far as to argue that Marie herself invented the genre of the narrative lay. Though scholarly debate in this area is still lively, most would reject Foulet's hypothesis as too extreme; there are courtly lays not by Marie, and even relative dates are difficult to establish for this period. Nevertheless, few modern critics would argue with Foulet's emphasis on the conscious art with which Marie shaped her material, wherever she may have found it. Each of the twelve lays is a carefully constructed whole; the tales are told with great economy of means, yet they include nuances of feeling and of moral character that can be quite delicate. Some critics, notably Edgar Sienaert, have seen a structure in the collection as a whole, and most will grant it a thematic unity, though there is disagreement on the nature and import of this unity. Because of the uncertainty about Marie's originality, nineteenth century critics tended to give her less than her due, but no contemporary scholar will deny that she was one of the major poets of her age.

BIOGRAPHY

Of the life of Marie de France, nothing can be said with certainty; her name is known because she included it in her works, but her identity is otherwise obscure. It is probable that she was born in France, in Île de France (the region of which Paris was the capital), and that she lived much of her life in England. She wrote in the Anglo-Norman dialect of Old French, which was spoken by the ruling class in twelfth century England, and knew English as well (she translated her *Fables* from an English original, now lost). It is unlikely that she would have identified herself by her place of origin if she had still been living there; moreover, the best manuscripts of *The Lais of Marie de France* and *Fables*

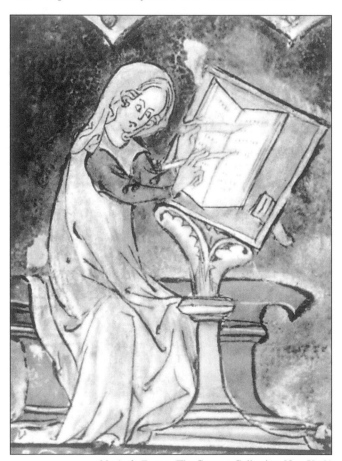

Marie de France (The Granger Collection, New York)

were found in England. It is also probable that she was a woman of noble birth, for she had noble patrons and even dedicated *The Lais of Marie de France* to a king; she may also have been a nun, for she knew Latin well (as can be seen from her translation of the teatise on Saint Patrick's purgatory) and was better educated than most laywomen would have had occasion to be.

Beyond this, all is speculation, and as Philippe Ménard has observed, the very number of proposed identifications indicates the tenuous character of the evidence. An attractive possibility—but only a possibility—is that she was Mary, abbess of Shaftesbury, an illegitimate daughter of Geoffrey Plantagenet and half sister to Henry II of England. This would account for her apparent familiarity with members of noble circles and with the courtly literature of which Henry's queen, Eleanor of Aquitaine, was an important patron.

ANALYSIS

Despite the volume of critical writing on Marie de France, and despite the limpidity of her own style, there is yet no clear scholarly consensus on how *The Lais of Marie de France* should be read. The age of the poems is undoubtedly one source of difficulty: Not only do they belong to a vanished cultural and intellectual milieu, but also much external evidence (such as sources and the means of accurate dating) that might have made their interpretation easier has been lost.

Two further difficulties recur in all discussions of *The Lais of Marie de France*. The first is a question of genre. The genre of the narrative lay is represented in surviving literature by only thirty-odd poems, and these are too diverse to suggest a clear-cut definition. What is more, Marie's own collection of twelve lays contains pieces that are quite disparate in theme and plot structure. The critic must thus seek unifying elements, and while most would agree that the theme of love runs through all the tales like a connecting thread, few agree on Marie's understanding of love or on her intention in portraying it.

The second major difficulty, which individual critics fail to acknowledge but which is evident from a review of the literature, is that the theme of love necessarily evokes subjective responses in readers, even when those readers are scrupulously "objective" critics. This is, of course, a danger in all criticism; it is exacerbated in Marie's case by the dearth of external evidence and by the intimate, almost seductive quality of some of her tales. Though it is important to consider the whole range of such responses, because each may have something to contribute to a full appreciation of the work, the most fruitful lines of research have been a new approach to the issue of genre and various efforts to see the lays in their original cultural and poetic context.

Thanks to important work by Sienaert, real progress has been made on the genre question; the unique and often puzzling emotional effects of the lays may plausibly be attributed to the ways in which they combine elements of two well-known genres, the fairy tale and the realistic *nouvelle*, or short story. At the same time, the lays have been shown to include didactic, courtly, and religious elements that reflect distinct tendencies of the age in which they were written. Marie is not content merely to entertain or "seduce" her readers; she has much to say about the real world and about the moral choices her characters are called upon to make in it.

MARIE'S CONCEPT OF LOVE

She also puts forward a conception of love that has at least something in common with the courtly love celebrated by her contemporaries the troubadours and trouvères. (Here it may be helpful to recall that Marie may have spent some time at the court of Henry II, whose wife, Eleanor of Aquitaine, was herself a Frenchwoman and the granddaughter of a troubadour.) As Emanuel Mickel has observed, Marie approves of love when it is elevated above concupiscence and self-seeking by a freely given pledge of loyalty. She differs from those courtly authors who celebrate one-sided love; in nearly every lay, the love portrayed is mutual. Though she often depicts such love as triumphing over obstacles, she also acknowledges that it may result in great suffering for the lovers. Her appeals to explicitly Christian values can be unorthodox, and she combines romantic love with Christian charity in unexpected ways, but she does not hesitate to condemn those who

betray trusting spouses—or feudal lords or vassals—out of calculated self-interest. The concluding lay of the collection also suggests that romantic love can serve as a bridge to the more complete love of God. Marie's chief interest, however, is unquestionably in the depiction of mutual romantic attachment and its various outcomes.

If there is still disagreement about Marie's thematic focus, her stylistic gifts are scarcely in doubt. In a reversal of earlier assessments, later critics have seen in her an accomplished storyteller and poet, suiting the length of each tale to its content, using dialogue to great effect, and endowing key objects with symbolic value so that they epitomize the themes of individual tales. The shortest of the tales—"Laüstic" ("The Nightingale") and "Chèvrefeuille" ("The Honeysuckle")—have even been seen as essentially lyric poems, so dominated are they by the central symbols of the nightingale and the honeysuckle entwined with the hazel. However, even these lays have plots, as Sienaert does well to recall. Though Marie translated her *Fables* from an English original that has been lost, these, too, display poetic and narrative skill (especially in the phrasing of dialogue) that must be attributed, at least in part, to the translator.

THE LAY AS GENRE

Sienaert's description of the lay as a mixed or intermediary genre is based on the work of folklorists, notably Vladimir Propp and Max Lüthi, who have identified (independently of one another) the basic structure of the European folktale. One of the most striking features of the folktale, or fairy tale (Sienaert's term for the genre is *conte merveilleux*: a tale with a happy ending, in which the "marvelous" is paramount) is that the identities and motivations of characters may be freely altered from one version to another, whereas the plot sequence, and the roles characters may fill in it, are rigidly maintained. The mainspring of the fairy-tale plot is not the motivated action of its characters but rather the intrusion of the marvelous, and although the working out of the plot satisfies deep human desires, its conclusion is not attained by human effort but by magic (a potion, a ring) or by a deus ex machina (a fairy, a speaking animal). It has long been recognized that there were affinities between the fairy tale and *The Lais of Marie de France*, but these affinities had remained somewhat vague, limited to the happy ending (which does not apply to a number of lays) and an ill-defined "charm." As Sienaert has shown, however, the lays sometimes follow the fairy-tale pattern in which motivation is not linked to plot. Thus, the knight Eliduc, for example, scarcely earns his happiness; it comes to him in spite of the bad faith he has shown his wife and his young lover. At the same time, though, and in the same tales, the motivation of Marie's characters can be essential to the outcome; thus, Eliduc's wife, by her unexampled generosity, makes possible for her husband the happy ending he had deserved to forfeit. Sometimes it even happens that a realistically motivated character *forestalls* the expected happy ending, as does the young man in "Les Dues Amanz" ("The Two Loves"), who refuses to drink the magic potion that would restore his strength. Finally, there are a few stories from which the fairy-tale plot is completely missing. "Equitan" has been compared to a fabliau (a more consistently realistic, generally coarse and cynical, short narrative genre contemporary to the lay) because of its realistic and cautionary plot of betrayal, attempted crime, and punishment; while falling within the scope of the medieval exemplum, or tale with a moral, it resembles the modern short story in linking the outcome to the character and actions of the central figures. Sienaert argues that Marie deliberately placed it second in her collection, after a tale that has many affinities with the fairy tale, to mark the two poles between that her pieces would move.

As will become apparent from a closer look at several lays, this approach to the genre question can be extremely useful. Its chief drawback is its degree of abstraction—it cannot account for the thematic content of the collection.

"LANVAL"

"Lanval" is a good example of a lay using a straightforward fairy-tale plot. Lanval, a "foreign" knight at King Arthur's court, is slighted by the King until a beautiful fairy maiden approaches him, offering both her love and riches if he will keep her existence secret. This he does, until one day the Queen likewise offers him her love, and he reveals the fact that he already loves another, whose least handmaiden surpasses the Queen in beauty and accomplishments. At this, the Queen denounces him to the King as having accosted

her, nor will the fairy-lover come at his call, since he has revealed her existence. When he is put on trial, however—more for insulting the Queen's beauty than for allegedly accosting her—the fairy relents, first sending her handmaidens and then arriving in person so that all can see the truth of Lanval's boast. The tale ends as Lanval rides off with her to the otherworldly Avalon, to live happily ever after.

This lay epitomizes a tendency of many of Marie's tales to fuse Celtic folk motifs with the courtly love theme. As Jean Frappier has observed, there is an analogy between the "otherworld" of Celtic mythology, to which the "marvelous" properly belongs, and the privileged condition of courtly lovers, whose experience of love (open only to a small, elect group), gives them a taste of paradise on earth. Avalon thus becomes an allegory for the state of mutual love, where the "foreigner" Lanval finds his true home after rejecting, and being rejected by, the flawed world of Arthur's court (where the king has slighted him and the queen accused him of her own infidelity). As Sienaert would add, however, the motivations of the characters—even of the fairy, who relents in her punishment of Lanval—are fully humanized and linked to the outcome. The lay is thus emotionally satisfying, not only for its fairy-tale ending but also for its vindication of mutual love—though it should also be noted that the "real world" is seen as hostile to that love, which can flourish only in a land of its own. In this respect, "Lanval" is perhaps the most frankly escapist of the lays.

"THE TWO LOVERS"

"The Two Lovers," by contrast, creates the expectation of a fairy-tale ending only to reverse it at the last moment. A widowed king, unwilling to part with his sole daughter, invents a trial in which he thinks no suitor can succeed: To win her hand in marriage, the suitor must carry her to the top of a mountain without pausing to rest. To help a young man whom she favors, the girl sends him to her aunt in Salerno, who provides him with a potion that can restore strength. During the trial, however, the young man feels strong enough to do without the potion; he resists the girl's repeated pleas that he drink it and reaches the summit only to collapse—his heart has given out. The distraught girl spills the potion, which causes medicinal herbs to spring up on the mountainside, and herself dies of grief on the spot, where the two are buried together.

Of all the lays, this one has perhaps evoked the greatest diversity of interpretation. It has been seen as a tragedy, a cautionary tale, even a satire. Here, Sienaert's insights are especially helpful, accounting for the diversity of critical (and emotional) response without explaining it away. The story is indeed tragic insofar as it reverses the carefully created expectation of a happy ending, and it is cautionary insofar as Marie stresses the *démesure* (lack of moderation) that leads to the boy's death. However, there is also something positive about the ending: After rejecting the magical means to success, the boy accomplishes the feat (though none of his predecessors had come close), and the girl's love, because it equals his, unites them in death. The boy's decision is flawed, as Marie herself observes: "I fear [the potion] will do him little good/ For he had in him no moderation." As Emanuel Mickel points out, the potion is not merely a magical expedient but a symbol of the potential strength and fruition to which the couple's love might have come; thus, the good herbs it causes to flourish on the mountainside might have been the couple's good deeds (as in "Eliduc") or those of their heirs. Nevertheless, it is hard not to sympathize with the boy's desire to prove himself or with the girl's anguished sense of what she has lost. Both characters are brought to vivid life in the scene on the mountain, as Marie endows them with fully human motives.

"EQUITAN"

"Equitan," the "realistic" lay mentioned above, offers yet another perspective on love; it is also one of the most carefully structured of the lays, making expert use of dialogue, symbolism, and irony. Equitan is a king who seems to possess all the knightly virtues. It soon emerges, though, that, like the boy in "The Two Lovers," he has no sense of moderation in love; what is more, he prefers pleasure to his responsibilities and often leaves the administration of justice to his seneschal while he goes hunting—literally and metaphorically, for he is fond of the ladies. (The hunt was frequently used by medieval authors as a metaphor for the pursuit of a woman's favors.) As it happens, the seneschal has a wife who is among the most beautiful women of the realm; hearing her praised, Equitan goes to hunt on the seneschal's lands, succeeds in meeting her, and falls passionately in love with her. Though he recognizes (in a soliloquy) that it means breaking faith with his loyal deputy, the king persuades himself by specious arguments to pursue the woman. At first she objects, but only on the grounds that his rank will make for inequality in their love; he assures her that—in accordance with the courtly convention—he will be her servant and she his lady. As Marie makes plain, this is what literally happens. Urged by his subjects to marry, Equitan refuses, assuring his lover that he would marry her if she were free; she then proposes that they murder her husband, and the king agrees to every detail of her plan. The hunt has become lethal, but this time Equitan is destined to become the quarry. Caught by the seneschal in his lady's arms, Equitan leaps into the boiling bath prepared for the murder. The irony is complete as the seneschal, to whom Equitan had delegated his own judicial responsibilities, proceeds to complete the punishment by throwing his wife in the bath after her lover. As might have been expected, those nineteenth century critics who were chiefly impressed by the "charm" of lays like "Lanval" found "Equitan" shockingly sordid; it seemed, moreover, to give a different and unfavorable account of the courtly love celebrated in many of the lays. Clearly, Marie does not disapprove of courtly love per se. As the ending of "Lanval" indicates, however, it is not always possible to reconcile the state of love—that "otherworld" to which Lanval and his mistress retreat—and the "real world," which makes claims of its own on the lovers. The fidelity of Equitan and his lady might in itself be admirable, but because it is grounded in the infidelity of both to the seneschal, it leads them to crime. Because it is also characterized by *démesure*, it also leads to death. In contrast to the *démesure* of the boy in "The Two Lovers," which is excusable because of his youth and which has a dimension that may be considered heroic, the *démesure* of Equitan is a form of slavery to appetite, which is all the more demeaning in the light of Equitan's rank as well as his responsibilities.

As Sienaert observes, "Equitan" is an extreme case—a worst case, in *The Lais of Marie de France*, where adulterous love is concerned. Marie frequently treats of courtly love that is also adulterous, and she is often sympathetic to the lovers. This is especially true of the three lays "Guigemar," "Yonec," and "The Nightingale," in which the female protagonist is a *mal mariée*—a woman married against her will, usually to a much older man who treats her as his property and shows her no love. Though the protagonist's love for another is portrayed sympathetically in each case, the stories end in very disparate ways: In the most realistic, "The Nightingale," the husband succeeds in separating the lovers by an act of cruelty (killing the bird that gave the wife an excuse to stand at the window from which she could see her lover); in the most fairy-tale-like, "Guigemar," the husband simply disappears from the story as the wife escapes and rejoins her lover in his distant homeland.

"ELIDUC"

The most complex case of adulterous love, however, is that seen in "Eliduc," the longest of the lays and the last in the manuscript that Sienaert takes to reflect Marie's own ordering of the tales. When the story opens, Eliduc has been happily married for some time; he decides to leave home because envious men have slandered him to the Breton king whom he faithfully serves. Crossing to England, he offers his services to the king of Exeter, who is hard-pressed by enemies, and wins a signal victory. The king's daughter, Guilliadun, hearing only good spoken of Eliduc, asks to meet him, and the two fall in love. Though Eliduc restrains himself to the extent that he does not sleep with the girl, he accepts her gifts and kisses and does not tell her of his wife. When his original sovereign, hard-pressed in turn, sends for him, he feels duty-bound to go and refuses to abduct the princess (who wants to go with him) on the grounds that he would be showing disloyalty to her father; yet he promises to return for her when his contract with her father will have expired. He does so—still without telling her of his wife—and during a storm on the channel, she learns the truth from a frightened sailor who thinks Eliduc's adulterous love has caused the storm. At the news, Guilliadun falls in a faint, and thinking she is dead, Eliduc throws the sailor overboard. The ship reaches land safely, and Eliduc, who cannot yet bring himself to bury the girl, hides her in a chapel on his estate. Worried by his obvious grief, his wife, Guildeluec, has him followed and discovers the

girl's body; far from showing envy or hatred, she revives Guilliadun with the aid of a magic herb and says she wishes to enter a convent so that Eliduc can marry the girl. After living for some time in "perfect love," the couple in turn enter religious life, and Guildeluec, now an abbess, welcomes Guilliadun "as her sister."

Once again, Sienaert's observations offer a useful line of approach to this puzzling tale. Like other courtly lovers in *The Lais of Marie de France*, Eliduc would like to keep his love in a world apart, safe from the interference of real life; when the sailor tries to call him back to reality, he blindly kills the man. (It should be noted, however, that the sailor scarcely speaks for Marie; he wants to do away with the innocent Guilliadun.) Unable to resolve his own dilemma, Eliduc is saved by the action of his wife, whose unparalleled generosity takes the place of the magical resolution one would expect in a fairy tale. What this approach cannot account for, however, is the care and the sheer length devoted to the developing love between Eliduc and Guilliadun. If, as Sienaert claims, Guilliadun's swoon represents the impotence of the courtly ethic (and even of a "fairy-tale princess") to deal with the moral dilemmas of the real world, why is such care devoted to the portrayal of her love for Eliduc, and above all, why does she and not Guildeluec win him back?

Mickel has observed that there is a correspondence between the lengths of individual lays and their plot structures: The shorter lays all end unhappily, whereas the longer ones end with the reunion of the lovers (or, as in "Yonec," with their vindication). Mickel attributes this characteristic to Marie's preference for faithful love, which must develop and be tested over time, yet it is Guildeluec who has loved Eliduc longest. Given the care with which Marie describes the growth of the adulterous love (it occupies 431 of 1,184 lines, or more than a third of the poem), it seems hard to avoid the conclusion that Marie meant her audience to be caught up in it. Though Eliduc is clearly acting in bad faith at some level, he never allows this to reach his awareness in his dealings with Guilliadun; he is a confused man, but not a bad one at heart. Because both lovers are essentially good, and can see the good in each other, their mutual love (in which they manage to observe some *mésure*) is more than mere concupiscence. This is why it can lead them to a life of shared good works, and ultimately to the love of God. Despite the decisive role of Guildeluec's selfless love and the fact that all three protagonists learn to love in her way, it seems wrong to read the entire lay as an exemplum. There is a real difference between romantic and Christian love, and Guildeluec is the first to recognize it. Romantic love must be mutual and cannot be learned; it is, as has been observed, akin to the "marvelous." Thus, Guildeluec makes her decision on the basis of Guilliadun's exquisite beauty, whose power she herself feels. Though Marie admits, in "Equitan," that such love can lead the partners to evil, she prefers stories in which it ennobles them, whether through shared happiness or shared suffering. She is thus both a didactic and a thoroughly courtly poet.

MARIE AS STORYTELLER

Because Marie is a narrative poet, her literary art is primarily that of the storyteller; thus, critical studies have emphasized her choice of significant detail, her use of dialogue, and above all, her skill in the ordering and pacing of plots. It is important to remember, however, especially if one reads her in a prose translation (and there are no verse translations in English), that she is also a poet, writing in rhymed octosyllabic couplets. Far from interrupting the flow of her narrative, this form contributes to its spare and vigorous quality. In contrast to the romances being written by her contemporaries in the same meter, the lays are anything but digressive. This is especially striking in the shorter lays, where not a line is wasted. *Fables*, though not an original work, deserves to be mentioned in this context because it demonstrates the same skill of compression to an even greater degree: The longer of the fables are of the same length as the shorter of the lays. The moral with which each fable concludes is particularly compressed (between four and eight lines long), and the rhymes are carefully chosen to bring home the point with special force.

IMAGERY AND SYMBOLISM

The other specifically poetic skill Marie displays is in the use of controlling images, which in her narrative context are usually symbolic objects (although she can also use metaphor, as in the tale of Equitan, "the hunter hunted"). Such objects loom especially large in two of the shortest lays, "The Nightingale" and "The Honeysuckle"; in both cases, they are related to the love theme

central to the collection. Though the nightingale is on one level a pretext that the woman uses to see her lover, it also symbolizes mutual love as something alive and beautiful. Though the husband can kill it and thus prevent the lovers from seeing each other, he cannot obliterate its memory; thus, the lover, to whom the woman sends the bird's body, has it encased in a jeweled box, which he carries about with him always.

The honeysuckle, which twines itself about the hazel until neither can stand alone, is a related symbol of love as a beautiful living thing. Though the bird and the plant are themselves vulnerable, the fidelity of the lovers in each case holds out a hope that human love may be more durable. In "The Honeysuckle," which describes a meeting between Tristan and Iseult, Tristan himself uses the symbol in this sense. In a passage that is a true lyric fragment (and that may be the message, inscribed on a hazel stick, alerting Iseult to her lover's presence), he exclaims, "Fair love, so it is with us:/ Neither you without me, nor I without you." Deservedly one of Marie's most famous couplets, it captures both her spare, direct style and the ideal of mutual fidelity embodied in so many of her lays.

BIBLIOGRAPHY

Bloch, R. Howard. *The Anonymous Marie de France.* Chicago: University of Chicago Press, 2003. Argues that Marie de France was a writer of profound importance and significance, a "[James] Joyce of the twelfth century." Includes notes and an index.

Burgess, Glyn S. *The "Lais" of Marie de France: Text and Context.* Athens: University of Georgia Press, 1987. A detailed study of the twelve lays contained in the British Library. The study notes thematic and textual parallels in the lays, with the author's hope that they will help scholars in future evaluations of the authorship of these works. Burgess discusses the problem of internal chronology and focuses attention on key terms in Marie's use of language. Includes extensive notes for further study, a bibliography, and an index.

_____. *Marie de France: An Analytical Bibliography.* Supplement no. 3. Woolbridge, Suffolk, England: Tamesis, 2007. A bibliography of the works by and about Marie de France, with critical analysis.

McCash, June Hall. "The Swan and the Nightingale: Natural Unity in a Hostile World in the *Lais* of Marie de France." *French Studies* 49 (October, 1995): 385-396. Discusses Marie's symbolic and mimetic depiction of nature in *The Lais of Marie de France*. Notes that although she uses a wealth of symbolic associations of birds, she does not alter their natural functions.

Maréchal, Chantal, ed. *In Quest of Marie de France: A Twelfth-Century Poet*. Lewiston, N.Y.: Edwin Mellen Press, 1992. Contains fifteen articles by established medievalists: three articles on the *Fables*, six general articles on *The Lais of Marie de France*, and six with a narrower focus. Of special interest is the editor's introduction, which offers a chronological approach to critical assessment of Marie through the centuries.

_____. *The Reception and Transmission of the Works of Marie de France, 1774-1974*. Lewiston, N.Y.: Edwin Mellen Press, 2003. A collection of essays that look at how Marie de France's works have been received and transmitted through time.

Mickel, Emanuel J. *Marie de France*. New York: Twayne, 1974. A good, full-length study of Marie, her works, and the intellectual background of the twelfth century for the general reader and for the student of medieval literature. Contains individual chapters on Marie's identity, the narrative lays, sources and plot summaries for the various lays, an interpretation, and the structure and style of *The Lais of Marie de France*. Includes a chronology of the time period, useful notes and references for further study, a select bibliography, and an index.

Semple, Benjamin. "The Male Psyche and the Female Sacred Body in Marie de France and Christine de Pizan." *Yale French Studies*, no. 86 (1994): 164-186. Discusses the first of Marie's lays, "Guigemar," and Christine de Pizan's *Livre de la cité des dames*; argues that the image of humanity that emerges from the texts, like the mystical vision, invites us to contemplate the essential paradox of a body that is at once sexual, intellectual, and ethical.

Sethurman, Jayshree. "Tale-Type and Motif Indexes to the *Fables* of Marie de France." *Le Cygne: Bulletin of the International Marie de France Society* 5 (Spring, 1999): 19-35. A table of folktale types linking Marie's *Fables* to the compilations of universal folktale motifs classified and cataloged by Antti Arne and revised and expanded by Stith Thompson.

Whalen, Logan E. *Marie de France and the Poetics of Memory*. Washington, D.C.: Catholic University of America Press, 2008. This study of Marie's poetry looks at all works ascribed to her and analyzes them. Also provides a table of extant medieval manuscripts.

Lillian Doherty

GIAMBATTISTA MARINO

Born: Naples (now in Italy); October 18, 1569
Died: Naples (now in Italy); March 25, 1625
Also known as: Giambattista Marini

PRINCIPAL POETRY

Le rime, 1602 (*Steps to the Temple*, canto 1 only, 1646)

Il ritratto del serenissimo Don Carlo Emanuello Duca di Savoia, 1608

La lira, 1615

Il tempio, 1615

Epitalami, 1616

La galeria, 1619

Egloghe boscherecce, 1620

La sampogna, 1620

L'Adone, 1623

La Murtoleide, 1626

La strage degli innocenti, 1632 (*The Slaughter of the Innocents*, 1675)

Gerusalemme distrutta, 1633 (unfinished)

L'Anversa liberata, 1956 (unfinished)

Adonis, 1967 (selections from *L'Adone*)

OTHER LITERARY FORMS

The voluminous production of Giambattista Marino (mah-REE-noh) is almost entirely in poetical form. In 1617, while he was in France, Marino wrote an invective against the enemies of the Catholic Church, *La sferza, invettiva a quattro ministri della iniquitá* (the whip: invective against four ministers of iniquity), which was first published in Paris in 1625. In addition, Marino's copious correspondence, included in *Lettere* (1627) and published in a modern edition, *Epistolario* (1912), is very important, for it provides revealing glimpses of his moral and aesthetic values.

ACHIEVEMENTS

Thematically and stylistically, Giambattista Marino is considered one of the greatest Italian poets of his age and also, perhaps, the most representative man of letters of Baroque Europe. His impact was felt immediately, not only in the various literary circles of Italy but also in France, where he produced his masterpiece, *L'Adone* (Adonis), and whence his fame spread throughout the Continent. Echoes and imitators of the Marinesque style are indeed to be found everywhere, from the Slavic world (Miklós Zríny, Dżivo Bunić-Vucić, Igniat Djordjić, Jan Andrzej Morsztyn) to seventeenth century England (Edward Herbert, Thomas Carew, Andrew Marvell, Richard Crashaw, Samuel Daniel, Edward Sherburne, Thomas Stanley, and so on).

Although Spanish literature of this period was to produce an equally influential figure in Luis de Góngora y Argote (who was to lend his name to Gongorism, an aesthetic current that paralleled Marinism), Spanish poets such as Juan de Tasis, Luis de Carrillo y Sotomayor, and Francisco Gómez de Quevedo y Villegas became admirers and imitators of Marino, and Lope de Vega Carpio expressed his admiration for the Italian poet by dedicating one of his comedies to him. It was undoubtedly in France, however, where Marino lived for some eight years as a favorite of Queen Marie de Médicis, that his influence was most powerfully felt. Poets as diverse as Antoine-Girard de Saint-Amant, Théophile de Viau, Tristan L'Hermite, Georges de Scudéry, Vincent Voiture, Jean de La Fontaine, Claude de Malleville, and Pierre Le Moyne betray a significant debt to Marino, and it was from France that Marinism radiated all over Europe.

BIOGRAPHY

Giambattista (Giovan Battista) Marino (or Marini, as it is often written), one of seven children, was born in Naples on October 18, 1569, the son of Giovan Francesco Marino. The elder Marino was a lawyer and hoped that his son would follow in his footsteps, but the young Marino was more interested in literary studies than in embracing a legal career. Having disappointed his father, Marino was unceremoniously asked to leave the paternal household, but his reputation as a spirited and bright young poet and man of letters was already sufficient to open to him the doors of several aristocratic houses, and in 1592, he entered the service of Matteo di Capua, prince of Conca, as a poet and a secretary.

As a young man, Marino led a dissolute life and was twice imprisoned: first in 1598, for having taken part in the rape of a young woman (probably a nun), and again in 1600, for having falsified some documents to prepare the escape from prison of his friend, Marc Antonio d'Alessandro, who had been condemned to death. Although Marino was freed from prison, he was forced to flee to Rome, where he found protection with the influential Monsignor Melchiorre Crescenzio. In 1601-1602, Marino traveled to Venice to oversee the publication of his first two volumes of *Le rime*, later incorporated in *La lira*. Upon his return to Rome, he found employment with Cardinal Pietro Aldobrandini, the nephew of Pope Clement VIII, and in 1606, after the pope's death, Marino followed Aldobrandini to his seat at Ravenna.

Enjoying a growing reputation as a poet, Marino accompanied Aldobrandini to Torino in 1608 to attend the marriage of two daughters of Duke Carlo Emanuele I of Savoy, and Marino seized the occasion to write *Il ritratto del serenissimo Don Carlo Emanuello Duca di Savoia* (the portrait of the most serene Don Carlo Emanuele, duke of Savoy), a panegyric in honor of the duke. The duke reciprocated by conferring on him the order of the knighthood of Saints Maurizio and Lazzaro—the title of "Cavaliere," of which Marino always felt especially proud and that he henceforth always prefixed to his name.

In 1609, the duke's secretary, Gaspare Murtola— himself a poet, jealous of Marino's rapidly rising status at the court of Turin—fired a pistol at Marino, hitting instead another man who was a favorite of the duke. Murtola was condemned to death, but at Marino's request, the sentence was commuted to exile. In 1611, Marino himself was sent to prison for fourteen months. The charges are not known, but presumably he had offended the duke with some satirical verses. Marino was freed in 1612, and in 1614, he published in Venice the result of years of creative labor: part 3 of *La lira*, later reprinted in a collected edition together with *Le rime* and the *Dicerie sacre* (holy discourses). In 1615, he received permission to go to the royal court in Paris, where he had been invited first by Marguerite de Navarre and then by Marie de Médicis, who had become Queen Regent after the death of her husband, Henry IV.

In Lyon, as soon as he set foot on French territory, Marino published a laudatory poem, *Il tempio* (the temple), in honor of the queen. Marino stayed in Paris, where he became a court favorite, until 1623, enjoying enormous popularity and receiving many honors. While in Paris, he published a volume of ten nuptial odes, *Epitalami* (epithalamia); a collection of six hundred poems celebrating various works of art, real and imagined, *La galeria* (the gallery); a gathering of poems on mythological and bucolic subjects, *La sampogna* (the shepherd's pipe); and finally, in April, 1623, his masterpiece, *L'Adone*, which he dedicated to Louis XIII. Immediately after the publication of the twenty cantos of *L'Adone*—a work more than twice as long as Dante's *La divina commedia* (c. 1320; *The Divine Comedy*, 1802) or Torquato Tasso's *Gerusalemme liberata* (1581; *Jerusalem Delivered*, 1600)—Marino, at the very peak of his popularity, decided to return to his native land to savor the triumphs that inevitably would be accorded to him as the greatest living Italian poet. In Rome, he found immediate protection at the household of Cardinal Ludovico Ludovisi, the nephew of Pope Gregory XV; was feted with a banquet held in his honor by the Roman Senate; and was elected prince of the Academy of the Umoristi, of which he had been a member for several years. While in Rome, he witnessed as a special guest the ceremonies for the election of the new pope, Urban VIII (previously Cardinal Maffeo Barberini).

Arriving in May, 1623, in his native Naples, Marino entered the city as a triumphant conqueror. A statue in his honor was unveiled there, and he was welcomed by the Spanish viceroy and by the various literary academies (the Academy of the Oziosi also made him a prince). In 1624, however, his stay in Naples was marred by the unwelcome news that his *L'Adone* had been placed on the Church's Index. Perhaps tired by his many public appearances and commitments and by the pressure to complete his religious epic, *The Slaughter of the Innocents*, he became ill, initially with a slow fever and then with a painful case of strangury. Before his death on March 25, 1625, he burned many of his sensual and profane writings. By order of the Neapolitan archbishop Cardinal Decio Carafa, Marino's burial took place during the night.

ANALYSIS

True to the spirit of his time, Giambattista Marino wrote a number of panegyrical poems, among them *Il ritratto del serenissimo Don Carlo Emanuello Duca di Savoia, Il tempio*, and *Epitalami*, a collection of ten very sensual nuptial odes patterned after traditional models, largely mythological in content, and written to celebrate the weddings of various princes and kings. Marino was equally at ease with religious subjects, which he treated with a certain emotional detachment. In 1614, he published *Dicerie sacre*, an important work that included three lengthy and elaborate metaphorical sermons on painting, music, and Heaven, inspired respectively by the "Sindone" (Christ's shroud), the seven last words of Christ, and the orders of Saints Maurizio and Lazzaro. In 1617, while in France, Marino wrote *La sferza, invettiva a quattro ministri della iniquitá*, an invective against the enemies of the Catholic Church.

Among Marino's other writings worthy of mention are his pastoral *Egloghe boscherecce* (sylvan eclogues), first published in 1620, although the only extant copies are dated 1627, and the famous *La Murtoleide* (the deeds of Murtola). *La Murtoleide*, published in 1626 but dating back to Marino's Turin period, consists of eighty-one *fischiate* (boos), satirical sonnets written against his rival, the mediocre court poet Gaspare Murtola, who had attacked Marino in a libelous *Abridgement of the Life of Cavalier Marino*. Rather predictably, Murtola retorted by writing a *Marineide* (the deeds of Marino), which consisted of thirty-two *risate* (laughs); he also tried, unsuccessfully, to kill Marino, shooting at him with a pistol.

A well-known tercet that is said to epitomize the quintessence of Marino's poetics is to be found in the thirty-third *fischiata* of *La Murtoleide*: "The goal of the poet is to cause wonder/ (I am speaking about excellent poets and not clumsy ones):/ Those who do not know how to astonish should go to the stables."

Marino also tried his hand at composing serious epic poetry, and great admirer of Tasso that he was, he attempted to deal with two themes much in the Tassian tradition: *Gerusalemme distrutta* (Jerusalem destroyed) and *L'Anversa liberata* (Antwerp delivered). Both of these poems, however, were left unfinished and were published posthumously, the first in 1633 and the second only in 1956.

L'Adone

Marino's masterpiece, *L'Adone*—an extremely long poem of twenty cantos, first published in Paris in 1623—displays his seemingly unlimited verbal and rhetorical virtuosity as well as his ability to use a surprising array of sources and themes.

Although some of the episodes in *L'Adone* can be traced to Dante, Ariosto, and Tasso, the bulk of the work derives from classical sources, particularly book 10 of Ovid's *Metamorphoses* (c. 8 C.E.; English translation, 1567). In a sense, *L'Adone* can be seen as a marvelous poetic catalog of a mythological world where the myths and Arcadian adventures of the classical deities, Satyrs, and nymphs are syncretically evoked against a lavishly sensual Baroque setting.

The plot begins unfolding when Cupid, rather ill disposed toward his mother Venus, seeks vengeance by making Adonis—the handsome prince born out of an incestuous relation between Mirrah and her father—arrive in Cyprus and fall in love with the goddess. Readily reciprocating Adonis's love, Venus takes the young prince to her palace and guides him through the Garden of Pleasure, divided into five sections that symbolize the various senses as they are engaged by lovemaking. Afterward, still guided by his pagan, unspiritual "Beatrice," Adonis experiences the pleasures of the mind. Joined by Mercury—clearly reminiscent of Dante's Vergil—Adonis visits Apollo's fountain, symbolizing poetry, and ascends to the first three Ptolemaic

spheres, those of the Moon, Mercury, and Venus. There, after some adulatory verses in honor of various royalties, he learns of the most advanced scientific notions and meets some of the most representative figures of the sixteenth century.

Unfortunately, Jealousy informs Mars of Venus's new passion, and Adonis is forced to flee before the enraged god, beginning a long series of adventures. Adonis falls into the hands of the lascivious and wicked fairy Falsirena, who, after unsuccessfully trying to seduce him, transforms him into a parrot and forces him to witness love scenes between Venus and Mars. Following other fantastic encounters, Adonis finally manages to return to Cyprus, where he is elected king of the island and can once more enjoy the favors of the goddess. On a hunt, however, Adonis is killed by a wild boar aroused against him by the disgruntled Falsirena and Mars. The poem ends with Adonis's funeral and with a description of the games held in his honor, as well as with a final series of classical myths dealing with love and death.

In a dazzling display of bravura, Marino's thin treatment of the theme of life, death, and rebirth is overpowered by the pageant of sensory delights that he presents to the reader. In a changing world filled with religious upheavals and sociopolitical tensions, Marino's ornate, brilliant display of rhetorical and poetic devices and his unrestrained celebration of life and sensual love offered an escape into the unreal realm of fables and myths. Marino's exuberant affirmation of the *meraviglia* (the astonishing, the marvelous) was judged by later critics as representative of the Baroque at its worst, its most excessive, yet his virtuosity has never been questioned. His masterly use of rhetorical figures remains unsurpassed. Indeed, the abundant use of metaphors by Marino and other Baroque poets went beyond the mere rhetorical exigencies of poetry or even the desire to display exceptional creative ability. Rather, it expressed a deeply felt if unconscious need to interpret their confusing and rapidly changing world.

Other major works

NONFICTION: *Dicerie sacre*, 1614; *La sferza, invettiva a quattro ministri della iniquitá*, pb. 1625 (wr. 1617); *Lettere*, 1627 (modern edition, *Epistolario*, 1912).

BIBLIOGRAPHY

Brand, Peter, and Lino Pertile, eds. *The Cambridge History of Italian Literature*. Rev. ed. New York: Cambridge University Press, 1999. Contains a chapter on the Baroque period and a section on Marino and his followers.

Guardiani, Francesco, ed. *The Sense of Marino: Literature, Fine Arts, and Music of the Italian Baroque*. New York: Legas, 1994. A critical interpretation of selected poetic works and an introduction the history of Italian poetry of the seventeenth century.

Mirollo, James V. *The Poet of the Marvelous: Giambattista Marino*. New York: Columbia University Press, 1963. A biography of Marino. Includes texts in Italian and English of "La canzone dei baci," "La maddalena di Tiziano," and an extract from "La pastorello."

Segel, Harold B. *The Baroque Poem: A Comparative Survey*. New York: Dutton, 1974. A survey of 150 texts from English, American, Dutch, German, French, Italian, Spanish, Mexican, Portuguese, Polish, Modern Latin, Czech, Croatian, and Russian poetry, in the original languages and accompanying English translations.

Roberto Severino

MARTIAL

Born: Bilbilis, Hispania (now near Calatayud, Spain); March 1, c. 38-41 C.E.
Died: Hispania (now in Spain); c. 103 C.E.

PRINCIPAL POETRY

Liber spectaculorum, c. 81 C.E. (also known as *Epigrammaton liber*; *On the Spectacles*, 1980)
Xenia, c. 84 C.E.
Apophoreta, c. 85 C.E.
Epigrammata, 86-98 C.E. (*Epigrams*, 1860)

OTHER LITERARY FORMS

Martial (MAHR-shuhl) is unknown to have written anything beyond the fifteen thousand short poems and epigrams that appeared in his published work.

ACHIEVEMENTS

Martial brought the centuries-old art of the epigram to new heights, perfecting the witty, barbed, quotable "zinger" while providing intimate glimpses of everyday life in Rome. Part vulgar gossip columnist, part ancient blogger, and always a keenly observant and skilled versifier, Martial was one of the most popular social commentators of his day during a volatile time—the first century C.E.—in which the Roman Empire greatly expanded, Christianity was introduced, and emperors rose and fell, sometimes violently.

Martial was active for more than thirty years in the midst of the world's most powerful military, political, and cultural force. A financially strapped survivor capable of a vast range of styles (fawning appeals to the wealthy, clever topical lists, straightforward reports of historical events, crude pornography), Martial moved across all social strata, rubbing elbows with the famous and infamous, and achieved nobility. His short poems record snapshot-like impressions in well-composed verse featuring every variation of human behavior witnessed first-hand in all settings imaginable, from the lowest dives to the court of the imperial palace. In the course of his life and work, Martial reinvented the style of the epigram, giving it a surprise ending, a "sting in its tail." Nearly two thousand years after his death, modern wits, public speakers, politicians, and poets still follow Martial's example of driving home a point in the last line to lend extra emphasis to what they say or write.

BIOGRAPHY

Marcus Valerius Martialis was the son of ordinary Roman citizens living in Spain, a colony of the Roman Empire. His parents were Fronto and Flaccilla, one of whom was of Celtic-Iberian heritage. His given name, Marcus, celebrates his birth on March first, probably late in the reign of the insane, ill-fated emperor, Caligula. Martial received a liberal education at home, and in 64 C.E., he journeyed to Rome with the intention of making his living as a poet.

Upon his arrival in the capital, Martial was welcomed into the literary circle of two fellow Spaniards, as well as into the patronage system that permitted starving artists of all disciplines to work under the financial sponsorship of the wealthy and powerful. Seneca the Younger, an elderly and noted dramatist, philosopher, and statesman, and Lucan (Seneca's nephew), a rising young epic poet about Martial's age, introduced the newcomer to Gaius Calpurnius Piso, a wealthy, influential senator. With such support, Martial's future seemed secure. However, in 65 C.E., Seneca, Lucan, and Piso were implicated in a conspiracy against reigning Emperor Nero and were forced to commit suicide. For the next fifteen years, Martial eked out a living, probably soliciting the rich to write occasional, ephemeral verse in the hope of landing a permanent, well-heeled patron.

Martial's earliest surviving work is *On the Spectacles*, a collection of epigrammatic poems written to celebrate the completion of the Colosseum in 80 C.E. Several years later, he published a pair of companion epigram collections, *Xenia* and *Apophoreta*. The first volume of his best-known work, *Epigrams*, appeared in 86 C.E. Due to the apparent popularity and notoriety of his work, he brought out a fresh collection of new poems every year or two.

Although Martial never gained a fortune from his writing, he did eventually achieve a measure of fame. He could count among his acquaintances the emperors Titus and Domitian, aristocrat-soldiers such as Frontinus, and many of the leading literary lights of the day, including poet-satirist Juvenal, letter-writer extraordinaire Pliny the Younger, rhetorician Quintilian, historian Tacitus, and epic poet Silius Italicus. Martial, relying on patronage for his subsistence for most of his working life, inherited a small farm near Nomentum, and in his mid-fifties acquired a modest house in Rome. He was granted a nominal imperial annual stipend and was made an honorary tribune of the equestrian order.

Late in life, with the financial assistance of Pliny the Younger, Martial returned to the town of his birth in Spain and spent his last years on a farm that a female patron, Marcella, had given him, and probably died there. He apparently never married and left no legitimate heirs.

ANALYSIS

Like many writers across the ages, before Martial made his mark on literature, he learned to compose by following the examples of earlier authors. Martial was an outspoken admirer of Catullus, a Roman poet of the previous century, and used his mentor's techniques to carve his own literary niche.

Throughout an effective—if not especially lucrative—working career spanning several decades in the heart of bustling, scandalous, fascinating first century Rome, Martial built a loyal following for well-crafted, sharp-pointed, often eyebrow-raising verse. Borrowing freely from the stylistic toolbox employed by Catullus and other epigrammatists, Martial made deft use of elegiac couplets (dactylic hexameter/dactylic pentameter, expressing a complete thought in as few as two lines), with occasional hendecasyllables (eleven-syllable lines) and choliambics (also known as scazons, which reverse the iambic meter in the last foot of a line) for rhythmic variety. Like Catullus, Martial achieved broad readership dealing with small, everyday, easily understood subjects and real contemporary figures, rather than mammoth epics of gods and heroes past. His direct, epigrammatic poetry drilled through the tumult of events, hammered home truths, and skewered individual behavior. His craftsmanship in constructing memorable two-liners (a set-up followed by a meaningful punch line) is still evident and still inspires to this day.

Although he may have attempted other types of writing, every extant work of Martial is in verse. Virtually all are of epigrammatic nature, most commonly of two to twelve lines, and seldom more than twenty lines long.

From the beginning of his career, Martial demonstrated both an eye for telling detail and a talent for marketing. His first known work, *On the Spectacles*—an eyewitness account of the first games held in the newly completed Colosseum—colorfully describes gladiatorial contests and battles among various species of animals. *On the Spectacles* opened with a poem boasting of the new facility's splendor, comparing it favorably to the pyramids of Egypt, the hanging gardens of Babylon, and other world wonders. This was followed by a dedication to the emperor before Martial launched into a series of brief, exciting glimpses of the action from the games.

Xenia and *Apophoreta* were likewise produced in timely fashion to capitalize on the celebration of Saturnalia (in 84 or 85 C.E.), a major weeklong celebration in December when masters and slaves reversed roles, gifts were given, and there was considerable merrymaking. Martial's elegiac couplets in *Xenia*—also prefaced with a sycophantic dedication to the emperor—were intended as clever tags to accompany gifts of food and wine, as though following course after course of a fabulous banquet. *Apophoreta*, containing couplets that occasionally use hendecasyllables, provides mottoes for more general Saturnalia gifts—artwork, books, animals, and other items.

EPIGRAMS

Martial's tour de force, and the work for which he is best remembered, is *Epigrams*, the collections of short poems he released between 86 and 98 C.E. A dozen of these books were produced during Martial's lifetime, and his earlier works, *Xenia* and *Apophoreta*, similar in structure and content, were later incorporated into the collection, as books 13 and 14, respectively. During his age and afterward, Martial earned a reputation for providing quality and quantity: Each book offered at least a hundred well-crafted epigrams. There was something for every taste: formal dedications, clever observations, gentle reminders, epitaphs and eulogies, friendly advice, birthday greetings, love poems, couplets in praise of the living and the dead, blatant appeals for patronage, scurrilous attacks, and crude scatological material—all in polished verse best appreciated in the original Latin. (Translations of Martial vary widely: Some preserve the meter and flavor of the poems, others gloss over the more sexually explicit of Martial's couplets.)

Book 1 of the *Epigrams* established the pattern that later entries would follow. In the opening poem, Martial addresses the reader, claiming, tongue-in-cheek, that he has exercised self-control and downplaying the significance of his poems, calling them merely jests. He summons the memory of previous epigram writers—Catullus, Marsus, Pedo, Getulicus—to justify the nature of the collection, apologizes in advance for sometimes blunt language, and cautions against reading too much meaning into his words. Other introductory material includes an obligatory dedication to the current emperor, Domitian, and the emperor's sup-

posed reply—also in terse epigram form. Martial demonstrates a very modern sense of promotion, claiming in successive poems that he is known worldwide for his humorous work and informing interested readers exactly where his books (published on parchment in small, handheld editions, the precursor of nineteenth century "penny dreadfuls" and twentieth century paperbacks) can be purchased.

Though there are occasional poems concerning places ("On Regulus") and nonhuman subjects ("To a Hare"), the bulk of book 1, like each subsequent entry in the *Epigrams* series, consists of short pieces aimed at specific individuals (for example, "To Maximus," "To Decianus," "On Gemellus and Maronilla," "On Accerra"). These are intended to illuminate and poke fun at a particular human characteristic, behavior, or activity. Though it may be presumed that Martial had an actual acquaintance in mind for every pointed barb, the living objects of his scorn are disguised behind a generic precognomen (otherwise, he would have provided full names, as in Marcus Valerius Martialis). This was undoubtedly done to avoid potential legal action for libel or defamation of character, which, for a man of modest means, could have been ruinous.

The use of such pseudonyms allowed Martial the freedom to write with impunity about whatever caught his fancy, without worrying about the consequences. Thus he could lampoon a certain Sextilianus's excessive drinking, mock a miser called Tucca who put cheap wine in casks labeled for an expensive vintage, insult a Fidentius who is accused of plagiarizing from Martial, or ridicule Laevina, who left her husband for a younger man.

Martial's work, in the twelve books of *Epigrams* and in the two posthumous inclusions of his earlier writings, ranges far and wide, and its content has a timeless quality that still resonates. The outstanding epigrammatist of his time covers, like no one before him and few afterward, the full panoply of foibles—pride, envy, greed, lust, gluttony, sadism, selfishness, and the other flaws all humans exhibit—demonstrating once again the aphorism first noted more than two millennia ago in Ecclesiastes, that there is nothing new under the sun.

BIBLIOGRAPHY

Califf, David J. *A Guide to Latin Meter and Verse Composition*. London: Anthem Press, 2002. Focuses on the different types of classical meter employed to achieve specific purposes, using examples from Latin literature to demonstrate how ancient writers used rhythm and nuance to achieve subtle effects.

Conley, Thomas M. *Toward a Rhetoric of Insult*. Chicago: University of Chicago Press, 2010. Examines Martial's epigrams, along with the work of many other writers, for their insulting qualities.

Fain, Gordon L. *Writing Epigrams: The Art of Composition in Catullus, Callimachus, and Martial*. Brussels: Editions Latomus, 2008. Examines how Martial and two other writers wrote epigrams.

Fitzgerald, William. *Martial: The World of the Epigram*. Chicago: University of Chicago Press, 2007. Focuses on Martial's body of work, demonstrating how the poet's epigrams, addressed to an ancient audience, also speak to modern readers.

Garthwaite, John. "*Ludimus Innocui*: Interpreting Martial's Imperial Epigrams." In *Writing Politics in Imperial Rome*, edited by William J. Dominik, J. Garthwaite, and P. A. Roche. Boston: Brill, 2009. Examines the political aspects of Martial's epigrams.

Howell, Peter. *Martial*. London: Bristol Classical Press, 2009. Contains biographical information on Martial and analysis of the epigrams.

Nauta, Ruurd R., Harm Jan van Dam, and Johannes J. L. Smolenaars, eds. *Flavian Poetry*. Boston: Brill Academic, 2005. This collection of scholarly papers deals specifically with the literature produced during the late first century reign of the Flavian emperors, under whom Martial lived and worked.

Rimell, Victoria. *Empire and the Ideology of Epigram*. New York: Cambridge University Press, 2009. This study examines Martial's poetic style and themes in the context of ancient Roman literature, culture, and history.

Wills, Garry. *Martial's "Epigrams": A Selection*. New York: Viking Adult, 2008. Presents Martial's most memorable short poems, newly translated, including about 150 examples from across the full range of his work.

Jack Ewing

HARRY MARTINSON

Born: Jämshög, Sweden; May 6, 1904
Died: Stockholm, Sweden; February 11, 1978

PRINCIPAL POETRY
Spökskepp, 1929
Nomad, 1931
Natur, 1934
Passad, 1945
Cikada, 1953
Aniara: En revy om människan i tid och rum, 1956 (*Aniara: A Review of Man in Time and Space*, 1963)
Gräsen i Thule, 1958
Vagnen, 1960
Dikter om ljus och mörker, 1971
Tuvor, 1973
Wild Bouquet, 1985
The Procession of Memories: Selected Poems 1929-1945, 2009

OTHER LITERARY FORMS

In addition to his poetry, Harry Martinson (MAHR-teen-sawn) published impressionistic travelogues as well as two autobiographical childhood recollections and a novel. They are all centered on the major symbol in his work, the "world nomad," the restless traveler, and form one coherent poetic bildungsroman in which initial bitterness over strong social handicaps and anguish at a world without love are superseded by the protagonist's—that is, the poet's—search for tenderness and acceptance. Martinson's later essay collections—sketches, meditations, and prose poems—in which concrete nature observation is blended with philosophical speculation, mark a departure from the autobiographical realm. Martinson insists, however, on drawing parallels between life in nature and human life. This approach leads him to a scathing criticism of modern civilization in the Rousseauian tradition, climaxing in his reports from Finland's Winter War of 1939-1940 against Russia.

ACHIEVEMENTS

The immediate and acclaimed breakthrough that Harry Martinson experienced with his collection *No-*

mad was unique in Swedish literature. The critics unanimously agreed in acknowledging an unusually gifted writer who combined sharp intellect and concise power of observation with an almost visionary ability to perceive a cosmic unity behind the fragmentation of modern thought, qualities that Martinson's later writings confirmed.

In Swedish literary history, Martinson belongs chronologically to the 1930's. For a time, he joined the group of young radical poets who rejected morality and modern civilization as too inhibiting in favor of an unrestricted worship of spontaneity and instinctive forces in life. However, in spite of his contributions to the anthology *Fem unga* (1929), Martinson is only in part related to the nature of that decade's D. H. Lawrence-inspired vitalism and primitivism. Nor does he belong to the exclusive and self-centered school of T. S. Eliot-inspired modernists of the 1940's. Already during his lifetime, he was accepted as a classicist, a classicist distinguished through linguistic imagination and a highly developed associative and myth-creating imagination. Also notable is his continuous endeavor to search for coherence in a chaotic world and—for the sake of troubled humanity—to warn against abusing the achievements of modern technology.

It is, however, impossible to place Martinson in a specific school or trend. Indeed, after his epic poem *Aniara*, a tremendous critical and public success, he emerged as one of the most independent yet compassionate humanists in twentieth century Scandinavian literature. In 1959, when *Aniara* premiered as an opera, with libretto by another prolific Swedish poet, Erik Lindegren, and music by Karl-Birger Blomdahl, it received international recognition. In 1949, Martinson was elected to the Swedish Academy as its first self-taught proletarian writer. In 1954, he received an honorary doctorate from the University of Gothenburg, and, in 1974, he shared, together with Eyvind Johnson, the Nobel Prize in Literature.

BIOGRAPHY

Harry Edmund Martinson was born on May 6, 1904, in Jämshög in the southeastern province of Blekinge, Sweden. His father, a captain in the merchant marines and later an unsuccessful businessman, died when Martinson was five. One year later, his mother emigrated to the United States, leaving her seven children to be cared for by the local parish. As a child, Martinson escaped from harsh reality into nature and into a fantasy world nourished by his reading (in particular the works of Jack London), and he dreamed of going to sea. He spent two years as a vagabond throughout Sweden and Norway before going to sea as a stoker and deckhand. He spent the next six years on fourteen different vessels, with extended periods in India and South America, before he finally returned to Sweden, having contracted tuberculosis.

The year 1929 proved to be a turning point in Martinson's life. He made his literary debut and also married the writer Moa Martinson, beginning a stimulating partnership that lasted until 1940. During the early 1930's, Martinson was tempted to pursue a career as a professional artist. His favorite subjects were factory workers, the jungle, and underwater scenes executed in a colorful and naïve style. In August, 1934, he participated in the Soviet Writers' Congress in Moscow, an experience that disillusioned the former Communist sympathizer. The outbreak of World War II was seen by him as the result of the "civilization of violence." In 1939, after Finland was attacked by the Soviet Union, Martinson joined the Finnish side as a volunteer. He wrote a book about his experiences, partly a glorification of rural Finland and its deep-rooted traditions as well as the country's courageous battle against the war machine from the east, partly direct reportage from the front, the "unequivocal idiot-roaring grenade reality." In 1942, Martinson married Ingrid Lindcrantz and settled in Stockholm, where he died on February 11, 1978.

ANALYSIS

From the very outset, it was Harry Martinson's intention to change the world. He embodied this intention in his utopian figure of the altruistic "world nomad" who represents humanity's search for a better world. The nomadic concept must be understood both concretely, in a geographical sense, and symbolically, as a journey into the realms of fantasy, dream, and the ideal future. Thus, dynamism and a moral intent emerged as the two basic qualities that were to characterize everything he wrote.

Martinson's own life as a sailor was the obvious point of departure for this expansion, which in his earliest poems is mainly depicted as daydreaming without specific direction: "Our thoughts are seabirds and they always fly away from us." They were written at sea on paper bags, Rudyard Kipling and Robert Burns being their models. Nevertheless, these texts, in particular those written with a free rhythmical and rhymeless structure, are characterized by a unique melodious softness and a ballad-like flow hitherto unknown in Swedish literature. In addition, Martinson's own experiences abroad add a quality of reliability and concreteness, which also became a personal trademark of his later writing.

Other literary models, Walt Whitman and Edgar Lee Masters, are noticeable in Martinson's contributions to the anthology *Fem unga*. His poetry, however, increasingly relies on memories from his childhood and impressions from the world of nature and of the sea, guided by the poet's vivid associative power: "Out at sea you feel a spring or summer only like a breeze./ The drifting Florida seaweed sometimes blossoms in the summer,/ and on a spring night a spoonbill stork flies towards Holland." A simultaneous striving for brevity and concentration, influenced by the Old Norse Eddic poetry, occasionally leads to a syntactic complexity and obscurity of thought. These characteristics are particularly present in his third collection, *Natur*, in which some of his most successful texts take on a surrealist quality inspired by Vladimir Mayakovski and contemporary art.

PASSAD

Martinson, in his progression from concrete detail to an almost mystical experience of a pantheistic unity, never loses sight of humankind in his writing. Satire can be found in "Rhapsody," the portrayal of a scientist who hunts for birds with a machine gun while at the same time recording bird songs. Usually—and in particular in the volumes *Passad* and *Aniara*—Martinson focuses on humanity in general, treating it in conjunction with the travel motif. In *Passad*, he creates a grandiose vision of the fundamental division of Western civilization pictured in the two travelers, Ulysses and Robinson Crusoe. One is the humanist and poet, the other the empiricist and scientist, and

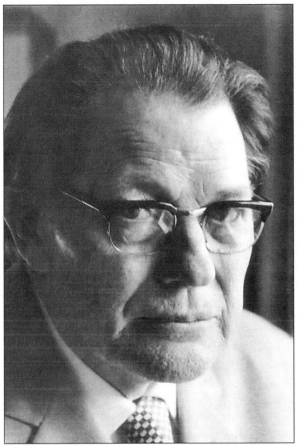

Harry Martinson (©The Nobel Foundation)

Martinson sees modern humanity's tragedy in the fact that these two personalities have not been synthesized. The trade wind, the "passad," becomes the symbol of the search for such a unity and harmony, which can only be discovered within oneself: "But new and wise explorers I have met/ have pointed inward . . . and I have listened to them/ and sensed/ a new trade wind." A fictional representative of Martinson's worldview is the persona of Li Kan, introduced in *Passad*, evincing Martinson's preoccupation with Chinese poetry and Asian philosophy, Daoism in particular. Li Kan's media are terse, almost aphoristic maxims, in which a tone of resignation and melancholy counterbalances Martinson's otherwise optimistic message of universal harmony.

ANIARA

Achieving this harmony becomes increasingly problematic in Martinson's works in the period after 1950.

This was a time in which his cosmic expansion and escaping dreams offered little consolation, a time overshadowed by nuclear bombs, wars, and political uprisings. Initially expressed in twenty-nine poems or songs, included in the collection *Cikada*, this misanthropy comes to its full expression in the verse epic *Aniara*, expanded to 103 songs. For years, Martinson had taken a keen interest in mathematics, physics, and astronomy. This expertise formed the background for his account of the giant spaceship *Aniara*, which in the year 9000 takes off with eight thousand evacuees from planet Earth following a nuclear catastrophe. The passengers seek consolation from the Mima, a supercomputer, which shows pictures from Earth and from other planets. Soon, however, the journey is no longer one of discovery but of horrible certainty, a travel toward ultimate extinction. After twenty-four years in space, the passengers die, and the *Aniara*, now a giant sarcophagus, continues on its way out of the galaxy. The *Aniara* is meant to be an image of civilization, and the characters aboard, prisoners indeed, represent a world steadily departing further from humanity toward still greater technological, impersonal sterility. Life aboard the spaceship offers a cross section of contemporary society, its different aspects and attitudes. Martinson goes beyond the social and political realm to an analysis of humanity's moral and spiritual decay. Thus, the *Aniara* becomes an image of humans and their doomed situation as they desperately attempt to avert catastrophe through artistic expression, rituals, and idolatry. Against this ship of fools, Martinson contrasts an ideal life of simplicity and harmony with nature as portrayed in an exquisite scene from the forests of Finnish Karelia. A beam of hope is lit through the various female characters, who together strive for nothing less than the Platonic ideals of truth, beauty, and goodness: "The eternal mystery of the firmament/ and the miracle of the celestial mechanics/ are laws but not the Gospel. Charity sprouts in the ground of life."

The style of *Aniara* is remarkable. Martinson's associative technique allows him to create a futuristic language composed of a flow of literary allusions ranging from the Bible to contemporary popular songs, hidden quotes, as well as a unique terminology based on self-coined technical words. With *Aniara*, Martinson cre-

ated what may be the only epic in Swedish literature judged to have significant artistic value.

Subsequently, Martinson returned to a simpler poetic form closer to that of his earlier works. In collections of lucid and artless poetry, he protested the exploitation and destruction of nature and continued to reject the modern lifestyle marred by commercialism, superficiality, and rootlessness.

It is important to remember that Martinson's view of nature is strictly unsentimental and anti-idyllic. His skepticism is not aimed at technology per se but at humankind's inability to cope with its advances and to make it subservient to humanity. Instead, the products of civilization are threatening humankind's dreams and imagination—the airplane is being used to drop bombs on civilians, and the radio has become an instrument for political propaganda. Hence also Martinson's prevailing hope that humankind can avoid the fate of the *Aniara* and its passengers, a hope that in some poems takes on a metaphysical dimension: "We have a foreboding that what we call space . . ./ is spirit, eternal spirit, untouchable,/ that we have lost ourselves in the sea of the spirit."

Martinson's vision is probably wider than that of any modern Swedish poet. His visionary and mystical approach is counterbalanced by the clarity and simplicity of his poems about childhood and nature; his sophisticated analyses of modern technology are counterbalanced by an intuitive delving into the fantasies and hopes of the human mind. He has created an entirely new poetic language and imagery, inspired by modern technology and the pictorial arts, the boldness of which makes him a modernist in the forefront of his art. At the same time, his humanist message establishes bonds that reach back to a long historical tradition.

OTHER MAJOR WORKS

LONG FICTION: *Vägen till Klockrike*, 1948 (*The Road*, 1955).

PLAYS: *Lotsen fran Moluckas*, pb. 1938; *Tre knivar från Wei*, pb. 1964.

NONFICTION: *Resor utan mål*, 1932; *Kap Farväl*, 1933 (*Cape Farewell*, 1934); *Nässlorna blomma*, 1935 (autobiography; *Flowering Nettle*, 1936); *Vägen ut*, 1936 (autobiography); *Svärmare och harkrank*, 1937;

Midsommardalen, 1938; *Det enkla och det svåra*, 1939; *Verklighet till döds*, 1940; *Utsikt från en grästuva*, 1963 (*Views from a Tuft of Grass*, 2005).

BIBLIOGRAPHY

Barnie, John. *No Hiding Place: Essays on the New Nature and Poetry*. Cardiff: University of Wales Press, 1996. Martinson's life and work are discussed at length in this thoughtful study. Includes bibliography.

Graves, Peter, and Philip Holms. "Harry Martinson." In *Essays on Swedish Literature from 1880 to the Present Day*, edited by Irene Scobbie. Aberdeen, Scotland: University of Aberdeen, 1978. A good introduction to Martinson, with a thorough analysis of *Aniara*.

Hall, Tord. Introduction to *Aniara: A Review of Man in Time and Space*, by Harry Martinson. Adapted and translated by Hugh McDiarmid and Elspeth Harley Schubert. New York: Avon Books, 1976. Praises *Aniara* as a unique blend of science, science fiction, and poetic expression.

Nordström, Lars. Introduction to *The Procession of Memories: Selected Poems, 1929-1945*, by Harry Martinson. La Grande, Oreg.: Wordcraft of Oregon, 2009. In this introduction to a bilingual edition of selected early poem by Martinson, Nordström describes the poet's life and the influences that shaped his life and work.

Sandelin, Stefan. *Harry Martinson, Nässlorna blomma*. Hull, England: Department of Scandinavian Studies, University of Hull, 1987. A critical assessment of Martinson's autobiography.

Smith, Scott Andrew. "The Role of the Emersonian 'Poet' in Harry Martinson's *Aniara: A Review of Man in Time and Space*." *Extrapolation: A Journal of Science Fiction and Fantasy* 39, no. 4 (Winter, 1998): 324-337. A close analysis of *Aniara* indicates that the work deserves far more critical attention than it has received.

Sven H. Rossel

MELEAGER

Born: Gadara, Syria (now Umm Qays, Jordan); c. 140 B.C.E.
Died: Cos, Greece; c. 70 B.C.E.
Also known as: Meleager of Gadara; Meleagros

PRINCIPAL POETRY

Stephanos, c. 90-80 B.C.E. (*Fifty Poems*, 1890; best known as *Garland*)

OTHER LITERARY FORMS

Meleager (mah-LEE-gur) specialized in collecting and writing epigrams, as understood in the original meaning of the word: short, pithy phrases intended to be chiseled on monuments and temples to commemorate important events, religious celebrations, or the lives of political and military leaders. He is known to have engaged in literary forms other than epigrams and short poetry, particularly satires in the style of his countryman Menippus (fl. third century B.C.E.), whom he admired, but these have not survived.

ACHIEVEMENTS

Meleager's chief claim to fame is his invention of the concept of the poetry anthology, both in form and in name; a later compiler called such collections anthologies, from the Greek words *anthos*, meaning "flower," and *logia*, meaning "gathering," preserving both the intent and definition of Meleager's the *Garland*. The idea of the anthology has been extended to cover collections of short stories, novels, comic strips, and other literary works.

Though others before him had collected witty sayings and poetical inscriptions, Meleager was the first to put together a comprehensive, systematic collection of significant writings gleaned from buildings, statuary, and cemeteries that attributed the words to their proper authors. His *Garland* gathered the encapsulated ideas and well-turned phrases from Greek writers, encompassing the work of predecessors from past centuries, as well as the work of contemporaries. In the process, Meleager demonstrated that epigrams were a literary form in their own right and need not be confined solely to engravings on stone.

Although the manuscript of the *Garland* has been lost, it has formed the basis for later anthologies. In 917, Constantinus Cephalas, a Byzantine official in Constantinople, compiled an anthology that included Meleager's *Garland* with collections made by other poets. However, Cephalas's anthology survives only in the *Greek Anthology*, discovered in a library in Heidelberg in 1606. In modern editions, the fifteen-volume *Greek Anthology* contains thirty-seven hundred epigrams from the Archaic through the Byzantine periods, grouped by themes.

BIOGRAPHY

Meleager was born in Gadara, the major metropolis of a Macedonian colony between the Sea of Galilee and the Jordan River then in Syria. The ruins of the ancient settlement—referred to as the land of the Gadarenes in the New Testament—can be found near modern-day Umm Qays, Jordan. Meleager was the son of Eukrates and may have had a Syrian mother. He probably grew up speaking Aramaic and undoubtedly learned Greek and Phoenician. At some point, he became enamored of the work of Cynic poet and satirist Menippus, a fellow Gadarene.

At the age of twenty, Meleager moved north to the ancient cosmopolitan Phoenician port city of Tyre (now in Lebanon), where he received his higher education. While biographical details are scarce, it is supposed that Meleager followed Cynic philosophy, shunning fame and fortune, and lived in self-sufficient poverty. He began writing poetry and satires in Cynic style, combining the elements of the serious and the frivolous in his work. It is presumed that while residing in Tyre, he began recording the inscriptions of his Greek predecessors from cemeteries, monuments, statues, and buildings; it is unknown how far afield he may have traveled to add to his collection. When he had sufficient material, Meleager published his anthology, the *Garland*, probably as a papyrus scroll, the usual form for literary works of the time—typically produced in small quantities, since each copy had to be made by hand. Meleager probably published other writings, but they, like the *Garland*, have since been lost.

Late in life, Meleager continued migrating north and settled on the Greek island of Cos, a few miles off the southwestern shores of Turkey, where he died. It is unknown whether he married or produced heirs.

ANALYSIS

Although the original no longer exists, Meleager's *Garland* is nonetheless significant for several reasons. It is considered the first true poetry anthology and as such is the prototype for countless anthologies that followed—including at least five different versions of what is now called the *Greek Anthology*—that incorporate parts of the *Garland*. Prefaced with another first, the thematic introduction, the collection presents the work of early and contemporary Greek poets, both major and minor, many of whom would otherwise be unknown. The *Garland* preserves a peculiarly Greek art of expression, the epigram: a brief, often witty or poignant poetic statement that can be committed to memory and perpetuated by recital. As reproduced in later anthologies, the *Garland* is the only extant source of Meleager's own poetry.

Although in modern times any short, memorable, well-phrased statement (such Mark Twain's wry observations, Ambrose Bierce's sly definitions, Oscar Wilde's *bon mots*, or Dorothy Parker's clever witticisms) can be called an epigram, in Meleager's day, the rules of composition were more formal. Epigrams were traditionally composed in hexameter, in rhyming couplets. Ideally, a single couplet was sufficient for expressing a complete, memorable idea, though slightly longer poems consisting of three or four elegiac couplets that expanded a poetic conceit also found favor. Epigrams were originally an outgrowth of *spoudaiogeloion* (from the Greek words for "serious" and "comical"), a satirical form employed from the time of Aristophanes (c. 450-c. 385 B.C.E.), combining high-flown subject matter with playful style. The serious-comedic blend was particularly appropriate for simple-living Cynics like Meleager, who could criticize specific aspects of society in terse verse, while including enough humor so as not to give undue offense.

Though it is unknown exactly how many individual epigrams were included in the original manuscript of the *Garland*, it presented the works of some forty-eight poets, including Meleager, who incorporated more than one hundred of his own epigrams. Meleager presented the epigrams in alphabetical order (from alpha to omega of the Greek alphabet) and included poets from the seventh to the first centuries B.C.E. The subject matter is diverse; however, most poems could be grouped under a few general headings: odes to nature, paeans to the gods, praise of the famous, epitaphs for departed humans and pets, musings on fate and death, celebrations of historical events, and verses dealing with the intricacies of love.

Meleager's particular forte was in the last category: Of some 140 of his epigrams that have survived, about 80 percent comment on the author's intimate relationships. Meleager may have lived a no-frills existence as a Cynic, rejecting wealth, recognition, and power, but he apparently led a rich love life. The poet addressed epigrams to a profusion of women (such as Heliodora) and to a succession of young men and boys (such as Alexis). Meleager was skilled at capturing elusive, almost inexpressible emotions through extended metaphor, invoking bees, gnats, arrows, lamps, and other commonplace beings and items in making subtle, imaginative comparisons to his feelings.

This ability is most evident in Meleager's introduction to the *Garland*, in which he compares each poet in the anthology to an appropriate flower or plant that might be woven into a celebratory floral display. Meleager, in a few pointed words, makes a critical comment on each entry, which can be better understood through a knowledge of the ancient symbolism of the selected botanical specimen. An egalitarian, he incorporates a fair number of female poets. The more recognizable names that have come down to the present, and the garden item with which they are linked include: Anyte (lilies), Sappho (roses), Simonides (vine blossom), Alcaeus (hyacinth), Erinna (crocus), Plato (golden bough), Callimachus (myrtle berry), Anacreon (honeysuckle), Leonidas of Tarentum (ivy clusters), and Antipater of Sidon (Phoenician cypress).

THE GREEK ANTHOLOGY

That the work of Meleager exists at all is courtesy first to another Greek writer of epigrams. Philippus of Thessalonica, more than a century after the death of Meleager, produced a collection of short poems incorporating the *Garland*, adding to it the writings of a dozen Greek poets—from the intervening years between the two editions—deemed worthy of inclusion. Philippus was allegedly the first epigram compiler to use the term "anthology" for his collection. Unfortunately, this cannot be proved, since Philippus's work, like his mentor's, has been lost to time.

A century later, Diogenianus of Heracleia selected the satirical lines from the work of Meleager and Philippus, added examples of contemporary wit, and produced a fresh offshoot of the original. Likewise, in the third century, Straton of Sardis gleaned homoerotic verse from all previous anthologies for his *Mousa paidike* (also known as *Musa puerelis*; "boyish muse"; *Puerilities*, 2001). In the fourth century, a collection of Christian epigrams—and less offensive samples from prior works—appeared. In the following century, poet and historian Agathias of Myrina, re-edited and updated the *Greek Anthology*, including about a hundred of his own epigrams.

The definitive edition of the *Greek Anthology*, containing most of the earlier collections of epigrams as well as new material, was compiled in 917. It was the work of Cephalas, a Byzantine official, who divided the material by subject. The entire fifteen-book manuscript is preserved in the Palatine Library at the University of Heidelberg, thus it is often referred to as the *Palatine Anthology*. This is to distinguish it from the bowdlerized, augmented *Planudes Anthology*, the work of fourteenth century monk Maximus Planudes. Many editions of each of these anthologies have since been published, in many different languages. Both versions have served as inspiration to generations of writers seeking instruction in the art of concision.

BIBLIOGRAPHY

Branham, R. Bracht, and Marie-Odile Goulet Cazé. *The Cynics: The Cynic Movement in Antiquity and Its Legacy*. Berkeley: University of California Press, 2000. A collection of essays with appendices, this work traces the history, development and influence of the Cynical tradition since its inception to the present, from social, ethical, and cultural perspectives.

Clack, J. *Meleager: The Poems*. Mundelein, Ill.: Bolchazy-Carducci, 1992. An overview of the poet, this text reproduces and discusses 132 of Meleager's epigrammatic verses—more than 90 percent of his known works.

Greene, Ellen, ed. *Women Poets in Ancient Greece and Rome*. Norman: University of Oklahoma Press, 2005. This is a collection of scholarly essays focusing on the work of many of the female Greek writers from Meleager's original *Garland*, including Sappho, Erinna, Moero, Nossis, and Anyte.

Gutzwiller, Kathryn J. *A Guide to Hellenistic Literature*. Malden, Mass.: Blackwell, 2007. Presents the full panoply of literature from Greece's Golden Age against the backdrop of history, showing how events shaped the form and function of writing. Many of the poets from the *Garland*—Posidippus of Pella, Erinna of Teos, Asclepiades of Samos, Callimachus, Meleager, and others—are discussed. The indexed work is supplemented with illustrations, maps, and chronologies.

_____. *Poetic Garlands: Hellenistic Epigrams in Context*. Berkeley: University of California Press, 1998. Beginning with a reconstruction of Meleager's *Garland*, Gutzwiller fully examines the development of the epigram as a literary medium throughout three centuries of the Hellenistic era following the death of Alexander the Great.

Hine, Darryl, trans. *Puerilities: Erotic Epigrams of "The Greek Anthology."* Princeton, N.J.: Princeton University Press, 2001. This collection presents, in original Greek with English translations, the anthology of Straton of Sardis, which incorporates many sexually oriented epigrams that first appeared in the *Garland*, including a number by Meleager, a master of the form.

Skinner, Marilyn B. *Sexuality in Greek and Roman Culture*. Malden, Mass.: Wiley-Blackwell, 2005. This study examines ancient Greek and Roman attitudes toward such permitted—and at times widely accepted—activities as homosexuality, pedophilia, and male and female prostitution. Skinner discusses sexuality in general and in the context of respective cultures, comparing ancient and modern civilizations through the use of a wide range of examples from art, architecture, and literature, including epigrams from Meleager's *Garland*.

Jack Ewing

HENRI MICHAUX

Born: Namur, Belgium; May 24, 1899
Died: Paris, France; October 17, 1984

PRINCIPAL POETRY

Fables des origines, 1923
Les Rêves et la jambe, 1923
Qui je fus, 1927
Écuador: Journal de voyage, 1929 (includes essays and diary; *Ecuador: A Travel Journal*, 1970)
Mes propriétés, 1929
Un Certain M. Plume, 1930
Un Barbare en Asie, 1933 (includes essays and diary; *A Barbarian in Asia*, 1949)
La Nuit remue, 1935
Lointain intérieure, 1938
Plume: Précédé de lointain intérieur, 1938
Peintures, 1939
Arbres des tropiques, 1942 (includes drawings)
Je vous écris d'un pays lointain, 1942
Exorcismes, 1943 (includes drawings)
L'Espace du dedans, 1944 (*Selected Writings: The Space Within*, 1951)
Épreuves, exorcismes, 1940-1944, 1945
Peintures et dessins, 1946 (expanded version of *Peintures*, includes drawings)
Nous deux encore, 1948
La Vie dans les plis, 1949
Mouvements, 1951 (includes drawings)
Face aux verrous, 1954
Paix dans les brisements, 1959 (includes drawings)
Poems, 1967
Selected Writings of Henri Michaux, 1968
Émergences-Résurgences, 1972 (*Emergences-Resurgences*, 2000; includes writings and drawings)
Chemins cherchés, chemins perdue, transgressions, 1982

OTHER LITERARY FORMS

Apart from his verse and prose poetry, Henri Michaux (mee-SHOH) has written travelogues, essays, drama, and fiction. He is, however, equally well known as a painter. Often merging forms and genres, Michaux's works traverse the boundaries of real and imaginary worlds, moving from outer to inner space with a constant focus on visual impressions while analyzing the experience. Michaux's writing cannot be divorced from the visual arts, and several of his foremost collections are combinations of original drawings (gouaches, water-colors, inks, acrylics) and texts. The poems are not merely accompanied by illustrations; rather, the two are simultaneous expressions of analogous themes.

Michaux also wrote a one-act play, *Le Drame des constructeurs* (pb. 1930; the builder's drama), which again reflects his interest in the visual arts. The setting is a lunatic asylum where various inmates, named A, B, C, D, E, F, G, and H, play "construction" games. Their guards can be seen in the background; every time one appears, the "builders" disperse. Law and order, Michaux implies, destroy imagination and deprive humanity of its ability to exist. Furthermore, the character "God" is aligned with the lunatics, whom he absolves and liberates. Ironically, the inmates continue their imaginary building, the guards remain, and nothing changes.

Another literary form that Michaux expertly handles is the aphorism. In *Tranches de savoir* (1950; slices of knowledge), 234 aphorisms, short-circuited proverbs, are posited. These brief phrases, in the French tradition of François La Rochefoucauld, are both sinister and amusing, for they scramble traditional sayings and reflect the themes and clichés found throughout literature. One can easily discover Molière, Jean de La Fontaine, and Charles Baudelaire reworked and answered across time and space in succinct one-line summaries of the human condition.

Michaux is especially well known for his introspective, scientific, and informative prose accounts of his experiences with mescaline and other hallucinogenic drugs. His period of drug usage lasted sixteen years (from 1955 to 1971) and produced five major essays: *Misérable miracle, la mescaline* (1956; *Miserable Miracle, Mescaline*, 1963), *L'Infini turbulent* (1957; *Infinite Turbulence*, 1975), *Connaissance par les gouffres* (1961; *Light Through Darkness*, 1963), *Vents et poussières* (1962; winds and dust), and *Les Grandes Épreuves de l'esprit et les innombrables petites* (1966;

The Major Ordeals of the Mind and the Countless Minor Ones, 1974). What distinguishes Michaux's investigations from those of the historical line of French writers who have created while under the influence of drugs is his objectivity. While he appreciates the liberating effect of hallucinogens, he found them to be more revelatory than creative. His prose accounts are not "automatic writings," in the tradition of the Surrealists, but reasoned, after-the-fact analyses of the feelings of fragmentation, alienation, energy, and elasticity of the persona.

ACHIEVEMENTS

Henri Michaux's achievements integrate both his literary and his artistic worlds. The poetry collection *Qui je fus*, Michaux's first work published in France, received considerable critical acclaim. Although he began painting in the mid-1920's, his first book of drawings and paintings did not appear until 1936. During the next several years, Michaux became a presence in the French world of art, and his premiere exposition of paintings and gouaches was held in the Galerie Pierre in Paris in 1938. In 1941, André Gide published, in booklet form, the controversial panegyric *Découvrons Henri Michaux*, which revealed the modernity and complexity of Michaux's creative process. In 1948, the Galerie René Drouin exhibited Michaux's first collection of wash drawings and, in 1954, his premiere exposition of ink designs. In 1960, he received the Einaudi Award in Venice.

Michaux turned to yet another medium in 1963 and created, with Eric Duvivier, a film titled *Images du monde visionaire*. The Musée National d'Art Moderne de Paris honored Michaux with a grand retrospective of his works in 1965; in the same year, he was featured by Geneviève Bonnefoi and Jacques Veinat in the film *Henri Michaux ou l'espace du dedans*. Also in 1965, Michaux was voted to receive the Grand Prix National des Lettres, which he decided not to accept. Both to acknowledge his literary works and to honor his refusal, the committee then chose not to award the prize that year. In 1966, a special issue of the journal *L'Herne* was dedicated to Michaux, and in 1976, the Fondation Maeght mounted another major retrospective exhibition of Michaux's drawings.

BIOGRAPHY

Henri-Eugène-Guislain Michaux's life, like his works, was cosmopolitan. He was born in Namur, Belgium, on May 24, 1899, and was reared in Brussels. Because of his delicate health and obstinate temperament, he was sent to a boarding school in Putte-Grasheide. After five years in the country, which was for him a time of solitude and refusal of societal norms, Michaux returned to Brussels in 1911 for the remainder of his formal education. He graduated from his *lycée* in 1916, but because of the German Occupation, he could not immediately enroll in a university. During this period, Michaux studied literature voraciously, learning about the lives of the saints and discovering the writings of mystics such as Jan van Ruysbroeck, Leo Tolstoy, and Fyodor Dostoevski. Refusing to believe that literature alone held the key to the essence of life, Michaux, in 1919, enrolled in medical school, but he later abandoned his studies there as well.

At the age of twenty-one, Michaux embarked upon the first of a series of voyages that greatly influenced his life and writing. He first became a sailor on a five-masted schooner at Boulogne-sur-Mer; then he joined the crew of the ten-ton *Victorieux* at Rotterdam. He explored the civilizations bordering the Atlantic, including the United States and South America. Michaux stayed in Marseilles, France, for a year, then returned to Brussels, where his first volumes—*Fables des origines* (fables on origins) and *Les Rêves et la jambe* (dreams and the leg)—were published. He was, however, dissatisfied with life in Belgium, particularly with his family's view of his "failure," and had already moved to Paris when the two works appeared.

The Parisian artistic scene of the 1920's had a tremendous impact on Michaux. Introduced to the Surrealists and to plastic art—primarily the paintings of Paul Klee, Max Ernst, and Giorgio de Chirico—he became interested in design. As early as 1927, he experimented with his own ideograms (*signes*), a mixing of the literary (the alphabet) and the plastic arts. Furthermore, the publication of *Qui je fus* in 1927 marked his break with parental and cultural authority. He traveled to South America with the poet Alfredo Gangotena and spent a year in Quito, Ecuador. In 1929, both of Michaux's parents died, and he journeyed to Turkey, Italy, and North Africa in an effort to erase the remaining psychological influences of both his homeland and his family. The year 1930 marks the appearance of Michaux's best-known fictional character, the humorous and pointedly emotionless Plume.

From 1930 to 1939, Michaux traveled extensively: to India, Ceylon (Sri Lanka), Malaya, Indonesia, China, Korea, Japan, Portugal, Uruguay, and Brazil. These were years of important literary production, and they included Michaux's first painting exhibition. During World War II, Michaux continued to write and draw. He experimented with various artistic techniques (watercolor and gouache) and published several volumes with original artwork. To escape the German Occupation of Paris, Michaux moved to Saint-Antonin and then to Lavandou, where he married in 1941.

His well-known anthology *Selected Writings: The Space Within* was published in 1944 during a time of personal tragedy. Michaux's brother had recently died, and his wife had contracted tuberculosis. Throughout 1947, Michaux traveled in order to help his wife convalesce, but in 1948, she died from burns received in a terrible accident. Despair moved him to compose the haunting *Nous deux encore* (still the two of us), and in the following years, he published several significant literary collections. There was also at that time a dramatic change in Michaux's creative direction. Removed from all family ties, he returned to his point of departure, the alphabet-sign. He wrote less and painted much more. The album *Mouvements* demonstrates his increased devotion to design and his personal voyage from one art form to another.

In 1955, Michaux became a naturalized French citizen. When, in 1957, he lost the use of his right hand, he trained himself to use his left hand to paint; he also embarked upon a new travel experience—the systematic use of hallucinogens to explore the inner self. The result of this experimentation was a series of essays devoted to the clinical analysis of drug-induced activity. It is important to note that during these same years, Michaux received international plaudits for his painting, and he revised and republished his major literary collections. He died in Paris on October 17, 1984, at the age of eighty-five.

ANALYSIS

Few modern French poets have equaled the range and scope of Henri Michaux. Often contrasted with René Char, who represents a positive vision and affirmation of the creative force, Michaux is known for his humor, his destructive power that renders all generic and structural barriers useless, and his ongoing investigation of the inner self and rejection of the outer world's conventions. Michaux's poetry transcends national boundaries and defies specific literary schools. His strong belief in the will makes his poetic images strong and intense. Michaux is also an enigma, an ethereal go-between from one world to the next. It is through this paradox—attack countered by whimsy, delicacy balanced by audacity, the pen in tandem with the brush—that each of Michaux's poems comes alive.

This paradox in Michaux's writing is displayed in his use of traditionally nonpoetic literary forms—artistic commentary, drama, travelogue, proverb, and essay—as a background for his poetry. Flux, rhythm, alliteration, litany, and repetition of sounds and words may be found in any Michaux text. Furthermore, all of Michaux's creations are self-referential and could never be considered objective nonfiction.

ECUADOR

Michaux's travelogues are a poetic voyage through both real and imaginary countries and creatures. *Ecuador* is the unique journal of Michaux's travels through South America and is not to be mistaken for a traditional guidebook. Rather, it is about Michaux's own self-discovery, a first-person narration that skips from vague, sensory perception to the specific notations of a diary, incorporating twenty-two free-verse poems, several prose essays, and entries recorded by hour and day. The importance of *Ecuador*, however, lies not in what Michaux sees and does, in the conventional approach to travel literature, or in the novel approach to traditional literary exoticism, but, instead, in Michaux's explorations of his self in an effort to expand his knowledge and feeling.

A BARBARIAN IN ASIA

Similarly, *A Barbarian in Asia* reveals a subjective view of Michaux's travels in the Far East. Here, Western man is revealed to be a barbarian—ignorant and unschooled, especially when faced with the refinement of Eastern civilization. In a series of short poetic essays, a "naïve" Michaux examines not "facts" but "style, gestures, accent, appearance, and reflexes" and also discovers that the Chinese originated the ideogram, his particular obsession.

IMAGINARY COUNTRIES

Michaux has also created in his poetry/travelogue form extensive accounts of imaginary countries and characters, the best of which—*Voyage en Grande Garabagne* (1936; trip to Great Garabagne), *Au pays de la magie* (1941; in the land of magic), and *Ici, Poddema* (1946; here, Poddema)—are grouped together in the collection *Ailleurs* (1948; elsewhere). Great Garabagne is a complete civilization; it has tribes, distinct geographical locations, and social and religious customs. In these accounts, Michaux is not concerned with Utopian visions but with a reordering of reality.

He continues in the same vein with the *Portrait des Meidosems* (1948; *Meidosems: Poems and Lithographs*, 1992), in which are presented personages whom Malcolm Bowie, in his 1973 study, *Henri Michaux*, has accurately defined as "me-images": shifting, self-propelled forms living in a world of continual flux.

I AM WRITING TO YOU FROM A
FAR-OFF COUNTRY

In another form of imaginary travelogue, *I Am Writing to You from a Far-Off Country* (from *Lointain intérieure*, the far-off inside), Michaux wrote twelve prose-poem segments, supposedly from a feminine writer to a desired partner, thus creating both the author and the reader of the text, who interjects his own commentary. While the faraway country does not exist, its sea, waves, and unusual fauna seem real because they are described personally and because the writer is trying to persuade her companion to meet her on this imagined plane of existence. This preoccupation with travel between real and make-believe worlds permeates all Michaux's works.

THE PLUME PERSONA

In his travelogues, as in all his works, Michaux refuses to imitate the world, preferring to turn it upside down. His first fictional character, Plume (whose name means both "feather" and "pen"), is indeed a lightweight, often pathetic, creature. His form varies from text to text; he has no firm characteristics and little awareness of the world around him. As a representative of modern man, Plume symbolizes the desperate and suffering yet resilient and matter-of-fact person existing in the bleak, often hostile, world of reality. Plume is the antithesis of Michaux's ideal; he is a victim who does not intervene, a dupe. Michaux uses humor in the Plume prose poems both to distort and to give relief. Plume cannot laugh—or at least, he does not—but the reader laughs at Plume, enjoys mocking him, and anticipates his destruction with glee.

"A TRACTABLE MAN"

In "Un Homme paisible" ("A Tractable Man"), Plume awakens to a series of disasters. The first time, he cannot find the walls of his room because ants have eaten them. Unperturbed, he falls back to sleep until his wife screams that the house has been stolen. Plume expresses disinterest and dozes off. Shortly afterward, he thinks that he hears a train, but again sleep overtakes him. When he awakens, he is very cold, covered with blood, and surrounded by various pieces of his wife. Expressing mild displeasure that the train passed by so quickly, he once more falls asleep and is abruptly disturbed by the voice of a judge who cannot decipher the mystery of Plume's apathy. Plume does not offer a defense, and when the judge plans Plume's execution for the following day, Plume pleads ignorance of the whole affair, excuses himself, and goes back to bed.

Michaux makes it clear that Plume richly deserves to be judged, condemned, and punished for not taking an active part in life. Each time Plume falls asleep, he repeats the Fall of Man, but Plume's sin is far worse, because he refuses to act. Michaux's use of the past tense in this poem expresses pessimism; man was born into a state of guilt (sleep), so he accepts his condemnation (falls back to sleep). Michaux calls upon the reader to attack Plume, to make fun of him—in short, not to identify with Plume's "peaceful" behavior but, instead, to take charge of life. One can feel no pity for the condemned man who has faced life with total passivity. The reader's laughter signifies his recognition of the absurdity of life and his alienation from Plume's apathy. Michaux encourages man to struggle, to fight for existence, even though it may be a futile battle with a hostile and absurd world.

"My King"

The theme of resistance and the attitude of scorn for man's paralysis are reiterated in the prose poem "Mon Roi" ("My King"), in the collection *La Nuit remue* (night on the move). Night, a time of apparitions and hallucinations, is the traditional period of sleep (bitterly attacked in the Plume pieces) and is a static and noncombative time for humanity, which is defeated at night. Michaux wishes to stir humankind to motion, to agitate people, to force them to participate. In the poem, it is during the night that an unnamed first-person narrator attacks a character he calls "my King," the figure of a super proprietor who is unique and powerful. The narrator strangles and shakes the King, laughs in his face, throws him on the ground, slaps him, and kicks him. However, the King does not move, his blue visage returns to normal, and every night he returns to the chamber of the narrator. The King is always seemingly victorious, but he cannot exist without a subject, while his subject, who is also a victim, cannot rid himself of the King. Like Albert Camus's Sisyphus, the narrator can acquire dignity and purpose only when in continual motion and revolt.

Michaux uses the present tense in "My King" to indicate that humanity's struggle never ends. This is the human condition wherein liberty is both necessary and impossible; the battle itself is what counts. Michaux's violent style, his use of the shock technique, and his refusal to reproduce the real constitute his call to action, his attack on society, and his indictment of humanity, which contains within itself two spirits: one, domineering and parasitic; the other, impotent and inert, a mere spectator of life. Humanity must not be resigned to this dilemma, Michaux asserts, for the only promise of salvation is in action.

"Clown"

The poem "Clown" (in the collection *Peintures*) is a brilliant summary of Michaux's poetic vision. A clown is a fool, a jester who paints on a ridiculous face, the caricature of a human being. What amuses the spectator about a clown, as he performs his zany antics, is the viewer's own superiority to the buffoon's mishaps, clumsiness, and inability to cope with the world. The clown exists in an absurd universe. He trips, he fumbles, he uncovers the unexpected, he pops in and out of boxes too small to contain human beings. His ludicrous nature, the "laughable," is dependent upon a reaction from the viewer; likewise, the spectator's appreciation and self-importance rest on the existence of the clown, his victim. People's laughter is therefore grotesque. On the other hand, the clown is not known as an individual but as a force. He is free in that he breaks with convention and logical order, going about the "expected" in his own way. Clowns make life more bearable by the creative energy of their destruction. Michaux's clown states that he will "chop off, upset, break, topple and purge" the "miserable modesty, miserable dichotomy" of his shackles.

Michaux's use of future tense in this poem is extremely important. In addition to lending urgency and a sense of power, it underscores the intolerable present and the interdependency of clown and audience. The jester must rid himself of his "worthy fellow-beings," his "look-alikes," to find the essence of a new and incredible freshness and purity (*rosée*). The sound of the word *rosée*, however, reveals a layer of deep pessimism and sets the tone for the ambiguous conclusion of the poem. A *rosé* is also a wine, potent as well as a cross between red and white, suggesting the very duality that the clown hopes to escape. Furthermore, Michaux indicates that the final revelation is *nul* (void) *et ras* (and blank) *et risible* (and ludicrous, laughable). After finally marshaling the strength and determination to discover what he might attain, the clown may find nothing but a vacuum—the final laugh.

OTHER MAJOR WORKS

FICTIONAL TRAVELOGUES: *Ailleurs*, 1948 (includes *Voyage en Grande Garabagne*, 1936; *Au pays de la magie*, 1941; and *Ici, Poddema*, 1946); *Portrait des Meidosems*, 1948 (*Meidosems: Poems and Lithographs*, 1992).

PLAY: *Le Drame des constructeurs*, pb. 1930 (one act).

NONFICTION: *Entre centre et absence*, 1936 (writings, drawings, and paintings); *Passages, 1937-1950*, 1950 (collected articles); *Tranches de savoir*, 1950 (aphorisms); *Misérable Miracle, la mescaline*, 1956 (*Miserable Miracle, Mescaline*, 1963); *L'Infini Turbulent*, 1957 (*Infinite Turbulence*, 1980); *Connaissance*

par les gouffres, 1961 (*Light Through Darkness*, 1963); *Vents et poussiéres*, 1962; *Les Grandes Épreuves de l'esprit et les innombrables petites*, 1966 (autobiographical essays; *The Major Ordeals of the Mind and the Countless Minor Ones*, 1974); *Idéogrammes en Chine*, 1975 (*Ideograms in China*, 1984); *Saisir*, 1979 (*Grasp*, included in *Stroke by Stroke*, 2006); *Par des traits*, 1984 (*Stroke by Stroke*, 2006).

MISCELLANEOUS: *Darkness Moves: An Henri Michaux Anthology, 1927-1984*, 1994.

BIBLIOGRAPHY

Bowie, Malcolm. *Henri Michaux*. Oxford, England: Clarendon Press, 1973. A critical study of Michaux's literary works. Includes bibliographic references.

Broome, Peter. *Henri Michaux*. London: Athlone Press, 1977. A short critical assessment of the works of Michaux. Includes an index and bibliography.

Hellerstein, Nina S. "Calligraphy, Identity: Scriptural Exploration as Cultural Adventure." *Symposium* 45, no. 1 (Spring, 1991): 329. A critical comparison of the works of Paul Claudel and Michaux traces each writer's fascination with Chinese and Japanese writing systems.

Kawakami, Akane. "Barbarian Travels: Textual Positions in *Un Barbare en Asie*." *Modern Language Review* 95, no. 4 (October, 2000): 978-991. *A Barbarian in Asia* is not so much a collection of Michaux's views on Asia as the trace of his passage through it. There is a complex relationship between Michaux and these Asian cultures that requires a more subtle explanatory model than the dualistic one of hegemony.

La Charité, Virginia A. *Henri Michaux*. Boston: Twayne, 1977. An introductory biography and critical study of selected works by Michaux. Includes bibliographic references.

Parish, Nina. *Henri Michaux: Experimentation with Signs*. New York: Rodopi, 2007. Examines Michaux's use of signs in the works *Mouvements*, *Par le voix des rhythmes*, *Saisir*, and *Par des traits*.

Rigaud-Drayton, Margaret. *Henri Michaux: Poetry, Painting, and the Universal Sign*. New York: Oxford University Press, 2005. The author argues that

Michaux's work, both verbal and graphic, is a quest for a universal language or sign.

Rowlands, Esther. *Redefining Resistance: The Poetic Wartime Discourses of Francis Ponge, Benjamin Peret, Henri Michaux, and Antonin Artaud.* New York: Rodopi, 2004. Presents a critique of linguistic resistance in the poetic texts compiled between 1936 and 1946 of Michaux, Ponge, Peret, and Artaud.

Katherine C. Kurk

MICHELANGELO

Born: Caprese, Tuscany, Republic of Florence (now in Italy); March 6, 1475

Died: Rome, Papal States (now in Italy); February 18, 1564

PRINCIPAL POETRY

Rime di Michelangelo Buonarroti, 1623 (*The Sonnets*, 1878)

Le Rime di Michelangelo Buonarroti, 1863 (Cesare Guasti, editor)

The Sonnets of Michel Angelo, 1878

Sonnets of Michel Angelo, 1905

Rime di Michelangelo Buonarroti, 1960

The Complete Poems of Michelangelo, 1960

Michelangelo: Self-Portrait, 1963

OTHER LITERARY FORMS

Michelangelo (mi-kuh-LAN-juh-loh), the renowned painter and sculptor, creator of the statue of David and the epic paintings of the Sistine Chapel's ceiling, also left a literary legacy. Along with his poetry, he wrote some five hundred letters that, though never intended as publishable literature, are a rich source of psychological and biographical material. Michelangelo's letters are largely concerned with money, contracts, the difficulties of dealing with popes, family quarrels and obligations, real estate deals and speculations, politics (very obliquely referred to), premonitions, and setting his worthless brothers up in business. Rarely, if ever, does he discuss the art that was his sole reason for exis-

tence. When he completed the paintings in the Sistine Chapel after four years of hard labor, all he wrote to his father was:

> I have finished the chapel I have been painting; the Pope is very well satisfied. But other things have not turned out for me as I'd hoped. For this I blame the times, which are very unfavorable to our art. . . .

ACHIEVEMENTS

By all accounts, Michelangelo reigned as the most important and most gifted sculptor of the Renaissance. When his *Pietà*, commissioned for Saint Peter's Basilica and carved when Michelangelo was barely twenty, was unveiled, it caused a great flurry of excitement, and when his *David* was presented less than a decade later, there was little doubt that his work would define the standards for the highest period of the Italian Renaissance. Throughout his life, he was sought after by both the Papacy and the patriarchs of Florence, not only for his talents as a sculptor but also for his gifts as an architect and a military engineer.

Michelangelo's allegiance was always to his art, and he was able to produce commissioned works as great as the Sistine Chapel or the Medici tombs without falling prey to the political rivalries between Rome and Florence—a feat in itself, attesting the esteem in which he was held by the ruling class. Four centuries after his death, Michelangelo is revered by popular opinion; his most famous works, especially the *Pietà* of Saint Peter's Basilica, the *David*, and the Sistine Chapel, draw tens of thousands of people every year and are among the most popular tourist attractions in Europe. In addition, critics have reevaluated Michelangelo's poetry, establishing its merit not simply as a sidelight to his sculpture but as an innovative and important body of work in its own right.

BIOGRAPHY

Michelangelo di Lodovico Buonarroti Simoni's attainments as a poet can be understood, both thematically and aesthetically, only against the background of the artist's life in the service of six popes of the Italian Renaissance and his colossal achievements in all the visual arts—sculpture, painting, and architecture.

Brought to Florence from Caprese while still an infant, Michelangelo was sent to nurse with a stone-cutter's wife in Settignano, where, he later liked to say, he imbibed marble dust with his wet-nurse's milk. When he was still a child, his mother died, leaving her husband, Lodovico, with five young sons. Lodovico remarried in 1485, and about that time, Michelangelo returned to Florence to live in the Santa Croce quarter with his father, stepmother, four brothers, and an uncle. Of the brothers, only Buonarroto, two years younger than Michelangelo, married and left progeny. The eldest brother, Leonardo, became a Dominican monk; the youngest brothers, Giovansimone and Sigismondo, passed their lives in trade, soldiering, and farming. Undoubtedly the untimely death of his mother and the overwhelmingly male household in which the artist spent his early years are important clues to certain aspects of Michelangelo's personality. He never married, asserting that his art was sufficient mistress for him; his nudes are characterized by a blurring of distinctly male and female attributes, a projection of a race whose physiognomy and physiology would seem to partake of the qualities of both sexes. Similar qualities are manifest in his poetry.

Michelangelo's correspondence with his father and brothers reveals the artist's deep, almost morbid attachment to his family, despite the fact that comprehension of, or even interest in, Michelangelo's art was entirely lacking on their part. Throughout their lives, his father and brothers looked on Michelangelo only as a source of income or as a counselor in their various projects. Although in his letters Michelangelo frequently refers to his financial affairs, he never discusses art with his family and rarely indeed with anyone else.

As a boy, Michelangelo cared little for the traditional Latin and Humanist studies; his inclination to draw led his father, despite his scorn for art, to enroll him (on April 1, 1488) as a student apprentice in the workshop of Domenico Ghirlandaio, then the most popular painter in Florence. A year later, however, Michelangelo left that master to study in the Medici gardens near San Marco, where Lorenzo the Magnificent had gathered a collection of ancient statues and had assigned Bertoldo di Giovanni, a follower of Donatello, to train young men in sculpture. A faun's head (now lost) that Michel-

angelo had freely copied from a classic fragment attracted Lorenzo's attention, and Michelangelo, then fifteen years old, was taken to live almost as a son in the Medici Palace, first with Lorenzo de' Medici, then briefly with his son Piero. It was during these impressionable years that the youthful artist absorbed the Neoplatonic ideas of Lorenzo's famous circle of Humanists, Poliziano, Marsilio Ficino, and Giovanni Pico della Mirandola. Undoubtedly, Michelangelo's notion of reality as an essence underlying, or contained within, an enveloping substance was derived from conversations he heard in Lorenzo's "academy." The sculptural art of "taking away"—that is, revealing the figure already contained within the block—is analogous to ascending the Platonic ladder to a preexistent Form. At Poliziano's suggestion, the young sculptor carved a relief, the *Battle of the Centaurs*, that showed indications of his mastery of the nude as the ideal vehicle of expression. The Neoplatonism that Michelangelo absorbed in the Medici Palace is one of the major themes of his poetry, especially the contrast between carnal and ideal love.

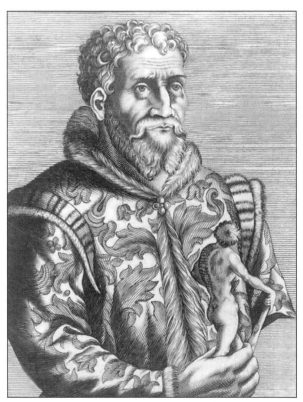

Michelangelo (Library of Congress)

After the death of Lorenzo the Magnificent on April 8, 1492, his unworthy son Piero showed little interest in Michelangelo's genius, assigning the sculptor such tasks as making a snowman. Subsequently, fearing the imminent invasion of the French under Charles VIII and the threatened fall of the Medici, Michelangelo and two companions fled to Venice and then returned to Bologna. Several times during the artist's life, unpredictable flights of this kind occurred, resulting apparently from nameless fears.

Michelangelo remained in Bologna from the fall of 1494 until the beginning of 1495 as a guest of Gianfrancesco Aldovrandi, a wealthy merchant, to whom Michelangelo read Dante, Petrarch, and other Tuscan poets. During his lifetime, Michelangelo had the reputation of being a profound scholar of Dante's *La divina commedia* (c. 1320; *The Divine Comedy*, 1802). A harsh exaltation informs the work of both Tuscans, and in Michelangelo's own poetry, the intellectual power of Dante is matched, if not his graceful style and fertile imagery.

In 1495, Michelangelo returned to Florence, where he carved in marble a *San Giovannino* and a *Sleeping Cupid* (both lost). The Cupid was such a skillful imitation of classical sculpture that it was sold to a Roman art dealer, who in turn sold the counterfeit as an authentic antique to Cardinal Raffaello Riario. Discovering the deception, the cardinal summoned Michelangelo to Rome in June, 1496, thinking to order other works from the astonishing young talent. Although the cardinal's patronage ultimately proved unrewarding, Michelangelo remained in Rome for five fruitful years. During this period, he completed a *Bacchus* in marble for the Roman banker Jacopo Galli and the *Pietà* that is now in Saint Peter's Basilica for the French cardinal Jean Villiers de la Groslaye. This first sojourn in Rome resulted in great fame for the youthful sculptor. Sharply revealed in his *Bacchus* and *Pietà* at this time are two of the main contrasting themes that served Michelangelo all his life: pagan exaltation of the nude male figure and love-pity for the Christ. Both of these works, however, in their combination of naturalistic detail, high finish, and rather cold classical beauty, still hark back to the earlier fifteenth century Florentine sculptors. A comparison of this *Pietà* with a *Pietà* from his last years shows how far the artist moved from this early, vigorous naturalism to an abstract spiritualization of form and material.

Three months before Michelangelo signed his contract for the *Pietà*, Girolamo Savonarola was burned at the stake (May 23, 1498) after his condemnation by the Borgia Pope Alexander VI. The martyrdom of the Dominican deeply affected Michelangelo, who continued to read Savonarola's sermons throughout his life. The prophetic nature of the friar was probably also a factor that led the artist to assiduous reading of the Old Testament. Nevertheless, the years of Savonarola's domination had been unfavorable to art, and it was perhaps the more propitious atmosphere that had come about in Florence, as well as the repeated urgings of his father, that drew Michelangelo back to his native city. When Michelangelo returned from Rome in 1501, he was already a famous sculptor. He was deluged with commissions, most notably for the gigantic *David*, a fourteen-foot nude extracted from a single, awkwardly shaped block of Carrara marble (1501-1504).

This colossal *David* was, both in dimension and conception, Michelangelo's first truly heroic work. The frowning hero is the first expression of the *terribilità* for which the sculptor later became so famous. In the disproportionate right hand and the strained position of the left hand holding the sling bag at the shoulder, the artist was already moving away from the more literal naturalism of his earlier work. The huge hand is an apotheosis of *la man che ubbidisce all' intelletto*— "the hand that serves the intellect." The fierce frown plays an odd counterpoint against the relaxed pose, a typical Michelangelo equilibrium between contrary forces, a coexistence of contrarieties frequently found also in his poetry.

In 1505, Pope Julius II summoned Michelangelo to Rome, assigning him the task of creating the pope's mausoleum. The project, which involved more than forty life-size figures, seemingly lacked any trace of religious spirit, and would have been a suitable secular glorification of the worldliness of the Renaissance papacy.

The intention was to place the mausoleum in the new apse then being constructed in the old basilica of Saint Peter's. The project threatened to dwarf the existing church and thus suggested to Julius the idea of reconstructing the entire basilica on a new, immense scale. It may therefore be said that the colossal dimensions of Michelangelo's plans for the tomb were an indirect cause of the construction of the new Saint Peter's. The fickleness of the pope and his failure to pay Michelangelo for the expense of carting the marble, as well as a nameless presentiment that his life was in jeopardy, caused the hypersensitive artist to depart unexpectedly for Florence on April 17, 1506, the day before the laying of the cornerstone of the new Saint Peter's. Followed in vain by messengers and threats from the pope, who sent three peremptory briefs to the Signory of Florence, Michelangelo fiercely refused to return to Rome. Several violent sonnets addressed to Pope Julius probably date from this period. Eventually Michelangelo was persuaded to attempt a reconciliation. In November, 1506, Michelangelo, "with a rope around my neck" (the traditional symbol of submission), came to Julius at Bologna, which the old pope, marching at the head of his troops, had just reconquered from the local tyrant, Giovanni Bentivoglio. In a stormy meeting, Julius pardoned Michelangelo and assigned him a new task—to cast a huge bronze statue of the pope to be set over the main portal of San Petronio in Bologna.

The bronze finished, Michelangelo returned home, planning to complete many assignments; Julius, however, summoned him again to Rome. Michelangelo sought in vain to free himself from the pope's insistence that Michelangelo fresco the vault of the Sistine Chapel instead of resuming work on the tomb. Again, the Florentine found himself engaged in a craft that he did not consider his own. Nevertheless, once Michelangelo undertook the assignment, he set to work with typical fury and confidence, resolved to surpass all other achievements in the art of fresco. Six assistants whom he had summoned from Florence were soon dismissed by the fiercely individualistic artist. Except for some manual help in preparing the plaster grounds and perhaps in painting some portions of the architectural setting, the entire stupendous task of decorating a barrel vault 128 feet long and 45 feet wide, 68 feet from the pavement, together with lunettes over twelve windows, was carried out by Michelangelo alone. From May 10, 1508, until October, 1512, with some interruptions, he worked on a special scaffolding, painting at great personal discomfort with the brush over his head "dripping a rich pavement" on his chest:

> I've already grown a goiter from this toil,
> as water swells the cats in Lombardy
> or any other country they might be,
> forcing my belly to hang under my chin.
> My beard to heaven . . .

After describing the grotesque distortions his body must assume, painting the vault 68 feet above the pavement, the poet-artist cries out:

> Therefore, fallacious, strange
> the judgment carried in the mind must fly,
> for from a twisted gun one shoots awry.
> My dead picture defend
> now, Giovanni, and also my honor,
> for I'm in no good place, nor I a painter.

Eventually the huge surface was covered with a vast panorama comprehending the story of Genesis up to the Flood and three episodes from the life of Noah. The choice of subject was Michelangelo's own, but it harmonized with the themes treated in the fifteenth century lateral-panel frescoes already in the chapel, which dealt with parallel episodes in the lives of Moses and Christ. Undoubtedly the most awesome pictorial achievement of the High Renaissance, the Sistine Chapel ceiling is the fullest expression of Michelangelo's genius in employing the human form and face in their manifold attitudes and attributes. The Sistine ceiling balances pictures from the Old Testament and nude Greek youths, pre-Christian prophets and pagan sibyls, pagan Humanism and orthodox Christianity.

Michelangelo, however, had never ceased to think of resuming work on Julius's mausoleum. Even during the creation of the most stupendous piece of painting in Western art, he had signed his letters "Michelangelo, sculptor in Rome." He had already arranged for the purchase, later concluded, of a house in Rome on the Macel de' Corvi near the area of the Trajan Forum, where he could collect and work the marble. On February 21, 1513, however, Pope Julius died, and then began the litigation with Julius's heirs, the abandonment of Michelangelo's first grand idea, the successive diminutions of the project to the present mediocrity in San Pietro in Vincoli. This much-reduced version has as its chief attraction Michelangelo's sculpture *Moses*. In the menacing *Moses*, with its hyperbolic beard and strained posture, left foot drawn back, the *terribilità* of the artist reached volcanic expression. Michelangelo was inspired more often by the heroes, prophets, and judgmental Jehovah of the Jews than by the Gospels. Only in the drawings and poems of his extreme old age does the Crucifixion appear as a theme.

In 1516, while Michelangelo was at Carrara gathering marble for the mausoleum, he had to return to Rome, where Pope Leo X (elected March, 1513) ordered him to construct and decorate with statues the facade of San Lorenzo in Florence. Thus, the artist again found himself deflected from the vast project on which he had set his heart, and once again he found himself in the service of the Medici. Leo, indeed, had known Michelangelo as a boy when they had sat together, almost as brothers, at the table of Lorenzo, Leo X's father. The pope was exactly Michelangelo's age, forty-one years old, a pleasure-loving man famous for his remark: "Let us enjoy the Papacy, since God has given it to us." Although he commissioned Michelangelo on the basis of competitive drawings and models, the contract was soon broken. Probably Leo found the sweeter and softer-natured Raphael more to his liking than the litigious and austere sculptor. At any rate, Michelangelo produced more during his tempestuous relationship with the "terrible" Julius than with the epicurean Leo.

In 1527, Rome was sacked by Emperor Charles V. At the news, the Florentines once again evicted the Medici (May 17, 1527) and restored the Republic. In July of the next year, Michelangelo's favorite brother, Buonarroto, died in his arms of the plague, and the cares of the widowed family fell on the sculptor's shoulders. When the armies of Clement VII and the reconciled Charles V moved against the city, Michelangelo was named magistrate of the Committee of Nine of the Florentine Militia, and a few months later, he was appointed governor and procurator general of the city's fortifications. Almost against his will, he participated in the defense of his city, executing missions of a military character at Pisa, Livorno, and Ferrara and fortifying the hill at San Miniato.

After the fall of Florence (August 2, 1530), the Medici returned. Pardoned by Clement VII, the artist continued working on the Medici tombs while attending to other assignments heaped on him by the pope. Then, distrusting Duke Alexander, the new Medici ruler of Florence, and desirous of concluding work on the tomb of Julius according to the last contract, Michelangelo returned to Rome to his house at Macel de' Corvi. He alternated his Rome sojourn with long stays at Florence, where he was needed for work on the library and the tombs. This was the period of his fervent friendships with the young Tommaso Cavalieri at Rome and the young Febo di Poggio at Florence. Many of Michelangelo's most beautiful poems are addressed to Cavalieri. In 1531, Michelangelo's father died at the age of ninety, prompting a touching poem of filial affection.

With the deaths of his favorite brother and father, his native city under a ruler unsympathetic to him, and feeling the urgency to free himself of what had become the incubus of the Julius mausoleum, the artist left Florence in September, 1534, never to return. Michelangelo arrived in Rome two days before the death of Clement VII. The new pope, Paul III, did not hesitate to assign work to the master, forcing him once again to reduce the part that still remained to be executed on the tomb.

Paul set Michelangelo immediately to work on the project of painting in fresco *The Last Judgment* on the wall of the Sistine Chapel (1534-1541). Thus, after having evoked on the vault the beginning of the universe, the artist depicted its end. The violence and disequilibrium of this swirl of nude bodies rising from the grave to Paradise, or descending to Hell, spiraling around a central figure of Christ the judge, a Christ with the body of a Heracles and the face of an Apollo, is in startling contrast to the luminous, floating balance of the ceiling. The abundant and violent nudity, the athletic Christ, the angels without wings, all stirred violent condemnation during the artist's lifetime and resulted in subsequent painting of loincloths over most of the nudities, in the first instance by Michelangelo's pupil Daniele da Volterra, who thereby won for himself the nickname Il Brachettone (the breeches maker).

Some critics see in *The Last Judgment* a reflection in

plastic terms of the crisis of Reformation and Counter-Reformation set off by Martin Luther's theses. Certainly, the artist, who grew increasingly religious with the years, was deeply troubled by the civil war in the body of Christianity. He was an intimate member of a reform Catholic movement centering on the poet Vittoria Colonna, whom the artist had met in 1536 and with whom he maintained a passionate platonic relationship until her death in 1547. He made many drawings for the poet, with whom he also exchanged poetry and discussed theological questions, some of which are expressed in intricate and ambiguous verse.

While working on *The Last Judgment*, Michelangelo had been named in 1535 architect, sculptor, and painter of the Apostolic Palace, wherein from 1541 to 1550, he frescoed the Pauline Chapel with the *Conversion of St. Paul* and the *Crucifixion of St. Peter*, thus completing his last paintings at the age of seventy-five. In 1547, Michelangelo was named architect of Saint Peter's. From then on, he was primarily involved with architecture: The disturbances and disequilibrium that still raged within the artist's soul found plastic expression in the broken pediments, recessed columns, blind niches, and frequently grotesque, abstract architectural forms.

Michelangelo's appointment as architect of Saint Peter's was reconfirmed by Julius III (1552), Paul IV (1555), and finally Pius IV (1559). Michelangelo resisted the insistent demands of the Medici Cosimo I that he return to Florence. More than eighty years old, Michelangelo was obsessed above all with the desire to push ahead the construction of Saint Peter's.

During these last years, the artist's thoughts dwelt constantly on the theme of death. It is probable that many of his finest sonnets and the last great drawings of the Crucifixion were executed during this time. After his seventy-fifth year, Michelangelo had begun work on the tragic *Pietà* now in the Duomo of Florence, in which the artist portrays himself as Nicodemus, the Pharisee who came to Jesus by night and raised troubled questions: "How can these things be?" According to biographer Giorgio Vasari, his contemporary, the work was intended for Michelangelo's own tomb.

At the end, Michelangelo seems to have broken through his suffering, gone beyond it into that tranquil yet tragic realm of his last two *Pietà* sculptures. The Rondanini *Pietà* leaps out of the Renaissance entirely, in two directions, one might say. The slender verticality—mother and Son merged—looks back to the column statues of Gothic portals and forward to the abstraction of Constantin Brancusi's *Bird in Space*—an almost macabre reduction of tragedy to pure essence.

ANALYSIS

Michelangelo's tomb in Santa Croce symbolizes his titanic achievements as a sculptor, painter, and architect. Curiously, the fourth crown of laurel is missing, despite the fact that he is currently recognized as the greatest Italian lyric poet of the sixteenth century. Michelangelo himself refused to take seriously the verses that (especially from his sixtieth year on) he was forever scribbling and revising on the backs of letters, on sheets of drawings, or any other odd scraps of paper at hand. After all, he was not the only artist of his day who wrote poetry. The Renaissance ideal was *l'uomo universale*, the universal man, not the specialist.

Thus, the fact that Michelangelo wrote poetry is not surprising; what is surprising is the extraordinary quality of the best of his work. His contemporaries recognized it. The poems circulated in manuscript; a number of his madrigals were set to music by celebrated Italian and foreign composers, including Jakob Arcadelt; and in 1546, the Humanist Benedetto Varchi lectured on one of Michelangelo's sonnets before the Academy of Florence. Michelangelo was even persuaded to gather a selection of his verses for publication.

The unforeseen death of his friend, the banker Luigi del Riccio, who had been the patron for such a collection, dissuaded the artist from continuing the project. As it turned out, the poems were not published until 1623 in a corrupt edition misedited by Michelangelo's great-nephew, a Florentine academician. Fearful for his ancestor's reputation, the younger Michelangelo committed mayhem on the text, bowdlerizing anything remotely questionable, turning masculine into feminine, making elegant what was rough, and rewriting images. Not until Cesare Guasti's edition of 1863 did a responsible text appear. Individual poems have been translated by such well-known English and American poets and writers as William Wordsworth, Robert

Southey, Henry Wadsworth Longfellow, Ralph Waldo Emerson, George Santayana, and Robert Bridges.

SONNETS, MADRIGALS, FRAGMENTS

The poetic works comprise 343 pieces—everything from sonnets and madrigals to fragments. Many of them appear to be a personal journal; others, such as the fifty epitaphs written at Riccio's request to commemorate the death of his nephew, serve some social purpose. The bulk of the verses seem to be the musings of an old man, although some love poems, full of conventional mannerisms, probably are earlier. All dating of the poems is speculative, deductive, but the assumption that very little of the earliest poetry has survived is supported by the fact that in 1518 the artist, in a burst of ire, burned many of his poems and drawings.

Michelangelo was particularly fond of the sonnet. Within its small space, as from a constricted block of marble, he hammered out harsh Dantesque lines that profoundly express his agony of spirit, now and again lightened by bursts of rough humor. Recurrent themes are the war of himself against himself; repentance for a nameless guilt; art as a symbol of the relationship of God to man; exalted platonic love; and a religious exaltation of death as liberation.

CONFLICTS REVEALED

Despite frequent obscurities and abstract knotted metaphors, Michelangelo's poetry is striking for its ultimate confessional power, a nakedness of soul akin to his nudes in the visual arts. "Be silent! Enough of pallid violets and liquid crystals and sleek beasts," the poet Francesco Berni, a contemporary of Michelangelo, cries out in exasperation against the facile Petrarchan warblers of the time. "He speaks things, and you speak words." Berni struck to the core: "Ei dice cose . . ." ("He speaks things"), and in this, Michelangelo is rare not only among Italian poets. His lines seem to struggle out of the matrix of language as his "prisoners" struggle out of the rock. Seldom mellifluous, frequently imageless (or making use of conventional conceits), Michelangelo's verse derives its power from a texture of language that seems to be reproducing the very contours of thought itself: its spurts, its exaltations, its hesitations, its withdrawals. Sometimes ungrammatical, these strained, hammered lines are undoubtedly those of a sculptor. The combination of idealism, harshness,

and crude jest reminds Italian readers of Dante. English readers, however, will be reminded of John Donne; there is the same love of paradox, the same coexistence of contraries, the same conflict between sensuality and austerity, the same mannered and overextended conceits, the same war of self against self: "Vorrei voler, Signor, quel ch'io non voglio . . ." ("I would want to want, O Lord, what I do not want . . .").

Just as in Michelangelo's sculpture (and in the painted sculpture that is the vault of the Sistine Chapel) *terribilità* coexists with melancholy resignation, so in these poems all the varieties of love—of God, of man, of woman, of art, of country—are celebrated in a grappling of ardor and ashes, the power to do anything frozen at the brink of a desire to do nothing.

Michelangelo was nourished on Dante, whose poetry he knew intimately; indeed, among his contemporaries, he was extolled as a Dante scholar. In Donato Giannotti's *Dialogues* on Dante, the artist figures as a major protagonist. However, if Michelangelo's spirit vibrated to that of his fellow Florentine, Dante, the forms and imagery of his verse were derived from the fashionable neo-Petrarchianism of the first half of the sixteenth century. The result is that Dantesque vigor and Michelangelesque spiritual suffering sometimes burst the fragile and stereotyped Petrarchan container. When these elements are in balance, the poetic achievement is of the very first order.

TENSION AND SUFFERING

Michelangelo's poems are those of a man deeply ill at ease with himself and with his world, and it is this tension that makes them seem so neurotically modern. Like a salamander, Michelangelo is always living in flame; like a phoenix, he is always being reborn from the ashes of his suffering: "A single torment outweighs a thousand pleasures." Indeed, there is something masochistic, passive, feminine in many of his curious images. Like gold or silver, the poet's desire must be melted by the fires of love, and then poured into him "through such narrow spaces" to fill his void. As a goldsmith or silversmith must break the form to extract the work, so he must be broken and tortured to draw forth the perfect beauty of his lady. In another poem, one whose effectiveness is destroyed by its exaggerations, love enters through the eyes like a bunch of sour grapes forced into a narrow-necked bottle, and swelling within, is unable to escape.

Elsewhere, Michelangelo compares himself to a block of stone that, being smashed, reveals its inner sparks, and then, pulverized and re-formed, is fire-baked to a longer life.

> So in love with the stone, in which it lies,
> Is fire, that, soon drawn forth, with its quick blaze
> It binds it, burns it, breaks it, and in new guise
> It makes it live in some immortal place.
> And that same stone, when baked, can brave and face
> All seasons, and acquires a higher price,
> Just like a soul that soars to blessèd days
> After the flames that cleanse while they chastise.
> Thus, if it is my fate that I soon must
> Be dissolved by this fire that hides in me,
> My new life shall be vast and manifold.
> Therefore, if I am now but smoke and dust,
> Cleansed by this flame, eternal I shall be:
> No iron chisel carves me—one of gold.

The imagery of the first six lines, relating to the preparation of a ground for fresco-painting, is typically masochistic: Suffering, being smashed, pulverized, is a necessary condition for the creation and rewards of art. In swift transition, the poet goes on to compare such purgation to the ascension of souls from Purgatory to Heaven and immediately returns to his central metaphor: Suffering enriches. Suffering is the fiery furnace for the creation of the most precious values.

NEOPLATONISM

The initial quatrain of another sonnet expresses with remarkable concision Michelangelo's entire Neoplatonic aesthetic and throws light on his technique of stone carving as well:

> The greatest artist has no single concept
> Which a rough marble block does not contain
> Already in its core; *that* can attain
> Only the hand that serves the intellect

Just as Plato's transcendental forms or ideas exist before their specific manifestations on earth, so the statue, fully formed, exists within the block of marble; there, it awaits the liberating hand of the artist, who finds it by stripping away the excess (*superchio*). Such a liberating hand does not function merely by instinct: It is guided to its goal by intelligence (*la man che ubbidisce all' intelletto*). Thus, the artist is a discoverer in the strictest etymological sense of the word.

ARTISTIC CONSISTENCY

What is so fascinating is that Michelangelo is always the same artist, whether he is twisting an idea or twisting David's right wrist, whether he is trying to fit all the ancestors of Christ into a spandrel of the Sistine Chapel or trying to fit too much concept into too little language. Just as the last great *Pietàs* and drawings have almost been dematerialized in the effort to render pure Idea, so in many of Michelangelo's poems language is being smashed, distorted, pulverized, almost as if the artist were trying to dispense with it.

The same poet addressed punning lines to a courtesan named Mancina, "Left-Handed"; lashed out at the bellicose Pope Julius, who was more devoted to the cult of Mars than to the Prince of Peace; and wrote stupendous sonnets to Night, whose dominions may be warred against by a single firefly; at the last, he held out his hands to Christ, longing for death to liberate him as he himself had liberated the perfect forms sleeping within the stone:

> Painting nor sculpturing no more will allay
> The soul turned toward the divine love
> Which opened to us its arms upon the cross.

OTHER MAJOR WORKS

NONFICTION: *I, Michelangelo, Sculptor: An Autobiography Through Letters*, 1962; *The Letters of Michelangelo*, 1963.

MISCELLANEOUS: *Complete Poems and Selected Letters of Michelangelo*, 1963.

BIBLIOGRAPHY

Barolsky, Paul. *The Faun in the Garden*. University Park: Pennsylvania State University Press, 1994. Barolsky's "analysis of poetic imagination" deeply relates Michelangelo's poetry to his artistic works and his contemporary biographies. He used all three to weave a fabrication of his "self" as creator and man.

Cambon, Glauco. *Michelangelo's Poetry: Fury of Form*. Princeton, N.J.: Princeton University Press,

1985. A specialized study of the diverse talents of Michelangelo.

Forcellino, Antonio. *Michelangelo: A Tormented Life.* Malden, Mass.: Polity, 2009. This biography, translated from the Italian, begins by describing Michelangelo's struggle with the powerful figures in his life, and how after his death they began to build a myth around him.

Gilbert, Creighton. *Michelangelo: On and Off the Sistine Ceiling.* New York: George Braziller, 1994. A specialized study of the diverse talents of Michelangelo.

Hallock, Ann Hayes. *Michelangelo the Poet.* Palo Alto, Calif.: Page-Ficklin, 1978. Hallock presents a reading and contextualizing of the *Rime*, emphasizing his "drive toward the essential." She uncovers elements of this in his use of language and "nuclei" (themes) of *patria*, family, friends, soul, and life and death. Often complicated language and no English translations.

Ryan, Christopher. *The Poetry of Michelangelo: An Introduction.* Madison, N.J.: Fairleigh Dickinson University Press, 1998. This introduction to the poet and poems emphasizes the individual works and the corpus itself, as it attempts to clarify the intricacies of both. Ryan lays the works out chronologically, in stages, providing relevant historical and biographical background. Translations are the author's.

Wallace, William E. *Michelangelo: The Artist, the Man, and His Times.* New York: Cambridge University Press, 2010. Wallace used Michelangelo's letters and poems for insight into the man in writing his biography, so there is more discussion of the poetry than in most biographies.

Sidney Alexander

ADAM MICKIEWICZ

Born: Zaosie, Lithuania; December 24, 1798
Died: Burgas, Turkey; November 26, 1855

PRINCIPAL POETRY

Ballady i romanse, 1822

Grażyna, 1823 (English translation, 1940)

Dziady, parts 2, 4, 1823, and 3, 1832 (*Forefathers' Eve*, parts 2, 4, 1925, and 3, 1944-1946)

Sonety krymskie, 1826 (*Sonnets from the Crimea*, 1917)

Sonety, 1826

"Farys," 1828 ("Faris")

Konrad Wallenrod, 1828 (English translation, 1883)

Pan Tadeusz: Czyli, Ostatni Zajazd na litwie historia Szlachecka zr. 1811 i 1812 we dwunastu ksiegach wierszem, 1834 (*Pan Tadeusz: Or, The Last Foray in Lithuania, a Tale of Gentlefolk in 1811 and 1812, in Twelve Books in Verse*, 1917)

Poems by Adam Mickiewicz, 1944

Selected Poetry and Prose, 1955

Selected Poems, 1956

The Sun of Liberty: Bicentenary Anthology, 1798-1998, 1998

Treasury of Love Poems by Adam Mickiewicz, 1998

OTHER LITERARY FORMS

In the last twenty years of his life, Adam Mickiewicz (meets-KYEH-veech), the national bard and prophet of Poland, wrote only a handful of poems, turning instead to religious and political works and to literary criticism. The messianic fervor of Mickiewicz's prose is exemplified by *Ksiegi narodu polskiego i pielgrzymstwa polskiego* (1832; *The Books of the Polish Nation and of the Polish Pilgrims*, 1833, 1925), a tract written in a quasi-biblical style. Mickiewicz's lectures given at the Collège de France in Paris, where from 1840 to 1844 he held the first chair of Slavic literature, fill several volumes of his complete works.

ACHIEVEMENTS

Adam Mickiewicz embodied in his work the soul of the Polish people. Through his poetry, he symbolized the land, history, and customs of Poland. Starting as a classicist and then quickly becoming a Romantic, he portrayed the everyday life of the Polish people and, at the same time, gave voice to visions and prophecies. His poems, written to be understood by the common man, brought him instant popular acclaim but also exposed him to attacks from many critics, who condemned his Romanticism and his provincial idioms.

The first volume of Mickiewicz's poetry was published in Wilno in an edition of five hundred copies. It contained ballads and romances, genres of poetry then unknown in Poland, and portrayed the common people in a simple but eloquent manner. A second volume followed in 1823, containing *Grażyna*, a tale in verse, and parts 2 and 4 of a fragmentary fantastic drama, *Forefathers' Eve*. With the publication of these works, followed by the narrative poem *Konrad Wallenrod*, set in medieval Lithuania, Mickiewicz became the founder of the Romantic movement in Polish literature. During his greatest creative period, in the years from 1832 to 1834, Mickiewicz published part 3 of *Forefathers' Eve*, which seethed with the eternal hatred felt by the Poles for their Russian conquerors. With its publication, Mickiewicz became a national defender, proclaiming that Poland was the Christ among nations, crucified for the sins of others. Like a prophet, he predicted that Poland would rise again. *Pan Tadeusz*, Mickiewicz's masterpiece, was also written during this period. An epic poem in twelve books depicting Polish life in Lithuania in 1811 and 1812, it is the greatest work of Polish literature and perhaps the finest narrative poem in nineteenth century European literature. Devoid of hatred or mysticism, it warmly and realistically depicts the Polish land and people and embodies a firm faith in their future.

BIOGRAPHY

Adam Bernard Mickiewicz was born on December 24, 1798, on the farmstead of Zaosie, near Nowogródek, a small town in Lithuania. After the Tartars' savage destruction of Kiev in 1240, the area previously known as Byelorussia and the Ukraine were annexed by the warlike Grand Duchy of Lithuania. In four centuries, however, the Lithuanian gentry was almost completely Polonized, and after the union with the Polish Crown in 1386, Lithuania's territory was greatly reduced. In the district of Nowogródek, while the gentry was predominantly Polish (old immigrants from Mazovia), the peasants were Byelorussian. Mickiewicz's father, Mikolaj, was a lawyer and a small landowner. His mother, Barbara (Orzeszko) Majewska, was also from the middle gentry. Both families had a strong military tradition.

It is noteworthy that Mickiewicz, the national bard of Poland, the ardent patriot who gave such superb literary expression to the life and aspirations of the Polish people, never even saw Poland proper nor its cultural centers, Warsaw and Krakow. Moreover, during his lifetime, Poland did not exist as a sovereign state, for Mickiewicz was born after the so-called Final Partition of 1795, when Poland was divided among Russia, Prussia, and Austria-Hungary.

Mickiewicz, one of five sons, started his education at home and then continued at the Dominican parochial school in Nowogródek. Later, he studied philology at the University of Wilno, where he excelled in Latin and Polish literature. He was greatly influenced by a liberal historian, Joachim Lelewel, who later became a leader in the Insurrection of 1830-1831. At the university, Mickiewicz was one of the six founders of the Philomathian Society, a secret society that emphasized Polish patriotism and tried to influence public affairs. After spending a short time in Kowno as a district teacher of Greek and Latin, Polish literature, and history, Mickiewicz returned to Wilno, where he maintained close relations with his friends in the Philomathian Society. In 1823, Mickiewicz and several of his friends were arrested by the Russian authorities for plotting to spread "senseless Polish nationalism" and were confined in the Basilian Monastery in Wilno, which had been converted to a prison. After their trial on November 6, 1824, Mickiewicz and his friend Jan Sobolewski were sent to St. Petersburg to work in an office.

In 1819, before his imprisonment and deportation, Mickiewicz met and fell in love with Maryla Wereszczaka, the daughter of a wealthy landowner. Maryla, however, complying with the wishes of her family, refused to marry Mickiewicz, who was only a poor student, and married the rich Count Puttkamer instead. Partially inspired by his unrequited love for Maryla, Mickiewicz turned to writing Romantic poetry and, with the publication of two small volumes of poetry in 1822 and 1823, became the founder of the Romantic school in Poland. His earlier writing shows the influence of the pseudoclassical style then prevalent in Poland.

Mickiewicz stayed in Russia almost four years and wrote his *Sonety* and *Sonnets from the Crimea* there as well as *Konrad Wallenrod* and "Faris," an Arabian tale. He lived in St. Petersburg, Odessa, and Moscow, where he was warmly accepted into literary circles, befriended by Alexander Pushkin and others, and made a welcome guest in the literary salon of Princess Zenaida Volkonsky (herself an accomplished poet, whom Pushkin called "tsarina of muses and beauty"). He often improvised there, gaining the admiration of Pushkin, who called him "Mickiewicz, inspired from above."

In 1829, Mickiewicz secured permission to leave Russia and lived for a time in Switzerland and then in Rome. The Polish Insurrection broke out in 1830, and Mickiewicz tried in vain to join the revolutionists in August, 1831. After the defeat of the insurrection, Mickiewicz settled in Paris, where he spent most of his remaining years. In 1834, he married Celina Szymanowski, the youngest daughter of Maria Szymanowski, a famous concert pianist, whom he had met while still in Russia. The marriage was unhappy because of her mental illness, and her early death left Mickiewicz with several small children. During this period, he wrote part 3 of *Forefathers' Eve*, a mystical and symbolic dramatic treatment of his imprisonment at Wilno by the Russian authorities. The poem embodied the anti-Russian feeling of the Polish people and intensified their hatred of their oppressor. Mickiewicz's next poem was his masterpiece, *Pan Tadeusz*, which glorifies the rustic life of the Polish gentry in picturesque Lithuanian Byelorussia and praises the Napoleonic invasion of Russia as symbolic of Poland's hope for liberation ("God is with Napoléon, Napoléon is with us"). *Pan Tadeusz* is a true national epic.

After the publication of his masterpiece, Mickiewicz fell under the influence of Andrzej Towiański, a charismatic figure who preached that a new period in Christianity was at hand and that he himself was its prophet. Unconditionally accepting Towiański's claims, Mickiewicz was compelled to give up his professorship at the Collège de France when he used his position to advance the doctrines of Towiański's sect. Mickiewicz spent his last years working for Polish independence and aiding fellow exiles. In 1855, following the outbreak in the previous year of the Crimean War, which he hailed as a prelude to the liberation of Poland, Mickiewicz went to Constantinople. He contracted cholera and died on November 26, 1855. His body was first sent to Paris; in 1890, it was brought to Wawel Castle in Krakow, where it now rests with Tadeusz Kościuszko and the Polish kings.

ANALYSIS

The Romantic movement had unique features in Poland, where it did not begin until the 1820's, some thirty years later than in England and Germany. The most prominent literary figure of Romanticism in Poland was Adam Mickiewicz, whose poetry grew out of his formative years in Lithuanian Byelorussia. Mickiewicz wrote poems that had universal as well as regional and national significance. A poet of genius, he raised Polish literature to a high level among Slavic literatures and to a prominent place in world literature.

Although he was in many respects the quintessential Romantic poet, Mickiewicz eludes categorization. There is a strong classical strain running throughout his oeuvre, evident in the clarity of his diction and the precision of his images. He combined meticulous observation of the familiar world with an evocation of spiritual realms and supernatural experience. His concerns as a poet went beyond poetry, reflecting a responsibility to his beloved, oppressed Poland and to humanity at large. As he was a spokesperson in exile for Polish freedom, so he remains a spokesperson for all those who share his hatred of tyranny.

FROM CLASSICISM TO ROMANTICISM

Mickiewicz's work in philology at the University of Wilno instilled in him the values of eighteenth century classicism. Accordingly, his first significant poem, "Oda do młodości" ("Ode to Youth"), reflected the tradition of the Enlightenment, but it also contained some of the pathos of Romanticism. In the ballad "Romantyczność" ("The Romantic"), this pathos becomes the dominant tone. The poem concerns a woman who is mocked and regarded as insane because, in despair, she talks to the ghost of her beloved. Mickiewicz treats her sympathetically, concluding: "Faith and love are more discerning/ Than lenses or learning." Revealing a Slavic preference for faith and feeling rather than Western rationalism, Mickiewicz returned to these youthful ideas in his later, more complex works.

Mickiewicz's shift toward a thoroughgoing Romanticism was influenced by his reading of Italian, German, and English literature, by his study of early Lithuanian history, and by his love for Maryla Wereszczaka. With his first two volumes of poetry Mickiewicz raised the stature of Polish poetry. His first volume contained short poems, mainly a group of fourteen "ballads and romances" prefaced with a survey of world literature. "The Romantic," the programmatic poem of the Polish Romantic movement, expresses his faith in the influence of the spirit world on man.

FOREFATHERS' EVE, PARTS 2 AND 4

The second volume of Mickiewicz's poems contained the second and fourth parts of the incomplete fantastic drama, *Forefathers' Eve*, a short poem, "The Vampire," connected with that drama; and a short tale in verse, *Grażyna*. The genre of the fantastic drama was in fashion at the time. *Forefathers' Eve*, complete with ghosts and demons, was based on a folk rite that involved serving a meal to the spirits of the departed on All Souls' Day. Part 2 of *Forefathers' Eve* (the first part of the poem to be written) is an idealization of this rite, in which Mickiewicz probably had participated as a boy in Lithuanian Byelorussia. He explained that Forefathers' Eve is the name of a ceremony celebrated by the common folk in memory of their ancestors in many parts of Byelorussia, Lithuania, Prussia, and Courland. The ceremony, once called the Feast of the Goat, originated in pagan times and was frowned upon by the Church.

In the first part of *Forefathers' Eve*, for which he only completed a sketch, Mickiewicz appears in the guise of Gustav, a name taken from *Valérie* (1803), a sentimental novel by Baroness von Krüdener. Gustav kills himself, disappointed in his love for Maryla. In a revised version of part 2 of *Forefathers' Eve*, Mickiewicz added a section expressing his love for Maryla. He depicts Maryla as a "shepherdess in mourning dress" whose lover, Gustav, has died for her. His spirit appears and gazes on the shepherdess and then follows her as she is led out of a chapel. In the fourth part of the poem, his ghost appears at the house of a priest and delivers passionate, sorrowful monologues, pouring out his sad tale of disillusioned love while casting reproaches upon Maryla. He recommends to the priest the rites of Forefathers' Eve and finally reenacts his own suicide. Gustav is Mickiewicz's version of the self-dramatizing Romantic hero, but he is also a tragic hero in the Aristotelian sense, since he is defeated by a mistake in judgment—his overwhelming love for a person who proves to be unworthy.

GRAŻYNA

Mickiewicz wrote *Grażyna*, an impersonal narrative poem, at about the same time he wrote the highly personal and passionate *Forefathers' Eve*. *Grażyna* resembles the tales or "novels" in verse characteristic of the Romantic movement in Western Europe but lacks the supernatural elements and the exoticism that distinguish such works. The poem concerns the Lithuanians' struggle in the fourteenth century against the German Knights of the Cross. Mickiewicz was inspired by the ruins of a castle near Nowogródek, by his study of early Lithuanian history, and by his reading of Torquato Tasso, Sir Walter Scott, and Lord Byron. In the narrative, the Lithuanian prince, Litavor, plans to join the Teutonic Knights against Duke Witold. These traitorous intentions are foiled by Grażyna, Litavor's brave and patriotic wife. Dressed in her husband's armor, she leads the Lithuanian knights in battle against the Teutons instead of accepting their help against her compatriots. Mickiewicz modeled his heroine on Tasso's Clorinda and Erminia, although the type goes back to Vergil's Camilla and ultimately to the Greek tales of the Amazons. This stately narrative reveals Mickiewicz's extraordinary gift for vivid characterization, even though the poet himself did not attach much importance to the work.

SONNETS FROM THE CRIMEA

At the end of 1826, Mickiewicz published his first cycle of sonnets, the so-called love sonnets. There were few Polish models in the sonnet form, and he turned for a model to the Petrarchan sonnet, with its elaborate rhyme scheme and rigid structure. His second cycle of sonnets, *Sonnets from the Crimea*, was vastly different in thought and feeling and was met with hostile criticism from Mickiewicz's classically minded contemporaries.

While in Russia, Mickiewicz had made a trip of nearly two months through the Crimea, and it was this journey that produced the eighteen poems that constitute the *Sonnets from the Crimea*. He made the trip with, among others, Karolina Sobański, with whom he had an ardent love affair; critics have speculated that the three sonnets "Good Morning," "Good Night," and "Good Evening" reflect their relationship. With his *Sonnets from the Crimea*, Mickiewicz introduced to Polish literature the Romantic poetry of the steppe, the sea, and the mountains, as well as the Oriental elements of European Romanticism, represented by Byron and Thomas Moore in England and by Pushkin in Russia. The sonnets express an attitude toward nature that is characteristically Romantic and at the same time "modern": Nature is valued for its own sake as well as for its symbolic reflection of the poet's psychological states. The sonnets are further distinguished by their exotic vocabulary, the fruit of Mickiewicz's study of Persian and Arabic poetry, mainly in French translation. (Near Eastern and Oriental literature was popular throughout Europe toward the end of the eighteenth century.) The rigid structure demanded by the sonnet form enabled Mickiewicz to communicate his psychological experiences with utmost conciseness, and these poems are among his finest.

KONRAD WALLENROD

Mickiewicz had conceived the idea of his next major work, *Konrad Wallenrod*, while in Moscow in 1825. Like *Grażyna*, the poem is set in medieval Lithuania during the conflict between the Lithuanians and the Knights of the Cross. *Konrad Wallenrod* is both longer and more powerful than *Grażyna*, however, and, although the poet modified and altered history to some extent, it is mainly based on actual historical events; Mickiewicz himself described the work as "a story taken from the history of Lithuania and Prussia." A tale in verse in the Byronic style, the poem relates the trag-

edy of a Lithuanian who is forced by fate to become a Teutonic Knight. The hero, in an effort to save his people from annihilation, sacrifices all that is dear to him, including his own honor. Mickiewicz changed the historical Wallenrod, an ineffective Grand Master of the Knights of the Cross, to a Lithuanian who, captured as a youth, has been reared by the Germans and then gains influence and authority over the Teutonic Knights in order to destroy them. To capture the aura of intrigue, Mickiewicz studied Machiavelli and read Friedrich Schiller's *Die Verschwörung des Fiesco zu Genua* (pr., pb. 1783; *Fiesco: Or, The Genoese Conspiracy*, 1796). The poem reverts to the somber and Romantic atmosphere that Mickiewicz had temporarily abandoned in his sonnets; it is Byronic in type, and Mickiewicz evidently used *The Corsair* (1814) and *Lara* (1814) for inspiration. Mickiewicz's Wallenrod, however, differs markedly from the Byronic hero: Above all, he is a patriot, rather than a mysterious outsider. Indeed, so clear is the political allegory that underlies *Konrad Wallenrod* that it is surprising that the Russian censors allowed the poem to be published.

"FARIS"

In St. Petersburg in 1828, Mickiewicz wrote "Faris," a poem depicting an Arab horseman's extravagant ride through the desert. Mickiewicz had developed an interest in Arabic poetry through his contact with the Oriental peoples in the south of Russia. The Arabic word *faris* means "horseman" or "knight." Mickiewicz's special affection for the poem is often attributed to its story of a proud, strong will that triumphs over great obstacles; perhaps Mickiewicz saw himself in this light.

FOREFATHERS' EVE, PART 3

Mickiewicz wrote his greatest works, part 3 of *Forefathers' Eve* and *Pan Tadeusz*, in a brief period from 1832 to 1834. Part 3 of *Forefathers' Eve* is only loosely connected with parts 2 and 4, published almost ten years earlier. It is the longest, the most enigmatic, and certainly the most famous of the three parts. The poet went back for his subject matter to his Wilno days in 1823, when the Russian authorities arrested him and other members of the Philomathians. Using his personal experience in the Romantic manner, Mickiewicz sought to justify the actions of a loving God in allowing a devout Roman Catholic country such as Poland to be partitioned by three cruel neighbors, each "on a lower moral level than their victim."

While in Rome, Mickiewicz had been intrigued by Aeschyulus's tragedy *Prometheus desmōtēs* (date unknown; *Prometheus Bound*, 1777), with its presentation of the Titan who rebels against Zeus in the name of love for humanity, and Aeschylus's influence is apparent in part 3 of *Forefathers' Eve*. The story of Prometheus attracted many Romantic writers, including Percy Bysshe Shelley and Johann Wolfgang von Goethe. Mickiewicz, who had considered writing his own poetic drama about Prometheus, may have been influenced by these authors as well in composing the third part of *Forefathers' Eve*.

Part 3 of *Forefathers' Eve* consists of a prologue, nine scenes, and a final sequence of six long poems about Russia. This sequence, titled "Ustcp" ("Digression"), constitutes a second act or epilogue. In the prologue, Maryla's lover, Gustav, a young prisoner, is seen in his cell in the Basilian Monastery, watched over by good and evil spirits. He takes the name Konrad, suggesting an affinity with Konrad Wallenrod. The first scene, a description of the life of the student prisoners, is followed by the improvisation—the foundation of the whole drama—in which Konrad arrogantly challenges God's justice, charging him with an absence of feeling or love in spite of his strength and great intellect. Konrad declares that he himself is greater than God, since he loves his nation and desires her happiness. The improvisation and the following scenes reflect the fulfillment of Mickiewicz's previous plan of writing a tragedy with the Prometheus theme adapted to a Christian setting. Konrad's arrogant pride, although inspired by love for Poland and a sense of divinity within himself, is blasphemous. Father Peter, who represents mystic humility just as Konrad represents mystic pride, receives in a vision an understanding of the source of Konrad's torment—the problem of the fate of Poland, an innocent victim crushed by cruel foreign powers. He sees Poland as the Christ among nations, who, crucified by Prussia, Russia, and Austria, will rise again. The promised hero who will bring about the resurrection of Poland is probably Mickiewicz himself, although in the work there is reference only to a hero whose name is "Forty and Four." With this notion

that Poland is the Christ among nations, Mickiewicz became the founder of Polish messianism, a mystic faith that helped to define "Polishness" for generations and that is not without influence in Poland even today.

PAN TADEUSZ

In November, 1832, Mickiewicz began work on *Pan Tadeusz*, a narrative poem that was to become his masterpiece. He worked on the poem until February, 1834. *Pan Tadeusz*, a stately epic of 9,712 lines, is a story of the Polish gentry. The poem's twelve books present the whole of Polish society in Lithuanian Byelorussia during a highly significant period of history, the time of Napoleon's campaign in Russia, in 1811-1812, a time when Polish society appeared to have achieved a temporary harmony, stability, and order. Mickiewicz stresses the value of ritual, order, and ceremony, and his characters are courteous, modest, and patriotic.

The subtitle of *Pan Tadeusz—Or: The Last Foray in Lithuania, a Tale of Gentlefolk in 1811 and 1812, in Twelve Books in Verse*—is significant: Mickiewicz's use of the word "tale" may indicate, as some critics have argued, that *Pan Tadeusz* is not an epic or narrative poem at all, although it is connected to these genres, but a blending together of a number of genres to achieve the poet's artistic purpose in a truly Romantic style. The word "last" in the subtitle implies the disappearance of a traditional way of life, as exemplified in the "foray" or ritualistic execution of justice. Mickiewicz's two main themes, the recapture of the past and the conflict between reality and appearance, are classic themes in Western literature, and the poem thus attains a certain universality in spite of its intense concern with a specific cultural and historical tradition.

The plot concerns Tadeusz, an impressionable young man recently graduated from the university; his love for Zosia; and a feud over a castle between the Soplicas and the Horeszkos: Tadeusz is a Soplica, while Zosia is a Horeszko (a premise that recalls William Shakespeare's *Romeo and Juliet*, pr. c. 1595-1596). To add to the conflict, the father of Tadeusz has killed Zosia's grandfather. The plot becomes more involved later in the work when an emissary of Napoleon turns out to be Tadeusz's father disguised as a monk, Father Robak. (In constructing his plot, Mickiewicz was influenced by Sir Walter Scott.) Mickiewicz chose for his setting rural Lithuanian Byelorussia, the land of his childhood, to which he longed to return. The real hero of the poem is Jacek Soplica, who wants to marry Eva, the daughter of an aristocrat, the Pantler Horeszko. When he is rejected, Jacek kills the Pantler in a fit of anger, under circumstances that falsely suggest collusion with the Russians. Jacek spends the rest of his life humbly serving his country. He becomes a monk and works as a political agent urging Poles to join Napoleon in his campaign against Russia and so to contribute to the restoration of Poland in an indirect manner. Mickiewicz united in Jacek the conflicting motives of pride and humility, represented in part 3 of *Forefathers' Eve* by Konrad and Father Peter. In *Pan Tadeusz*, Mickiewicz is no longer a prophet and teacher, appearing rather as a kindly, genial man who is proud of the glorious past of his country and has faith in her future. He is once more the jovial companion of his Wilno days and no longer the leader of Polish exiles who were haunted by their own misfortunes and those of Poland. He is a realist who sees the faults of his countrymen but still loves them.

It is difficult to believe that part 3 of *Forefathers' Eve* and *Pan Tadeusz* were written by the same poet within a period of two years. In the latter, the poet is moved by childlike wonder: He sees beauty in even the most commonplace scenes in Poland, such as a young girl feeding poultry in a farmyard. The period about which he was writing embodied the whole life of Old Poland—its people, its customs, and its traditions. While the action of *Pan Tadeusz* develops in the country among rural people, set against a background of vibrant descriptions of nature and animals, all classes of the gentry are described, including the wealthy, the aristocratic, the middle class, and the poor gentry, and there are representatives of a number of old offices, such as chamberlain, *voyevoda*, pantler, cupbearer, seneschal, judge, and notary. In addition, there are representatives of other classes and nationalities, including the peasants (rather incompletely presented, however), a Jew, and various Russians.

In *Pan Tadeusz*, Mickiewicz describes nature in a manner that has never been equaled in Polish literature. He paints verbal pictures of the forest, meadows, and ponds at different times of the day and night in different lights and in myriad colors; he describes sunrises and sunsets, and the world of plants and animals, all with acute perception. Mickiewicz also meticulously describes a mansion, a castle, a cottage of the provincial gentry, an inn, hunting parties, the picking of mushrooms, feasts, quarrels, duels, and a battle—an extraordinary range of settings and experiences.

The masterpiece of Polish literature, *Pan Tadeusz* is regarded by many as the finest narrative poem of the nineteenth century. "The smile of Mickiewicz" reflected in the kindly humor of the poem, the radiant descriptions, and the dramatic truth of the characters, all contribute to its excellence. *Pan Tadeusz* is known and loved throughout Poland, by peasants as well as university professors. With this masterpiece, Mickiewicz reached the summit of his literary career. It is unfortunate that the total effect of the poem, which is derived from a close interaction of diction, style, and word associations, the portrayal of marvelously drawn characters, the presentation of setting, and the creation of a dynamic atmosphere, cannot be conveyed in all its beauty in translation.

OTHER MAJOR WORKS

PLAYS: *Jacknes Jasinski, ou les deux Polognes*, 1836; *Les confédérés de Bar*, 1836.

NONFICTION: *Ksiegi narodu polskiego i pielgrzymstwa polskiego*, 1832 (*The Books of the Polish Nation and of the Polish Pilgrims*, 1833, 1925); *Pierwsze wieki historyi polskiej*, 1837; *Wyklady Lozanskie*, 1839-1840; *Literatura slowianska*, 1840-1844 (4 volumes).

BIBLIOGRAPHY

Debska, Anita. *Country of the Mind: An Introduction to the Poetry of Adam Mickiewicz*. Warsaw: Burchard, 2000. A biography of Mickiewicz that also provides literary criticism, particularly of *Pan Tadeusz*.

Gross, Irena Grudzinska. "How Polish Is Polishness: About Mickiewicz's *Grażyna*." *East European Politics and Societies* 14, no. 1 (Winter, 2000): 1-11. Mickiewicz has been enshrined as an icon, his work classic and his vibrant presence is felt strongly in Polish culture. Gross examines Mickiewicz's poem *Grażyna* and the nationalism in it.

Kalinowska, Izabela. "The Sonnet, the Sequence, the

Qasidah: East-West Dialogue in Adam Mickiewicz's Sonnets." *Slavic and East European Journal* 45, no. 4 (Winter, 2001): 641. Looks at Orientalism in the sonnets Mickiewicz published in 1826.

Koropeckyj, Roman. *Adam Mickiewicz: The Life of a Romantic*. Ithaca, N.Y.: Cornell University Press, 2008. This biography of Mickiewicz examines his entire life as well as his major works.

_____. *The Poetics of Revitalization: Adam Mickiewicz Between "Forefathers' Eve," Part 3, and "Pan Tadeusz."* Boulder, Colo.: East European Monographs, 2001. This work focuses on two works, *Forefathers' Eve*, part 3, and *Pan Tadeusz*, and the author's development between them.

Welsh, David. *Adam Mickiewicz*. New York: Twayne, 1966. An introductory biography and critical study of selected works by Mickiewicz.

John P. Pauls and La Verne Pauls

CZESŁAW MIŁOSZ

Born: Šeteiniai, Lithuania; June 30, 1911
Died: Kraków, Poland; August 14, 2004
Also known as: J. Syruć

PRINCIPAL POETRY

Poemat o czasie zastygłym, 1933
Trzy zimy, 1936
Wiersze, 1940 (as J. Syruć)
Ocalenie, 1945
Światło dzienne, 1953
Traktat poetycki, 1957 (*A Treatise on Poetry*, 2001)
Król Popiel i inne wiersze, 1962
Gucio zaczarowany, 1964
Wiersze, 1967
Miasto bez imienia, 1969 (*Selected Poems*, 1973)
Gdzie wschodzi słońce i kędy zapada, 1974
Utwory poetyckie, 1976
Bells in Winter, 1978
Poezje, 1981
Hymn o perle, 1982
Nieobjęta ziemia, 1984 (*Unattainable Earth*, 1986)

The Separate Notebooks, 1984
The Collected Poems, 1931-1987, 1988
Provinces, 1991
Facing the River: New Poems, 1995
Wiersze wybrane, 1996
Piesek przydrozny, 1997 (*Road-side Dog*, 1998)
Poezje wybrane—Selected Poems, 1998
To, 2000
New and Collected Poems, 1931-2001, 2001
Second Space: New Poems, 2004
Selected Poems, 1931-2004, 2006
Wiersze ostatnie, 2006

OTHER LITERARY FORMS

Although it was the poetry of Czesław Miłosz (MEE-wohsh) that earned for him the 1980 Nobel Prize in Literature, his work in other genres is widely known among the international reading public. One of his most important nonfiction works is the autobiographical volume *Rodzinna Europa* (1959; *Native Realm: A Search for Self-Definition*, 1968). Unlike most autobiographies, this volume emphasizes the social and political background of the author's life at the expense of personal detail. For example, Miłosz makes but two passing references to his wife in the course of the entire work. Despite such lacunae, it is a work of the utmost personal candor and is indispensable for anyone endeavoring to fathom Miłosz's poetic intent. Similarly helpful is the novel *Dolina Issy* (1955; *The Issa Valley*, 1981), the plot of which focuses on a young boy's rites of passage in rural Lithuania during and after World War I. An understanding of the Manichaean metaphysics that inform this work as well as *Native Realm* is fundamental to a reading of Miłosz's poetry.

In an earlier novel, *Zdobycie władzy* (1953; *The Seizure of Power*, 1955), Miłosz presented a series of narrative sketches dealing with the suppression of the insurrection in Warsaw by the Germans in 1944, the Red Army's subsequent advance through Poland, and the eventual seizure of power by pro-Soviet Polish officials. Miłosz also analyzed Communist totalitarianism in a work of nonfiction, *Zniewolony umysł* (1953; *The Captive Mind*, 1953). A large part of this book is devoted to the fate of four writers in Communist Poland and provides a moving account of their gradual descent into spiritual slavery under the yoke of Stalinist oppression. Although Miłosz designates these men only by abstract labels—Alpha, the Moralist; Beta, the Disappointed Lover; Gamma, the Slave of History; and Delta, the Troubadour—their real identities are easily surmised by anyone familiar with postwar Polish literature.

Some of Miłosz's nonfictional works were originally written in English, notably *The History of Polish Literature* (1969, enlarged 1983). A large section of this volume is devoted to contemporary literature, and it is instructive to read Miłosz's critical evaluation of his own stature as a Polish poet. Another valuable work originally written in English is *Świadectwo poezji* (1983; *The Witness of Poetry*, 1983), which gathers Miłosz's Charles Eliot Norton lectures, given at Harvard University during the 1981-1982 academic year. Throughout these lectures, Miłosz argues that poetry should be "a passionate pursuit of the real."

More than half of the essays contained in *Emperor of the Earth: Modes of Eccentric Vision* (1977) are also written in English. Most of the pieces in this collection are devoted to Polish and Russian writers with whom the author shares a spiritual affinity. Among the essays included are two chapters from Miłosz's monograph on Stanisław Brzozowski, *Człowiek wśród skorpionów* (1962; man among scorpions), which was published on the occasion of the fiftieth anniversary of the death of this controversial Polish writer. (These two chapters were translated by the author himself, as were some of the other essays that were originally written in Polish.) The "Emperor of the Earth" referred to in the title is a character in a Russian work of science fiction who poses as a benefactor of humankind but who in reality is the Antichrist, a wolf in sheep's clothing. Miłosz thus underscores his belief that a religion of humanity often paves the way for totalitarian rule. If there is any thematic unity among the disparate essays included in *Emperor of the Earth*, it is to be found in the author's longstanding fascination with the problem of evil.

Miłosz also published two important collections of essays and what he called a "spiritual autobiography," *Ziemia Ulro* (1977; *The Land of Ulro*, 1984). In these volumes, Miłosz is inclined toward historical speculation and takes a deeply pessimistic view of contemporary society. The title *The Land of Ulro* is derived from the poetry of William Blake, where Ulro represents the dehumanized world created by materialistic science. Just as the inhabitants of Blake's Ulro are destined one day to experience a spiritual awakening, so Miłosz is hopeful regarding humanity's ultimate redemption.

Kontynenty (1958; continents) is a collection of works in various genres, including poems, literary essays, diary excerpts, and translations of poetry from several languages. Later, Miłosz published a similar potpourri, *Ogród nauk* (1979; the garden of knowledge). This volume is divided into three parts: The first section consists of essays; the second part presents verse translations (with commentary) of French, Yiddish, English, and Lithuanian poetry; and the third and final subdivision contains a translation of the biblical Ecclesiastes together with a stylistic analysis of biblical discourse and its relevance to the modern age.

Miłosz was very active in translating works from other languages into Polish. His most important translations from French include the poetry of his cousin Oscar de L. Miłosz and that of Charles Baudelaire. In 1958, while in exile in Paris, Miłosz edited and translated selected writings of Simone Weil from French into Polish. Having taught himself English in Warsaw during the war years, he later put his talents to good use by translating works of English-language poets such as Walt Whitman, Carl Sandburg, and T. S. Eliot. It was Miłosz, in fact, who produced the first Polish version of Eliot's *The Waste Land* (1922) in 1946. To promote the fortunes of contemporary poets from Poland, Miłosz translated from Polish into English. For this purpose, he issued an anthology in 1965 titled *Postwar Polish Poetry*. He also produced English versions of many of his own poems, working either independently or in collaboration with his students and fellow poets. Working from the original Greek and Hebrew, he rendered the Gospel According to Saint Mark, the book of Ecclesiastes, and the Psalms into Polish, with the goal of translating the entire Bible into a Polish that is modern yet elevated, sharply distinct from the debased journalistic style of many modern translations of the Bible.

ACHIEVEMENTS

Prior to receiving the 1980 Nobel Prize in Literature, Czesław Miłosz had already won a number of other prestigious awards and honors. When his novel *The Seizure of Power* was published in France in 1953 under the title *La prise du pouvoir*, he received the Prix Littéraire Européen (jointly with German novelist Werner Warsinsky). In 1974, the Polish PEN Club in Warsaw honored him with an award for his poetry translations. He was also granted a Guggenheim Fellowship in 1976 for his work as both poet and translator. He received honorary doctorates from the University of Michigan in 1977 and from Catholic University in Lublin, Poland, in 1981, when he finally returned to his native country after thirty years. In 1978, he was selected as the fifth recipient of the biennial Neustadt International Prize for Literature by a panel of judges assembled under the auspices of the editorial board of *World Literature Today* (formerly called *Books Abroad*). Miłosz accepted the award in public ceremonies held at the University of Oklahoma on April 7, 1978.

In a written tribute to his candidate for the 1978 Neustadt Prize, Joseph Brodsky, the eminent Soviet émigré writer and Nobel laureate, declared that he had no hesitation whatsoever in identifying Miłosz as one of the greatest poets of his time, perhaps the greatest. Miłosz's preeminence as a poet in no way stems from any technical innovations to be found in his poetry, as he was actually quite indifferent toward avant-garde speculation pertaining to aesthetic form, and the greatness of his poetry lies in its content. The most remarkable aspect of Miłosz's poetry is that, despite his having experienced first hand the depths of humankind's depravity in the form of Nazi barbarism and Soviet tyranny, it still affirms the beauty of this world and the value of life. From the Commonwealth Club of California, he received two Silver Medals (1988, 1991) and one Gold Medal (2001). He won three Northern California Book Awards in poetry (1984, 1991, 1995), the Robert Kirsch Award from the *Los Angeles Times* (1990), and a PEN Center USA Literary Award for poetry (1992).

One of Miłosz's most impressive achievements was that he continued to produce outstanding new work after the age of eighty. In 1997, he published two volumes of a memoir, *Abecadlo Milosza* (1997; *Miłosz's ABCs*, 2001), written in a distinctively Polish genre called *abecadlo*, an alphabetical arrangement of entries on people, places, and events from an individual's life. His collection of aphorisms, anecdotes, musings, and observations, *Road-side Dog*, won the 1998 Polish Nike Literary Prize. In 2002, the Northern California Book Awards presented a Special Recognition Award for distinguished contirbution to literature and culture to Miłosz.

BIOGRAPHY

Czesław Miłosz was born to Aleksandr Miłosz and Weronika (Kunat) Miłosz in Šeteiniai, which is located in the Kédainiai province of Lithuania. This area of Europe is a place where Polish, Lithuanian, and German blood intermingled over the centuries, and the ancestry of Miłosz himself was a mixed one. It can, however, be established through legal documents that his father's ancestors had been speakers of Polish since the six-

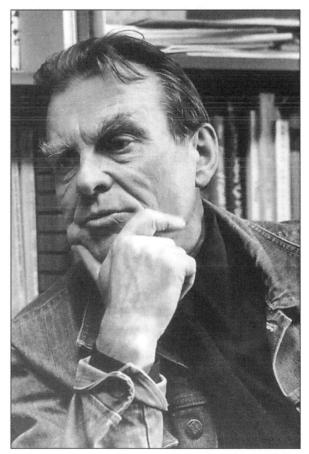

Czesław Miłosz (©The Nobel Foundation)

teenth century. Nevertheless, Miłosz had great pride in his Lithuanian origins and even took perverse pleasure from the fact that Lithuania was the last country in Europe to adopt Christianity. The lateness of this conversion, which occurred in the year 1386, permitted the survival of pagan attitudes toward nature on the part of the peasantry, and the influence of this pagan heritage can be detected in much of Miłosz's poetry as well as in his novel *The Issa Valley*.

Like much of Poland itself, Lithuania was part of czarist Russia's empire at the time of Miłosz's birth. Miłosz's father, a civil engineer by profession, made a yearlong trip to Siberia in 1913 under government contract and was accompanied by his wife and son. Shortly after their return home, when World War I broke out, his father was drafted into the Russian army as a military engineer and once again took his family to Russia, where they remained for the duration of the conflict. In these years, Miłosz imbibed Russian to such a degree that proficiency in that language became second nature to him and never deserted him in subsequent years.

After the Bolsheviks seized power in Russia, the Miłosz family returned to the newly independent Baltic states for a few years but finally decided to settle down in the city of Wilno. This city, although once the capital of ancient Lithuania, had long been a predominantly Polish-speaking municipality and was then incorporated into a fully restored Poland. In Wilno, Miłosz entered a Roman Catholic high school at the age of ten. There, he received exceptionally thorough training in religion, science, and the humanities over the course of eight years. It was also there that Miłosz received his first exposure to the Gnostic and Manichaean heresies that were to profoundly alter his outlook on life. Nothing in his home life could be said to have inspired the religious rebelliousness that he manifested in high school. His father was actually indifferent toward any form of worship, and his mother, although a devout Catholic, was quite tolerant of other faiths. Miłosz's religious revolt, however, stopped far short of atheism, for he lived in a state of constant wonder at the mystery of life and kept expecting an epiphany to occur at any moment.

In 1929, Miłosz matriculated as a law student at the King Stefan Batory University in Wilno and soon published his first poems in its literary review, *Alma Mater Vilnensis*. Here, he also became affiliated with a group of young poets who referred to themselves as Żagary (brushwood) and who subsequently founded a journal bearing the same name. While still a student, Miłosz published a slim volume of verse called *Poemat o czasie zastygłym* (a poem on congealed time), for which he received the poetry award from the Polish Writers Union in 1934. In the same year, Miłosz obtained a master's degree in law from the University of Wilno as well as a fellowship in literature from the Polish government, enabling him to study in Paris during the years of 1934 and 1935.

Miłosz had already been in France on one prior occasion when he and two other students from the university made an excursion to Western Europe in the summer of 1931. One of the highlights of that junket was his meeting with Oscar de L. Miłosz (1877-1939), a cousin of his from Lithuania and a highly accomplished poet in the French language. As a result of Miłosz's obtaining his fellowship, the two cousins were able to see each other often, and the older man exerted a profound influence on his young relative from Poland. Oscar de L. Miłosz especially enjoyed indulging in prophetic visions of a catastrophe that was about to befall Europe. His cousin's prophecies struck a responsive chord in Miłosz, whose own psychological state was somewhat chaotic at this time. When Miłosz returned to Poland after his fellowship year in France, he published a collection of poems titled *Trzy zimy* (three winters), in which the theme of personal and universal catastrophe is expressed. Oscar de L. Miłosz also helped to shape his young cousin's views on the craft of poetry and fostered his commitment to a poetry anchored in religion, philosophy, and politics.

Miłosz went on to obtain employment with the Polish Radio Corporation at its station in Wilno. He was eventually ousted from his post as programmer because of pressure exerted by local rightist groups, who considered him to be a dangerous left-winger if not an actual Communist. Although Soviet-style Communism never attracted Miłosz, his attitude toward Marxist dialectical and historical materialism was a decidedly favorable one at that time. It is also true that Miłosz did little to conceal his intense dislike for the reactionary politicians who controlled Poland after the death of Marshal Pilsudski in 1935. Fortunately, a sympathetic director of Polish Radio in Warsaw offered him a comparable post in that city, and after touring Italy in 1937, Miłosz settled down to a successful administrative career in broadcasting. This phase in Miłosz's life came to an abrupt halt when the Germans attacked Poland on September 1, 1939. Miłosz put on a uniform in time to join units of the Polish armed forces in a retreat to the eastern part of the country. This region was soon to come under Soviet occupation as a result of an invasion by the Red Army that was initiated on September 17, 1939, and Miłosz eventually returned to Wilno.

Wilno had changed drastically since Miłosz last saw it, for the Soviets chose to award the city to Lithuania as a gesture of goodwill shortly after capturing it. The Soviets, however, gradually increased their control over Lithuania and finally coerced it into becoming a Soviet Socialist Republic in the summer of 1940. When Lithuania was officially annexed to the Soviet Union, Miłosz concluded that its servitude would, in all likelihood, prove to be permanent, and he resolved to return to Warsaw. At great personal peril, Miłosz made several border crossings to get back to the part of Poland that the Germans had designated as the Government General.

Despite the horrendous conditions in Warsaw, Miłosz continued to write poetry and clandestinely published a new volume of verse called *Wiersze* (poems) in 1940 under the pseudonym J. Syruć. This was probably the first literary work to be printed in occupied Warsaw. It was run off on a ditto machine and laboriously sewn together by Janina Dluska, whom Miłosz married in 1944 and by whom he was subsequently to become the father of two sons. When the Germans decided to rearrange the holdings of Warsaw's three largest libraries, Miłosz managed to get himself hired as a laborer loading and transporting the packing cases, and he spent the next few years engaged in this interminable project. Some form of opposition to the German occupiers was a moral imperative, and he soon became active as a writer in the Resistance movement. In 1942, Miłosz edited a clandestine anthology of anti-Nazi poetry that appeared under the title *Pieśń niepoldlegla* (the independent song) and also provided the under-

ground press with a translation of Jacques Maritain's anticollaborationist treatise *À travers le désastre* (1941). Almost as an act of defiance toward the German oppressors, Miłosz began an intensive study of the English language and derived spiritual sustenance from reading poems such as Eliot's *The Waste Land*. Eliot's poem surely must have made appropriate reading at the time of such tragedies as the Warsaw Ghetto uprising in the spring of 1943.

A revolt against the Germans on a much grander scale occurred in the latter half of 1944 as the Red Army reached the outskirts of the Polish capital. The underground Home Army, whose hierarchy was controlled by the London-based government-in-exile, sought to take charge in Warsaw prior to the arrival of the Russian forces and launched an attack on the Germans stationed within the city. Not surprisingly, the Russian response to the insurrection was to cease all military activity against the Germans on the Warsaw front, and the Home Army was left to its own resources to do battle with the vastly superior Nazi forces. Miłosz himself was not a member of the Home Army because he had no desire to see the restoration of the political establishment that had governed Poland before World War II. Then, as later, he considered the rising to be an act of folly. The bitter struggle lasted more than two months and cost more than two hundred thousand Polish lives. After the surrender of the Home Army, the Germans forced the evacuation of the surviving populace and then systematically destroyed the city, block by block. Caught completely unawares by the outbreak of the rising, Miłosz and his wife were seized by the Germans as they attempted to leave Warsaw, but after a brief period of detention in a makeshift camp, they were released through the intercession of friends. Thereafter, they were to spend the next few months wandering about as refugees until the Red Army completed its annihilation of the German forces and Poland was at last liberated after more than five years of Nazi rule.

Since Warsaw had been almost totally destroyed, the center of literary activity in Poland had gravitated to Kraków, and it was there in 1945 that a collection of Miłosz's wartime poetry was issued in a volume titled *Ocalenie* (rescue). This work was one of the very first books to be published in postwar Poland. Because of his prominence as a poet, Miłosz was selected for service in the diplomatic corps and was posted as a cultural attaché at the Polish Embassy in Washington, D.C., from 1946 to 1950. He then was transferred to Paris, where he was appointed first secretary for cultural affairs. In 1951, shortly after the practice of Socialist Realism became mandatory for all Polish writers, he decided to break with the home government in Warsaw and to start life anew by working as a freelance writer in France. The next decade proved to be remarkably productive for Miłosz. His reasons for breaking with the Warsaw regime were fully set forth in the nonfictional study *The Captive Mind* as well as in the political novel *The Seizure of Power*. At the same time, he continued to create poetry of the highest order. His novel *The Issa Valley* also dates from this period, as does his long poem *A Treatise on Poetry*.

In recognition of these literary accomplishments, Miłosz was invited to lecture on Polish literature at the University of California, Berkeley, during the academic year 1960-1961. In 1961, he decided to settle in Berkeley after he was offered tenure as a professor of Slavic languages and literatures. He became a naturalized American citizen in 1970 and eventually retired from active teaching in 1978 with the rank of professor emeritus. Just as he retained his creativity during his years in exile as a freelance writer in Paris, so too did Miłosz manage to maintain his literary productivity within an academic environment in the United States. Fully one-third of the works included in the edition of Miłosz's *Utwory poetyckie* (collected poems), which was printed under the aegis of the Michigan Slavic Publications in 1976, were written in the United States. His lifetime achievement as a poet received acknowledgment when he was selected as the winner of the Nobel Prize in Literature in 1980.

In June, 1981, Miłosz returned to Poland for the first time since his self-imposed exile in 1951. The Polish government, still under Communism, now claimed him, although his Nobel Prize acceptance speech was published only after the anti-Communist sentiments were edited out. Polish presses were now able to publish his poetry, at last making it available in Polish to his native people, many of whom had never heard of their newly crowned national bard. With the declaration of martial law in December, 1981, however, his work was again banned by the government, although some of it remained available in *samizdat*, or underground, publications. Upon his return to America, Miłosz began a series of lectures as the Charles Eliot Norton Professor at Harvard University for the academic year 1981-1982. These lectures were later published in *The Witness of Poetry*.

Miłosz was incredibly prolific in his twilight years, publishing several collections of poetry, essays, and criticism: As he entered his nineties, Miłosz continued to publish. His wife, Janina, died in 1986 after a ten-year battle with Alzheimer's disease. Miłosz married again and divided his time between Berkeley and Kraków until his death in 2004.

ANALYSIS

The principal group of Polish poets in the period between the two world wars was known by the name "Skamander," after the title of its official literary organ. The Skamander group consisted of a number of poets with very disparate styles and diverse interests, and its members included such renowned literary figures as Julian Tuwim, Kazimierz Wierzyński, Jaroslaw Iwaszkiewicz, Antoni Słonimski, and Jan Lechoń. Since the Skamanderites were viewed as belonging to the literary establishment, younger poets formed movements of their own in opposition. A group now designated as the First Vanguard was centered in the city of Kraków during the 1920's and derived much of its aesthetic program from the ideas propounded by the Futurists in Italy. Around 1930, many new literary groups sprang up in various parts of Poland, and these groups are today known collectively as the Second Vanguard. Building on the formal innovations of the First Vanguard, its members generally sought to intensify the social and political dimensions of poetry.

The Żagary group of poets, to which Czesław Miłosz belonged while a student at the University of Wilno, was part of the Second Vanguard. Because of the apocalyptic premonitions expressed in their poetry, the Wilno group soon came to be labeled "catastrophists."

POEMAT O CZASIE ZASTYGŁYM

Miłosz's first published book, *Poemat o czasie zastygłym*, represents a youthful attempt to write civic poetry and is often marred by inflated political rhetoric as well as by avant-garde experimentation in both language and form. Apparently, Miłosz himself recognizes its overall shortcomings, since he chose to exclude the work from the edition of his collected poems published at Ann Arbor in 1976.

TRZY ZIMY

His next work, *Trzy zimy*, is largely free from the defects of the previous one and constitutes a decided advance in Miłosz's development as a poet. Despite his continued reliance on elliptical imagery, these poems frequently attain a classical dignity of tone. This quality is even present when Miłosz gives vent to forebodings of personal and universal catastrophe. One of his finest poems in this vein is called "Do ksiedza Ch." (to Father Ch.) and is passionate and restrained at the same time. Here, after describing a world being destroyed by natural calamities as a result of humanity's sinfulness, Miłosz ends his poem on a note of reconciliation. Shared suffering will, he says, reunite longtime antagonists, and the last pagans will be baptized in the cathedral-like abyss.

OCALENIE

Such premonitions of catastrophe turned into reality after the outbreak of World War II. The poems that Miłosz wrote during the war years in Poland were gathered together and published in 1945 under the title *Ocalenie*. Among the works in this collection are two outstanding poems that deal with the destruction of the Warsaw Ghetto. The first is "Campo di Fiori" and begins with a description of this famous square in modern-day Rome. The poet recalls that Giordano Bruno was burned at the stake on that very spot before a crowd that resumed its normal activities even before the flames were completely extinguished. The scene then shifts to Warsaw, where the crowds also carry on with mundane matters on a beautiful Sunday evening even while the ghetto is ablaze. The loneliness of the Jewish resistance fighters is then likened to the solitary fate suffered by Bruno. The poet, however, resolves to bear witness to the tragedy and to record the deeds of those dying alone, forgotten by the world.

The second poem is called "Biedny chrześcijanin patrzy na getto" ("A Poor Christian Looks at the Ghetto"). Here, the poet watches as bees and ants swarm over the ruins of the Ghetto. He then spots a tunnel being bored by a mole, whose swollen eyelids remind him of those of a biblical patriarch. Guilt overwhelms the poet as he wonders if in the next world the patriarch will accuse him of being an accomplice of the merchants of death. This guilt is less that of a survivor than of one who regrets that he was unable to help a fellow human being in his hour of need.

Many other poems in the collection focus on purely personal themes, but it is in his role as a national bard that Miłosz is most impressive. Although Miłosz's poetic style is generally modern in character, the reader frequently encounters traces of the diction and phraseology associated with great Romantic poets such as Adam Mickiewicz, Juliusz Słowacki, and Cyprian Norwid. Any avant-garde preoccupation with finding new modes of linguistic expression could only have appeared trivial in the light of the horrendous events that overwhelmed the poet and his nation during the war years.

ŚWIATŁO DZIENNE

While in exile in France during the years 1951 to 1960, Miłosz published two important volumes of verse: *Światło dzienne* (daylight) and *A Treatise on Poetry*. In the first of these works, the poet dwells on political grievances of various sorts. One of the best of these political poems is titled "Dziecie Europy" ("A Child of Europe"). After a bitterly ironic opening section in which the poet reminds those who managed to live through the war how often they sacrificed their honor as the price of survival, he goes on to ridicule the belief in historical materialism and implies that the doctrine of the inevitability of socialism rests more on the use of force against all classes of society than on the laws of history. To those who are compelled to live in a communist state, he offers a counsel of despair: If you wish to survive, do not love other people or the cultural heritage of Europe too dearly.

A TREATISE ON POETRY

In his *A Treatise on Poetry*, Miłosz surveys the development of Polish poetry in the twentieth century and discusses the role of the poet in an age of crisis. A work of about twelve hundred lines, it is unrhymed, except for a few rhymed insertions, and employs a metrical line of eleven syllables with a caesura after the fifth syllable. The meter is quite familiar to Polish readers because of its previous appearance in major literary works by Mickiewicz and Słowacki. Even so, Miłosz's style here is classical rather than Romantic. A dissertation of this kind that employs verse has, to be sure, a number of contemporary counterparts, such as W. H. Auden's *The Double Man* (also known as *New Year Letter*; 1941) and Karl Shapiro's *Essay on Rime* (1945), but the genre had not been used in Polish literature since the Renaissance. *A Treatise on Poetry* is, therefore, considered to be in the nature of an innovation in Miłosz's homeland. For this and other reasons, it is ranked very highly among the poetical works in Miłosz's oeuvre.

KRÓL POPIEL I INNE WIERSZE

The publication of Miłosz's *Król Popiel i inne wiersze* (King Popiel and other poems) in 1962 was closely followed by a second volume of verse titled *Gucio zaczarowany* (Bobo's metamorphosis) two years later. In both works, all formal features associated with poetry are minimized. Stanza, rhyme, and regular meter tend to disappear, and the poet veers toward free verse. The title poem in the first work tells the story of Popiel, a mythical king from the time of Polish prehistory who was said to have been devoured by mice on his island fortress in the center of a large lake. In recounting this legend, Miłosz makes the reader aware of the narrow mode of existence that must have been the lot of Popiel and his kingly successors, for whom possession of territory and material objects was of overriding importance and to whom all cosmological speculation was alien. The pettiness of Popiel's end mirrors the pettiness of his thought.

GUCIO ZACZAROWANY

Much longer and much more complex is "Gucio zaczarowany" ("Bobo's Metamorphosis"), the title poem of the subsequent collection. Miłosz, with the assistance of Richard Lourie, has himself translated the work into English and is thus responsible for its current title; a more literal rendition of the original Polish would be "enchanted Gucio." (Gucio is one of the diminutive forms of the name Gustaw.) The poem itself has eight sections; in the seventh, an individual called Bobo (Gucio) is transformed into a fly for a few hours. As a result of this experience, Bobo often has difficulty

adopting a purely human perspective on matters. All of the other sections of the poem likewise involve the problem of reconciling various perspectives. In the final section, the poet explores the psychological tensions that arise between a man and a woman as they mutually recognize the impossibility of penetrating the private universe of another person's mind. In place of understanding, they have no recourse but to posit humanity and tenderness. The dialectical tension in this poem, and its resolution, is quite typical of Miłosz's cast of mind, for he intuitively looks at the world in terms of contrary categories such as stasis and motion or universal and particular. Similarly, in many of his poems, a sense of apocalypse is juxtaposed to a feeling of happiness.

MIASTO BEZ IMIENIA

In *Miasto bez imienia* (city without a name), a collection of verse published in 1969 and translated in the 1973 collection *Selected Poems*, Miłosz does much to clarify his view of poetry in the works titled "Ars poetica?" ("Ars Poetica?") and "Rady" ("Counsels"). The opening lines of "Ars Poetica?" are used by the author to proclaim his desire to create a literary form that transcends the claims of either poetry or prose. Nothing short of this, he declares, is capable of satisfying the demoniac forces within the poet that inspire the content of his work. There can, however, be no assurance that the *daimon* will be an angel, for a host of Orphic voices compete for possession of a poet's psyche. Over the years, so many invisible guests enter a poet's mind that Miłosz likens it to a city of demons and reminds the reader how difficult it is for anyone who writes poetry to remain only one person. Still, he personally eschews the morbid and expresses his disdain for confessional poetry of the psychiatric variety. Miłosz is committed to the kind of poetry that helps humankind to bear its pain and misery, and he underscores this belief in "Counsels." Younger poets are hereby cautioned against propagating doctrines of despair. This earth, Miłosz insists, is not a madman's dream, nor is it a stupid tale full of sound and fury. He himself concedes that this is a world wherein justice seldom triumphs and tyrants often prosper. Nevertheless, Miłosz argues that Earth merits a bit of affection if only because of the beauties it contains.

Neither in "Counsels" nor elsewhere in his poetical oeuvre does Miłosz ever hold God to be the cause of the misfortunes that humans inflict on other humans, and he likewise absolves the deity of responsibility for any of the other evils that befall human beings in this world. His conception of God has much in common with that to be found in the writings of the Gnostics and Manichaeans, for which he first developed a partiality while still a high school student in Wilno. Hence, Miłosz is frequently tempted to view God as a perfect being who is completely divorced from all forms of matter and who is, therefore, not responsible for the creation of the material universe. In that light, everything that has a temporal existence can be said to be under the control of a Demiurge opposed to God. Miłosz does, however, advise his readers not to assume a divine perspective in which humanity's earthly tribulations are to be seen as inconsequential. In "Do Robinsona Jeffersa" ("To Robinson Jeffers"), a poem included in his essay collection *Widzenia nad zatoką San Francisco* (1969; *Visions from San Francisco Bay*, 1982), Miłosz objects to the way in which Jeffers, in some of his poetry, demotes the stature of humanity by contrasting people's pettiness with the immensity of nature. Miłosz prefers to remain true to his Slavic and Baltic heritage, in which nature is anthropomorphized, rather than to adopt an inhuman view of the universe such as the one propounded by Jeffers.

GDZIE WSCHODZI SŁOŃCE I KĘDY ZAPADA

The free-verse style of *Gdzie wschodzi słońce i kędy zapada* (from where the sun rises to where it sets) sometimes borders on prose. The author, in fact, freely juxtaposes passages of verse and prose in the title poem, an explicitly autobiographical work that is almost fifty pages long. In the seven sections of this poem, Miłosz moves between past and present in a spirit of free association and contemplates the nature of an inexplicable fate that has brought him from a wooden town in Lithuania to a city on the Pacific coast of the United States. True to his dialectical frame of mind, Miłosz's attitudes alternate between forebodings of death and affirmation of life. "Dzwony w zimie" ("Bells in Winter"), the final section, contrasts the Wilno of his youth, where he was usually awakened by the pealing of church bells, with the city of

San Francisco, whose towers he views daily across the bay in the winter of his life. The entire poem is an attempt to bridge the gap between his expectations as a youth in Poland and the realities of his old age in America.

"YOU WHO HAVE WRONGED"

Bridge-building in the reverse direction occurred when Polish workers belonging to the Solidarity movement selected some lines from one of Miłosz's poems to serve as an inscription on the monument erected outside the shipyards in Gdańsk for the purpose of commemorating the strikers who died during demonstrations against the government in 1970. These lines are taken from the poem "Który skrzywdziłeś" ("You Who Have Wronged"), included in the collection *Światło dzienne*, and run as follows:

> You, who have wronged a simple man,
> Bursting into laughter at his suffering . . .
> Do not feel safe. The poet remembers.
> You may kill him—a new one will be born.
> Deeds and talks will be recorded.

For a poet in exile, it must have been a source of profound satisfaction to learn that his words had been chosen by his countrymen to express their own longing for a free and independent Poland. Verse that previously had been circulated clandestinely in *samizdat* form could now be read by everyone on a public square in broad daylight.

THE COLLECTED POEMS, 1931-1987

Like the other long serial poems, "La Belle Époque" from "New Poems, 1985-1987," which appears at the end of *The Collected Poems, 1931-1987*, mixes verse and prose, speaks in multiple voices, and moves freely in time, along the way pointing out the intersections of personal fate with history. The poem returns over its seven sections to a few central characters. The poet's father and the beautiful teenage Ela seem to represent for the poet the inevitable human tendency toward empathy and connection; he identifies so closely with each that he feels he "becomes" them. However, such feeling is terrifyingly fragile in the face of catastrophe, whether natural catastrophes or the everyday catastrophe of human mortality. Miłosz relates with necessary, quiet detachment, for instance, the fact of the execution of Valuev and Peterson, train passengers engaged in a debate over mortality, each feverishly in pursuit of his own truth. The poem's final section asserts the fragility of not only the individual human, but also the entire belle époque and its nearsighted optimism with the sinking of the *Titanic*.

"La Belle Epoque," with its harsh pessimism, is not the conclusion to "New Poems, 1985-1987." Rather, in the last poem, "Six Lectures in Verse," with characteristic insight, Miłosz goes beyond the contradiction of mortality to a new recognition: that the facts of history and mortality are forgotten in that moment when sensuous reality is far more present and more "real" than any concept we have of it.

FACING THE RIVER

From the mid-1980's to the mid-1990's, Miłosz's poetry underwent a profound change. The poem "Realism," in the collection *Facing the River*, gives some indication of the source and direction of his poetic goals. Admitting that the language humans use to tame nature's random molecules fails to capture eternal essences or ontological reality, Miłosz still insists on a realm of objectivity embodied in the still life. Abstractionism and pure subjectivity are not the final prison for the triumph of the ego, and Miłosz recalls Arthur Schopenhauer's praise of Dutch painting for creating a "will-less knowing" that transcends egoism through "direct[ing] such purely objective perception to the most insignificant of objects." So Miłosz proceeds in "Realism" from the still life to the idea of losing himself in a landscape:

> Therefore I enter those landscapes
> Under cloudy sky from which a ray
> Shoots out, and in the middle of dark plains
> A spot of brightness glows. Or the shore
> With huts, boats, and on yellowish ice
> Tiny figures skating. All this
> Is here eternally, just because once it was.

This is remarkable because the preceding poem, "The Garden of Earthly Delights: Hell," completes the series of meditations—written more than a decade earlier and published in *Unattainable Earth*—on Hieronymous Bosch's terrifying painting of the same title. In moving from the scene of worldly hell to the Dutch still

life and landscape, Miłosz conveys his desire to move beyond the tragic and egocentric to the sensuous, yet peaceful and eternal.

"The Garden of Earthly Delights: Hell" is, in fact, one of the most frightening poems in this, the most hell-haunted of all of Miłosz's work. This is the "missing panel" of Miłosz's meditation on Bosch's painting, *The Garden of Earthly Delights*. Sensitive to such details in the painting as "a harp/ With a poor damned man entwined in its strings," one feels Miłosz's own painful skepticism of the worth of a life in art. Here he takes one of the most painful jabs at his own endless pursuit of the real as hiding fear of death:

> Thus it's possible to conjecture that mankind exists
> To provision and populate Hell,
> The name of which is duration. As to the rest,
> Heavens, abysses, orbiting worlds, they just flicker
>   a moment.
> Time in Hell does not want to stop. It's fear and
>   boredom together
> (Which, after all, happens) And we, frivolous,
> Always in pursuit and always with hope,
> Fleeting, just like our dances and dresses,
> Let us beg to be spared from entering
> A permanent condition.

This is the ironic version of what he says in "Capri": "If I accomplished anything, it was only when I, a pious boy, chased after the disguises of the lost Reality." The question for Miłosz is when the "chasing" stops that carried him forward in time, out of his past, and now back into his past. Where is the final reality beneath "dresses" and "disguises," metaphors for the changing forms of history and of his own art?

SECOND SPACE

Second Space was published just after Miłosz's death. The title comes from the first poem in the collection, in which the author meditates on most people's loss of belief in the afterlife. Most of the other thirty-one poems in the collection have religious themes as well, although a few, such as "New Age" and "Late Ripeness" discuss old age, and "A Master of My Craft" is a salute to fellow poet Jaroslaw Iwaszkiewicz, a member of the Skamander group. The shortest poem with only five lines is "If There Is No God," an argument that even if God does not exist, there are still moral laws by which to live.

The longest poem in the collection, "Treatise on Theology," covers twenty pages. As the title indicates, it concerns Christianity, especially Catholicism. The narrator describes a young man, clearly based on Miłosz himself, who is a poet struggling with his religious beliefs and meditating on the mysteries of the Trinity, Original Sin, and Redemption. There are several references to Mickiewicz, a Polish poet who combined elements of the Enlightenment and romanticism; Jacob Boehme, a theologian who was burned at the stake for supporting the astronomical theories of Copernicus; Arthur Schopenhauer, a German philosopher known for his atheistic pessimism; Emanuel Swedenborg, a Swedish scientist who became a mystic and theologian; and Charles Darwin, the English scientist who developed the theory of evolution.

"Father Severinus" is a monologue by a Catholic priest who no longer believes in God, especially in the necessity of the Crucifixion, and feels guilty for consoling his parishioners with church doctrines in which he no longer believes. He wonders why Christians worship a man who bleeds and why they feel a need for Hell when life on Earth is bad enough. He is envious of the ancient Greeks, who worshiped gods such as Athena, Apollo, and Artemis. He thinks that if he had been at the Council at Nicea in 325, he would have voted against making the concept of the Holy Trinity a critical part of Christian doctrine. The name of the poem is a reference to the Roman Christian philosopher Boethius, whose full name was Anicius Manlius Severinus Boethius and whose best known work was *De consolatione philosophiae* (523; *The Consolation of Philosophy*, late ninth century).

"Apprentice" is an appreciation of Miłosz's distant cousin Oscar de L. Miłosz, and this poem is the most thoroughly footnoted work in this collection. Czesław Miłosz met his relative in Paris in 1931, developed a closer relationship with him, studied his poetry and catastrophism based on the Book of Revelations, studied Swedenborg under his guidance, and talked to other people who knew him. In this poem, Miłosz imagines what it must have been like to have been the other Miłosz and laments that Oscar would have been better off if he had not been born wealthy and lived in Paris for most of his adult life.

SELECTED POEMS, 1931-2004

Selected Poems, 1931-2004 contains more than one hundred poems arranged chronologically. The first poem in the collection is "Dawns," which belongs to his early period when, under the influence of Oscar de L. Miłosz, he was preoccupied with catastrophes. The last is "Orpheus and Eurydice," a modern retelling of the classic myth. In Miłosz's version, Orpheus has to deal with automobiles, elevators, and other modern devices on his journey to Hades. The underworld's entrance, a glass-paneled door, has a sidewalk in front of it, and Hades is several hundred stories below the ground in the form of a labyrinth. Orpheus still carries a nine-string lyre, and he uses his voice to persuade the goddess Persephone to free Eurydice. The poem does not change the ending, but afterward, Orpheus finds consolations in the scents, sounds, and textures of nature.

Other poems include "The World" (1943), which is written in the style of a nursery rhyme and follows a group of children coming home from school. Their mother feeds them soup, a boar's head comes to life and confronts them, they read poetry and picture books before going to play in the woods, and find reassurance from their father that the night's darkness will pass. The darkness symbolizes the Nazi occupation, and the children's father represents God. One year later, Poland was "liberated" by the Red Army, and the Communists replaced the Nazis. In "Mid-Twentieth-Century Portrait" (1945), he portrays a Communist Party official as a hypocrite.

Over the years, Miłosz wondered whether poetry was a worthy pursuit, and even when he decided it was, he wondered whether he was worthy of it. In "Song of a Citizen" (1943), the speaker wonders whether poetry is worthwhile. "With Trumpets and Zithers" (1965) celebrates life, but the poet despairs over whether he can adequately describe it. In "Secretaries" (1975), Miłosz compares the work of a poet to a secretary who merely transcribes what other people say.

Miłosz was always interested in philosophical issues. "Encounters" (1936) argues that mediation is not enough when responding to the world. Whimsical metaphysical questions concern "Magpiety" (1958). When the poet sees a magpie in France, is it improbable that it is the same magpie he had seen years before in Lithuania. In the tradition of Plato, he tries to grasp the essence of the magpie, which he calls "magpiety." In "To Raja Rao" (1969), Miłosz traces his development from youthful visionary to a more mature man who rejects both Western rationalism and Eastern mysticism. In "Bypassing Rue Descartes" (1980), Miłosz rejects rationalism in the tradition of René Descartes.

In "Slow River" (1936), Miłosz uses multiple voices to show how difficult it is for people to accept nature's beauty on its own terms. "From the Rising of the Sun" (1973-1974) is a fifty-page poem using not only multiple voices, but also multiple languages, including Polish, Lithuanian, and Byelorussian.

OTHER MAJOR WORKS

LONG FICTION: *Zdobycie władzy*, 1953 (*The Seizure of Power*, 1955); *Dolina Issy*, 1955 (*The Issa Valley*, 1981).

NONFICTION: *Zniewolony umysł*, 1953 (criticism; *The Captive Mind*, 1953); *Rodzinna Europa*, 1959 (autobiography; *Native Realm: A Search for Self-Definition*, 1968); *Człowiek wśród skorpionów*, 1962 (criticism; *The History of Polish Literature*, 1969 (enlarged 1983); *Widzenia nad zatoką San Francisco*, 1969 (*Visions from San Francisco Bay*, 1982); *Prywatne obowiązki*, 1972; *Emperor of the Earth: Modes of Eccentric Vision*, 1977; *Ziemia Ulro*, 1977 (*The Land of Ulro*, 1984); *Nobel Lecture*, 1981; *Świadectwo poezji*, 1983 (criticism; *The Witness of Poetry*, 1983); *Zaczynając od moich ulic*, 1985 (*Beginning with My Streets: Essays and Recollections*, 1991); *Rok myśliwego*, 1990 (*A Year of the Hunter*, 1994); *Legendy nowoczesności*, 1996 (*Legends of Modernity: Essays and Letters from Occupied Poland, 1942-1943*, 2005); *Abecadło Milosza*, 1997 (*Miłosz's ABCs*, 2001); *Striving Towards Being: The Letters of Thomas Merton and Czeslaw Milosz*, 1997; *Zycie na wyspach*, 1997; *To Begin Where I Am: Selected Essays*, 2001; *Rozmowy Czesław Miłosz: Aleksander Fiut "Autoportret przekorny,"* 2003; *Czesław Miłosz: Conversations*, 2006.

EDITED TEXTS: *Pieśń niepoldlegla*, 1942; *Postwar Polish Poetry*, 1965; *With the Skin: Poems of Aleksander Wat*, 1989; *A Book of Luminous Things: An International Anthology of Poetry*, 1996.

MISCELLANEOUS: *Kontynenty*, 1958; *Ogród nauk*, 1979.

BIBLIOGRAPHY

Davie, Donald. *Czesław Miłosz and the Insufficiency of Lyric*. Knoxville: University of Tennessee Press, 1986. The poet Davie examines the poetry of Miłosz, paying attention to technique.

Fiut, Aleksander. *The Eternal Moment: The Poetry of Czesław Miłosz*. Translated by Theodosia S. Robertson. Berkeley: University of California Press, 1990. A comprehensive examination of the artistic and philosophical dimensions of Miłosz's oeuvre. Fiut analyzes the poet's search for the essence of human nature, his reflection on the erosion of the Christian imagination, and his effort toward an anthropocentric vision of the world.

Grudzinska-Gross, Irena. *Czesław Miłosz and Joseph Brodsky: Fellowship of Poets*. New Haven, Conn.: Yale University Press, 2010. Examines the relationship between these two poets and compares and contrasts them.

Ironwood 18 (Fall, 1981). Special Miłosz issue. Published a year after Miłosz received the Nobel Prize, this issue's self-proclaimed purpose was to "help Americans absorb and assimilate his work." Offers a broad range of responses to Miłosz's work from his American and Polish contemporaries, many well-known and admired poets themselves, such as Robert Hass, Zbigniew Herbert, and Stanisław Barańczak.

Malinowska, Barbara. *Dynamics of Being, Space, and Time in the Poetry of Czesław Miłosz and John Ashbery*. New York: P. Lang, 2000. A discussion of poetic visions of reality in the works of two contemporary hyperrealistic poets. In its final synthesis, the study proposes the comprehensive concept of ontological transcendence as a model to analyze multidimensional contemporary poetry. Includes bibliographical references.

Miłosz, Czesław. Interviews. *Conversations with Czesław Miłosz*. Edited by Ewa Czarnecka and

Aleksander Fiut. Translated by Richard Lourie. New York: Harcourt, 1987. Incredibly eclectic and illuminating set of interviews divided into three parts. Part 1 explores Miłosz's childhood through mature adulthood biographically, part 2 delves more into specific poetry and prose works, and part 3 looks at Miłosz's philosophical influences and perspectives on theology, reality, and poetry. It is especially interesting to hear Miłosz's interpretations of his own poems.

_____. Interviews. *Czesław Miłosz: Conversations*. Edited by Cynthia L. Haven. Jackson: University Press of Mississippi, 2006. Part of the Literary Conversations series, this collection of interviews examines the poet's views on literature and writing.

Mozejko, Edward, ed. *Between Anxiety and Hope: The Poetry and Writing of Czesław Miłosz*. Edmonton: University of Alberta Press, 1988. Although these seven articles by accomplished poets and scholars are not focused around any one theme, some topics that dominate are catastrophism and the concept of reality in Miłosz's poetry and his place in Polish literature. Also shows Miłosz's ties with Canada in an article comparing his artistic attitudes to those of Canadian poets and an appendix describing his visits to Canada.

Nathan, Leonard, and Arthur Quinn. *The Poet's Work: An Introduction to Czesław Miłosz*. Cambridge, Mass.: Harvard University Press, 1991. The first book by an American to serve, as Stanisław Barańczak puts it in the foreword, as a "detailed and fully reliable introduction . . . to the body of Miłosz's writings." This work by two of Miłosz's Berkeley colleagues (Nathan was also a cotranslator with Miłosz of many of his most challenging poems) benefits from the authors' lengthy discussions of the texts with the poet himself.

Victor Anthony Rudowski; Tasha Haas;
Robert Faggen
Updated by Thomas R. Feller

EUGENIO MONTALE

Born: Genoa, Italy; October 12, 1896
Died: Milan, Italy; September 12, 1981

PRINCIPAL POETRY

Ossi di seppia, 1925 (partial translation, *The Bones of Cuttlefish*, 1983; full translation, *Cuttlefish Bones*, 1992)
Le occasioni, 1939 (*The Occasions*, 1987)
La bufera, e altro, 1956 (*The Storm, and Other Poems*, 1978)
Poems by Eugenio Montale, 1959
Eugenio Montale: Poesie/Poems, 1965
Selected Poems, 1965
Provisional Conclusions: A Selection of the Poetry of Eugenio Montale, 1970
Satura, 1962-1970, 1971 (English translation, 1998)
Diario del '71 e del '72, 1973 (partial translation in *New Poems*, 1976)
New Poems: A Selection from "Satura" and "Diario del '71 e del '72," 1976
Quaderno di quattro anni, 1977 (*It Depends: A Poet's Notebook*, 1980)
L'opera in versi, 1980
Diario postumo, 1991-1996 (2 volumes; *Posthumous Diary*, 2001)
Collected Poems, 1920-1954, 1998
Selected Poems, 2004

OTHER LITERARY FORMS

In addition to his several volumes of verse collected by R. Bettarini and G. Contini in a critical edition, *L'opera in versi*, Eugenio Montale (mohn-TAH-lay) wrote the obliquely autobiographical short stories of *Farfalla di Dinard* (1956; *Butterfly of Dinard*, 1971). His critical essays on literature were collected by G. Zampa in *Sulla poesia* (1976; on poetry) and those on broadly cultural or social topics in *Auto da fé* (1966). To them should be added the travelogues and interviews of *Fuori di casa* (1969; abroad), which arose from the practice of journalism, and the musical reviews posthumously reprinted in book form: *Prime alla Scala* (1981; premieres at La Scala), edited by G. Lavezzi. The revealing intellectual diary of 1917, *Quaderno genovese* (pb. 1983), also deserves mention.

ACHIEVEMENTS

Eugenio Montale won the Premio dell'Antico Fattore (1932), the Premio Manzotto (1956), Italy's Dante Medal (1959), the Feltrinelli Prize from the Accademia dei Lincei (1963, 1964), Paris's Calouite Bulbenkian Prize (1971), and honorary degrees from the Universities of Milan, Rome, Cambridge, Basel, and Nice. In 1967, he was named senator of the Italian Republic. In 1975, he won the coveted Nobel Prize in Literature.

BIOGRAPHY

The youngest of five siblings, Eugenio Montale was born in Genoa on October 12, 1896, to Giuseppina

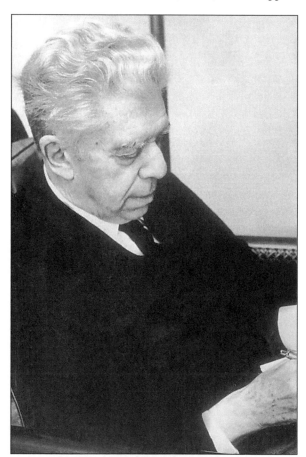

Eugenio Montale (©The Nobel Foundation)

Ricci and Domingo Montale, a well-to-do businessman who shared with two first cousins the ownership and management of a firm for the importation of turpentine and other chemicals. Poor health forced Montale to withdraw from school as a ninth-grader; henceforth, only his insatiable curiosity for books and the unfailing assistance of his sister Marianne—a philosophy student—were to sustain him in the pursuit of a broad cultural education, ranging from Italian, French, and English literature to modern philosophy. Entering the family firm or a bank, as his brothers did, was out of the question from the start for the dreamy adolescent, who, sharing with his family a great love for opera, soon began to train for baritone singing with Ernesto Sivori. This fine teacher's death in 1916 put an end to Montale's plans for an operatic career but not to his lifelong interest in musical theater. In 1917, Montale joined the army and soon was serving as an infantry officer on the Trentino front against the Austrians.

During the years immediately following World War I, Montale's contributions to literary journals and the limited if solid success of *Cuttlefish Bones* were not enough to earn a living, and in 1927, he moved to Florence, where he found work first with Bemporad, a publishing firm, and then as curator of the Vieusseux rare books library in the employ of the city administration. He was to lose that congenial position in 1938 for political reasons, but he remained in Florence through the war years as a freelance translator and an acknowledged leader of the literary scene until 1948, when he moved to Milan as contributing editor to the leading daily *Il corriere della sera*. Long before he received the 1975 Nobel Prize in Literature, he was made a senator for life by the president of the Italian Republic. The death in 1963 of his wife, Drusilla Tanzi, affected him deeply, as the "Xenia" sequence in *Satura* shows; from then on, the old poet was entrusted to the devoted care of their housekeeper, Gina Tiossi. Much earlier, two other women had left a durable imprint on his art: a visiting American scholar in the 1930's (who became the unnamed angelic figure of many poems in *The Occasions* and the Clizia of *The Storm, and Other Poems*) and, in the late 1940's and early 1950's, an Italian poetess (who inspired the "Volpe," or "Vixen," poems in *The Storm, and Other Poems*). Montale's funeral in mid-September, 1981, was attended by the Italian chief of state and many other prominent figures of public and artistic life.

ANALYSIS

Emerging from the welter of experiments and iconoclasms that had marked the decade before World War I, Eugenio Montale's intense lyrics set the tone for the interwar period in Italian poetry. Giuseppe Ungaretti's verse, jotted down in the Carso trenches and first published in 1916, had already pointed the way to a new poetics of elliptical imagery, inward essentialness, modern diction, and deconstructed meter that had distilled Futurist exuberance into noiseless immediacy. Montale's first collection, *Cuttlefish Bones*, discovered the untapped possibilities of a venerable tradition, which, purged of academic sclerosis and vatic posturing or bombast, could best articulate the dilemmas, the self-criticism, and the yearning for authentic values that variously haunted so many of the war's survivors. The starkness of style of this first book sharpened into thinly veiled prophetic denunciation with Montale's next collection, *The Occasions*, which registered the gathering of a new storm. In his third collection, *The Storm, and Other Poems*, Montale responded to World War II and its aftermath in an unfashionable vein of visionary lyricism. His books of the 1970's, from *Satura* on, approach the threshold of prosiness, in keeping with the prevalently satirical and gnomic bent of his later years. The Nobel laureate of 1975 became the poetic conscience of the generation that had groped for truth in the dark times between two world wars; he showed that the best way for a writer to be modern was not to discard a tradition which went all the way back to Dante but instead (in Ezra Pound's words) to "make it new."

CUTTLEFISH BONES

Cuttlefish Bones displays simultaneously the alert richness of youth and maturity's searching control. Scrupulous attention to the formal resources of the word, far from foundering into aesthetic complacency, bespeaks an ingrained commitment to cognitive values, and since there can be no final certainty about these values, the persona wavering between sudden contemplative rapture and unappeased doubt transcends the merely autobiographical level to become as memorable a spokesperson for the modern human condition as T. S. Eliot's Prufrock or Pound's Mauberley. It was no accident that the author of *Cuttlefish Bones* should eventually become a friend of Pound (politics apart) and try his hand at translating one short section of *Hugh Selwyn Mauberley* (1920) as well as three of Eliot's "Ariel Poems," while Eliot, for his part, published "Arsenio," chronologically the last poem of *Cuttlefish Bones*, in a 1928 issue of *The Criterion*. "Arsenio," the most lucidly despondent and subtly modulated monologue in *Cuttlefish Bones* (the poem first appeared in the collection's third edition), was translated by Mario Praz, and it was Praz who, two decades later, identified certain formal and thematic affinities between Eugenio Montale's and Eliot's poetry.

The affinities are there, if one but thinks of the wasteland-like component in Montale's style and worldview, but they should not overshadow the differences and, above all, Montale's independence from the Eliotic paradigm. Montale's poetics of dryness, which found an early embodiment in "Meriggiare pallido e assorto" ("The Wall"), stems from the Dantesque leanings first recognized by Glauco Cambon in 1956 and openly confirmed by the poet himself many years later.

In "The Wall," written several years before the publication of *The Waste Land* (1922), Montale's characteristic tone is already evident.

> . . . e andando nel sole che abbaglia
> sentire con triste meraviglia
> comè tutta la vita e il suo travaglio
> in questo seguitare una muraglia
> che ha in cima cocci aguzzi di bottiglia.

> . . . and walking on under the blinding sun
> to feel with sad amazement
> how all of life's painful endeavor is
> in this perpetual going along a wall
> that carries on its top sharp bottle shards.

The familiar sight of such walls protecting gardens and orchards in the northern Italian upland countryside has elicited an unmistakable emblem of the burdensome human condition which the stoic Montalian persona repeatedly faces. The emblem, whether in the same form or in the guise of cognate imagery, pervades

Montale's poetry. In one of *Cuttlefish Bones*'s most cryptic and tensest lyrics, "Crisalide" ("Chrysalis"), it reaches its symbolic acme: "e noi andremo innanzi senza smuovere/ un sasso solo della gran muraglia" ("and we shall go right on without dislodging/ even a single stone of the huge wall"). Perhaps, the poem continues, we humans shall never meet on our way "la libertà, il miracolo,/ il fatto che non era necessario!" ("freedom, miracle,/ the fact that was not shackled by necessity!").

That cry of the heart and of the whole mind against the seeming barrier that reality opposes to humankind's need for knowledge and deliverance voices the central concern of the Montalean persona and propels his utterance beyond whatever seductions the lavish landscape of sensuous experience may offer. "The mind investigates, harmonizes, disjoins," as Montale writes in "I limoni" ("The Lemon Trees"), the first poem of *Cuttlefish Bones* after the epigraph lyric; it is a question of finding "a mistake of Nature,/ the dead point of the world, the loose chain-ring,/ the thread to be unravelled" which will finally "place us in the midst of a truth." Remarkably, and understandably, the search for truth can take place only as an attempt to disrupt the opaque compactness of existence. The revolt against closure, the distrust of intellectual systems that claim to explain everything, marks Montale's imagery and thought from beginning to end and accounts for his interest in Émile Boutroux's contingentist thought, which openly challenged the still prevalent determinist philosophies of science.

Montale is a thinking poet, a "poet on the edge" in Rebecca West's apt words; he cannot take phenomenal reality for granted but must forever question it. Denial is his concomitant gesture. With Arthur Schopenhauer (and Giacomo Leopardi), Montale at times sees and feels existence as sheer suffering. The "pain of living" can be escaped only in a kind of Buddhist "divine indifference," the privilege of the noon-haloed statue in the garden, of the floating cloud, of the high-soaring hawk—or else, acme of negations, in the Nirvanic ecstasy of the sunflower "impazzito di luce" (maddened with the light). The "glory of outspread noon" rules over Liguria's seething sea and rocky, olive-tree-studded slopes, a fierce beauty not to be forgotten by

the war-tried persona who revisits the landscape of his childhood.

It was an Eden, now lost forever, as stated in "Fine dell'infanzia" (end of childhood). Here the persona, confronting the numinous turbulences and calms of the Mediterranean, rehearses what had been his initiation to poetry and self-knowledge, in self-differentiation from, and reimmersion in, the godlike native element. Alternatively, he contemplates, in the person of the lithe swimmer Esterina ("Falsetto"), the momentary bliss that immersion in the welcoming bosom of her "divine friend" can bestow, though the contemplator himself remains "on dry land," apart from that alien joy. The "Mediterraneo" ("Mediterranean") series at the center of the book has been faulted by some critics (Gianfranco Contini, Silvio Ramat, and the author himself) as a relapse into suspect exuberance from the terse spareness achieved by "Cuttlefish Bones," the eponymous series that precedes "Mediterranean" in the collection. "Mediterranean," however, with its nearly Whitmanesque expansiveness, counterpoints the systole of "Cuttlefish Bones" and thus makes the entire book pulsate with a vitality of its own.

THE OCCASIONS

When that vitality subsides into the mournfulness of "Arsenio" (a piece added to the third edition of *Cuttlefish Bones* in 1928), the stage is set for the next cycle of poems, *The Occasions*, which disappointed a friendly critic, Pietro Pancrazi; in Pancrazi's opinion, Montale with this new book had turned to abstruse "metaphysical" poetry instead of staying with the "physical" concreteness of *Cuttlefish Bones*. Actually, what occurred was no involution but a deepening of style and vision into the kind of clipped writing that can evoke an innermost reality from the barest outline of factual detail. The relative colorfulness of the sunstruck earlier book yields to a gray monochrome. The diction becomes even more conversational, the tone more low-key yet amenable to sudden soarings in elliptical concentration, and metric patterns tend to disintegrate as far as stanza form goes, even if the lines as such stay mostly within the regular cast of the hendecasyllable and alternative shorter verse types. *The Occasions*, accordingly, evinces a less literary and more penetrating voice than its predecessor, from which it nevertheless takes seminal motifs. The epistemological urge turns from the cosmic to the personal and historical, political sphere, facing the precariousness of individual existence to denounce (in guarded yet ultimately transparent allegory) the evils of Nazi and fascist totalitarianism, the threat of impending war. Liuba, in "A Liuba che parte" ("For Liuba, Leaving"), is a Jewess forced to flee persecution, carrying her household gods (a cat in a hatbox) like a diminutive Noah's ark that will tide her over the flood of "the blind times." In "Dora Markus," the title figure, an Austrian Jewess whose very "sweetness is a storm," recalling "migratory birds that crash into a lighthouse," withstands time's (and the times') ordeal by the mere strength of her womanly amulets, while it get "later, ever later"; in the teeth of Nazism's "ferocious faith," she refuses to "surrender/ voice, legend or destiny." An unnamed girl from Liguria who died young (a poem of the last years will identify her as Annetta) haunts the persona's memory in "La casa dei doganieri" ("The Shorewatcher's House"), where she will never return, while "the compass spins crazily at random" and "there is no reckoning the dice's throw." The persona's interlocutor in "Barche sulla Marna" ("Boats on the Marne") shares with him a peaceful Sunday on that French river which nevertheless conjures in his mind the fateful meandering of human history away from the dreamed possibility of a just, serene, and happy life on Earth.

In another holiday setting, the English bank holiday in "Eastbourne," the persona strolling on the beach descries dark omens; "evil is winning, the wheel will never stop," and perhaps not even the countervailing force of love, which holds the world together, will manage to stem the tide. It is a force coming from, and oriented toward, his absent beloved, who thereby acquires mythic, not to say godlike, status; the stirring hyperbole recalls Dante's myth of Beatrice in a different, if equally apocalyptic, context. No less apocalyptically, the same transfigured lady from the Atlantic's other shore battles the forces of obscurantism on a chessboard which clearly figures forth the contemporary world under the gathering storm ("Nuove stanze"), and she dawns on the persona's mind to exorcize those forces in "Elegia de Pico Farnese" (elegy for Pico Farnese) and in "Palio" (Palio at Siena), where the

clamoring crowd and the wheeling horses in the folk event of worldwide renown evoke the mass hysteria and the apparent ineluctability of sinister political developments in the late 1930's.

At the heart of *The Occasions*, the Beatrice-like American woman dominates the twenty "motets" addressed to her by a modern troubadour who effortlessly renews the medieval worship of Eros in the very act of confronting a bleak modern reality. Descanting on the vicissitudes of love from afar, Montale attains a poignancy attuned to the contrapuntal polyphony of Orlando di Lasso, Giovanni Pierluigi da Palestrina, and Carlo Gesualdo:

> Un ronzìo lungo viene dall'aperto.
> Strazia com'unghia ai vetri. Cerco il segno
> smarrito, il pegno solo ch'ebbi in grazia
> da te.
> E l'infernoè certo.
>
> A long whir comes from the outside.
> It grates like a nail on windowpanes. I seek the sign
> lost, the one pledge I had as a grace
> from you.
>   And hell is certain.

Even though, as Montale later saw fit to reveal, this particular motet and the two following ones were inspired by another lady (a Peruvian visitor) and not by the one whom he was to call Clizia, the Ovidian girl metamorphosed into a sunflower in *The Storm, and Other Poems*, it serves as a perfect opening to the whole series, with which it thematically and tonally coalesces.

THE STORM, AND OTHER POEMS

The "I-thou" rhetorical stance, the repudiation of the irrational times, and the persistent conversation with absent Clizia across the ocean—all these obviously link *The Occasions* to *The Storm, and Other Poems*, which at the same time shows new developments in style and theme. The first part of this book, with the title "Finisterre," had been published in Lugano, Switzerland, by Bernasconi in 1943, and one climactic poem, "Primavera hitleriana" ("The Hitler Spring"), protesting Hitler's official visit to Florence in 1938, could not appear in print before the end of the war. "Finisterre" pushes emblematic allusiveness to a truly hermetic point, covertly indicating the war unleashed by the Axis powers. The diction is melodiously stylized, there is a tendency toward legato as opposed to the earlier staccato and related percussive alliterations, and the very fact that three of the poems happen to be sonnets (albeit treated with deft sprezzatura) signals an unprecedented Petrarchan leaning—openly avowed by the author in "Intenzioni, intervista immaginaria" (intentions, an imaginary interview) of 1946, a poem later reprinted in *Sulla poesia*. These "Finisterre" lyrics are germane to the coeval translation of three sonnets by William Shakespeare, to be found in *It Depends: A Poet's Notebook*.

Family memories, a moving poem to Montale's wife (who was briefly hospitalized during the last days of the battle for Florence in August, 1944), and a series of madrigals to the poetically gifted lady addressed under the code name of the "Volpe" (Vixen), contribute to the uniqueness of *The Storm, and Other Poems*, a book also characterized by the frequent naming of God (a novelty in Montale) and by the joyous vitality that the poems to the Vixen and the breathtaking dithyramb "L'anguilla" ("The Eel"), ostensibly addressed to Clizia, hymnically convey. The two poems in the last section, "Conclusioni provvisorie" ("Provisional Conclusions"), provide a dark antiphon by casting a saturnine eye on the disappointing postwar world, where the dominant mass ideologies of Stalinism and Christian Democracy ("red" and "black clerics") seem equally unacceptable to the devotee of a humanist faith in the dignity of humankind. The impending extinction of Western civilization is allegorized in a "shadowy Lucifer," though the persona still clings to his dream of love for Clizia.

SATURA

Satura (the Latin title means "satire" but also connotes a medley of offerings) picks up those somber clues in a prosaic register which would persist down to the last of Montale's books. A Lucifer-like god darkens by his very absence the allegorized historical scene of "Botta e risposta I" (thrust and riposte I), where the persona, reviewing what preceded and followed the latest catastrophe, decries the fact that Italy's liberation by the Allied armies failed to bring about a permanent cleansing of the Augean stables, public life being now repulsively shapeless. A bracing antiphon to that de-

pressing message and tone rings out in "Xenia," and much else in *Satura*—especially "Angelo Nero" (black angel)—shows Montale's old mettle, even in the new, exceedingly deflated style. The books of the 1970's comment discursively on public issues or private events and memories, and if an aggressively flat chattiness seems at times to take over, the epigrams and some satirical pieces have a sharpness of their own. All in all, these last collections constitute the uneven aftermath of the great poetry that had reached its lyric climax in *The Storm, and Other Poems*.

OTHER MAJOR WORKS

NONFICTION: *Farfalla di Dinard*, 1956 (short articles, prose poems, memoirs; *The Butterfly of Dinard*, 1970); *Auto da fé*, 1966; *Fuori di casa*, 1969; *Nel nostro tempo*, 1972 (*Poet in Our Time*, 1976); *Sulla poesia*, 1976; *Prime alla Scala*, 1981; *The Second Life of Art*, 1982; *Quaderno genovese*, pb. 1983 (wr. 1917).

BIBLIOGRAPHY

Brook, Clodagh J. *The Expression of the Inexpressible in Eugenio Montale's Poetry: Metaphor, Negation, and Silence*. New York: Clarendon Press, 2002. Locating Montale firmly within European modernism, this book examines the struggle with language that is central to his work. In its unraveling of the inexpressibility paradox, Brook offers his reading of Montale's early verse and discusses ways in which Montale gives insight into both his poetics and the whole process of expression.

Butcher, John. *Poetry and Intertextuality: Eugenio Montale's Later Verse*. Perugia: Volumnia, 2007. This analysis of Montale's poetry concentrates on the works he produced in later years, including *Satura*.

Cambon, Glauco. *Eugenio Montale's Poetry: A Dream in Reason's Presence*. Princeton, N.J.: Princeton University Press, 1982. A critical assessment of Montale's career as a poet. Includes bibliographical references and indexes.

Cary, Joseph. *Three Modern Italian Poets*. Chicago: University of Chicago Press, 1993. Cary presents striking biographical portraits and provides an understanding of the works of Umberto Saba, Giuseppe Ungaretti, and Montale. In addition, Cary guides readers through the first few, difficult decades of twentieth century Italy. Includes chronological tables, bibliography.

Huffman, Claire Licari. *Montale and the Occasions of Poetry*. Princeton, N.J.: Princeton University Press, 1983. A collection of the author's essays and lectures about Montale's life and works. Includes bibliographical references and index.

Montale, Eugenio. *Selected Poems*. Translated by Jonathan Galassi, Charles Wright, and David Young. Edited with an introduction by David Young. Oberlin, Ohio: Oberlin College Press, 2004. This collection of poems, translated by three well-known Montale translators, contains an introduction that provides biography and analysis of Montale's works.

Sica, Paola. *Modernist Forms of Rejuvenation: Eugenio Montale and T. S. Eliot*. Florence, Italy: L. S. Olschki, 2003. Sica examines modernism through the works of Montale and Eliot.

West, Rebecca. *Eugenio Montale: Poet on the Edge*. Cambridge, Mass.: Harvard University Press, 1981. The well-known novelist's critical interpretations of some of Montale's major works. Includes bibliographic references and an index.

Young, David. *Six Modernist Moments in Poetry*. Iowa City: University of Iowa Press, 2006. This discussion of modernism looks at Montale's "Mediterranean" as well as poems by Rainer Maria Rilke, William Butler Yeats, Wallace Stevens, William Carlos Williams, and Marianne Moore.

Glauco Cambon

CHRISTIAN MORGENSTERN

Born: Munich, Germany; May 6, 1871
Died: Untermais, near Meran, Austro-Hungarian Empire (now Merano, Italy); March 31, 1914

PRINCIPAL POETRY

In Phanta's Schloss, 1895
Auf vielen Wegen, 1897
Horatius travestitus, 1897
Ich und die Welt, 1897
Ein Sommer, 1900
Und aber ründet sich ein Kranz, 1902
Galgenlieder, 1905 (*The Gallows Songs*, 1963)
Melancholie: Neue Gedichte, 1906
Einkehr, 1910
Palmström, 1910
Ich und Du: Sonette, Ritornelle, Lieder, 1911
Wir fanden einen Pfad, 1914
Palma Kunkel, 1916
Der Gingganz, 1918
Stufen, 1918
Epigramme und Sprüche, 1919
Klein Irmchen, 1921
Mensch Wanderer: Gedichte aus den Jahren 1887-1914, 1927
The Moonsheep, 1953
The Daynight Lamp, and Other Poems, 1973
Gesammelte Werke in einem Band, 1974
Lullabies, Lyrics, and Gallows Songs, 1995

OTHER LITERARY FORMS

Christian Morgenstern (MAWR-guhn-shtehrn) was an active translator of Scandinavian literature. Among his translations are August Strindberg's *Inferno* in 1898; a large number of plays and poems for the German edition of Henrik Ibsen's work; and Knut Hamsun's *Aftenrøde* (1898) in 1904 as *Abendröte*, and his *Livets spil* (1896) in 1910 as *Spiel des Lebens*. Morgenstern also translated the works of Frederick the Great. There are two editions of his letters, *Ein Leben in Briefen* (1952) and *Alles um des Menschen willen* (1962). Otherwise, Morgenstern is known chiefly for his poems.

ACHIEVEMENTS

Christian Morgenstern began to write serious and humorous verse while still in school. By 1894, he was contributing to various magazines, and in the following years, he began to travel extensively. In 1903, he became a reader for publisher Bruno Cassirer and edited *Das Theater*. The serious side of his nature was stimulated by the lectures of Rudolf Steiner, and in 1909, he became a member of the Anthroposophical Society. The German Schiller Society made him the recipient of an honorary stipend in 1912, and in November, 1913, he was honored at a Morgenstern festival in Stuttgart.

BIOGRAPHY

Christian Otto Josef Wolfgang Morgenstern was born just as the Franco-Prussian War ended, and he died shortly before the outbreak of World War I. His life span covers a long interval of peace in the history of modern Germany. The lack of external political problems may have been responsible in part for his attention to that which ailed the country from within, particularly the crass materialism he perceived and the callousness of the upper class with regard to the plight of the worker.

Morgenstern was the only child of Carl Ernst Morgenstern, a landscape painter, and his wife, Charlotte, née Schertel. Both parents came from artists' families. Because of the frequent changes of residence necessitated by his father's profession, Morgenstern's education was erratic. He changed schools frequently and sometimes received private tutoring. After the death of his mother in 1881 of tuberculosis—a disease from which he also suffered, requiring frequent sanatorium visits—he was sent to his uncle's family in Hamburg. This arrangement proved to be unsuitable, and when his father married again, Morgenstern was sent to a boarding school in Landshut. The strict, oppressive environment there, which included corporal punishment, was unbearable for him, and his bitter complaints to his father resulted in his removal from the school after two years. In March, 1884, he joined his parents in Breslau and attended a local *Gymnasium* for four years. Although Morgenstern's schooling was not a positive experience, he began to write poetry and became acquainted with the philosophy of Arthur Schopenhauer and medieval German mystics such as Meister Eckhart and Johannes Tauler. Shortly before entering a military academy in 1889, he met Friedrich Kayssler, who became an actor and Morgenstern's best and lifelong friend. It quickly became obvious that Morgenstern was not suited for the military life; in 1890, he entered the *Gymnasium* in Sorau, and after his graduation in 1892, he became a student of economics and political science at the University of Breslau. The following two years brought some personal upheavals that culmi-

nated in his estrangement from his father. In the summer of 1893, his tubercular condition became more severe, requiring an extensive period of rest. He began reading Friedrich Nietzsche, to whose mother he sent his first book of poetry. Meanwhile, his father had divorced his second wife, remarried, and refused to finance his son's further schooling. In the spring of 1894, Morgenstern left for Berlin.

Newly independent, Morgenstern was briefly employed at the National Gallery. He then began to contribute to a number of different journals, among them the *Neue Deutsche Rundschau* and *Der Kunstwart*. For the latter magazine, he wrote theater reviews. This activity brought him in contact with Max Reinhardt, the famous theatrical producer, who became one of Morgenstern's friends. In 1895, his first volume of poetry, *In Phanta's Schloss*, was published. Morgenstern characterized it as humorous and fantastic, but it contains lyrics with mythological and mystical elements engulfed in pathos. Even as a sixteen-year-old, he had written a poem on reincarnation, and during the winter of 1896-1897, he had several dreams that he transformed into a cycle of lyric poems. They became part of *Auf vielen Wegen*. Between 1897 and 1903, Morgenstern translated a large number of plays and poems by Ibsen, whom he met in 1898 on a journey to Oslo. Morgenstern always had a sense of urgency about his work—a conviction that his time was limited. He traveled extensively to Scandinavia, Switzerland, Italy, and within Germany, always writing, always battling his deteriorating health. While vacationing in Dreikirchen in the Tirol, he met and became engaged to Margareta Gosebruch von Liechtenstern in 1908; they were married in 1910.

At this point in his life, Morgenstern was seriously ill and had to spend considerable time in hospitals and sanatoriums. After learning of the spiritualist and occultist research being done by Rudolf Steiner, the couple attended his lecture in January, 1909, on Leo Tolstoy and Andrew Carnegie. Steiner had written studies on Johann Wolfgang von Goethe and Nietzsche as well as on mysticism in Christianity. After having outlined his philosophy in *Philosophie der Freiheit* (1894; *Philosophy of Freedom*, 1964) and in his *Theosophie* (1904; *Theosophy*, 1954), he published a work in 1909 outlining his method of attaining a knowledge of the occult. Morgenstern became a member of his Anthroposophical Society in May, 1909, and attended Steiner's lectures in Oslo, Budapest, Kassel, and Munich. During the last years of his life, Morgenstern's longing for communication with a world beyond that of his present existence took shape in a number of poems of a meditative nature. Two weeks before his death, he determined that the last collection of his lyrics was to be called *Wir fanden einen Pfad* (we found a path). After being removed from a sanatorium in Gries to private quarters in Untermais, Morgenstern died on March 31, 1914.

ANALYSIS

Christian Morgenstern himself considered his serious lyrics paramount in his poetic oeuvre, although he is best known for his humorous poems. He has been compared to contemporaries such as Stefan George, Hugo von Hofmannsthal, and Rainer Maria Rilke, with whom he shared a sense of poetic mission and a certain melodiousness of verse. Morgenstern's poetry is considerably less complicated both linguistically and metaphorically than Rilke's, although it expresses emotion sincerely. Only a few of his serious poems have been translated into English, and German audiences were more receptive to his grotesque humor than to the expressions of his religious convictions or metaphysical thought. Although Morgenstern considered his light and provocative verse to be *Beiwerke* (minor efforts), it is in this area that he anticipated trends that were later exploited more extensively in Dadaism and concrete poetry. He experimented with visually and acoustically innovative techniques, presented a satirical view of a philistine society in his verse, and playfully created new and sometimes nonsensical word constellations that appear to mock both the advocates of a *poésie pure* and the efforts of those who, thirty years after his death, attempted a reconstruction of his poetry with ciphers and absolute metaphors. Satire, religious fervor, humor, and mysticism found in Morgenstern an expressive spirit.

THE GALLOWS SONGS

Morgenstern's frivolous verse is the foundation of his fame, notwithstanding his protestations. His most popular collection was *The Gallows Songs*, which ran

through fourteen editions in his lifetime and by 1937 had sold 290,000 copies. Critics persisted in reading hidden meanings into these witty lyrics, so that he felt compelled to render mock explanations in *Über die Galgenlieder* (1921; about the gallows songs). The first group of these whimsical lyrics were composed when Morgenstern was in his twenties. On the occasion of an outing with some friends, they arrived at a place referred to as Gallows Hill. Being in a bantering mood, they founded the Club of the Gallows Gang, Morgenstern contributing some frivolous poems that another of the group later set to music. These poems obviously attest Morgenstern's lighter side, and no attempt should be made to imbue them with a depth that they do not have and that was not intended, yet it will not detract from the reader's pleasure if the spirit of innovation and the subtle humor that pervade them are pointed out.

Morgenstern's raw material is the sound, the structure, the form, and the idiomatic usage of the German language. The nineteenth century saw an abundance of grammarians and linguists who attempted to regulate and explain linguistic phenomena and to limit expression to precisely defined and carefully governed modes of communication. Morgenstern perceived this approach to be hopelessly dull, "middle-class safe," and philistine. A degree of arbitrariness is an essential element of language, and he proceeded to point this out by confusing the complacent and satirizing the pedants. He accomplished this on the semantic, grammatical, and formal levels in his poems. In "Gruselett" ("Scariboo"), he created what has come to be known as a nonsense poem:

> The Winglewangle phlutters
> through widowadowood,
> the crimson Fingoor splutters
> and scary screaks the Scrood.

By arranging essentially meaningless words according to a familiar syntactical pattern within the sentence and by adding a number of adjectives and verbs that stimulate lexical memory, Morgenstern coerces the reader into believing that he has grasped the sense of what has been said. It must be pointed out here that most of the translations of Morgenstern's poems have not been literal and have frequently deviated greatly from the original to preserve a semblance of the poet's intention (the use of puns, untranslatable idioms, grammatical constructions not found in English, and so on).

"THE BANSHEE"

Proper inflection, punctuation, and use of tense also come under attack by Morgenstern, who freely admitted that his teachers had bored and embittered him. His poem "Der Werwolf" ("The Banshee") reflects the eagerness, gratitude, and eventual disillusionment of the pupil, as well as the futility and uselessness of that which is taught by smug grammarians. When the banshee requests of an entombed teacher, "Inflect me, pray," the teacher responds:

> "The banSHEE, in the subject's place;
> the banHERS, the possessive case.
> The banHER, next, is what they call
> objective case—and that is all."

The banshee, delighted at first, then asks how to form the plural of "banshee":

> "While 'bans' are frequent," he advised,
> "a 'she' cannot be pluralized."
> The banshee, rising clammily,
> wailed: "What about my family?"
> Then, being not a learned creature,
> said humbly "Thanks" and left the teacher.

The teacher's wisdom is depicted as severely limited and out of touch with reality. His linguistic expertise extends only to abstractions.

"AMONG TENSES" AND "KORF'S CLOCK"

Time, that element which is "money" to the businessperson and is "of the essence" to the philistine, is only relative to Morgenstern. He satirizes the preoccupation of humanity with the temporal in several ways, one of them grammatical. In the poem "Unter Zeiten" ("Among Tenses"), past and future are on equal terms in the present: "Perfect and Past/ drank to a friendship to last./ They toasted the Future tense/ (which makes sense)./ Futureperf and Plu/ nodded too." The clock, the object that enslaves humanity because it measures every minute and every hour and restlessly reminds us that "time flies" (*tempus fugit*), is reinvented to improve on the fatal flaw. "Die Korfsche Uhr" ("Korf's

Clock") not only deprives time of its sovereignty but also recalls those people who, while still existing in the present, seem to live forever in the past:

> When it's two—it's also ten;
> when it's three—it's also nine.
> You just look at it, and then
> time gets never out of line,
> . . . .
> time itself is nullified.

A counterpart to Korf's clock, and one with yet greater flexibility and sophistication, is Palmström's clock ("Palmströms Uhr"): It heeds requests and slows or quickens its pace according to the individual's wishes. It "will never/ stick to petty rules, however," and is "a clockwork with a heart." For those who are incurably enslaved by time and who permit it to upset their equilibrium grievously, Morgenstern suggests a cure: Since time is not a matter of reality but merely of habit, it is useful to read tomorrow's paper to find out about the resolution of today's conflicts.

"THE FUNNELS" AND "FISH'S LULLABY"

Morgenstern's visual verse is a forerunner of concrete poetry. It expresses graphically in the poem what is described linguistically in the choice of words. Max Knight translates the poem "Die Trichter" ("The Funnels") in the singular:

> A funnel ambles through the night.
> Within its body, moonbeams white
> converge as they
> descend upon
> its forest
> pathway
> and
> so
> on

The funnel in effect becomes its own pathfinder as it streamlines the moonlight through its neck and directs it like a flashlight on the dark path. Although this poem is meant to be humorous, it contains an element of Morgenstern's own undaunted search for cosmic (divine) direction and communication, which is very evident in his serious poetry. As a final example of Morgenstern's humorous verse, the visual poem "Fisches Nachtgesang" ("Fish's Lullaby"), may suffice:

```
            -
           ~ ~
          - - -
         ~ ~ ~ ~
          - - -
         ~ ~ ~ ~
          - - -
         ~ ~ ~ ~
          - - -
         ~ ~ ~ ~
          - - -
           ~ ~
            -
```

Fish, as mute creatures, can express lyrical sentiments only wordlessly, by rhythmically opening and closing their mouths. The unverbalized song is formally recorded by Morgenstern as a series of dashes that leave the content to the imagination of the reader.

"EVOLUTION" AND "THE EIGHTEEN-YEAR-OLD"

A large part of Morgenstern's work is serious prose, much of it dealing with profound matters, such as the search for truth, and with humanity's position in the universe and in relation to God. Not only did Morgenstern write deeply religious verse in the Christian tradition, but also he developed poems involving the concepts of pantheism and reincarnation. Although his basic philosophical tenets may not have changed significantly, a change in style, a greater facility and fluency in writing, is evident in a comparison of portions of his early with his late work. This may be perceived in the opening stanzas of two poems dealing with reincarnation, one of which, "Der Achtzehnjährige" ("The Eighteen-Year-Old"), was written in 1889, while the other, "Evolution," was written shortly before Morgenstern's death. "The Eighteen-Year-Old" begins:

> How often may I already have wandered before
> on this earthly sphere of sorrow,
> how often may I have changed
> the substance, the form of life's clothing?

The formal aspects of this poem in the German are scrupulously observed: iambic meter with four feet, regular *abab* rhyme scheme. The first two strophes posit the fundamental question (rhetorically), and the last one answers it with the metaphor of the ever-changing waves of the sea. The finality of the answer is sententious. Despite the use of enjambment, the poem grinds along with the deadening regularity that is one of the pitfalls of iambic meter, and it does so because the metric stress coincides almost perfectly with the syllabic emphasis of the words.

Thus, the prosodic perfection becomes somnolent and detrimental to the poem's overall effect. The single place (in the second stanza) in which the word "order" is reversed for the sake of the rhyme causes the verse to sound contrived and strange. It may be argued that the monotony of the verse is intentional, thereby underscoring the repetitiousness of life, death, and rebirth inherent in the concept of reincarnation. While such a theory is certainly plausible, other early poems by Morgenstern with different topics show a similar emphasis on the regularity of rhyme and meter and thereby reveal the style to be a sign of poetic immaturity and inexperience.

The difference between "The Eighteen-Year-Old" and the poem "Evolution" is striking. The latter begins:

> Barely that that, which once separated itself from Thee,
> recognized itself in its special entity,
> it immediately longs to return to its element.

The excessive pathos and the sententiousness that characterized the first poem are missing here. The certainty, too, is absent: There are no answers in "Evolution," only ambiguity, longing, and the realization that this yearning cannot yet find fulfillment. The easy solutions of youth have mellowed into a peaceful submission, a quiet recognition and acceptance of the inevitable unfolding of individual and collective destiny. The formal presentation is also different. Although the poem in its entirety retains a formal meter (iambic pentameter) and a regular rhyme scheme (*aba bcb c*), there is a natural flow of rhythm akin to that inherent in prose: The monotony of the iambs is broken by the deliberate placement of semantically significant syllables on metrically unstressed ones, and vice versa. The interlocking rhymes facilitate the smooth flow of verse, and the third strophe is not a glib retort but a reduction, a one-line confrontation with an unfathomable phenomenon.

Morgenstern's serious poetry is not without beauty

and merit, although it has been neglected both by the reading public and by the critics. There is a certain dogmatism, a religious and mystical undercurrent inherent in it that limits its appeal and precludes the kind of universal acceptability that, for example, the lyrics of Rainer Maria Rilke possess. Morgenstern's lighter verse, which exemplifies the cheerful side of his personality, not only requires less empathy from the reader but also stimulates the reader's intellect without engaging the personal prejudices that he might have. It is an art worthy of pursuit.

Other major works

NONFICTION: *Ein Leben in Briefen*, 1952; *Alles um des Menschen willen*, 1962.

TRANSLATIONS: *Inferno*, 1898 (of August Strindberg's novel); *Abendröte*, 1904 (of Knut Hamsun's play *Aftenrøde*); *Spiel des Lebens*, 1910 (of Hamsun's play *Livets spil*).

MISCELLANEOUS: *Über die Galgenlieder*, 1921.

Bibliography

Bauer, Michael. *Christian Morgensterns Leben und Werk*. Munich: R. Piper, 1941. The standard biography, illustrated. In German.

Forster, Leonard. *Poetry of Significant Nonsense*. New York: Cambridge University Press, 1962. A brief treatment of Morgenstern in the context of Dada and nonsense verse.

Hofacker, Erich P. *Christian Morgenstern*. Boston: Twayne, 1978. A good English-language introduction to Morgenstern's life and works.

Knight, Max, trans. Introduction to *The Daynight Lamp, and Other Poems*, by Christian Morgenstern. Boston: Houghton Mifflin, 1973. The translator's introduction to this slim collection casts light on Morgenstern's poetics.

Scott, Robert Ian. "Metaphorical Maps of Improbable Fictions: The Semantic Parables of Christian Morgenstern." *Et Cetera* 52, no. 3 (Fall, 1995): 276. Scott argues that Morgenstern made absolute faith in words "obviously ridiculous" in demonstrating that the world does not follow human logic. He examines a number of Morgenstern's poems.

Helene M. Kastinger Riley

Eduard Mörike

Born: Ludwigsburg, Württemberg (now in Germany); September 8, 1804
Died: Stuttgart, Germany; June 4, 1875

Principal poetry

Gedichte, 1838, 1848, 1856, 1867 (*Poems*, 1959)
Idylle vom Bodensee oder Fischer Martin und die Glockendiebe, 1848

Other literary forms

Although Eduard Mörike (MUR-ree-kuh) is famous for his poetry, and many of his poems have been set to music, he was not primarily a poet. His first publication was a three-hundred-page novella in two parts, *Maler Nolten* (1832; *Nolten the Painter: A Novella in Two Parts*, 2005). He also wrote seven shorter works; the most well-known is *Mozart auf der Reise nach Prag* (1855; *Mozart's Journey from Vienna to Prague: A Romance of His Private Life*, 1897). Of particular significance for his poetry are his translations of classical poetry that retain the stanza form of the original. His editorial work attests to his interest in the works of contemporary Swabian poets and novelists, as well as in Greek and Roman poetry.

Achievements

During Eduard Mörike's lifetime, very few German literary awards were being awarded, as most awards were not established until the twentieth century. For that reason, the recognition he received carries all the more weight. In 1847, Mörike won the Tiedge Prize for his *Idylle vom Bodensee oder Fischer Martin und die Glockendiebe*. In 1852, he received an honorary doctorate from the University of Tübingen, and in 1862, the king of Bavaria awarded him the Order of Maximilian for Arts and Sciences. In 1864, Mörike was awarded the Knight's Cross First Class of the Württemberg Order of Friedrich.

Biography

Eduard Mörike spent his entire life in southwest Germany, in what is now the state of Baden-Württemberg.

He is sometimes referred to as a Swabian poet, because Swabian is the dialect spoken in that region. The family's standard of living was severely reduced when Mörike's father, a physician, suffered a massive stroke in 1815 and died two years later. Although Mörike was not a good student, an influential uncle arranged for him to attend the theological seminar in Urach and then to study theology in Tübingen. Mörike subsequently served reluctantly as a Protestant clergyman in numerous posts. He was not convinced of the doctrine he was required to preach and was not appreciated by his parishioners. In 1834, he was appointed pastor in Cleversulzbach and brought his mother and younger sister Klara to live with him there. It was his last position with the church. In 1843, two years after his mother's death, Mörike took early retirement.

The Mörikes were a close-knit family. Eduard Mörike was devastated when his younger brother August died of a stroke in 1824 and commemorated him in the poem "To an Aeolian Harp." Three years later, his older sister Luise died at age twenty-nine, and Mörike had to take several months' leave of absence. His own health was delicate, and he was often overextended financially because he felt obliged to help his siblings. Mörike was apolitical, and was shocked by the interrogation he underwent after his brother Carl was jailed for political protest.

In 1823-1824, during Mörike's student years, he was briefly infatuated with an attractive transient, Maria Meyer. Then, believing she had deceived him, he refused to see her again, a decision that caused him considerable emotional suffering. That relationship is the subject of his five "Peregrina" poems. He was engaged to Luise Rau from 1829 to 1833 but was also working on *Nolten the Painter* at the time, and Rau left him for someone better able to provide for her. Mörike did not marry until he was forty-seven. It is indicative of his open-mindedness in intolerant times that his wife, Margarethe Speeth, was a Roman Catholic. Their two daughters, Fanny and Marie, were born in 1855 and 1857. Mörike supported his family, which still included his sister Klara, by teaching from 1851 to 1866 at the Katharinenstift, a girls' school in Stuttgart.

Throughout Mörike's life, a friend from student days, Wilhelm Hartlaub, was a constant source of companionship and support. Mörike's poem "To Wilhelm Hartlaub" describes how Hartlaub's piano playing could transport him into other worlds. Hartlaub had what Mörike longed for, a sense of fulfillment as a clergyman and a peaceful domestic life. Mörike was estranged from his wife and in financial straits during the last years of his life. He is buried in the Prague Cemetery in Stuttgart.

ANALYSIS

A glance at Eduard Mörike's 225 poems reveals his remarkable versatility as a poet. The influence of Greek and Roman poetry is evident in his sonnets, odes, and idylls, and in his frequent use of iambic hexameter. The Germanic influence is evident in the rhymed quatrains and simple folksongs. However, Mörike was not limited by any form: Some of his poems are just two verses long; others run for pages. In most cases, he uses rhyme, meter, and stanza structures only as artistically necessary. Many of his poems are in free verse. His writing is direct, often conversational in tone. The five "Peregrina" poems are one of only two groups of poems. (The other group, "Pictures from Bebenhausen," has been only partially translated.) Otherwise, each poem stands for itself. Mörike let a friend decide on their order of appearance when his poems were published.

Nothing in Mörike's poetry indicates that he lived in a time of political unrest; nothing indicates that he was a clergyman. Some of his contemporaries criticized him for not mentioning political or historical events, but ironically, it is his refusal to be governed by current events that has made his poetry timeless. Mörike focused on personal issues, everyday life, and the inner peace he experienced in the presence of friends or when beholding a "Beautiful Beech Tree" or an object, as in "On a Lamp." He could capture the moment and infuse it with meaning. Much of his poetry, though, has an undercurrent of dissonance, a dissonance Hugo Wolf transferred well to his musical settings of fifty-seven Mörike poems in the 1880's. Mörike shows that even "At Midnight," one is constantly reminded of the affairs of the day. He was aware of conflicting beliefs, changes brought with the passage of time, and the omnipresence of death.

"Peregrina" poems

Mörike wrote his five "Peregrina" poems between 1824 and 1828 and included versions of four of them in *Nolten the Painter*. These early poems—some rhymed, some unrhymed, some in regular stanzas, and some in free verse—derive from Mörike's intense love for and then loss of the migrant or peregrine Meyer. The male poetic persona experiences heartbreak because he still loves Peregrina, indeed will always love her, yet feels he had to send her away because of his desire to remain in respectable society.

Mörike portrays a dangerous struggle between emotion and reason, between sexual attraction and societal norms. The temptation is great. In the first poem, the speaker tells Peregrina of her powerful effect on him: "To set us both on fire with wild beguiling:/ Death in the cup of sin you hand me, smiling." The wedding scene in the second poem is far removed from any Christian context. The bride is dressed in explicitly sexual colors, with her black dress and scarlet headscarf, but the reader should remember that black and red are also the colors of traditional Black Forest costumes. The turning point is the third poem, in which the speaker realizes he has been deceived. He sends Peregrina away, but cannot stop thinking of her, and he wonders how he would react if she were to reappear. The fourth poem shows how thoughts of her still intrude and move him to tears in other surroundings. The fifth poem, a sonnet, has him longing for her return, while he remains convinced that she will never come back again.

In *Nolten the Painter*, the Peregrina figure is conflated with the gypsy Elizabeth and is portrayed as truly malign, bringing death to Nolten and any women who are interested in him. This change in her character may be seen as rationalization on the part of the author, making the object of his attraction seem worse than she was to justify his rejection of her.

"On a Christmas Rose"

"On a Christmas Rose," a two-part poem, was written in 1841. Mörike wrote to his friend Hartlaub on October 29 of that year that he and his sister Klara had found the rare flower they had been seeking in a churchyard. Known in English as the Christmas rose, the plant is actually *Helleborus niger*. Mörike describes its delicate fragrance and the green tint in its white petals.

Because he found it blooming on a grave in a churchyard and because of its common name, *Christblume*, Mörike first associates the flower with Christian imagery, mentioning an angel, the Virgin Mary, and the wounds of Christ. However, the purely Christian frame of reference was never adequate for Mörike. In the last stanza of part 1, he draws on the pre-Christian, Germanic belief in spirits of the forest by having an elf tiptoe past the flower. Mörike's poetry is rich in undercurrents because for him, many things could be simultaneously present.

Part 2 is a classic example of Mörike's inclusive vision, a fanciful superimposition of summer on winter. Commenting that a summer butterfly can never feed on the nectar of a Christmas rose that blooms in winter, Mörike then wonders if the butterfly's fragile ghost, drawn by the faint fragrance, may not still be present and hovering around its petals, although invisible to him.

"A Visit to the Charterhouse"

"A Visit to the Charterhouse (epistle to Paul Heyse—1862)," a long idyll in iambic hexameter, was one of Mörike's last poems and was recognized early on as one of his best. It refers to the Carthusian charterhouse or monastery between St. Gallen and Constance that Mörike visited in 1840.

In the poem, the speaker makes a return visit to the charterhouse after fourteen years and finds that the last monks have dispersed and the monastery building is now a brewery. The traveler falls into a reverie about the hospitable prior he met on his previous visit, and by virtue of his vivid description, the prior is present again, in the same way that the butterfly hovers around the Christmas rose.

An object then links the past with the present more tangibly. The traveler recognizes the prior's clock on the mantelpiece, a pewter clock engraved with the Latin memento mori: *Una ex illis ultima* (one of these hours will be your last). The realization that death will put an end to life is one of Mörike's main themes, as in "O Soul, Remember" and "Erinna to Sappho."

In "A Visit to the Charterhouse," thoughts of death are pleasantly interrupted. The local physician entertains the traveler with the story of the clock. The prior bequeathed it to the father steward, and when the father suffered a slight stroke, the clock disappeared. Years later, the brewer's wife found the clock wrapped up behind the chimney stack, with a label bequeathing it to the brewmaster. The poem is a tribute to companionship and conversation, the best means on earth to banish mortal fears.

OTHER MAJOR WORKS

LONG FICTION: *Maler Nolten*, 1832 (*Nolten the Painter: A Novella in Two Parts*, 2005); *Das Stuttgarter Hutzelmännlein*, 1853; *Mozart auf der Reise nach Prag*, 1855 (*Mozart's Journey from Vienna to Prague: A Romance of His Private Life*, 1897); *Die Historie von der Schöen Lau*, 1873 (illustrations by Moritz von Schwind).

TRANSLATION: *Theokritos, Bion und Moschos. Deutsch im Versmasse der Urschrift*, 1855 (with Friedrich Notter).

EDITED TEXTS: *Jahrbuch Schwäbischer Dichter und Novellisten*, 1836 (with Wilhelm Zimmermann); *Classische Blumenlese: Eine Auswahl von Hymnen, Oden, Liedern, Elegien, Idyllen, Gnomen und Epigrammen der Griechen und Römer*, 1840; *Gedichte von Wilhelm Waiblinger*, 1844; *Anakreon und die sogenannten Anakreontischen Lieder: Revision und Erzänzung der J. Fr. Dege'schen Übersetzung mit Erklärungen von E. Mörike*, 1864.

MISCELLANEOUS: *Iris. Eine Sammlungerzählender und dramatischer Dichtungen*, 1839; *Vier Erzählungen*, 1856.

BIBLIOGRAPHY

Adams, Jeffrey. "Eduard Mörike." In *Dictionary of Literary Biography. Nineteenth-Century German Writers to 1840*, edited by James Hardin and Siegfried Mews. Vol. 133. Detroit: Gale, 1993. A chronological overview of Mörike's life and works.

_____, ed. *Mörike's Muses. Critical Essays on Eduard Mörike*. Columbia, S.C.: Camden House, 1990. Of the eleven essays in the anthology, only seven provide English translations of the poems discussed. Mark Lehrer's interesting essay compares Mörike's implicit values with those of his contemporary Karl Marx. Contains Stern's translation of "A Visit to the Charterhouse."

Hölderlin, Friedrich, and Eduard Mörike. *Friedrich Hölderlin, Eduard Mörike. Selected Poems*. Translated by Christopher Middleton. Chicago: University of Chicago Press, 1972. Contains translations of thirty-six of Mörike's poems. Middleton has read all of Mörike's letters and has written an informative introduction and detailed notes about the poems. Includes the five "Peregrina" poems.

Mare, Margaret. *Eduard Mörike. The Man and the Poet*. London: Methuen, 1957. An excellent, classic biography with twenty illustrations consisting of art by Mörike and family portraits. Appendix 1 contains English translations of eight major poems.

Mörike, Eduard. *Mozart's Journey to Prague and a Selection of Poems*. Translated by David Luke. London: Penguin Classics, 2003. Contains translations of forty-three of Mörike's poems, a useful introduction, and notes on the poems.

_____. *Poems by Eduard Mörike*. Translated by Norah K. Cruickshank and Gilbert F. Cunningham. With an introduction by Jethro Bithell. London: Methuen, 1959. Translation includes a useful introduction and brief information about each of the forty translated poems. Includes "On a Christmas Rose."

Oxford German Studies 36, no. 1 (2007). This special issue on Mörike contains two excellent articles on his poetry. "Mörike and the Higher Criticism," by Ritchie Robertson, focuses on Mörike's combination of Christian and pagan elements in the poem "To a Christmas Rose." "Idyll and Elegy: Mörike's 'Besuch in der Carthause,'" by Ray Ockenden, draws on Mörike's knowledge of classical verse forms to lend deeper understanding to this previously neglected late poem.

Slessarev, Helga. *Eduard Mörike*. New York: Twayne, 1970. The long, well-organized chapter on Mörike's poetry places it in the context of his classical education and the events of his life.

Jean M. Snook

Alfred de Musset

Born: Paris, France; December 11, 1810
Died: Paris, France; May 2, 1857

Principal poetry

Contes d'Espagne et d'Italie, 1829 (*Tales of Spain and Italy*, 1905)
Rolla, 1833 (English translation, 1905)
Un Spectacle dans un fauteuil, 1833 (first series, 2 volumes; *A Performance in an Armchair*, 1905)
Poésies complètes, 1840 (*Complete Poetry*, 1905)
Poésies nouvelles, 1840; definitive edition, 1852 (*New Poetic Works*; definitive edition in *The Complete Writings*)
Premières Poésies, 1840; definitive edition, 1852 (*First Poetic Works*; definitive edition in *The Complete Writings*)

Other literary forms

The prose *contes* and *nouvelles* of Alfred de Musset (myoo-SEH) have sustained an appreciative audience, but it is his lyric verse and, above all, his dramas that truly endure. As Phillipe Van Tieghem has observed, Musset's theater is an admirable synthesis of the neoclassical tastes of seventeenth as well as eighteenth century theater with the passion and variety of Romantic trends. This synthesis also characterizes the best of Musset's verse.

Achievements

Henry James called Alfred de Musset "one of the first poets" of his day, a judgment that many modern critics would dispute. Although neither innovative nor influential, Musset's verse achieves a distinctive personal voice. Musset has been described as the supreme poet of love. Certainly, a handful of Musset's poems, both in the original French and in translation, maintain their vitality.

Biography

Born in Paris on December 11, 1810, Louis Charles Alfred de Musset lived the role of the Romantic artist with a self-destructive passion. His family traced itself

back to the twelfth century, numbering among its ancestors the great Renaissance poet Joachim du Bellay. Musset spent his childhood in an atmosphere of belleslettres. His father not only was responsible for an edition of the works of Jean-Jacques Rousseau but also wrote a critical and biographical study of Rousseau. Musset's mother held a salon attended by some of the noted literary figures of the day, and it was in this milieu that Musset took his first, faltering steps in verse.

Two important notes in the ground bass of Musset's life were sounded in the poet's youth—his emotional hypersensitivity and his dependency on his brother Paul. The latter, in his biography of Musset, has recorded an anecdote demonstrating both characteristics. A gun that Musset was handling accidentally fired a shot that narrowly missed Paul; perhaps as a result, Musset was stricken with a high fever. Indeed, "brain fever," as it was known in the nineteenth century, plagued the poet throughout his life.

Musset achieved literary celebrity with his first volume of verse, *Tales of Spain and Italy*. In the following decade, he produced a great number of plays, a fair

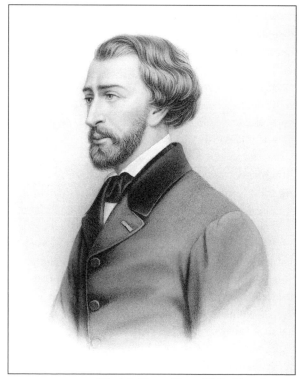

Alfred de Musset (Roger Viollet/Getty Images)

body of poetry, and a variety of work in other forms as well. In 1833, he began a stormy liaison with the novelist George Sand (who was then thirty years old to Musset's twenty-three). Both Musset and Sand wrote novels based on the affair: Musset's *La Confession d'un enfant du siècle* (1836; *The Confession of a Child of the Century*, 1892) and Sand's *Elle et lui* (1859; *She and He*, 1902); the latter prompted a rebuttal from Paul de Musset, the novel *Lui et elle* (1859; he and she). Alfred de Musset's liaison with Sand was only the most notorious of a number of love affairs in which he was involved. Among them, one of the most important was his relationship with the great tragic actress Rachel (Elisa Felix), who nourished his love for the neoclassical masterpieces of French, particularly the works of Jean Racine.

Musset's production dropped sharply in the 1840's and the 1850's, though he enjoyed several theatrical successes and was elected to the French Academy. The last years of his life were marred by alcoholism. Musset died in Paris on May 2, 1857.

ANALYSIS

Alfred de Musset's passion for neoclassical literature and femmes fatales offers a useful guide to his lyric poetry; in addition, to anyone with an essentially Anglo-American background in literature, the career of Lord Byron might offer a passport into that of Musset. Indeed, the neoclassical strain in the works of Musset is very like that in Byron. Both made solid contributions to a Romantic trend that they despised. In their best work, they looked to Greco-Roman classicism and French neoclassicism for their models. Musset's aesthetic, like Byron's, was neither Romantic nor neoclassical; rather, elements of the two were counterpoised in a balanced tension. Musset also resembles Byron in his posing and attitudinizing before what he regarded as the "infernal feminine." Both men took personal delight and gained poetic capital from the pains they suffered at the hands of a rather impressive number of women. Although both poets were masters of satire, neither indulged in didacticism—political or religious.

Although Musset later denied any direct influence from Byron, his first two collections of poetry are filled

with Byronic elements. *Tales of Spain and Italy* and *A Performance in an Armchair*, after their initial publication, were later authoritatively compiled in *First Poetic Works*. Beyond their biographical importance as juvenilia, these poems are of only slight significance.

In comparison to that of Lord Byron, the output of Musset was quite small; moreover, his most ambitious poems, such as *Rolla*, have fallen by the wayside. Musset the poet worked best in miniature, when he could keep his Romantic and his neoclassical impulses in perfect balance.

"MAY NIGHT"

Musset's growing mastery of poetic form became evident in "La Nuit de mai" (1835; "May Night"), composed in the year of his final separation from Sand, the year in which he came under the more benevolent influence of a Madame Jaubert. In this work, Musset's persona, the poet, has suffered from a love affair—presumably based on that of Musset and Sand. "May Night," which found its definitive place in the collection *New Poetic Works*, is the most frequently anthologized representative of Musset's less restrained Romantic side. Even this undeniably passionate work, however, is not without a certain restraint. The dialogue form permits the poet to maintain a certain distance from the personal subject matter, although such control is not sustained throughout the poem. Musset's failure to maintain aesthetic control of his material is reflected in the form of the verse: As the poem progresses, the caesura is often lost, and lines alternate randomly between ten and twelve syllables.

When the Muse first speaks to the poet, he cannot hear her; he can only sense her by hazy and indirect manifestations, which anticipate the mysterious auras pervading the Symbolist dramas of Maurice Maeterlinck. In his second speech, the poet bursts into a series of questions, seeking to unveil the secret behind the uncanny phenomena that surround him. Only in her third speech is the Muse able to penetrate the poet's torpid senses, reminding him of a bitter experience. The poet has only recently had his first sorrowful encounter with a woman; in the words of the Muse, "still a youth, you were dying of love." This youthful passion and sorrow, acted on by the same Spring that is transforming the landscape, forms the substance of which the poet's divine ecstasy is made: "the wine of youth ferments tonight in the veins of God."

In the Muse's fourth speech, Musset adopts the rhetorical flamboyance that the critic Henri Peyre has identified as characteristic of French Romanticism. Many of the lines, sometimes for five lines running, begin with a first-person-plural verb formulation (such as *chanterons-nous*). The rich images range from legendary Greece to Rome, from medieval to modern France. One important image in this veritable barrage is that of a hunter in the Middle Ages, who, after killing a deer, cuts out its still-beating heart and throws it to the dogs. The image, emblematic of the poet's act of self-immolation, prepares the way for the culminating symbol of self-immolation in the Muse's fifth speech.

The Muse, in this her final address, continues what has been fully established as the central theme of "May Night": that poetry grows from its creator's active confrontation of his human hurts. As the Muse says, "Nothing makes us so great as a great sorrow." Although in his final speech, which closes the poem, the poet rejects the Muse's advice and dismisses any poetry he might create as mere writing "on the sand," the existence of the poem itself demonstrates that Musset, as opposed to his persona, felt otherwise and followed the bidding of the Muse. Musset's creativity was encouraged, not thwarted, by his encounters with women.

"A Wasted Evening"

Equal to the influence exercised by Sand and Madame Jaubert on Musset's lyric creativity was that of the celebrated actress Rachel. "Une Soirée perdue" ("A Wasted Evening") is a meditation centering on a performance of Molière's *Le Misanthrope* (pr. 1666; *The Misanthrope*, 1709), referred to in the poem by the name of its protagonist, Alceste, at the Théâtre-Français, better known now as the Comédie-Française. Musset clearly had been aggravated by the poor attendance at the performance.

"A Wasted Evening" is a pastiche—but in the best sense of the word—of Molière's Alexandrines. In the main, the poem might be termed a critical dialogue between a persona who represents the popular taste of the day and another representing Musset's own views. The first ten lines of the poem are given to the representative

of the crowd, who observes that the play, after all, "was only Molière." This great playwright, judged by the melodramatic standards of the well-made play of the mid-nineteenth century, is a "great bungler" who seems unable "to serve a concluding scene cooked to perfection." Here, Musset's irony is a bit heavy-handed; the poet has changed his usual rapier for a broadsword.

In the eleventh line, the poet offers his rebuttal: "I, however, listened to this simple harmony/ And hear how common sense can make genius speak." In these lines, the neoclassical concepts of "simple harmony" and "common sense" have been joined with the Romantic notion of "genius." As if reverting to the fashionable view, the second speaker asks rhetorically if mere admiration for this play suffices. His reply is clearly in the Romantic camp, if on his own terms: He says that it is enough to attend this performance "in order to hear in the depths of the soul a cry of nature." He catches sight of a young woman whose intense absorption in the performance is clear proof of the play's entrancing qualities. He describes her by way of a synecdoche, speaking of her white neck and black hair, which he then compares with ebony encased in ivory. It is no accident that this image echoes lines of the neoclassical, if transitional, poet, André Chenier.

In the next stanza, Musset's spokesman calls for a return to neoclassical art, with its paradoxical capacity to combine frankness with subtlety. This he sees as the necessary replacement for the "muddy stage" of Victor Hugo and Alexandre Dumas, fils. The next stanza continues in the same vein: The poet calls on the satirical spirit of Molière, "master of us all," appealing for a renewed attack on inferior art and on the society that sponsors it.

In the last stanza, however, the speaker abruptly dismisses his dream of artistic triumph as "a foolish fancy." He then notices the young woman—now veiled—and follows her unconsciously, only to see her "disappear on the threshold of her home." The artistry with which Musset gradually introduces the young woman recalls the subtle clarity that he admires in French neoclassical literature. The woman is a symbol of the concrete beauty that distracts the poet from his public aspirations:

"Alas! my dear friend, that is the story of my life.
While my soul was seeking its will,
my body had its own and followed beauty;
and when I awoke from this reverie,
there only remained for me the sweet image."

"ON A DEAD WOMAN"

"Sur une morte" ("On a Dead Woman"), which deals out its wit with greater subtlety than does "A Wasted Evening," is unique in its combination of a rich lyricism of rhythm and imagery with a spirit of pure invective; only Catullus might offer a parallel. Here, Musset does not denigrate the object of his satirical attack; rather, he makes it clear that she is a formidable woman—clearly worthy of his wrathful energies. Musset makes her strength eminently clear in the opening stanza: She is compared to the impressively muscled virago called *Night* that Michelangelo sculpted on the tomb of Giuliano de' Medici. If the woman in question is beautiful, says the poet, then Michelangelo's *Night* "can be fair."

It is known that the poem was directed at the Princess Christine Trivulce de Begiojoso, whose great crime was to have resisted Musset's advances. In short, she was a strong woman—so strong, in fact, that in 1849, long after the poem had appeared, she wrote, with her pride undamaged, a gracious letter complimenting Musset on one of his plays that had recently been performed.

In the next three stanzas, the poet continues the attack by impugning the princess's salient traits: Her Christian charity and piety are viewed as hypocrisy; her intellectual aspirations, as the pretensions of a bluestocking. These stanzas are impressive, above all, for the concrete precision of their imagery. The princess's act of giving alms is reduced to the mere motion of "the hand casually opening and giving" and to "gold" given "without pity." Similarly, her intelligent conversation is presented as "the empty noise of a sweetly modulated voice," which in turn is compared to a "babbling brook." Most devastating of all, one can only consider her prayers to be such "if two fair eyes, now fixed earthward, now raised heavenward, can be called prayers." Here again, the feeling is inescapable: Such well-loaded siege guns suggest an impressive target.

"On a Dead Woman" crystallizes all the characteristic qualities of Musset's poetry. Typically, the poem was inspired by an encounter with a woman. Although motivated by a powerful emotion (here, anger), the poem is marked by a restraint that recalls the icy control of the neoclassicists.

OTHER MAJOR WORKS

LONG FICTION: *Gamiani, ou deux nuits d'excès*, 1835 (*Gamiani: Or, Two Passionate Nights*, 1908); *La Confession d'un enfant du siècle*, 1836 (*The Confession of a Child of the Century*, 1892).

SHORT FICTION: *Les Deux Maîtresses*, 1837 (*Two Mistresses*, 1905); *Emmeline*, 1837 (English translation, 1905); *Le Fils du Titien*, 1838 (*Titian's Son*, 1892); *Frédéric et Bernerette*, 1838 (*Frederic and Bernerette*, 1892); *Margot*, 1838 (English translation, 1905); *Histoire d'un merle blanc*, 1842 (*Adventures of a White Blackbird*, 1892); *Pierre et Camille*, 1843 (*Pierre and Camille*, 1905); *Les Frères Van Buck*, 1844; *Le Secret de Javotte*, 1844 (*Secret of Javotte*, 1905); *Mimi Pinson*, 1845; *La Mouche*, 1854 (*The Beauty Spot*, 1892).

PLAYS: *La Nuit vénitienne: Ou, Les Noces de Laurette*, pr. 1830 (*The Venetian Night: Or, Laurette's Wedding*, 1905); *À quoi rêvent les jeunes filles*, pb. 1833 (*Of What Young Maidens Dream*, 1905); *André del Sarto*, pb. 1833 (English translation, 1905); *Les Caprices de Marianne*, pb. 1833 (*The Follies of Marianne*, 1905); *La Coupe et les lèvres*, pb. 1833 (*The Cup and the Lips*, 1905); *Fantasio*, pb. 1834 (English translation, 1853); *Lorenzaccio*, pb. 1834 (English translation, 1905); *On ne badine pas avec l'amour*, pb. 1834 (*No Trifling with Love*, 1890); *Un Spectacle dans un fauteuil*, pb. 1834 (second series, 2 volumes); *Le Chandelier*, pb. 1835 (*The Chandelier*, 1903); *La Quenouille de Barbarine*, pb. 1835, revised wr. 1851, pr. 1882 (*Barbarine*, 1890); *Il ne faut jurer de rien*, pb. 1836; *Un Caprice*, pb. 1837 (*A Caprice*, 1847); *Il faut qu'une porte soit ouverte ou fermée*, pb. 1845 (*A Door Must Be Either Open or Shut*, 1890); *L'Habit vert*, pr., pb. 1849 (with Émile Augier; *The Green Coat*, 1915); *Louison*, pr., pb. 1849 (English translation, 1905); *On ne saurait penser à tout*, pr. 1849 (*One Can Not Think of Everything*, 1905); *Carmosine*, pb. 1850 (English translation, 1865); *Bettine*, pr., pb. 1851 (English translation, 1905); *L'Âne et le ruisseau*, pb. 1860 (wr. 1855; *Donkey and the Stream*, 1905); *Comedies*, pb. 1890; *A Comedy and Two Proverbs*, 1955; *Seven Plays*, 1962.

TRANSLATION: *L'Anglais mangeur d'opium*, 1828 (of Thomas de Quincey's *Confessions of an English Opium Eater*, 1821).

MISCELLANEOUS: *The Complete Writings*, 1905 (10 volumes).

BIBLIOGRAPHY

Bishop, Lloyd. *The Poetry of Alfred de Musset: Styles and Genres*. New York: Peter Lang, 1987. Focuses on Musset's poetry and provides valuable information on his life and literary output. Bibliography and index.

Levin, Susan M. *The Romantic Art of Confession: De Quincey, Musset, Sand, Lamb, Hogg, Frémy, Soulié*. Columbia, S.C.: Camden House, 1998. Levin's work on the confession literature of Romanticists such as Musset, Thomas De Quincey, James Hogg, George Sand, and Charles Lamb sheds light on the life of Musset, as revealed in his semiautobiographical novel. Bibliography and index.

Musset, Alfred de. *Comedies and Proverbs*. Edited by David Sices. Baltimore: The Johns Hopkins University Press, 1994. Although this edition of seven of Musset's comedies focuses on his drama, Sices's commentary provides insight into the poet as well.

Siegel, Patricia Joan. *Alfred de Musset: A Reference Guide*. Boston: G. K. Hall, 1982. A bibliography of studies of Musset.

Wakefield, David. *The French Romantics: Literature and the Visual Arts, 1800-1840*. London: Chaucer Press, 2007. Covers Romanticism in France, with chapters on Musset, Alfred de Vigny, and Victor Hugo.

Rodney Farnsworth

N

GÉRARD DE NERVAL

Born: Paris, France; May 22, 1808
Died: Paris, France; January 26, 1855

PRINCIPAL POETRY

Elégies nationales, 1826
Poésies allemandes, 1830 (translation)
Petits Châteaux de Bohême, 1853 (includes poetry and prose)
Les Chimères, 1854 (English translation, 1965; also known as *Chimeras*, 1966; best known as *The Chimeras*, 1982)
Fortune's Fool: Selected Poems, 1959

OTHER LITERARY FORMS

Gérard de Nerval (nehr-VAHL) tried his hand at drama, short fiction, and nonfiction. He wrote two dramas in collaboration with Alexandre Dumas, *père*. They are *Piquillo* (pb. 1837) and *Alchimiste* (pb. 1839). His other dramas include *Chariot d'enfant* (1850, with Joseph Méry), *L'Imagier de Harlem* (pr. 1851), and a translation of Johann Wolfgang von Goethe's *Faust: Eine Tragödie* (pb. 1808; *The Tragedy of Faust*, 1823) and *Faust: Eine Tragödie, zweiter Teil* (pb. 1833; *The Tragedy of Faust, Part Two*, 1838) in 1827 and 1840. Among his nonfiction prose works are *Voyage en Orient* (1851; *Journey to the Orient*, 1972); *Les Illuminés* (1852), and *Aurélia* (1855; English translation, 1932). A collection of his stories came out as *Les Filles du feu* (1854; *Daughters of Fire*, 1922).

ACHIEVEMENTS

During his lifetime, Gérard de Nerval was generally regarded as an enthusiastic but harmless eccentric, a writer of some genius whose best and freshest productions were marred by occasional lapses into obscurity. Because of his bouts with madness—both manic-depressive psychosis (or, in modern psychological language, cyclothymic depression) and schizophrenia—he struck most of his contemporaries as an oddity, a poet sometimes pathetic yet never dangerous except to his own well-being. Around him numerous legends accumulated, most of them ludicrous. Some of the more absurd stories were given wider circulation by Jules Champfleury in *Grandes Figures d'hier et d'aujourd'hui: Balzac, Gérard de Nerval, Wagner, Courbet* (1861) and by Arsène Houssaye in *Les Confessions: Souvenirs d'un demi-siècle* (1885, 6 vols.). In part as a result of such droll anecdotes, Nerval's reputation during the first half of the nineteenth century was that of a minor figure: a poet with close affinities with German Romanticism, a distinguished translator of Johann Wolfgang von Goethe's *Faust*, a moderately popular playwright and the author of sumptuously exotic travel literature, and a lyricist whose originality and vigor were evident but whose interests were too often attached to the curious and the extravagant. Later during the century, critics compared Nerval with Charles Baudelaire, treating both as psychologists of the aberrant. After the beginning of the twentieth century, commentators judged Nerval favorably in relation to the Symbolists, especially to Stéphane Mallarmé and Arthur Rimbaud. Still later, Nerval was appreciated as a forerunner of Guillaume Apollinaire and modernist experimentation. Since the 1920's, Nerval's achievements have been viewed independently of their connections with other writers or movements. Treated not as a precursor of greater talents but as a towering genius in his own right, Nerval has been examined as a seer, a mystic, a student of Hermetic doctrine and of alchemy, a poet of extraordinary complexit, resonance, and power. His most important works in prose and poetry—*Petits Châteaux de Bohême*, *Aurélia*, and *Daughters of Fire*—are among the glories of French literature.

BIOGRAPHY

Gérard de Nerval was born Gérard Labrunie, the son of Étienne Labrunie, a medical doctor, and of Marie-Antoinette Marguerite Laurent, daughter of a Paris draper. Nerval did not change his name until 1831, when he signed a letter "G. la Brunie de Nerval," taking the name from a property, Le Clos de Nerval, belonging to his mother's family. The name is also an

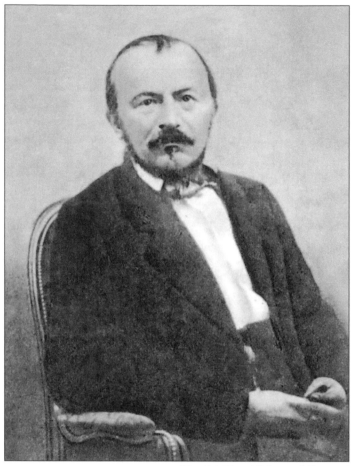

Gérard de Nerval (Library of Congress)

In November, 1827, Nerval published his translation of Goethe's *The Tragedy of Faust*, but under the publication date of 1828. This work was well received in Parisian literary circles, and Nerval became a disciple of Victor Hugo and joined his *cénacle romantique*. In the notorious dispute that followed the disruptive theatrical opening (February 25, 1830) of Hugo's play *Hernani* (pr., pb. 1830; English translation, 1830) however, Nerval sided with Gautier, and thereafter Nerval frequented Gautier's *petit cénacle*.

An inheritance from his maternal grandfather in 1834 allowed Nerval to give up his medical studies and pursue a literary career, much to his father's disapproval. In the fall of that year, Nerval visited Italy (Florence, Rome, and Naples), a trip that later proved invaluable to his writing. Upon his return to Paris in 1834, he met and fell in love with the actress Jenny Colon. In May of 1834, he founded the theatrical review *Le Monde dramatique*, dedicated to the glorification of Colon. For a brief time, Nerval enjoyed a life of prosperity, identifying himself with the "Bohème galante." When the review failed in 1836, however, financial difficulties forced Nerval to become a journalist, writing articles for *Le Figaro* and *La Presse*. He visited Belgium with Gautier in 1836 in an effort to forget his personal struggles for a time.

On October 31, 1837, Nerval's play *Piquillo* premiered in Paris with Colon in the lead role as Silvia. The play was a success, and Nerval was encouraged to declare his love for her. On April 11, 1838, however, Colon married the flutist Louis-Gabriel Leplus, an event that left the poet bitterly disillusioned. During the summer of that year, he traveled to Germany with Dumas, *père*, and from that time the two writers began a series of theatrical collaborations.

The next two years were ones of increasing mental instability and depression for Nerval. Though he published his translation of *The Tragedy of Faust, Part Two* in 1840, the strain of the work took its toll, and

anagram of his mother's maiden name, Laurent. It is known that Nerval hated his father, who served with Napoleon's Grande Armée as a field surgeon and who was, throughout the poet's life, an aloof, insensitive parent. Nerval's mother died when the boy was only two years old, and Nerval was sent to live with his great-uncle, Antoine Boucher, at Mortefontaine. Nerval later described these early years as the happiest of his life. He had free range of a library of occult books and discussed philosophy with his great-uncle, who may have served as a model for Père Dodu in Nerval's short story "Sylvie" (1853; English translation, 1922). When Nerval's father returned from the front in 1814, the boy joined him in Paris. In 1820, Nerval entered the Collège Charlemagne, where he began to exhibit a fondness for literary pursuits and began his lifelong friendship with the poet Théophile Gautier.

Nerval was hospitalized as a result of a nervous breakdown. The death of Colon in 1842 did nothing to restore his ailing spirits. In ill health and overcome with grief, he embarked in 1843 on a trip to Malta, Egypt, Syria, Cyprus, Constantinople, and Naples. He later published an account of his travels in *Journey to the Orient*. Nerval had discovered his psychological need to wander, a theme found in his major works.

Though his mental and physical health continued to deteriorate, Nerval struggled to support himself with his writing. Still hoping to establish himself in the theater, he wrote *Chariot d'enfant* with Méry, a production which premiered on May 13, 1850. In September, 1851, Nerval suffered an accident, followed by a serious nervous breakdown. Nerval believed that he would soon become incurably insane, a realization which made him increase his literary efforts. In 1852, he published *Les Illuminés*, a series of biographies on historical figures interested in mysteries of the occult and of alchemy. In 1853, he published a volume of nostalgic poems recalling a happier youth, *Petits Châteaux de Bohême*. In the summer of that year, Nerval published his best-known story, "Sylvie," followed by two other great works, *Daughters of Fire* and *The Chimeras*, in 1854. *Aurélia*, an account of his madness, appeared in 1855. Alone and destitute, Nerval hanged himself in an alley on January 26, 1855.

ANALYSIS

Gautier, who perhaps appreciated the fine qualities of Gérard de Nerval's character and art more than any other contemporary, once described his friend as an "apodal swallow." To Gautier, Nerval was

> all wings and no feet: At most he had perceptible claws; these enabled him to alight, at least momentarily, just long enough to catch his breath, then go on . . . to soar and move about in fluid realms with the joy and abandon of a being in his element.

Gautier's idealization of Nerval as an ethereal figure— a Percy Bysshe Shelley-like bird in flight who abjured the common terrestrial condition of humanity—is a valid judgment only to a limited degree. To be sure, a reader may approach Nerval on a superficial level as a poet of intense, vivid, direct intuition; a poet of

dreams and visions; a creator of myths and fantastic personal symbolic constructs that reach into the archetypal imagination.

Certainly, most of Nerval's poetry, much of his prose poetry, and a portion of his dramatic work can be appreciated according to the qualities of Impressionism. His work has, on a simple level of perception, an evocative, dreamy, otherworldly, melancholy vein that resembles the Impressionism of otherwise dissimilar poets such as Edgar Allan Poe and Paul Verlaine. One can enjoy the seemingly imprecise but hauntingly evocative imagery of a familiar Nerval poem such as "Le Point noir" ("The Dark Smudge") as though the writer were merely inducing an impression of malign fate. Reading Nerval for his surface characteristics of hauntingly sonorous music, vague but unsettling imagery, and technically perfect mastery of verse forms, one can accept Gautier's early evaluation of the poet as a kind of birdlike spirit—or, to use Baudelaire's image of a poet idealized as an albatross ("L'Albatros"), a creature free in the air but confined and crippled on the crass Earth.

Moreover, a reader who approaches Nerval's basic themes without first investigating their intellectual context is likely to appreciate their surface qualities of authentic feeling and simplicity of expression. Nerval is always concerned with human values, no matter that he may choose exotic subjects or complex methods to express them. His work is nearly always confessional. Although he rarely tends to be self-dramatizing in his poetry, he often places his persona—his other self—at the center of the theme in order to examine the psychological insights of a human life. An early verse, "Épître première" (first epistle), at once expresses his artistic philosophy and predicts his fate; he will, despite madness under the aegis of the moon, serve humanity with a generous desire. In his poems as well as in much of his prose and drama, Nerval appeals directly—without a reader's need for critical exegesis—to the human heart: to its courage, its idealism, its love. Although Nerval's subjects often appear to be odd, exotic, or perverse, the poet treats the flowers of his imagination not as "evil," as does the great poet of the next generation, Baudelaire, but as fragrant symbols of a mysterious, arcane harmony in the universe.

Indeed, Nerval is best appreciated as a mystic and a seer, a poet whose surface qualities of vague dreaminess conceal an interior precision of image and ideas. Reading a popularly anthologized lyric such as "Fantaisie" ("Fantasy"), for example, one tends to dismiss the poem as a piece influenced by German Romanticism, especially by the *Märchen*-like songs of Heinrich Heine or Goethe. A closer reading, however, will show that the seemingly vague images are not merely decorative; they are rendered with precision, although their precise significance as personal symbol is not clear. Nevertheless, the "green slope gilded by the setting sun" and the stone castle are objects, not atmosphere, and the mysterious theme of déjà vu is intended to be psychological truth, not fairy tale.

GERMAN ROMANTICISM

To appreciate Nerval fully, one should understand the poet's relationship to German Romanticism without treating him exclusively as a Romantic—or, indeed, exclusively as a pre-Impressionist, pre-Symbolist, or pre-modernist. Although his affinities to poets such as Heine and Goethe (Romantics), Poe and Verlaine (Impressionists), and Mallarmé and Rimbaud (Symbolists) are obvious—as are his temperamental affinities to Baudelaire—Nerval is best compared to two poets whose productions are similarly visionary and, in some respects, arcane: William Blake and William Butler Yeats. Like Blake, Nerval was a seer who searched into the heart of mysteries to discover the correspondence of opposites; a follower of the eighteenth century mystic Emanuel Swedenborg; and an originator of complex myths and symbolic systems. Like Yeats, Nerval was a student of theosophy and an adept of the religions of the East. He believed in magic and the occult, communicated with revealers of the spirit world, and—using the phases of the moon and similar cosmic symbols—created a complex system of psychological and historical types of personalities.

ARCHETYPAL IMAGERY

In addition, Nerval cultivated dream visions, experimented with drugs such as hashish, and was a student of the Kabbalah, alchemy, ancient mystery religions, Illuminism, Orphism, Sabbean astral worship, and the secrets of the Egyptian pyramids. If his abstruse researches were merely incidental to his work, much of

his thinking might be safely ignored as burdensome, esoteric, or irrelevant. Nerval, however, uses a great deal of his learning in his prose and poetry. An extremely careful writer, he placed layer upon layer of meaning, often mixing different systems that are not related historically into a single new system, within the texture of his poetic prose and his poetry. To ignore these layers of meaning is to neglect as well a great deal of Nerval's subtlety as an artist.

In *Aurélia*, for example, he used archetypal images that appear to emanate from the collective unconscious—among them the image of the *magna mater* (great mother). Included are manifestations of woman as loving, gentle, compassionate, noble-hearted; as vain, dissembling, inconstant; or as the dangerous fury who terrorizes a dreamer; or finally, as the temptress, the coquette. Also he includes, in various manifestations, the father archetype. In *Journey to the Orient*, the poet transmutes the legend of Solomon and Sheba from a biblical tale into a personal vision centering on the character of Adoniram, a "double" for the artist, the creator. In this book, Nerval exposes themes involving the story of Cain as well as the secrets of Hermetic lore and of the pyramids (Nerval actually visited the site of the Great Pyramid of Khufu, or Cheops, and descended into its depths).

SYMBOLISM AND HERMETICISM

Nerval's poetry is less obviously arcane than much of his symbolic prose; nevertheless, a careful student should understand that the poet uses language in a very special way. His constant endeavor was to express through symbolic language a unity that he perceived in the spiritual and the material elements of the universe. To grasp this language, a reader needs to know several concepts basic to Swedenborgian correspondence and Hermetic alchemy.

Nerval's research into these abstruse subjects began early in his life, notably from his interest in a tradition of thought known as Illuminism. This tradition affected writers from the middle of the eighteenth century until the end of the nineteenth century. Illuminists were fascinated with ancient Oriental manuscripts and with the tenets of Middle Eastern thinkers. Among the manuscripts that they studied were the *Corpus Hermeticum*, a collection of forty-two books attributed to Hermes

Trismegistus, perhaps the most important source of alchemical knowledge of the period. To these books were added the works of Paracelsus and his disciples.

These doctrines were cultivated by members of various secret societies (Rosicrucians, Freemasons, Martinists) which flourished at the end of the eighteenth century, particularly in France and in Germany. By means of such secret societies, Nerval came to acquire knowledge and appreciation of alchemy, while his visionary application of alchemical principles can be traced to the works of Swedenborg. In his study of the *Corpus Hermeticum* and of the Kabbala, Swedenborg had reached two conclusions that were to have a tremendous influence upon the literary world of the nineteenth century. The first of these conclusions was his idea of correspondence, the notion that every visible phenomenon has a direct opposite—upon which it depends—in the invisible and spiritual world. The second conclusion was his conception of a universal language in which these correspondences can best be expressed.

THE CHIMERAS

Nerval's poetry reveals his obsession with creating a new language, one that will allow for a communication between the visible and the invisible, the sensible and the spiritual. Such a language would permit a correspondence between the two orders. A corollary of this belief is the principle of the identity of contraries or opposites. Thus, in *The Chimeras*, Nerval establishes a syncretism of religious beliefs based upon compatibilities. His object is to demonstrate the oneness of religious thought; to achieve this high purpose, he selects a special language, using the metaphors of alchemy principally but not exclusively, as a vehicle to redeem humanity.

A reader may wonder whether a poet so learned as Nerval actually believed in the esoteric doctrines of alchemy. Certainly he used these doctrines, extracting from their classical and medieval origins a philosophical rather than pseudoscientific content, in order to construct his metaphors. In this sense, Nerval believed in alchemy as Blake believed in his visions and as Yeats believed in the symbolic constructs of his spiritual communicators. Nerval's poetry incorporates four basic alchemical principles: first, the theory of correspon-

dence; second, the act of imagining, which can bring about corporeal transformations; third, meditation, or an inner dialogue with the invisible, which requires a "new language"; and finally, the identity of opposites, whereby every image elicits by definition its contrary. In this complex scheme, Mercury (quicksilver) becomes the symbol of alchemy: liquid metal, or the embodiment of a contradiction.

To appreciate how deeply interfused with the surface dreaminess of Nerval's verse are his symbolic constructs of alchemy, one can examine the cycle of twelve sonnets titled *The Chimeras*. The number twelve is crucial in the alchemical system, since it represents the *coniunctio tetraptiva*, or the dilemma of three and four—the chimera being the archetype of the triad. It should also be noted that the structure of the sonnet itself is representative of the problem of three and four, but in reverse. If the chimera represents the triad in the *coniunctio tetraptiva*, the four symbolizes the union of persons, and this is the underlying matrix of *The Chimeras*. By a process known as *henosis*, a tetrasomia or synthesis of opposites is produced to create a unity.

"EL DESDICHADO"

The first sonnet of *The Chimeras* is probably Nerval's best-known poem, "El desdichado" (the title, meaning "the unhappy one," was borrowed from Sir Walter Scott's *Ivanhoe*, 1819). It focuses upon the descent into the abyss, the *nigredo* of the alchemist, or the opening stage of the process. The images used to describe this phase are all somber: images of death and of caves, and even of Hell (the Achéron and the evocation of Orpheus). More important, however, is Nerval's linking of these dark, demoniac images with traditionally positive images—the union of contraries being the functional principle in such expressions as *soleil noir* ("black sun"). The most powerful character in the poem, one who is there by implication and not by name, is Melusina, the absent-but-present feminine principle. Melusina also embodies the identity of contraries, possessing either the tail of a fish or that of a snake; sometimes she appears only as a snake. Her ability to metamorphose as well as to heal diseases and injuries makes her—in the mind of the alchemist and of the poet-seer—the feminine counterpart to Mercury. Thus, in "El desdichado," Nerval posits a synthesis of the medieval duality with the Greco-Roman duality, Hermes-Mercury.

"MYRTHO"

In the succeeding sonnet, "Myrtho," Nerval assesses the descent into the abyss. It is in this manner that one can achieve the light. Moreover, it is here that the black is an essential component of the gold: "Aux raisins noirs mêlés avec l'or de ta tresse" ("and black grapes mingled in your golden tresses"). In this descent into the interior world of the light, the poet-seer necessarily meets the sovereign of the underworld, Bacchus-Dionysus-Osiris. The final two lines announce the reconciliation of certain poetic visions: that of Vergil's neopaganism with the Illuminism of the eighteenth century. Like "El desdichado," then, "Myrtho" presents a unification of various systems of thought.

"HORUS"

The sonnet "Horus" concerns the Egyptian deity considered by the syncretists to be a prefiguration of Christ. Horus also symbolizes Hellenistic mysticism, providing a direct link with Hermes and, by association, with Hermes Trismegistus, the alchemist. Isis, Horus's mother, the symbol of nature's mysteries, is identified with Venus in the same manner that Hermes is linked with Osiris, leading to a form of Greco-Egyptian religious syncretism. In this system is to be found the "esprit nouveau," the result of which is a rainbow or the vision of colors, a necessary stage which precedes the appearance of gold in alchemy.

"ANTÉROS"

"Antéros" presents a vision of Hell, with Semitic overtones. To be of the race of Antéros (Antaeus) means to gather strength from the earth from which one has sprouted. This agrarian subtext is consistent with references to Cain, the keeper of the fields, and to Dagon, the Philistine agrarian god. The Satanic aspect is sustained in the mark of Cain and in the thrice-dipping into the Cocyte, one of the rivers of Tartarus. The sonnet projects the archetypal struggle of the vanquished giant who refuses defeat—here represented by the Amalekites, a nomadic tribe which was virtually exterminated by the Israelites during the time of David. These pagans are associated with the race of Satan and Cain. "Antéros" ends with a metaphor of rebirth, that of sowing the dragon's teeth in order to create a new race of gi-

ants. In alchemical terms, the sowing of the divine seed (*germinis divi*) provides the continuity necessary for the continual process of transformation which involves death and rebirth, descent and resurrection. The baptism of Hell is the equivalent of the baptism at the holy font.

"DELFICA"

In "Delfica," Nerval includes the trees most often discussed by alchemists as symbols for the human body. Daphne, who was transformed into a tree, is the personification par excellence of the desired synthesis of humanity and nature. The lemons which carry the imprint of her teeth are the natural equivalents in tree code to the metallic gold. Just as the *lapis philosophorum* (the philosopher's stone) holds the key to the mysteries at its center, so too the grotto holds the dragon, sign of the danger of the penetration into the mysteries and also carrier of the all-important seed, or seminal material, which now lies dormant. Ancient beliefs, Nerval suggests, have been overcome by Christianity, yet like the anima of Daphne in the tree, they remain essentially intact, awaiting a revival.

"ARTÉMIS"

"Artémis" begins with an invocation to the mysteries: the number thirteen, an indivisible number, joining the basis of oneness and of the Trinity (which is always One). Thirteen is also the symbol of death in the Tarot (Arcane XIII). The sonnet centers upon the alchemical mystique of the rose; Nerval follows the tradition whereby the rose symbolizes the relationship between king and queen. More important, the rose provides the essential alchemical link with Christ. As such, the rose must be blood-colored in order to be identified with the Redeemer and the Cross. The final line indicates that the descent into the abyss is a necessary step in the making of a saint.

In alchemical writings, the philosopher's stone represents the *homo totus*, which will shed a bloody sweat. In this way, the stone prefigures the agony of Christ. Indeed, the Evangelist Luke says of Christ: "and His sweat was as it were great drops falling down to the ground" (Luke 22:44). It should therefore come as no surprise that Nerval would follow "Artémis" with five sonnets dealing with Christ in the Garden of Gethsemene. In his final hours of agony, Nerval's Christ is truly human, doubting the existence of a supreme power. In the fifth sonnet of the series, he recalls the necessity of descent in order to ascend, the necessity of death in order to give life. Christ's death gives life to a new belief which spells death to the old gods, yet Nerval poses an interesting question: "Quel est ce nouveau dieu qu'on impose à la terre?" ("who is this new god who is being imposed on Earth?"). The answer is reserved for the Almighty, who blessed the children of Adam ("les enfants du limon"). As already noted, the lemon is symbolic of the alchemical gold—that is, the quest for perfection and transcendence that Christ represents.

"VERS DORÉS"

In "Vers doré" ("Golden Verses"), Nerval not only states his theory of correspondences but also offers his most compact statement concerning the role of alchemy in poetry. A new language is to be found—"À la matière même un verbe est attaché" ("even with matter there's a built-in word")—and a Divine Spirit is present in the darkness, waiting to shed his light. The last two lines describe the poet-seer as having opened his third eye; thus, he is able to strip away the layers of stone (the *lapis*) and finally attain the "gold" of the alchemist. Nerval's *The Chimeras*, therefore, achieves a synthesis of various manifestations of contrary elements, each time through the use of personification. "Vers dorés" symbolizes the achievement of the *coniunctio*, the realization of a new form of poetic inspiration and performance.

OTHER MAJOR WORKS

SHORT FICTION: *Les Illuminés*, 1852; "Sylvie," 1853 (English translation, 1922); *Les Filles du feu*, 1854 (*Daughters of Fire*, 1922).

PLAYS: *Faust*, pb. 1827, 1840 (translation of Johann Wolfgang von Goethe's play); *Piquillo*, pb. 1837 (with Alexandre Dumas, *père*); *Alchimiste*, pb. 1839 (with Dumas, *père*); *Léo Burckart*, pr., pb. 1839 (with Dumas, *père*); *Chariot d'enfant*, pb. 1850 (with Joseph Méry); *L'Imagier de Harlem*, pr. 1851.

NONFICTION: *Voyage en Orient*, 1851 (*Journey to the Orient*, 1972); *Promenades et souvenirs*, 1854-1856; *Aurélia*, 1855 (English translation, 1932).

MISCELLANEOUS: *Selected Writings*, 1957 (Geof-frey Wagner, translator); *Selected Writings*, 1999 (Richard Sieburth, translator).

BIBLIOGRAPHY

Behdad, Ali. "Orientalist Desire, Desire of the Orient." *French Forum* 15, no. 1 (January, 1990): 37-51. Useful background on the psychological implications of Nerval's fascination with the East. The story of Adoniram is discussed in relationship to its context in the storytelling tradition of Constantinople. The veiled women of the East symbolize another aspect of the separation between Nerval and the woman who represents his ideal, and the author sees this concealment as increasing desire.

Dubruck, Alfred. *Gérard de Nerval and the German Heritage*. The Hague, the Netherlands: Mouton, 1965. This study of German influences in Nerval's work cites E. T. A. Hoffmann, Johann Wolfgang von Goethe, and Heinrich Heine.

Ender, Evelyne. "A Case of Nostalgia: Gérard de Nerval." In *Architexts of Memory: Literature, Science, and Autobiography*. Ann Arbor: University of Michigan Press, 2005. In this chapter, Ender argues that the main theme in Nerval's writing is nostalgia, and that his writing predominantly involves memory.

Jones, Robert Emmet. *Gérard de Nerval*. New York: Twayne, 1974. This volume situates Nerval within the Romantic movement in France. Discusses his life and his poetry and prose.

Knapp, Bettina L. *Gérard de Nerval: The Mystic's Dilemma*. Tuscaloosa: University of Alabama Press, 1980. Knapp's study is organized as a biography and looks at mysticism in his works.

Lokke, Kari. *Gérard de Nerval: The Poet as Social Visionary*. Lexington, Ky.: French Forum, 1987. This thematic study uses Nerval's works to define the nature of his hallucinations and his concept of "the other."

MacLennan, George. *Lucid Interval: Subjective Writing and Madness in History*. Rutherford, N.J.: Fairleigh Dickinson University Press, 1992. A history of literature and mental illness with particular attention to the work of Nerval. Includes bibliographical references and index.

Rhodes, S. A. *Gérard de Nerval, 1808-1855: Poet, Traveler, Dreamer*. New York: Philosophical Library, 1951. This biography offers useful background on Jenny Colon and how Nerval linked her to the Queen of Sheba.

Rinsler, Norma. *Gérard de Nerval*. London: Athlone Press, 1973. This volume begins with a brief biography and goes on to cover his works.

Strauss, Jonathan. "Death-Based Subjectivity in the Creation of Nerval's Lyric Self." *Espirit Créateur* 35, no. 4 (Winter, 1995): 83-94. Strauss focuses on Nerval's lyric poetry, specifically his most famous sonnet, "El desdichado," in the context of the influence of Georg Wilhelm Friedrich Hegel. This discussion raises issues of the author's alienation from himself that illuminate the use of doubled characters in the short stories.

_____. *Subjects of Terror: Nerval, Hegel, and the Modern Self*. Stanford, Calif.: Stanford University Press, 1998. Despite the mention of Georg Wilhelm Friedrich Hegel in the title, this is a book about Nerval. The first two chapters deal with Hegel and other influences in order to put Nerval's madness in context in chapter 3, ending with an overview of *Daughters of Fire*. Chapter 4 focuses on "Les Faux Saulniers," an extract from "L'Abbé de Bucquoy" from *Les Illuminés*.

Leslie B. Mittleman

NOVALIS
Friedrich von Hardenberg

Born: Oberwiederstedt, Prussian Saxony (now in Germany); May 2, 1772

Died: Weissenfels, Saxony (now in Germany); March 25, 1801

PRINCIPAL POETRY

Hymnen an die Nacht, 1800 (*Hymns to the Night*, 1897, 1948)

Geistliche Lieder, 1802 (*Devotional Songs*, 1910)

OTHER LITERARY FORMS

The poetry alone does not even hint at the full scope of the literary activity of Novalis (noh-VOL-uhs) or his encyclopedic interest in philosophy, science, politics, religion, and aesthetics. While two seminal collections of aphorisms—*Blütenstaub* (pollen) and *Glauben und Liebe* (faith and love)—were published in 1798, the bulk of his work was published posthumously. Among these writings are six neglected dialogues and a monologue from 1798-1799; the essay *Die Christenheit oder Europa* (*Christianity or Europe*, 1844), written in 1799 but first published fully in 1826; and two fragmentary novels, *Die Lehrlinge zu Sais* (1802; *The Disciples at Sais*, 1903) and *Heinrich von Ofterdingen* (1802; *Henry of Ofterdingen*, 1842), begun in 1798 and 1799 respectively. As prototypes of the German Romantic novel, these two works comprise a variety of literary forms: didactic dialogues, poems, and literary fairy tales. Like so much of Novalis's work, these novels were first published by Ludwig Tieck and Friedrich von Schlegel in the 1802 edition of Novalis's writings. Insights into these literary works and into Novalis's poetics are provided by his theoretical notebooks and other papers, which include his philosophical and scientific studies and outlines and drafts of literary projects, as well as his letters, diaries, and professional scientific reports.

ACHIEVEMENTS

Novalis is perhaps best known as the creator of the "blue flower," the often trivialized symbol of Romantic longing, but his importance has a far more substantial basis than this. Within the German tradition, his Romanticism influenced important writers such as Joseph von Eichendorff, E. T. A. Hoffmann, and Hermann Hesse. As an innovative theorist and practitioner of the Romantic novel, Novalis prepared the way not only for the narrative strategies of Franz Kafka's prose but also for the themes and structures of Thomas Mann's major novels. As the poet of *Hymns to the Night* and as a theorist of poetic language, Novalis set the Orphic tone for German Romantic poetry and the aesthetic agenda for German Symbolists such as Rainer Maria Rilke and Stefan George.

Novalis's impact outside Germany is no less consequential. His evocative imagery, the prose poems included in *Hymns to the Night*, and his view of poetic language as musical and autonomous make him a major precursor of the French Symbolist poets. Among them, Maurice Maeterlinck was especially drawn to Novalis's philosophy of nature, and he translated *The Disciples at Sais* in 1895. Later, Novalis's imaginative poetics not only inspired André Breton, one of the founders of French Surrealism, but also had an impact, less widely known, on Chilean Surrealism via the poets Rosamel del Valle and Humberto Díaz Casanueva. In the English-speaking world, Novalis was first praised in 1829 by Thomas Carlyle, whose enthusiasm spread ultimately to writers as diverse as Ralph Waldo Emerson, George Eliot, Edgar Allan Poe, Joseph Conrad, and George MacDonald.

In the poetry anthology *News of the Universe: Poems of Twofold Consciousness* (1980), the American poet Robert Bly justly lauded Novalis as a prime shaper of modern poetic consciousness. Such an evaluation offers hope that Novalis will continue to gain recognition as an internationally important forerunner of both modern poetry and literary theory, especially as more of his literary and theoretical works become accessible in translation.

BIOGRAPHY

Novalis was born Georg Philipp Friedrich von Hardenberg, the first son of Heinrich Ulrich Erasmus von Hardenberg, a strict member of the pietistic *Herrnhut* sect, and Auguste Bernhardine von Bölzig. Throughout his life, Novalis attempted to reconcile the practical demands of his father with the poetic inspiration he claimed first to have received from his mother. Novalis's acquaintance with the popular poet Gottfried August Bürger in 1789 intensified his early literary aspirations, but encouraged by his father to pursue an administrative career, Novalis began the study of law at the University of Jena in 1790. Although his lyric output during his stay in Jena seems to have abated, he soon found his poetic proclivities rekindled and redirected by the poet Friedrich Schiller, who was then a professor of history at the university. Under Schiller's spell, the young Novalis became more introspective

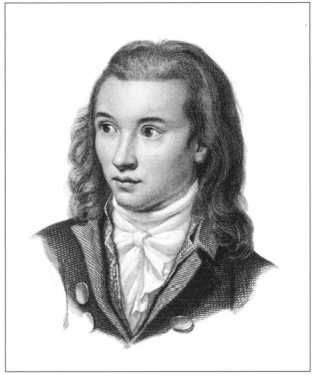

Novalis (Roger Viollet/Getty Images)

and sought a solid foundation for his life and poetry. With this new outlook, he bowed to paternal pressure and transferred to the University of Leipzig in 1791. His experience there once again only strengthened his literary and philosophical interests, however, for it was in Leipzig that he began his friendship and fruitful intellectual exchange with Schlegel, the brilliant theorist of German Romanticism. Only after taking up studies in Wittenberg did he receive his law degree, in 1794.

After several carefree months with his family in Weissenfels, Novalis was apprenticed by his father to Coelestin August Just, the district director of Thuringia, who lived in Tennstedt. It was during his first months there that Hardenberg came to know the twelve-year-old Sophie von Kühn of nearby Grüningen, who revived his active poetic imagination and became a central figure in his new poetic attempts. Within a year, they were engaged, but Sophie's serious illness led to her death in March, 1797. Sophie's death, followed by the loss of his brother Erasmus in April, shattered Novalis, and he turned inward to come to grips with the experience of death. This experience, certainly the most crucial of his life, helped him to articulate his mission to transcend the dual nature of existence through poetry. His confrontation with death did not weaken his will to live or cause him to flee from life, as is sometimes claimed; rather, it was a catalytic event that enabled him to reorient his life and focus his imaginative powers on the fusion of life and poetry.

With a new, clearly poetic mission before him, Novalis could commit himself to life; it was at this time that he assumed the pen name (meaning "preparer of new land") by which he is known. By the end of 1797, he had resumed his intense study of the Idealist philosophers Immanuel Kant and Johann Gottlieb Fichte. Novalis's interest in science grew also, and in December, he commenced studies at the Freiberg Mining Academy, which would later give him a career. In the next year, he not only published the philosophical aphorisms of *Blütenstaub* and *Glauben und Liebe*, but also attempted to articulate his own philosophical ideas in a novel, *The Disciples of Sais*. By December, 1798, his involvement in life embraced the domestic once again, and he became engaged to Julie von Charpentier.

Novalis had finally reconciled his poetic mission with the practical demands of life and career. During 1799, he not only worked on *Devotional Songs* and *Hymns to the Night*, which had grown out of the crisis of 1797, but also accepted an appointment to the directorate of the Saxon salt mines. Both his career and his literary endeavors flourished. In 1800, he worked on *Henry of Ofterdingen*, conducted a significant geological survey of Saxony, published *Hymns to the Night*, and wrote some of his best poems. However, illness had overpowered Novalis's resolve to live and fulfill his poetic mission. On March 25, 1801, Novalis died in the family home in Weissenfels. A few days before his death, he had said to his brother Carl: "When I am well again, then you will finally learn what poetry is. In my head I have magnificent poems and songs." These died with him.

ANALYSIS

The late eighteenth century in Germany was a time of new beginnings. The gradual change from a feudal to a capitalistic society bestowed a new importance on the individual, as reflected in the philosophy of German Idealism, which emphasized the primacy of the subjective imagination. At the same time, however, the weakening of the Holy Roman Empire gave rise to a new sense of German nationalism. German writers responded to these changes by seeking to initiate a new literary tradition, a new beginning that would free them from the tyranny of foreign taste and example. Understandably, in such a dynamic age, no single, unified movement emerged, and the literary pioneers—writers as diverse as Gotthold Ephraim Lessing, Friedrich Klopstock, and Christoph Martin Wieland—set out in many different directions. Nevertheless, by the end of the century, Schlegel would proclaim that he lived "not in hope but in the certainty of a new dawn of a new poetry."

Schlegel's optimism was based on his conviction that his contemporaries were on the verge of creating a new mythology, a new Romantic poetry in which the newly emerging self would examine its own depths and discover universal truths, ultimately achieving a synthesis of subject and object. Like the literature of the eighteenth century, the poetry of Novalis moved toward the realization of this Romantic goal. While he experimented with many styles in his early works, betraying his debt to various currents of the Enlightenment, he soon developed a personal Romantic voice and new mode of expression that marked the advent of a new poetic age. This development became more obvious after Sophie's death in 1797, but it is evident even in the poems of his literary apprenticeship (1788-1793). Indeed, many themes that preoccupied Novalis after the crisis of 1797 had already surfaced in his earliest poetry. The theme of death and the dual images of night and darkness, for example, find their initial expression in early poems, although at this stage his poetry was largely imitative. Only after his encounter with Schiller and his relationship with Sophie, which made him more introspective, did Novalis strike out on his own to record his own experiences and the changes that had taken place within himself. He was then able to create a consistent vision, a vision proclaiming the transforming power of love and raising personal experience to the level of mythology. In transforming his subjective experience into universal symbolism, Novalis created the Romantic mythology that Schlegel had proclaimed the *sine qua non* of the new poetic age. In his last poems, which envision the return to paradise brought on by the union of poetry and love, Novalis transcended his personal experience to create symbolic artifacts behind which the poet himself nearly disappears. In his lyric poetry, then, Novalis ultimately reveals himself not only as a pioneer of Romanticism but also as a precursor of Symbolism.

If Novalis's last poems are thematically consistent and anticipate the Symbolist movement, his early poems are endlessly diversified and echo the Enlightenment. In the poets of the eighteenth century, the young writer, searching for a poetic voice, found his models, limited only by his eclectic taste. Besides translations from classical poetry, Novalis composed serious political verse influenced by the work of Friedrich Stolberg and Karl Ramler, and in the bardic tradition of Klopstock; Rococo lyrics under the particular influence of Wieland; elegiac verse echoing Ludwig Christoph Heinrich Hölty and Schiller; and a spate of lyrics in the style of Bürger. The variety of these early attempts, the assorted literary models that they imitate, and the poems showing a young poet experimenting with traditional forms (such as the invented necrologues addressed to living family members) reveal a writer in quest of a suitable mode of expression.

"To a Falling Leaf"

While they do share some common concerns, many of which inform the later writings, the early poems lack the unified vision and unique perspective that would come later with Novalis's Romantic lyrics. Poems that foreshadow later developments also contrast significantly with the more mature poetry. The first version of the poem "An ein fallendes Blatt" ("To a Falling Leaf"), written in 1789, paints a melancholy scene in which the approach of winter storms is compared to the approach of death. The melancholy tone, however, is purposely undercut by a conclusion that affirms death as a joyous experience of the eternal that need not be feared. This view of death hints, perhaps, at the thanatopsis that Novalis would elaborate in *Hymns to the Night*, but it is merely a hint, for here the idea is actually no more than a common poetic cliché, and the poem as a whole lacks the visionary perspective that underlies the later works. This poem's persona, in fact, is barely

visible at all, and his emotional response to death's coming at the end of the poem is expressed impersonally: "Oh happy . . ./ One need not then fear the storm/ That forbids us our earthly life." The persona and his climactic emotional exclamation vanish behind the anonymous "one," and death—which had been only indirectly introduced through a comparison—loses not only its sting, as the poet intended, but its poetic bite as well.

"Evening"

The poem "Der Abend" ("Evening"), probably written in the same year as "To a Falling Leaf" but in many ways a more suggestive and complex work, not only has a more directly involved and visible persona but also links death and night in anticipation of *Hymns to the Night*. This poem's persona, who stands in a sympathetic relationship to a thoroughly personified nature, perceives and responds to a serene evening by wishing that "the evening of my life" might be "more peaceful still than this/ Evening of the countryside." The lovely yet decidedly rational comparison of the soul to nature is still far removed from the Romantic identification of self and nature that can be found in Novalis's last poems—for example, in "Der Himmel war umzogen" ("The Heavens Were Covered"). Moreover, despite the reflective mood that nature inspires in the persona, this is not an introspective poem like those found among Novalis's first truly Romantic poems. "Evening" does not yet focus primarily on the poetic self but on the eighteenth century ideal of bucolic harmony. Similarly, the persona's final wish, that his "soul might slumber over to eternal peace" in the same way that the weary farmer "slumbers over" toward the next day, only tentatively prefigures the ideas and vocabulary of *Hymns to the Night*. The link between death and sleep remains, after all, an eighteenth century cliché, and its one-dimensional appearance here only lightly foreshadows Novalis's later and much more complex symbol of the eternal and truly visionary "holy sleep."

This poem, like "To a Falling Leaf," is still controlled by a rationalistic poetic consciousness. Simile, not symbol, is the rhetorical means of linking humanity and nature; subject and object are linked, not synthesized. This is the overriding technique of the early poems. The transcendent vision based on deep self-reflection and the unifying power of the imagination is not found here. The poet of "Evening" is one step closer to the Romantic poet of *Hymns to the Night* than the poet of "To a Falling Leaf," but the Romantic poet whose feelings, perceptions, and very self are the basis of Romantic expression steps forward only tentatively. Before he could free himself from his Enlightenment models, focus his vision, and become the very subject of his Romantic art, Novalis would first need to know himself.

"On a Saturday Evening"

The experience of love and death in his relationship with Sophie was the catalyst that would initiate important changes in Novalis's writings, the lens through which he would ultimately bring into sharper focus the themes and images that had been hinted at in the early poems. Initially, however, the experience led to self-examination and the definition of a new, more Romantic voice. Much of the poetry from this period—and there is relatively little—records the changes that the Sophie experience caused in Novalis, and it is, consequently, largely confessional, reflective poetry in which the poet himself becomes the subject.

In the poem "Am Sonnabend Abend" ("On a Saturday Evening"), for example, the persona expresses his astonishment at the transformation that has taken place within himself since his relationship with Sophie: "Am I still the one who yesterday morning/ Sang hymns to the god of frivolity. . . ." This confession suggests not only the changes that had affected a once frivolous university student but also those poetic changes that had occurred in the former poet of lighthearted Anacreontic verse. Earlier, in 1791, Novalis had expressed similar reservations about his lifestyle and youthful verse in "A Youth's Laments," a poem written under the maturing influence of Schiller, but it was only after Novalis had met Sophie that his inner reorientation became complete and the poet could begin anew.

"Beginning"

In the poem "Anfang" ("Beginning"), Novalis analyzes the nature of Sophie's effect on him and argues that his new state of mind is not "intoxication" (that is, illusion) but rather "higher consciousness," which Sophie as a mediator had revealed. This aptly titled poem is in several ways profoundly significant for No-

valis's development as a Romantic poet. In the first place, its conclusion that higher consciousness not be mistaken for intoxication admits a new Romantic form of perception that is aggressively antirationalistic. Second, the characterization of Sophie, the embodiment of love, as a female mediator between visible and invisible worlds, not only marks the first use of this central Romantic image in Novalis's work but also signals the inception of a Romantic theory of Symbolism, which posits the fusion of the finite with the infinite. Finally, the intensely introspective persona, whose theme is his own consciousness ("the growth of a poet's mind," as William Wordsworth put it), places this poem directly into the Romantic tradition.

In "Beginning," Novalis's new vision, based on the higher consciousness inspired by Sophie, assumes a universal import transcending the initially personal experience. This is manifest in the last lines of the poem, where the private experience of the poet is superseded by a vision of humanity raised to a new level of existence:

> Someday mankind will be what Sophie
> Is to me now—perfected—moral grace—
> Then will its *higher consciousness*
> No longer be confused with the mist of wine.

The Stranger

The poems Novalis wrote in 1798 and 1799 in Freiberg after Sophie's death confirm this universalizing tendency. In fact, the relative paucity of poems written in the wake of the experience itself suggests that Novalis was not simply concerned with self-indulgent solipsistic effusions. (The one poem written shortly after Sophie's death in 1797, while Novalis was still in Tennstedt, is a humorous composition commemorating the Just family's purchase of a garden.) Similarly, it has been pointed out that Novalis probably chose the classical verse forms of the Freiberg poems as a more objective medium for his universal themes. One can also point to the objectifying perspective of the several poems that analyze the self from a point of view once removed. In both "Der Fremdling" ("The Stranger"), written in January, 1798, and "Der müde Fremdling ist verschwunden" ("The Weary Stranger Has Disappeared"), a fragment from one year later, Novalis—the stranger—analyzes his initial alienation after Sophie's death and then his self-rediscovery through a persona who "speaks . . . for him." This allows Novalis to remain in the introspective mode, making use of his experience, yet standing at an objective distance. As a consequence, the stranger symbolizes any individual who seeks the return of the paradise he has lost, "that heavenly land."

SELF-KNOWLEDGE

The major poems of the Freiberg period are inhabited by seekers who ultimately find themselves. Introspection leading to self-revelation is the goal and method of these poems, but the path inward does not lead to solipsism. Self-knowledge, as Novalis teaches in "Kenne dich selbst" ("Know Thyself"), results in a deep knowledge of nature's mysteries as well. Moreover, because his own path to self-knowledge, which had been prepared by the guiding spirit of love, led to higher consciousness, Novalis interprets his experience as a symbol. He imbues his introspective poems with a universal significance, as in these lines from "Letzte Liebe" ("Last Love"):

> As the mother wakes her darling from slumber with a
>   kiss,
> As he first sees her and comes to understand himself
>   through her:
> So love with me—through love did I first experience
>   the world,
> Find myself, and become what as a lover one becomes.

What *one*—anyone, not just Novalis—becomes when a lover, is a poet. The successful seeker of love and self-knowledge is called, like the poet addressed in "Der sterbende Genius" ("The Dying Genius"), to "sing the song of return," the myth of the return to paradise.

Having found himself again, Novalis defined for himself a Romantic mission: to transform his personal experience through poetry into a universal vision of love, which would lead others inward along the path to self-knowledge, higher consciousness, and rebirth: "Toward the East sing then the lofty song,/ Until the sun rises and ignites/ And opens for me the gates of the primeval world."

HYMNS TO THE NIGHT

In *Hymns to the Night*, the gates of eternity are opened not by the rising sun—the conventional symbol

of rebirth—but by the fall of darkness and night. This poetic work is Novalis's "lofty song," "the song of return," the clearest and most complete fulfillment of his Romantic mission. In it, Novalis transforms his personal experience of Sophie's death—to be precise, his ostensibly mystical experience at her graveside on May 13, 1797—into a universalized vision of death and night as a realm of higher consciousness and eternal love.

Hymns to the Night was not merely an immediate emotional response to Sophie's death. Although he might have begun work on an early version in the fall of 1797, Novalis resumed serious work on the cycle only in late 1799 and early 1800, when he was well over his initial grief and actively involved in life. Moreover, the textual changes that he made between setting down that version in manuscript and publishing a still later prose version in the journal *Athenäum* in 1800 show a conscious effort to rise above personal experience and indicate that his goal was not autobiography but symbolism.

Unlike the fragmentary verse epic of 1789, *Orpheus*, which uses a classical myth to examine the theme of death, *Hymns to the Night* makes personal experience the basis of a broad symbolism utilizing elements of various mythological systems (including the theme of Orpheus). Although the first three hymns describe principally the poet's own experience of "the holy, ineffable, mysterious night"—his own Orphic descent to the realm of death—the work begins significantly with a more universal reference to all living creatures in the world of light. Among these stands "the magnificent stranger" who is man himself. As in the Freiberg poems, the stranger symbolizes the universal seeker of a lost paradise. From this broad context, it becomes clear that the persona, himself a stranger in the rational world of light, is representative and his experience symbolic. This universality is reinforced in the fourth hymn when, for example, the symbol of the Cross, which at first signifies Sophie's death and links her to Christ, is finally called "the victory banner of our race." The fifth hymn continues to broaden the significance of the poet's experience by restating his subjective development toward an understanding of death in terms of humankind's changing relationship to death in history. In the sixth and final hymn, subjective experience coalesces completely with the universal. Not only is the mediating beloved explicitly identified with Christ, but also the poet's individual voice is transformed into a universal "we" singing a communal hymn of praise. The stranger, who in the Freiberg poems had given up his voice to the poet who spoke for him, here lends his voice to the chorus of humankind.

DEVOTIONAL SONGS

Devotional Songs, also written during the years 1799 through 1800, were similarly intended to raise personal experience to the level of universal—if not entirely orthodox—religious symbolism. This is evident not only from the symbols that the poems share with *Hymns to the Night*—for example, the eroticism of Christ the beloved—but also from the shared communal context and implications. Novalis had tentatively planned these songs as part of "a new, spiritual hymnal"; in them, the Sophie experience is so thoroughly transformed by virtue of the pervasive Christian imagery that many have been adopted (and sometimes adapted) for use in hymnals.

The songs, which are sometimes confessional, sometimes exhortative, are all informed by Novalis's self-conscious mission to reveal the role of love in the re-creation of the earth. The ninth song, for example, which proclaims the day of Resurrection to be "a festival of the world's rejuvenation," is more than a profession of religious faith in the coming of God's kingdom; it is a self-conscious profession of faith in the poet's mission to reveal that kingdom in humanity's midst:

> I say to each that he lives
> And has been resurrected
> That he hovers in our midst
> And is with us forever.
> I say to each and each says
> To his friends anon
> That soon everywhere
> The new kingdom of heaven will dawn.

In truly Romantic fashion, the voice of the prophet is first and foremost the voice of a poet, speaking out of his own experience but in the service of a still higher cause and announcing to all humankind the advent of a world renewed by love, which is made manifest in his words.

"THE POEM"

Novalis's last poems are almost exclusively concerned with the renewal of the universe and the return to the Golden Age; their vision is more explicitly secular and aesthetic than that which informs *Hymns to the Night* and *Devotional Songs*. Here, Novalis's belief that poetry itself can transform the world receives full expression, and many of these last works are indeed poems about poems, in which Novalis's personal experience is not the focus.

Such is the case in the significantly titled poem "Das Gedicht" ("The Poem"). The anonymous persona who speaks for humankind in its fallen state relates how "a lost page"—a poetic saga—inspires in the present a vision of the past Golden Age and keeps alive the hope for its return. Because it is able to unite past and future in the present and give form to the spirit of love, the poem itself temporarily re-creates the Golden Age. The paramount concern of "The Poem," then, is precisely what the title announces it to be: the poem—not simply the ancient saga and not even Novalis's poem in itself, but all poems, the poem per se. In its ability to unite subject and object, spirit and matter, every poem becomes a medium of higher consciousness and the salvation of the world.

"TO TIECK"

Once poetry becomes a major theme in Novalis's work, a new poetic voice emerges. The reflective persona that had spoken in the introspective poems of 1794 to 1799 is silenced. In "The Poem," for example, the reflective self is replaced by an essentially impersonal persona. This is no longer a case of a poet reflecting on himself but of poetry reflecting on itself. In the poem "An Tieck" ("To Tieck"), another anonymous persona narrates the tale of a child's discovery of an ancient book and an encounter with Jakob Boehme, which presage the coming of the Golden Age.

Despite the dedicatory title and autobiographical allusions in the poem (Tieck had introduced Novalis to Boehme's writings), the personal significance has been entirely transformed by the symbolism of the poem. The dominance of myth in these last poems precludes the need for a personal voice, as it does in the novel *Henry of Ofterdingen* of the same period. If early poems such as "To a Falling Leaf" resort to an anonymous voice because Novalis lacked experience, then the final poems do so because he succeeded in rising above his personal experience.

AUTONOMOUS LATE POEMS

The appearance of a first-person voice among the late poems does not contradict this conclusion. A number of poems in which the poet speaks in the first person were in fact intended for fictional characters in *Henry of Ofterdingen*. In some of these and in others not intended for the novel, the persona himself becomes part of an integrated mythos. Such poems are distinct from earlier reflective works such as "Beginning" and "Last Love."

Although the late poems also describe the changing consciousness of the persona, they do so in symbolic terms and not in the largely expository or intellectual manner of the earlier poems. Whereas the poet of "Beginning" simply states that Sophie has led him to higher consciousness, the speaker of "Es färbte sich die Wiese grün" ("The Meadow Turned Green") tells the story of his rebirth by narrating his experience of spring and love: During a walk deeper and deeper into the forest, the persona marvels uncomprehendingly at the transformation of nature; he then encounters a young girl and, hidden from the sun in deep shadows, suddenly understands intuitively the changes both in nature and within himself.

One can easily discern the same theme that dominated the Freiberg poems: The spirit of love, embodied by a female mediator, reveals the higher consciousness that leads to knowledge of self and of the external world. In this narrative plot, however, the theme has been thoroughly mythologized. The symbols which Novalis uses here and in all his late poems are autonomous, stripped of all but the most general personal relevance. The forest, the sun, the girl, springtime—all these derive their mythological significance from their shared archetypal context.

"The Meadow Turned Green" is autonomous, too, in that it reflects back upon itself. It is, after all, not merely a description of revelation and the path to higher consciousness; it is both the direct result of the poet's epiphany and the re-creation of it. The poem describes and mythologizes its own creation.

The process of objectifying and imbuing his personal experience with universal meaning that Novalis had begun in the poems of 1794 to 1799 was completed in his last poems, in which he totally transforms experience into myth, into symbols which have no fixed meanings outside themselves. This creation of a reflexive and fully autonomous poetry was a significant landmark on the road to nineteenth century symbolism. To reach this stage and to find his own poetic voice, it was not enough for Novalis that he free himself from Enlightenment models and create a poetry of the self. He also needed to rise above the self and to create a mythological poetry. For this, he needed a poetic voice that not only spoke from the core of his experience but also spoke in the universal language of symbolism. In achieving this goal, Novalis fulfilled the Romantic ideal of becoming like God the Creator, whose creative voice echoes eternally throughout his autonomous creation while he hovers silently above.

OTHER MAJOR WORKS

LONG FICTION: *Die Lehrlinge zu Sais*, 1802 (*The Disciples at Sais*, 1903); *Heinrich von Ofterdingen*, 1802 (*Henry of Ofterdingen*, 1842).

NONFICTION: *Blütenstaub*, 1798; *Glauben und Liebe*, 1798; *Das Allgemeine Brouillon*, 1798-1799 (*Notes for a Romantic Encyclopaedia*, 2007); *Die Christenheit oder Europa*, 1826 (*Christianity or Europe*, 1844); *Philosophical Writings*, 1997; *The Birth of Novalis: Friedrich von Hardenberg's Journal of 1797, with Selected Letters and Documents*, 2007.

MISCELLANEOUS: *Pollen and Fragments: Selected Poetry and Prose of Novalis*, 1989.

BIBLIOGRAPHY

Freeman, Veronica G. *The Poetization of Metaphors in the Work of Novalis*. New York: Peter Lang, 2006. This work examines mysticism and Romanticism in the works of Novalis and his use of metaphors.

Hodkinson, James R. *Women and Writing in the Works of Novalis: Transformation Beyond Measure?* Rochester, N.Y.: Camden House, 2007. Hodkinson examines how Novalis was affected by women, including Sophie von Kühn, and how this is evident in his writing.

Holland, Jocelyn. *German Romanticism and Science:*

The Procreative Poetics of Goethe, Novalis, and Ritter. New York: Routledge, 2009. Holland compares and contrasts the works of Novalis, Johann Wolfgang von Goethe, and Johann Wilhelm Ritter, paying particular attention to the idea of procreation.

Kennedy, Clare. *Paradox, Aphorism, and Desire in Novalis and Derrida*. London: Maney, for the Modern Humanities Research Association, 2008. Kennedy examines the themes of desire and paradoxes in the aphorisms of Novalis and philosopher-critic Jacques Derrida.

Molnár, Géza von. *Romantic Vision, Ethical Context: Novalis and Artistic Autonomy*. Minneapolis: University of Minnesota Press, 1987. Highly philosophical approach to the life and work of Novalis. Discussion of his work involves detailed expositions of Novalis's interpretations of Kantian and Fichtean philosophy. Also examines Novalis's relationship with Sophie von Kühn, his novel *Henry of Ofterdingen*, and his visionary poems in *Hymns to the Night*.

Neubauer, John. *Novalis*. Boston: Twayne, 1980. Excellent general introduction to Novalis, tailored to English-speaking readers. Interweaves the life and work to show the relationship between the two and also discusses Novalis both as a visionary and as a logical thinker. Includes discussions of Novalis's contributions to science, philosophy, the novel, poetry, politics, and religion. Includes bibliography and chronology.

Newman, Gail M. *Locating the Romantic Subject*. Detroit: Wayne State University Press, 1997. Complex interpretation of the life and work of Novalis in light of the modern object-relations theory of British psychologist D. W. Winnicott. Particular emphasis on Novalis's major novel, *Henry of Ofterdingen*, as a psychoanalytic case study.

O'Brien, William Arctander. *Novalis: Signs of Revolution*. Durham, N.C.: Duke University Press, 1995. Examines both the life and the work of Novalis with the purpose of contradicting "the myth of Novalis" as a dreamy, death-obsessed mystic. Sees Novalis as the quintessential early German Romantic. A chapter called "The Making of Sophie" brings new perspectives to Novalis's profound experience with the young Sophie von Kühn.

Donald P. Haase

O

BLAS DE OTERO

Born: Bilbao, Spain; March 15, 1916
Died: Majadahonda, Spain; June 29, 1979

PRINCIPAL POETRY
Cántico espiritual, 1942
Ángel fieramente humano, 1950
Redoble de consciencia, 1951
Pido la paz y la palabra, 1955
Ancia, 1958
Parler clair, 1959 (*En Castellano*, published in a
     French/Spanish edition)
Esto no es un libro, 1963
Blas de Otero: Twenty Poems, 1964
Que trata de España, 1964
Expresión y reunión: A modo de antología, 1969,
     1981 (as *Blas de Otero: Expresión y reunión*)
Mientras, 1970
*Selected Poems: Miguel Hernández and Blas de
     Otero*, 1972
Todos mis sonetos, 1977 (*All My Sonnets*, 1997)
Poemas de amor, 1987

OTHER LITERARY FORMS

Blas de Otero (oh-TAYR-oh) experimented with progressively freer verse forms. An evolution began with the collection *Pido la paz y la palabra* (I ask for peace and the right to speak) and continued until his poetry approached prose. In their brevity, their imagery, and their dependence on sound effects, the pieces collected in his only full-length book of prose, *Historias fingidas y verdaderas* (1970; false and true history), resemble poetry more than prose, as in "Andar" (walking): "And I saw the world as a sea churning with people, hanging on to one another as they went down; and the world just risen among broken tombs and inscriptions that lied."

As Geoffrey Barrow has noted, Otero's prose repre-sents a further slackening of poetic convention rather than an abjuration of poetry. The first section of *Historias fingidas y verdaderas* includes fifty-six pieces in which Otero meditates on his own personality. The next section comprises his thoughts on Spain, its long and tangled history and how it could profit from the Socialist revolution. The third section is devoted to speculation on the human condition in general. In contrast to the confidence that typified his writing of the previous decade, he raises doubts about the effectiveness of his role as a poet; it is now self-scrutiny rather than faith in the revolutionary potential of the majority that occupies him. Although no political theory of art emerges from his desultory observations, he attributes the social marginality he experiences as a poet to the written nature of the transference of his poetry. The secular millenarianism to which he subscribes, his belief in the imminent redemption of Spain and the world heralded by the Cuban revolution, betokens the incontrovertible romanticism of his revolutionary stance.

ACHIEVEMENTS

During his lifetime, Blas de Otero certainly did not lack recognition and praise. He was hailed as one of the most virile poets Spain had produced since its civil war; Dámaso Alonso placed his sonnet "Hombre" (man) in the company of the sonnets of Francisco Gómez de Quevedo y Villegas; and the social and metaphysical concerns of his poetry have prompted comparisons to the work of Miguel de Unamuno y Jugo, William Blake, Arthur Rimbaud, Gerard Manley Hopkins, and Robert Lowell. Otero was awarded the Premio Boscan in 1950 and later the Premio de la Critica and the Premio Fastenrath from the Real Academia Española de la Lengua. His works have been translated into many languages, and criticism of his work has appeared in all the major European languages.

BIOGRAPHY

Blas de Otero Muñoz was born in 1916 in the industrial city of Bilbao, Spain, that "dark lap" of his youth, a city "damp with rain and smoky with priests." His ancestry was Basque, and though he boasted of being a "universal Basque" and occasionally wrote poems to fellow Basques such as the poet Gabriel Aresti, his powerful love for Spain as a single entity precluded regional or ethnic partialities.

Otero was a laconic man who did not leave behind an abundance of biographical detail. "I write and am silent," he wrote in one of the most valuable autobiographical documents available, the poem "Biotz-Begietan"; when Otero was questioned on whether the poem were indeed autobiographical, he replied with one word: "Almost."

His early schooling in Bilbao was typically Basque: traditional, Catholic, and Jesuit in an environment of fear, severity, and intellectual repression that contributed to the distrust he felt toward priests and the Catholic Church. He began writing poetry at an early age; he tells the story of being struck at school by a priest who disliked some of his youthful verses. Although many of Otero's poetic anecdotes from childhood are painful, he speaks warmly of such things as the light of August streaming down upon the cherry trees of his grandmother's orchard, the happy days of his confused adolescence in Madrid, and the laughter of a youthful girl-

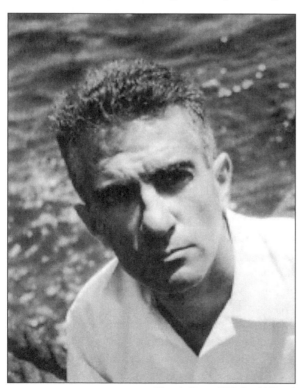

Blas de Otero (©F. Catalá Roca)

friend nicknamed Little Porcelain Jar. He graduated from high school in Madrid, earned a law degree at the University of Valladolid (although he never practiced law), and then began the study of literature at the University of Madrid. By the time he was nineteen, he had published several poems, including "Baladitas humildes" (humble little ballads) and "Cuerpo de Cristo, por mi amor llagado" ("body of Christ, by my love wounded"), in the *Revista de la Congregación (Kostkas) de Bilbao*. Then, the Spanish Civil War erupted, and Otero, apparently caught between shifting lines of battle, found himself fighting on one side and then the other. The postwar period was for Otero as painful as the war itself, and his desperate search for God, as it became more and more emotional, turned eventually into a desperate struggle with God. The poet who, in 1942, wrote, "oh beautiful God, oh flesh of my flesh and of my soul/ that, without You, would disappear like the fog," would write sarcastically in 1963, "What a shame there is not/ a god as excellent as they say."

Luis Romero describes Otero in 1946 as thin, ascetic-looking (although then not so much as he would later appear), ironic, a convincing polemicist, preoccupied, and looking more like a mystic or a philosopher than a poet. At this time, he lived on the Alameda Recalde in Bilbao with his widowed mother and an unmarried sister, of whom he rarely spoke. He earned his living as a tutor of private students, but this did not occupy much of his time.

Otero made his first trip outside Spain to Paris in 1951, where, according to his poem "Biotz-Begietan," he suffered "pangs of the spirit." Soon he became interested in Communism and for the rest of the 1950's was continuously preoccupied with leveling criticism at the Francisco Franco regime. If Otero lost interest in his search for God, he did not lose his sense of messianic purpose (his own life he called Calvary, and he titled a poem about himself "Ecce Homo"), which he transferred to his search for brotherhood among men. Even after his commitment to Marxism, his literary work expresses a longing for revolution in primarily moral and religious terms.

From 1955 to 1958, Otero lived in Barcelona; in 1959, he participated in the homage for Antonio Machado at the Sorbonne in Paris, where he read his poem "Palabras reunidas para Antonio Machado" (words put together for Antonio Machado). In 1963, he traveled to the Soviet Union and to China and had insuperable difficulties with the Spanish censors. *En Castellano* (in plain words), which was published in Paris in 1959 (*Parler clair*), was still not available in Spain, so Otero decided to permit its bowdlerized publication; when it came out, more than a hundred poems were missing.

Otero spent three years in Cuba, from 1965 to 1968, and returned to Spain with the word *guajiro* (Cuban peasant) in his vocabulary and with images of *los yanquis* (yankees) taking unfair advantage of everyone in the Americas. Soon after his return to Spain, he had a malignant tumor removed, a fact to which he refers in his chilling "Cantar de amigo" ("friend's song"): "Where is Blas de Otero? He's in the operating room, with his/ eyes open . . ./ Where is Blas de Otero? He is dead, with his eyes/ open." Throughout the 1970's, he continued assembling anthologies of his past work and writing new poetry which appeared primarily in magazines. In 1976, in ill health, he participated in commemorative services for Federico García Lorca at Fuentevaqueros. Apparently late in life, he was married to Sabina de la Cruz, who wrote the introduction to the posthumous edition of his anthology *Blas de Otero: Expresión y reunión*. Otero died in 1979 at his home in Majadahonda, outside Madrid.

ANALYSIS

Blas de Otero was fond of embedding his own name in his poems, and he did not shrink from acknowledging by name other poets whom he admired in his own work. The title *Ángel fieramente humano* (angel fiercely human) is admittedly taken from Luis de Góngora y Argote; *Esto no es un libro* (this is not a book) is from Walt Whitman; and *Historias fingidas y verdaderas* is from Miguel de Cervantes; Otero also makes ample use of epigraphs for his poems, taken from the Bible, popular Spanish songs, Saint John of the Cross, Machado ("A solitary heart is not a heart at all"), Francis Thompson, Augusto Ferrán, Rubén Darío ("Shall we be silent now in order to cry tomorrow"), and Luis de León.

Otero addresses poems to Machado, Quevedo, the Basque poet Aresti, Nobel Prize winner Vicente Aleixandre, the Turkish Communist poet Nazim Hikmet ("Considering how you have moved me/ at this time when tenderness is so difficult"), Paul Éluard, and Miguel Hernández, and recognizes by name as kindred spirits Pablo Neruda, the Bulgarian poet Nicolai Vaptzarov, Rafael Alberti, César Vallejo, Gabriel Celaya, and León Felipe.

Similarly, he made no secret of his scorn for the idea that poetry, not accessible to everyone, is for the "immense minority," as advanced by Juan Ramón Jiménez; thus was inspired his own commitment to the "immense majority." Otero was also vocal in denying Unamuno's influence on his thinking, an idea put forth by the critic Emilio Alarcos Llorach, and his attitude toward Cervantes and his knight errant is complicated by his resentment that both of them helped to perpetuate the myth of idealism.

LANGUAGE AND STYLE

As regards Otero's style, he is partial to words that convey violence and passion (such as *rasgar*, "to tear"; *arrancar*, "to wrench") and derivative verbs and participles using the prefix *des-* (such as *desterrar*, "to drive away"; *desarraigar*, "to uproot"; *desgajar*, "to wrench off"), the violence of which presents a striking contrast to the more positive condition of the word without the prefix (*terra*, "land"; *arraigo*, "stability"; *gajo*, "branch"). He commonly adds the suffix *-azo* to nouns, thereby incorporating the strong Castilian *th* pronunciation (as in *trallazo*, "whiplash"; *zarpazo*, "thud"). Among colors, yellow (*amarillo*) appears the most frequently, redolent of aging and decay.

In contrast, when moments of violence and anger give way to resigned melancholy and "when roses spring forth from the wall of grief," some of Otero's favorite words are *paz* (peace), *luz* (light), the neologism *frondor* (the lushness of fronds), and the names of various birds and flowers. Generally, Otero adheres to a basic Spanish vocabulary, almost colloquial, and for the most part, he avoids literary or unusual words. An exception is his delight in some of the more unusual designations for rugged terrain (such as *llambria, galayo, cantil*), whose very "difficulty" seems to mimic that which they denote.

Otero's conception of humanity as adrift in a vast abysmal ocean, straining to grasp some support, or as an island, floating with its flora of anxieties and its fauna of appetites, leads the poet to employ a full panoply of nautical terms, some of which are technical enough to sound awkward in English translation. The same is true of the poet's reliance on the imagery of directional winds, such as *cierzo* (cold northerly wind) and *galerna* (stormy northwest wind). The word *zafarrancho*, metaphorically "struggle," which Otero uses to sum up his life in a later poem, is another nautical term, originally referring to the drudgery of cleaning the deck of a ship.

Otero also creates new words, which he does by agglutination (as in the title "Españahogándose" / "Choking on Spain"), by blending (as in *Ancia*, composed of the first syllable of *Ángel fieramente humano* and the last syllable of *Redoble de consciencia* ("drumroll of conscience"), which also suggests *ansia*, "anguish," one of the key words in Existential philosophy), and by analogy ("alángeles y arcángeles," where the former is created on the model of the latter to denote another type of angel). Another feature of Otero's style is his tendency to freshen clichés and lines from other poets by making slight changes. Thus, the idiom "cogido de la mano" (hand in hand) is converted to "cogidos de la muerte": "You and I, linked by death" instead of "You and I, hand in hand." Otero takes a line from León, "espaciosa y triste España" (sad and spacious Spain), and recasts it as "esta espaciosa y triste cárcel" (this sad and spacious prison). A famous line from Gustavo Adolfo Bécquer, "While there exists one beautiful woman,/ there will always be poetry," becomes for Otero "Where there is in the world/ one single word,/ there will be poetry."

"DÉJAME"

To inculcate an idea, Otero does not avoid repeating the same or near-synonymous words (for example, "doors, doors, and doors. And more doors"). He is also fond of enjambment, which serves to speed up the rhythm of some of his poems or, conversely, to slow down their progress, as it does in the following lines from "Déjame" (leave me), where it suggests the uneven, ill-defined quality of the poet's relationship with God:

You do me harm, Lord. Take your hand
from upon my head. Leave me with my vacancy,
Leave me. For an abyss, with my own
I have enough. Oh God, if you are human,
take pity, remove your hand
from my head. It does me no good. It makes me cold
and scared.

Other noteworthy techniques operative in Otero's poetry are the hyphenation of words in such a way as to permit an ambivalence of meaning: frequent use of the rhetorical question and experimentation with unconventional punctuation.

WOMEN AND LOVE POETRY

Although Otero did not customarily write love poetry unmarred by the dark thoughts connected with one or another of his compulsive searches, he was not reluctant to name names, and he identifies in his poems a significant number of women important to him. In his earliest poems, he treats the desired woman as a virginal symbol and his potential union with her as a union of body and soul: "Mademoiselle Isabel," apparently his teacher of French as an adolescent, with her carnation-colored breasts and rose-colored body; "Little Porcelain Jar," who smelled of hyacinth; and "La Monse" reclining in a field of yellow flowers. A special case is Tachia, nickname of Conchita Quintana, who, little more than a teenager when she befriended Otero, then in his thirties, gave the poet some of the happiest moments of his life. In fact, it was Tachia who helped the poet to realize the futility of his marathon bout with God, and it was she who invited him to concern himself instead with the brotherhood of humankind: "You said: Entwine your grief with mine,/ like a long and jubilant tress;/ immerse your dreams in my kind; push aside/ your thirst for God. My kingdom is of this world."

In later poems, this ethereal love becomes tainted by the tantalizing pain caused by the body of a woman, and Otero's imagery becomes less dainty: The poet lifts the warm skirts of one woman to find a shadow, fear, and a "silent hole," and he writes cheerlessly of the impoverished Laura, who has a "little accordion/ between her legs." In the relatively late "La palmatoria de cobre" ("the copper ferule"), Otero avails himself of the appellation "sister," borrowed from the biblical Song of Solomon to address the consoling female subject of his poem. The consolation of love with women, however, is not enough to provide the poet with a permanent distraction from his *Weltschmerz*. In fact, one of the only times he speaks of women generically is in the form of a savage diatribe, where women are characterized as "Cunning, calculating, liars/ lily-white in public, notorious with their masks."

CÁNTICO ESPIRITUAL

Otero destroyed hundreds of early poems, or so he claims in "Es a la inmensa mayoría" (to the immense majority). His attempts to maintain his faith in God after the horrors of the Spanish Civil War are the theme of his first published work, *Cántico espiritual* (spiritual canticle), written in homage to Saint John of the Cross on the occasion of the fourth centenary of his birth (1942). These homage poems, which establish the relationship of God and humanity as the product of a violent meditation ("I moan and clamor for You like a sin"), Otero never allowed to be reprinted, and in comparison to his later poems, they seem rather less spontaneous.

ÁNGEL FIERAMENTE HUMANO

For the next eight years, Otero published in the Basque literary magazine *Egan* and began to acquire a following. In 1950, *Ángel fieramente humano* appeared, dedicated to the "immense majority" and bringing into sharper focus Otero's personal quarrel with God and his conception of the vacancy and loneliness to which humankind is subjected in this life. The Existentialism of these poems recalls Søren Kierkegaard; Otero's views during this period were influenced by discussions among the young Basque intellectuals connected with *Egan*. Otero speaks of the terrible silence of God, a silence made to seem even more terrible in the wake of the unnecessary killing (twenty-three million, by Otero's count) in World War II. When the poet raises his hand, God, clearly the angry God of the Old Testament rather than the loving Jesus of the New, lops it off; when he raises his eyes toward God, God gouges them out. If man is an angel in the image of God, then his wings are like chains. Nevertheless, there are still to be found in this work vestiges of Otero's deep religious feeling, as in "Salmo por el hombre de hoy" ("Psalm for the Man of Today"), written as a prayer: "Raise us, O Lord, above death./ Extend

and sustain our gaze/ so that it can learn henceforth to see You."

REDOBLE DE CONSCIENCIA

Otero's next collection, *Redoble de consciencia*, was devoted to the same theme and written mainly in free verse. The lament of Job that he was ever born serves as the epigraph of the sonnet "Tierra" (land), and Saint John's observation that the soft hand of God can weigh heavily on the soul of humans, serves to introduce "Déjame" (leave me). In the latter poem, Otero, equal in pride to God who made him, reaches the point of wishing he could kill God as God kills humans; a godless abyss without hope is thus preferable to an abyss reigned over by an oppressive God who tantalizes with a hope that is unattainable.

PIDO LA PAZ Y LA PALABRA

In *Pido la paz y la palabra*, Otero, heeding the advice of Tachia, devoted himself to the working class in poems which J. M. Cohen has called monotonous in their anger. Such apparently self-indulgent lines as "I have seen few Calvaries like the one I have" and "I am a man literally beloved by all sorts of ruin" are relieved somewhat by subsequent pledges to offer his life "to the gods/ who live in the country of hope" and "to leap up to the beautiful towers of peace," "sway other breezes," and "call at the doors of the world." One remarkable poem from this collection is "Hija de Yago" (daughter of Saint James), which depicts Spain on the map of Europe as its bloody heel which trod upon the face of a torpid America.

ANCIA

In 1958, Otero published *Ancia*, comprising a selection from *Ángel fieramente humano* and *Redoble de consciencia* as well as thirty-eight new poems, some of which were from the earlier periods of his life and among which is Otero's version of Matthew Arnold's "Dover Beach," a poem addressed to Tachia and titled "Paso a paso" (step by step). As the drum rolls from one side of Europe to the other, he begs his beloved to put death behind her; "The night is long, Tachia/ . . . Listen to the sound/ of daybreak/ opening its way step-by-step—between the dead."

EN CASTELLANO

En Castellano, which did not pass the Spanish censors and had to be published in France in a bilingual edition as *Parler clair* in 1959, contained Otero's most unconventional poetry to date. Here, Otero broke up his customary hendecasyllables by distributing the words of a single line over several lines or by introducing short lines of another measure. He was increasingly concerned with eliminating decorative rhetoric and achieving the most direct style possible. The collection includes this now-famous dictum: "Formerly I was—they say—an existentialist./ I say that I am a co-existentialist." Much of its content, however, was aimed at the Franco dictatorship and is of limited interest to the contemporary reader.

ESTO NO ES UN LIBRO

Esto no es un libro, so called because its poems deal with real people and places, was published in Puerto Rico in 1963. It is a thematic anthology containing poems from different periods of the poet's life as well as several poems he was forced to omit from *Que trata de España* (all about Spain), which was published in Barcelona the following year and is confined to expressing the beauty and the misery of Otero's native land. Although in this book he evokes memories by the mention of place-names (130 of them) or words for regional phenomena (such as *orvallo* and *sirimiri* for "rain"), and although many of the images are beautiful in their own right ("the mountains of Leon glitter/ like a blue sword/ waved in the mist"), Otero manages to insert social criticism into every poem, touching on everything from consumerism and agrarian reform to Vietnam and the United Nations. If he rhapsodizes about "bright Catalonia," "pure Leon," and "Segovia of ancient gold," he ends the poem with a tweak of conscience about "fertile Extremadura,/ where people and bread/ are parted unjustly."

QUE TRATA DE ESPAÑA

The original, uncut edition of *Que trata de España*, published by Ruedo Ibérico in Paris in 1964, contains 155 poems, subdivided thematically into five parts: "El forzado" (he who is forced), "La palabra" (the word), "Cantares" (songs), "Geografía e historia" (geography and history), and "Verdad comun" (common truth). The first section depicts the poet as the child of a miserable and beautiful mother and stepmother who is Spain, a proud country soaked by centuries of fratricidal bloodletting and disdainful of science and prog-

ress. It is to the people that Otero speaks, a people broken and burned beneath the sun, hungry and illiterate in their millenarian wisdom and "hospitable and good,/ as the bread they do not have."

The second section reflects the poet's admiration for simple words, especially for the simple, vivid (albeit sometimes ungrammatical) speech and eloquent gestures of the Spanish peasants. By this time, Otero had begun to realize that his poetry was not reaching the working person for whom it was written, and in defense of his original premise he added to one of his poems an epigraph (author unidentified): "In the condition of *our hemisphere* poetry is for the majority not because of the number of its readers, but because of its theme."

Spain has a richer inheritance of epic poetry and folk ballads than does any other European country, with the possible exception of England, and it was in appreciation of this inheritance that Otero named his third section "Cantares." All the poems included here have some link with the folk poetry of Spain or with folk-inspired modern poetry, such as that of García Lorca, and Otero's use of certain archaic variants of poetic words underscores this folk element. It is in this section that Otero launches a violent diatribe against the lie of literature and proffers the advice, "if you want to live peacefully,/ don't be corrupted by books."

In the fourth section, Otero paints more loving vignettes of Spain and probes deeply into the sad history of the country, invoking the aid of the painter Diego Rodriguez de Velázquez to forge an iron tongue on the anvil of truth; there is also a memorial poem to Machado and a collage poem on the death of Don Quixote. The final section attempts to join Spain with other countries of the world in a common hope for a better future: "we/ open our arms to life,/ we know/ another fall will come, heavy with gold,/ beautiful as a tractor in the wheat."

MIENTRAS

The collection *Mientras* (in the meantime), which the poet later wished to have incorporated into a larger work to be called "Hojas de Madrid con la galerna" (pages from Madrid with the northwest wind), contains poems written in Madrid after his return there from his three-year residence in Cuba and often shares metaphors, allusions, and symbols with the prose pieces of

Historias fingidas y verdaderas, published the same year. The poems are characterized by the subjectivity and reflectiveness of a dying man who reviews and evaluates the facts of his life. In "Morir en Bilbao" (to die in Bilbao), he observes that although he loves Moscow as he does his right arm, he is Bilbao with his entire body in a way he can never be Moscow. The burden of being so peculiarly Spanish, however, is no longer as oppressive as it was in the earlier poems; the poet concedes that in part, his wishes for peace have been granted, and the subject of death no longer inspires defiance in him.

Whether Otero was struggling against the dreadful aloneness of humanity, as in his earlier work, or against the evils of war and political dictatorship, as he did in his later work, he plied his trade with subtlety and power. The justice he sought for Spain, "disheveled in its grief" under fascism, he grew to demand for citizens of the entire world, even if within a political framework as extreme in the other direction as the fascism that he loathed. His voice is sometimes sarcastic and often bitter, but it never quavers, and it is never without hope for a tomorrow better than today.

OTHER MAJOR WORK

NONFICTION: *Historias fingidas y verdaderas*, 1970.

BIBLIOGRAPHY

Barrow, Geoffrey R. *The Satiric Vision of Blas de Otero*. Columbia: University of Missouri Press, 1988. A critical examination of Otero's work. Includes bibliographic references and an index.

Cannon, Calvin, ed. *Modern Spanish Poems: Selections from the Poetry of Juan Ramón Jiménez, Antonio Machado, Federico García Lorca, and Blas de Otero*. New York: Macmillan, 1965. A collection of twentieth century Spanish poetry with commentary by the editor. Contains a discussion of Otero.

Debicki, Andrew Peter. *Spanish Poetry of the Twentieth Century: Modernity and Beyond*. Lexington: University Press of Kentucky, 1994. Debicki examines the sweep of modern Spanish verse, which he situates in the context of European modernity, tracing its trajectory from the Symbolists to the postmodernists. Touches on Otero.

Mellizo, Carlos, and Louise Salstad, eds. *Blas de Otero: Study of a Poet*. Laramie: Department of Modern and Classical Languages, University of Wyoming, 1980. A collection of critical essays in English and Spanish. Includes bibliographic references and an index.

Winfield, Jerry Phillips, ed. *Twentieth-Century Spanish Poets: Second Series*. Vol. 134 in *Dictionary of Literary Biography*. Detroit: Gale Research, 1994. Contains an entry on Otero that provides background and criticism.

Jack Shreve

———

OVID

Born: Roman Empire (now Sulmona, Italy); March 20, 43 B.C.E.

Died: Tomis on the Black Sea, Moesia (now Constanţa, Romania); 17 C.E.

PRINCIPAL POETRY

Amores, c. 20 B.C.E. (English translation, c. 1597)

Ars amatoria, c. 2 B.C.E. (*Art of Love*, 1612)

Heroides, before 8 C.E. (English translation, 1567)

Medicamina faciei, before 8 C.E. (*Cosmetics*, 1859)

Remedia amoris, before 8 C.E. (*Cure for Love*, 1600)

Fasti, c. 8 C.E. (English translation, 1859)

Metamorphoses, c. 8 C.E. (English translation, 1567)

Epistulae ex Ponto, after 8 C.E. (*Letters from Pontus*, 1639)

Ibis, after 8 C.E. (English translation, 1859)

Tristia, after 8 C.E. (*Sorrows*, 1859)

OTHER LITERARY FORMS

Ovid (AHV-uhd) composed a tragedy, *Medea* (pr. before 8 C.E.), probably a rhetorical closet-drama in the manner of Seneca. Only two or three short fragments of this work remain.

ACHIEVEMENTS

Without any hostility toward Vergil, Ovid led Roman poetry away from the manner and technique of epic poems such as the *Aeneid* (c. 29-19 B.C.E.; English translation, 1553). Ovid was a poet of great talent whose works cover a vast range of types, including love poems, elegy, mytho-historical epic, handbooks on love, and a set of fictitious letters written by mythological heroines. He produced a voluminous body of poetry even though he had studied to be an advocate and government official.

Ovid's extensive influence began in his own lifetime. His poems were known throughout the Roman Empire, and they continued to be read through the Middle Ages. Ovid was a favorite author of the period of chivalry, and his works live again in Geoffrey Chaucer, Giovanni Boccaccio, Petrarch, and the whole circle of Italian Renaissance writers and painters, the *Metamorphoses* in particular providing many subjects for the artists. Later, Ovid was to influence Ludovico Ariosto, Desiderius Erasmus, Johann Wolfgang von Goethe, Pierre de Ronsard, Jean de La Fontaine, Molière, Edmund Spenser, William Shakespeare, John Milton, William Congreve, and Lord Byron. Early American literature has preserved a retelling of some of his stories in Nathaniel Hawthorne's *Tanglewood Tales for Boys and Girls* (1853). Ovid was not profound—he had none of the vision and greatness of Vergil—but he remains one of the most skillful writers of verse and tellers of tales that the Western world has ever known.

BIOGRAPHY

Publius Ovidius Naso was born at Sulmo in the Pelignian territory of Italy on March 20, 43 B.C.E., of wealthy parents. They were not particularly generous with their son while they lived but left him a comfortable inheritance on their death. Of equestrian, not aristocratic rank, but with good connections and great talents, Ovid was expected to devote himself to the duties of public life. At first, he studied law but had no interest in such a profession. He soon abandoned law in disgust and turned to rhetoric, studying at Rome under Arellius Fuscus and Porcius Latro. Then, according to the custom, he spent a short time in Athens; while he was in Greece, he took the opportunity to visit the renowned

cities of Asia Minor. He returned to Rome at the age of twenty-three or twenty-four and made a halfhearted beginning at a public career, holding such minor offices as triumvir and decemvir. The effort, however, was short-lived. He felt that he had neither the physical nor the mental stamina for a civic career, and he certainly lacked the interest. He finally abandoned politics and threw himself headlong into the life of a man-about-town. He joined the literary circle that included the love poets Aemilius Macer, Sextus Propertius, and Albius Tibullus. Ovid heard Horace recite and, although Ovid was not an intimate of Vergil, the two probably met.

Ovid soon made a name for himself, and before long, his elegant poems were being recited in the salons and streets of Rome. His literary career falls into three clearly defined periods. The first is marked by the composition of the *Amores*, the *Heroides*, and the brilliant but calamitous trio, the *Art of Love*, the *Cure for Love*, and *Cosmetics*. The *Amores* was a collection of short elegiac poems, addressed to an imaginary mistress, Corinna; the *Heroides* purported to be letters from famous ladies of heroic times to their lovers. (There are twenty-one epistles, but only the first fourteen are beyond all doubt Ovid's own.) The *Art of Love*, one of the most elegant pieces of seduction in all literature, was published in 2 B.C.E., to be followed shortly after by *Cure for Love*, which may have been intended as a recantation, and by a treatise on *Cosmetics*.

The next ten years constitute the second phase of Ovid's literary career. During this period, Ovid turned from amorous compositions to serious themes. His interest in Greek and Roman literature and mythology now had free rein. He wrote the *Fasti*, a poetic calendar of astronomical data, embellished with references to the historical, political, and social highlights of the Roman year. To this period also belongs the *Metamorphoses*, his great poem of transformations, and the greatest collection of mythology in any literature. This monumental work had been completed but had not received the master's finishing polish, when, in 8 C.E., like a thunderbolt from a blue sky, an imperial decree banished Ovid from Rome forever.

This shattering calamity marked the commencement of the third and final period of Ovid's life. The rest of his extant poetry was written after his banishment and includes *Sorrows*, an autobiographical poem, and *Letters from Pontus*, letters written in an attempt to induce Augustus to change the location of his banishment. Besides these works, Ovid wrote, while in exile, the *Ibis*, a vicarious piece of learned abuse. The *Fasti* is by far the most important product of Ovid's banishment, although the first books were probably composed before his exile. It is a versified Roman calendar for the first six months of the year. Several other poems by Ovid are now lost.

His banishment is one of the great mysteries of literature, for no explanation was ever given (at least to the public), and Ovid himself refers to the cause in only the vaguest of terms. It was generally believed that the reason was the emperor's anger at the immorality of the *Art of Love*. This is reasonable enough, because Augustus had tried very hard, even by legislation, to reduce the moral laxity prevailing in the capital. Ten years, however, had passed since the *Art of Love* was published, and it must be assumed that some more immediate cause had suddenly fanned the flames of this old resentment. Historians had not far to seek. The emperor's daughter, Julia, and his granddaughter (also named Julia) were both wanton and dissolute women, and their behavior in court circles had long been a source of anxiety, distress, and shame to Augustus. In the same year in which Ovid was banished, Augustus also banished his granddaughter from the court and the city of Rome. It has been surmised that Augustus knew (or suspected) that Ovid had been aware of some intrigues in the royal household involving the younger Julia that he neither prevented nor reported. In his autobiographical poem *Sorrows*, Ovid several times takes pains to deny any complicity. He says that he was merely an innocent witness of something he should not have seen and that the cause of his banishment was an error, not a crime.

The punishment, grievous though it was, was not as bad as it might have been. Ovid was banished, not exiled, and this apparently subtle distinction had tangible advantages, for he was allowed to retain not only his citizenship but also his property in Rome. Ovid's wife (his third—he had divorced the first two) did not accompany him. She remained in Rome at Ovid's request, possibly to look after his property and to en-

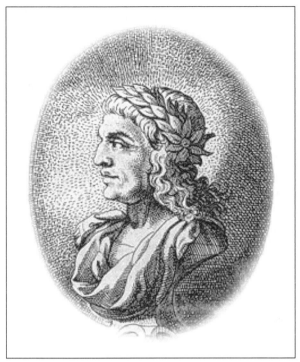

Ovid

deavor to persuade her influential friends to intercede for her husband. This was the brighter side of Ovid's disaster. The rest was a refinement of cruelty. Ovid, the genial, friendly, pleasure-loving poet, was ordered to Tomis on the Black Sea, a barbarous town on the very frontiers of civilization, peopled by long-haired, uncouth Sarmatians, chilled by interminable frost and snow, constantly attacked by savages, and utterly devoid of any culture, literature, or even intelligent conversation.

In anger and despair at the downfall of his hopes, Ovid, on leaving Rome, burned the unrevised manuscript of his *Metamorphoses*. Some friends, however, had kept a copy, and thus the masterpiece was preserved.

For nearly ten years, Ovid lived out a miserable existence that was one long apologia for his life. He defended himself, excused himself, and explained himself. He sorely missed the sights and sounds of Rome: They were always in his thoughts. One thing remained to him: the exercise of his poetic gift. He continued to pour out elegiac verses, but the sparkle had gone out of them. The lamp was burning low. Nine years of self-pity, self-reproach, abject self-abasement, prayers, tears, and, finally, total despair had taken their toll.

All this time, Ovid had never ceased to hope for a reprieve, but Augustus was unbending, and his successor Tiberius was equally adamant. Ovid bitterly realized that there is no pardon when a deity is offended. The gentle, self-indulgent spirit of the poet was broken. He pathetically pleaded that his ashes be brought home and that imperial malice not pursue him beyond the grave. In 17 C.E., Ovid, the playful singer of tender loves, was dead.

ANALYSIS

Ovid always maintained a decorous loyalty to language and sentiment in his poetry. He was not a propagandist but a man of letters, pure and simple. He produced mainly love poetry until he turned his attention to something on a larger scale, a quasi epic. His talents were not suited to long flights, such as the *Aeneid*. He was a thorough Alexandrian in that respect, as in his learning and high polish. It was with the poetry on amatory themes that Ovid first won his reputation, and he continued to work at them for some years, recasting and rearranging them.

AMORES

The existing poems of the *Amores* form three books containing, in all, forty-nine poems, none very long (they range from 18 to 114 lines). Most of them tell the story of the poet's relations with a certain Corinna. No one has ever succeeded in identifying her, and a careful reading of these charming trifles reveals Corinna to be a fantasy figure, whom Ovid could adorn with all his taste and ingenuity.

Love poetry as a genre in Roman literature already existed and had been developed by a whole generation of poets before him. Ovid employed two aspects of the genre developed by earlier poets: the autobiographical mode of composition and the devising of transitions from one traditional motif to another. Ovid's strength, however, lies in grace, not depth. The major pleasures of the *Amores* are their verbal and metrical dexterity. These poems have an epigrammatical quality; verbal dexterity has sharpened a point to precision but no mental picture is evoked. The result is, at times, a slight incoherence, characteristic of poetry that concentrates

more on effect than on expression. Ovid produces three effects in the *Amores*: neatness, ingenuity, and irony. Neatness is largely a matter of antithesis, balance, and contrast, both in thought and expression, supported often by verbal echoes. Ingenuity is evident in word order, brevity, compression, allusive periphrases, and deliberate ambiguity. Irony, often implied by antithesis, is enhanced by parentheses and asides. The diction is based on the stock amatory vocabulary, but Ovid does coin new words in moderation and skillfully manipulates different registers of diction against the poetic norm. Ovid calculates his effects with great precision and accuracy; imagery consequently plays a minor part in his poetry, in contrast to the various figures of balance and antithesis.

Like earlier Roman love poets, Ovid employs the autobiographical mode of composition. He does so not because he is trying to express inner feelings with the greatest attainable immediacy, but because, for Ovid, the autobiographical form has the advantage that characters and situation can be taken for granted; no explanation is needed. Ovid leaves little to the reader and only demands that he keep his sense of language and the subtle relationships of words at key pitch.

Ovid's love poetry is far easier to understand than that of his predecessors, because of his clearer transitions from one idea or emotion to another. Ovid's technique of composition is self-consciously concerned with the fine details of language and thought. This form encouraged him to use an extremely orderly, even rigidly logical process of exposition. Surprising leaps of thought and reversals of emotion are ruled out by a technique that leaves nothing unsaid that can be said.

The style of the *Amores* is not, of course, beyond criticism. Its brilliance is in a sense superficial; it lacks majesty and mystery; and it is too lucid to present real intellectual problems. Yet the *Amores* is not an entirely superficial work. The serious note in the poems on poetic immortality has long been recognized, and there is an underlying seriousness in Ovid's treatment of love and in his attitude to the Augustan regime. His attitude toward love is one of amused resignation, where the difficulties, follies, and deceptions of the lover are humorously magnified, cheerfully minimized, or positively welcomed. In a sense, Ovid is offering an alternative and perhaps more practical approach to love than the shapeless idealism of other love poets and the negative stance of the moralists. The work is saved from mere triviality by the warm humanity and psychological truth which underlie its ironic approach. At only one point, when he discusses abortion, does Ovid's genial banter seem to descend to callousness.

The technique and spirit of the *Amores* are basically Alexandrian, although in some cases the setting is clearly Roman rather than Greek. It was, however, impossible for a Roman of the Augustan Age to detach himself from the political and social conditions of his time. The *Amores* inevitably reflects Ovid's attitude to the regime of Augustus and its ideals. In Ovid's choice of love rather than any higher theme for poetry and in his evident enthusiasm for the life of a lover, he is clearly flying in the face of Augustus's attempts to reform marriage. Ovid is flippant about religion, the military ideal, and Augustus himself, but toward politics he reveals indifference rather than any positive stance. The *Amores* seems to be apolitical and not exactly what Augustus had in mind for the Roman literary scene.

ART OF LOVE AND CURE FOR LOVE

The *Art of Love*, along with its companion piece, the *Cure for Love*, is an adaption of the elegiac tradition to the didactic poem, a genre with a clearly defined tradition that had in Vergil a distinguished recent practitioner. Superficially, the *Art of Love* is on a par with practical poems such as that on hunting by Ovid's contemporary Grattius, but the use of the didactic form for such an untraditional subject as love creates a light, even comic atmosphere. Ovid establishes his place in the higher poetic form of the tradition by using the standard introductory (*principio*), transitional (*adde quod*), and hortatory (*accipe*) formulas of Lucretius and Vergil, and by employing the traditional ship and chariot metaphors for the progress of the poem. Nevertheless, the *Art of Love* lacks the dedication to a patron that is common in more serious works.

The poem, in which Ovid denies the traditional divine inspiration and claims that his poem is based entirely on experience, announces his ironic approach to the genre. When Ovid refers to his literary predecessors, it is not in a spirit of reverence, but rather to show how cleverly he can twist their serious themes to his own lighthearted purposes. Lucretius's passage on the birth of civilization is adapted to prove the susceptibility of women to love, and Vergil's instructions on seasons and types of soil become, with a little modification, instructions on how to find and win women. Ovid's most interesting adaptation of the genre is his creation of a humorous persona for the mentor of love, thus underlining the element of burlesque. This persona makes extravagant claims for his powers, seeing himself as a prophet or a pilot of the chariot of love. Thus, between the sophisticated poet and his sophisticated readers there is a fictitious mentor and the equally fictitious students to whom the work is addressed. In other words, the whole work is an elaborate literary game.

The *Art of Love*, like the *Amores*, makes extensive use of the themes of love poetry, but there is an essential difference between the two. The setting of the didactic poem is unmistakably contemporary Rome. The *Amores*, although Roman in some details, is set in the shadowy half-Roman, half-Hellenistic world of elegy. This contemporary element of the *Art of Love* has two aspects. First, it presents many glimpses of the more private aspects of Roman life. Second, it can hardly avoid making at least an implicit comment on Augustan society and on the ideals of the regime. The ideas hinted at in the *Amores* are now expressed much more strongly. For example, there is one passage in which Ovid explicitly rejects the idealization of the past and of rustic simplicity. Instead, he prefers the splendor of contemporary Rome and the life of refinement. The main theme of the *Art of Love*, a manual of seduction and intrigue, is clearly in conflict with Augustus's attempts to encourage marriage. Ovid's claims that he is not writing for married women does nothing to disguise this fact.

There are other ways in which Ovid seems to show little respect for Augustus and for the symbols of his prestige. His budding program, his public spectacles, his foreign policy, and his cults of the gods are all either treated frivolously or at least debased by being set in a frivolous context. All this does not turn Ovid into a political propagandist or imply that the main purpose of the *Art of Love* was to criticize Augustus and his regime. What is clear is that Ovid's natural impudence, irreverence, and sense of the incongruous were not inhibited by any feeling of veneration for the ideals of Augustus. Ovid no doubt expected to delight many of his readers by his daring, and he was not concerned if he shocked others. He himself brushed off criticisms of the _Art of Love_ in his _Cure for Love_, and in this he ultimately miscalculated. In the end, a jaded bureaucracy seized on the subversive aspects of the work, although its original purpose was surely humorous rather than political.

The basic style of the _Art of Love_ and the _Cure for Love_ is the style of the _Amores_, characterized by neatness and wit. This style is perfectly suited to the persona of the mentor of love. The most significant stylistic developments in the _Art of Love_ (apart from the adoption of didactic formulas and imagery) are the techniques of description and narrative, evident especially in the vignettes of Roman life and in the set-piece, mythological digressions. A careful analysis of the language of the descriptive passages (both of city life and in the many similes from nature) reveals an eye for detail and a sense of color and brightness, vigor and enjoyment, beauty and elegance. The narratives are technically accomplished; a single episode, the "Rape of the Sabines," includes the following devices: aphorism, wordplay, verbal repetition, antithesis, extended description with small details and hints of color and scent, similes from nature, focus on individuals, carefully varied rhythms, impudent reinterpretation of Roman history, and an aetiological conclusion. Here, undeniably, is the basis of the narrative style of the _Fasti_ and of the _Metamorphoses_.

The final question is whether the _Art of Love_ is anything more than a _jeu d'esprit_. It is right to emphasize that the main quality of these poems is wit and that their main appeal lies in their sophistication and ingenuity. As in the _Amores_, however, they are saved from triviality or mere frivolity by their underlying humanity and psychological insight. It has often been observed that Ovid draws on works of serious philosophy in framing his precepts: The instructions to women in book 3 of the _Art of Love_ share certain principles with Cicero's _De officiis_ (44 B.C.E.; _On Duties_, 1534); and the advice in the _Cure for Love_ echoes that of Cicero's _Tusculanae disputationes_ (44 B.C.E.; _Tusculum Disputations_,

1561). The aim of these borrowings may have been partly to show how cleverly Ovid could adapt other works to his own purposes; but the passages do not read like parody, and the effect is to give a backbone of human understanding to the poems. There was a basic decency with which the game of seduction and deception was to be played, and Ovid was not being entirely frivolous in his ideal of civilized life.

METAMORPHOSES

The course of Ovid's life allowed him only seven more creative years after the publication of his early works. This short span sufficed for the composition of the fifteen volumes of the _Metamorphoses_; only the final revision was lacking. It is, nevertheless, his masterpiece; it is one of the finest poems handed down from antiquity.

The writing of the _Metamorphoses_ meant a new departure for Ovid in several respects, and his poetic powers were to be exercised in fields where he had little previous experience. For one thing, his poetry had moved, so far, only in the given and natural world. Now, he was to conquer the province of the fabulous and miraculous. In his previous works, Ovid had been expressing emotional experiences, but now he had to cultivate concreteness. Definite characters had to be portrayed, their stories told in appropriate settings, and sceneries devised to fit plots. Ovid met the challenge and his invention was more than equal to the task. The epic style had to be handled by an author who had been writing elegiacs. Finally, Ovid had to overcome somehow a serious defect of his intellect: his inability to order his material systematically and to develop his ideas consistently. He compensated for this weakness with an inexhaustible ingenuity in improvisation. Ovid is constantly luring the reader on from one story to the next, and yet he is always arresting him with the present tale.

The main subject of the epic is the transformation of human beings or gods into animals, plants, stones, or constellations. The theme of metamorphosis provides a sense of continuity, reinforced by Ovid's ability to link the stories into groups and to create ingenious transitions between one story or group of stories and the next. He chose the theme because the fantastic and utopian character of the stories appealed to him and because it gave him scope for displaying many varieties of insecure and fleeting identity, of a self divided or spilling over into another self. Separation from the self usually means death, but not in a metamorphosis; Ovid's mild disposition avoided crushing finales. This is best illustrated by the Myrrha story. Myrrha cannot live on after a hideous sin that she has committed. She prays to the gods for a harsh punishment, a change in shape, denying her both life and death. Ovid intercedes in his own narrative and is not ashamed to betray how much it moves him; he feels relieved that Myrrha's prayer is answered and that she does not have to die. When he has reported how she was transformed into a myrrh tree, and how her tears were to be known in all ages as precious grains of incense, he even characterizes the metamorphosis as an honor rather than as a punishment.

In general, the character of the *Metamorphoses* is romantic and sentimental. A great many stories are concerned with the human experience of love. The poem is remarkable for its wide range in this regard: Pyramus and Thisbe, Iphis and Anaxarete, Cephalus and Procris, Ceyx and Alcyone, Baucis and Philemon, Pygmalion, Myrrha, Io, Callisto. Indeed, one of the outstanding elements of the poem is the breadth of human sympathy that is obvious despite the unrealistic atmosphere and the rhetorical elements of Ovid's style. The story of Io, the woman loved by Zeus and transformed by him into a cow, is a good example. Why, in spite of the fantastic plot, is the reader moved by the tale to feel concern for the cow woman? Everyone can understand what it means to try to escape from his own self. There is much in Ovid's fables that can easily be divested of the miraculous and translated into some everyday occurrence.

Another theme employed by Ovid in the *Metamorphoses* is the interplay between otherness and sameness. He explored this new frontier of experience in a great number of stories. One of his best is the tale of the narcissus that once upon a time was a young man. At the age of sixteen, between boyhood and manhood, Narcissus aroused the love of both men and women, but tender though his beauty was, it made him arrogant and hard; his heart remained unmoved. His punishment was to fall in love with himself. In the secluded solitude of a lush meadow deep in the woods, he lay down at the edge of a pond to drink, and the calm water mirrored his shape. Ovid describes at length the strong deception and enchantment with which Narcissus unwittingly desires himself. Then Ovid breaks into his narrative with a direct address. The poet, like an excited child in a theater who tries to help the hero, forgets his supposed aloofness and talks to his character to extricate him from error. Finally the truth dawns on Narcissus: "He is I." Narcissus longs for nothing but death, and he wastes away in physical and mental starvation. Self-love turns into self-destruction. When Narcissus is gone, his beauty is preserved by his metamorphosis into a flower as white and pink as he used to be, and as fine, proud, and useless as he was.

The *Metamorphoses* is too long and somewhat repetitious. The range of Ovid's creative imagination was great but not unlimited, and the poet overtaxed his inventive powers. After book 11, the epic changes its character and no longer is there a bounty of short, tender, sentimental fables. An ambition for grandeur develops, and Ovid begins to insert massive compositions, each devoted to a single subject. In the last four books, he competes with historical epic and recounts patriotic legends.

The style of the *Metamorphoses* is so rich and varied as to make generalization difficult. The essential qualities of Ovid's narrative style are speed and vividness. A lead-in is provided for each story by a swift transition, and little time is wasted in introducing the new characters. The scenic descriptions with which a number of stories begin contribute both to the vividness of the scene (with their typical pool, wood, cave, and pattern of light and shade) and to the atmosphere, but the apparently tranquil or innocent elements of the setting portend, and are even symbolic of, danger or sexuality. The narrative itself can be elliptical and syncopated, even abrupt; details are carefully selected and highlighted in what is almost a cinematic technique. Similes are carefully used to create vividness or to emphasize violence and emotion, but they are rarely developed at such a length as to distract from the stories. The final metamorphosis often comes as an abrupt conclusion, even though its details are described with curious fascination. The verse itself flows smoothly and easily; the diction is straightforward but never dull.

Words are coined in moderation, and examples of archaism or vulgarism are rare.

Another important aspect of the style is its pervasive humor. Humor is notoriously difficult to analyze, but Ovid's sense of humor is implicit in his treatment of his material and is often underlined by asides and parentheses. It can frequently be seen in his humanization of the gods, his exploitation of the paradoxes of divine and human behavior, and his ironic attitude toward the credibility of his own stories. Ovid's literary humor is largely based on incongruity and exaggeration, together with an element of audacity.

At the end of his epic, Ovid boldly asserts that he will prove to be no less immortal or divine than the deified emperors. He has dared the supreme worldly power and predicts that the *Metamorphoses* will triumphantly survive. It did.

OTHER MAJOR WORK
PLAY: *Medea* (pr. before 8 C.E., fragment).

BIBLIOGRAPHY

Barchiesi, Alessandro. *The Poet and the Prince: Ovid and Augustan Discourse*. Berkeley: University of California Press, 1997. A scholarly assessment of Ovid's *Fasti* that examines pro-Augustan and anti-Augustan readings of the poem. Bibliography, index, index locorum.

Davis, P. J. *Ovid and Augustus: A Political Reading of Ovid's Erotic Poems*. London: Duckworth, 2007. In this volume, Davis discusses how the sexual nature of Ovid's poetry caused Roman emperor Augustus to send him into exile. Davis examines all of Ovid's poems, particularly *Art of Love*, to show how they express Ovid's views of erotic love and how they conflict with Augustus' definition of morality. Each chapter is devoted to a single one of Ovid's works and contains clear and convincing arguments to support Davis's view of Ovid and Augustus and their philosophies.

Hardie, Philip, ed. *The Cambridge Companion to Ovid*. New York: Cambridge University Press, 2002. Chapters by well-known scholars discuss Ovid, his backgrounds and contexts, the individual works, and its influence on later literature and art. Includes bibliography and index.

Holzberg, Niklas. *Ovid: The Poet and His Work*. Ithaca, N.Y.: Cornell University Press, 2002. A fine and readable examination of Ovid and his oeuvre.

Johnson, Patricia J. *Ovid Before Exile: Art and Punishment in the "Metamorphoses."* Madison: University of Wisconsin Press, 2008. Johnson argues that *Metamorphoses* breaks with epic tradition and shows evidence of the censorship caused by a need to please those in authority.

Knox, Peter E., ed. *A Companion to Ovid*. Malden, Mass.: Wiley-Blackwell, 2009. This collection of essays covers most of his poetic works and compares Ovid to both ancient and later poets.

_____. *Oxford Readings in Ovid*. New York: Oxford University Press, 2006. This collection of twenty of the most important essays on Ovid written by Latin scholars in the previous thirty years covers the full range of Ovid's poetic works.

Reeson, James E. *Ovid, "Heroides" 11, 13, and 14: A Commentary*. Leiden, the Netherlands: E. J. Brill, 2001. Close interpretation of these three verse epistles, introduced by an examination of Ovid's use of his sources and the epistle form.

Spencer, Richard A. *Contrast as Narrative Technique in Ovid's "Metamorphoses."* Lewiston, N.Y.: Edwin Mellen Press, 1997. A good discussion of Ovid's style and use of narrative. Includes bibliographical references and an index.

Williams, Gareth D. *Banished Voices: Readings in Ovid's Exile Poetry*. New York: Cambridge University Press, 1994. Examines the exile poetry in close readings that reveal the irony and hidden meanings of these poems, particularly the rift between Ovid's overt despair over his declining talents and the reality of the artistry of the poems. Bibliography, indexes of authors, passages cited, and words and themes.

Shelley P. Haley

P

GIOVANNI PASCOLI

Born: San Mauro di Romagna, Kingdom of Sardinia
(now San Mauro Pascoli, Italy); December 31,
1855

Died: Bologna, Italy; April 6, 1912

PRINCIPAL POETRY

Myricae, 1891

Poemetti, 1897

Canti di Castelvecchio, 1903

Poemi conviviali, 1904 (*Convivial Poems*, Part I,
1979, Part II, 1981)

Primi poemetti, 1904

Odi e inni, 1906

Canzoni di Re Enzio, 1908-1909

Nuovi poemetti, 1909

Inno a Torino, 1911

Poemi italici, 1911

Poesie, 1912

Poemi del risorgimento, 1913

Traduzioni e riduzioni, 1913

*Ioannis Pascoli carmina recognoscenda curavit
Maria Soror*, 1914

The Poems of Giovanni Pascoli, 1923

The Poems of Giovanni Pascoli, 1927

Selected Poems of Giovanni Pascoli, 1938

*Poesie con un profilo del Pascoli e un saggio di
Gianfranco Contini*, 1968 (4 volumes)

OTHER LITERARY FORMS

Giovanni Pascoli (POS-koh-lee) dabbled in Dante
criticism, and between 1898 and 1902 he wrote *Minerva oscura* (1898; dark Minerva), *Sotto il velame*
(1900; under the veil), and *La mirabile visione* (1902;
the marvelous vision). His assertion that *La divina
commedia* (c. 1320, 3 volumes; *The Divine Comedy*,
1802) "is not a strong and living poetic organism, a harmonious whole . . . but a great ocean, in which the po-

etic moments are the pearls" was not well received, although he did influence the views of the scholar Luigi
Pietrobono. Pascoli's critical essays are more revealing
of Pascoli himself than they are of the works that he
attempts to interpret. In defense of Italian colonial activity in Africa, Pascoli wrote the essay "La grande
proletaria s'e mossa" (the great proletariat has moved)
in 1911.

In his famous essay "Il fanciullino" (the little boy),
written in 1897, Pascoli explains his theory of poetry,
derived from the story of the child who led the blind
poet Homer by the hand. A true poet, says Pascoli, listens to the child within him, to what the child sees and
perceives. The blind man's *fanciullino* strives not to become famous but only to be understood. In his endeavor to present as many objects as a child sees in a
world that is always new and beautiful, Pascoli found
fault with literary Italian, cramped by classical tradition and condemned to an extremely restricting "poetic" vocabulary, and he invented words and borrowed
many others from the nonliterary dialects of Italy.
Pascoli's devotion to the child's perception ruled out
much of what is generally thought of as poetry (love
poetry, for example, and meditative poetry), and was so
limiting that criticism came swiftly, from Benedetto
Croce among others. Croce, who emphasized ideas
over the mere words that describe them, found Pascoli's valorization of childhood particularly offensive
and attacked Pascoli's poetry for its sentimentality, affectation, and childish emotionalism, claiming that it
seemed "to oscillate perpetually between a masterpiece
and a mess."

Pascoli was active as a translator. He translated folk
and heroic ballads (Breton, Greek, Illyrian) from the
anthologies of Vicomte Hersart de la Villemarqué,
Franz Passow, and Niccolò Tommaseo; sections of
Homer's *Iliad* (c. 750 B.C.E.; English translation, 1611)
and *Odyssey* (c. 725 B.C.E.; English translation, 1614);
and a wide range of classical works. He rendered into
Italian some of the Latin poetry of Pope Leo XIII and
several poems by Victor Hugo, Eduard Bauernfeld,
Friedrich Schiller, and José Antonio Calcaño. In addition, Pascoli translated Percy Bysshe Shelley's "Time
Long Past," Alfred, Lord Tennyson's "Ulysses," and
William Wordworth's "We Are Seven," the latter a

poem of special significance to Pascoli because of his own childhood experience with the death of family members.

ACHIEVEMENTS

As one of the nineteenth century triad—Giosuè Carducci, Gabriele D'Annunzio, and Giovanni Pascoli—of Italian literary greats, in company with the other two triads of Italian literature (Dante, Petrarch, and Giovanni Boccaccio; Alessandro Manzoni, Ugo Foscolo, and Giacomo Leopardi), Pascoli is one of the sacred nine included in every survey of literature course offered to Italian students.

While not as assertive or outspoken as Carducci or D'Annunzio, Pascoli was ultimately more influential than either. Some modern critics are offended by his sentimentality, but other aspects of his poetry in one way or another anticipated almost all Italian poetry that was to follow: the work of Guido Gozzano, Sergio Corazzini, Marino Moretti, and that group of poets known as the *crepuscolari*; Filippo Tommaso Marinetti and the Futurists; the Hermeticism of Eugenio Montale; and the religious poetry of Carlo Betocchi and Paolo De Benedetti. By translating his sense of the mystery of life into images and sounds, he anticipated the neutral, grayish tones of consciousness elaborated by the *crepuscolari*. His use of onomatopoeia, when successful, pointed the way to Marinetti's less successful "tumbtumb" and the like. Umberto Saba was influenced by Pascoli's use of humble subject matter, as were such local color poets as the Sicilians Lucio Piccolo and Giuseppe Villaroel. The tone of his *Myricae* (tamarisks) poems, when uncluttered by sentimental excesses, even points in the direction of Italian realism, the school of literature that came to be dominant after World War II.

Pascoli greatly enlarged the basic store of Italian poetic vocabulary. Even some of the dialectal words he introduced into his poems were used by subsequent poets, as, for example *cedrina* ("lemon verbena"; compare with the standard Italian *limoncina*), used by both Gozzano and Montale. Pascoli's interest in the common people has been described as nothing less than a poetic revolution which shifted the thematic and linguistic focus from the bourgeois to the petit bourgeois.

This "lowering" of poetic language is evident in Pascoli's easy recourse to dialect and common words as yet unconsecrated by literary usage. Pier Paolo Pasolini, who wrote his graduate thesis on Pascoli, found in this practice a point of departure for his own theories concerning the "reduction of poetic language."

Pascoli died in 1912 and was mourned throughout the entire Italian peninsula. His death was part of the inspiration for the moving pages of D'Annunzio's *Contemplazione della morte* (1912; the contemplation of death), the first canto of a prose poem trilogy.

BIOGRAPHY

Giovanni Pascoli was born in 1855 in the village of San Mauro di Romagna (later renamed San Mauro Pascoli) in what was then the papal state of Romagna, the fourth of ten children born to Ruggero and Caterina Vincenzi Alloccatelli Pascoli. He was a sensitive child, and he thrived in an idyllic family situation until the age of twelve, when his father was murdered. Ruggero Pascoli, the bailiff of the La Torre estate of the princely Torlonia family, was driving his carriage home on August 10, 1867, when someone fired a shot from behind a hedge; his dapple-gray mare ("La cavalla storna" of Pascoli's poem of that title) brought him home a corpse. The unexplained and unpunished crime marked Pascoli for life. His first volume of verse, *Myricae*, was dedicated to his father and includes a poem that describes the incident, "X agosto" ("The Tenth of August"). He wrote, "Reader, there were men who opened that tomb. And in it a whole flourishing family came to an end." Later, in the preface to *Canti di Castelvecchio* (songs of Castelvecchio), he added, "Other men, who remain unpunished and unknown, willed the death of a man not only innocent, but virtuous, sublime in his loyalty and goodness, and the death of his family. And I refuse. I refuse to let them be dead."

In 1868, the oldest Pascoli child, Margherita, died of typhoid at sixteen, and within a month, Pascoli's mother followed. Three years later, Luigi, Pascoli's next older brother, died of meningitis, and shortly after that Pascoli's fiancé died of tuberculosis. Five years later, his oldest brother, Giacomo, died, and then Giacomo's two small children. At the age of twenty-one, Pascoli became the head of a family consisting of his two younger brothers and two younger sisters, the latter still in a convent school. He possessed such a thorough familiarity with death that the worlds of life and death assumed for him a kind of parity, and he always numbered both the living and the dead when he counted the members of his family.

Despite the disintegration of his family, Pascoli was able to continue his studies with the brothers of the Scolopi Order at Urbino; later, he attended high school at Rimini and Florence. In 1873, he entered a competition for a scholarship to study at the University of Bologna, and the judges, among whom was Carducci, who later acted as Pascoli's mentor, awarded him first place. In 1879, he participated in a Socialist demonstration and spent three months in jail. As a result, he lost his scholarship, but he was able to regain it later. He took his degree in Greek literature in 1882 and went to teach at a *lycée* in far-off Matera in southern Italy, transferred to Massa in northern Tuscany, and then spent eight years at Leghorn. In 1895, he was able to purchase a comfortable home in the Serchio Valley among the Tuscan mountains at Castelvecchio di Barga and set up a household with his devoted sister, Maria. This was to be his home for life. Here he always returned to spend summers and whatever other free time he had; here he entertained such friends as composer Giacomo Puccini and author D'Annunzio; and here he shared his life with his dog Gulì, who often figures in his verse.

In 1895, Pascoli became a probationary teacher at the University of Bologna, and in 1897, he was appointed professor of Latin literature at Messina, in Sicily, where he remained until 1903. From there, he went on to Pisa and, upon the death of Carducci in 1907, was invited to assume Carducci's chair in Italian literature at Bologna.

From 1891 to 1911, Pascoli entered his own Latin poems in the yearly *Certamen poeticum hoeufftianum* (a competition in memory of the Dutch scholar Jacob Hoeufft) at the Amsterdam Academy of Sciences, and in thirteen of these years he won the highest award.

Pascoli remained a bachelor. His health began to fail in 1908 after he developed a tumor, and four years later, as he feverishly strove to complete unfinished projects, he died. He was buried in a chapel next to his home at Castelvecchio. His sister Maria, his lifelong devoted companion, was his literary executrix. The book Maria wrote about her brother, *Lungo la vita di Giovanni Pascoli* (1961; about the life of Giovanni Pascoli), appeared after her death in 1953.

ANALYSIS

Much of Giovanni Pascoli's poetry is autobiographical and touches upon his family, his home, the simple maritime and peasant folk he knew, his patriotism, his pessimism, and his obsession with death. His was a child's world of small actualities, and he wrote tenderly of children themselves. Predictably, some of his work borders on, or even crosses over into, the realm of the unabashedly sentimental.

Unlike Carducci, who unequivocally rejected Christianity, Pascoli called it "the poetry of the universe" and kept a candle lit before the Virgin's picture above his hearth. His attitude toward the Christian religion has been characterized by Ruth Shepard Phelps as indulgent rather than devout; she points out that when his dead speak to him, as in "Il giorno dei morti" ("All Souls' Day"), they address him from the tomb and not from Heaven. Nevertheless, he does not shy away from traditionally Christian themes: "La buona novella" ("The Good News"), appropriately placed at the end of his Hellenic *Convivial Poems*, heralds the age of a new humanitarianism and spares pagan Rome, "drunk with blood," no embarrassing details. In his Latin poetry especially, persecuted Christians figure prominently, as does Christ himself. In "Centurio," for example, an old centurion who has returned to Rome is surrounded by boys begging for tales of adventure; instead, he tells them of the four times he saw and heard one whom he last saw nailed upon the Cross.

Pascoli's classical interests are evident throughout his work, but his devotion to Greece and Rome functions not so much as a proud material possession, as it was for Carducci, or as a means to self-aggrandizement, as it was for D'Annunzio, but more as a wistful vision of a lost Eden to be recovered by a strategy as simple as assembling and savoring in a single work those Italian words that clearly mirror their Greek and Latin origins. As much as he loved the classical heritage of Greece and Rome, he could write in "Il fanciullino": "In our literary style we have taken the

Latins for our model, as they did the Greeks. This may have helped to give concreteness and dignity to our writings, but it has suffocated our poetry." Despite a few isolated attempts to pattern his verse on Greek and Latin cadences, Pascoli generally adheres to the prosody of Italian, excelling in his treatment of the traditional hendecasyllable.

Romantic love did not interest Pascoli (it is not love of beautiful women, he wrote in "Il fanciullino," that interests the child but rather tales of adventure: "bronze shields and war-chariots and distant journeys and storms at sea"), nor was he concerned with politics, his own psychology, or syllogistic reasoning. In place of romantic love, Pascoli substitutes love of nature and concerns himself with the entire gamut of natural phenomena, observing and interpreting their varying states with the touch of a master. This emphasis on the natural world sometimes involves a vein of mysticism, and despite his avowal that philosophy is too adult a matter for poetry, such poems as "Il ciocco" ("The Blockhead"; literally, "the log") and "La vertigine" ("Vertigo") are philosophical poems of cosmic imagination.

Much of his verse follows the pattern of common speech in its simplicity, novelty, and hesitation, and could be rewritten as prose. His unconventional rhythms resemble in some respects the poetry of Alexander Pushkin and the sprung rhythm of Gerard Manley Hopkins. Pascoli enjoyed using familiar forms but felt equally comfortable with forms of his own invention. He used alliteration and assonance extensively. Characteristic of his syntax (regarded at the time as daringly modern) is his oxymoronic pairing of contradictory words or ideas, such as "glauco pallore" (greenish pallor) or "la Vergine Maria piange un sorriso" (the Virgin Mary weeps a smile).

Pascoli stands out in the Italian poetic tradition for the quality of his language and for the individual words which he savored with the delight of a lexicographer. He does not hesitate to identify the humbler things of life by their even humbler dialectal designations, and he makes bold use of archaic Italian words and Latinate borrowings for special effect, of the pidgin Italian of returning emigrants, of childlike expressions, and of onomatopoeia. In the preface to the second edition of *Canti di Castelvecchio*, Pascoli thought it necessary to add an

apologia for his use of so many dialectal words, insisting that the peasants speaking their dialects "speak better than we do," with their crude and pithy utterances. Pascoli thus anticipated by half a century the more extreme indulgences of descriptive linguistics.

Birds are important in the poetry of Pascoli—not only the romantic species such as larks and nightingales, but also the more plebeian sparrows, wrens, kites, plovers, shrikes, robins, and finches. Pascoli rendered bird and animal sounds as he heard them, from the charming *ku kuof* of the turtledove, *uid uid* of the lark, and *tri tri* of the cricket to the ridiculous extremes of the *tellterelltellteretelltell* of the sparrow, the *zisteretetet* of the titmouse, and the *addio addio dio dio dio dio* of the nightingale. In the poem "Un ricordo" (a memory), a scene of great poignance, describing the last time his mother sees his father before the latter's murder, is staged against a backdrop of brooding turtledoves making *hu hu* sounds; even in recounting such a moment, Pascoli could not forgo his fondness for onomatopoeia.

MYRICAE

Pascoli began to write poetry before 1880, but his first collection of poems, called *Myricae*, patterned on the eclogues of Vergil and symbolic of the humbler forms of rural poetry, was not published until 1891. The poems portray the minute distinctions of form or sound or action that the poet liked to observe, and in *Myricae*, as later in the *Canti di Castelvecchio*, there is an intimation of death, as though the tragic mourning of the poet was always there behind every vision. In the preface to *Canti di Castelvecchio*, he justified this obsession with death: "Life without thought of death, this is to say, without religion, which is what distinguishes us from the animals, is a madness, either intermittent or continuous, either expressionless or tragic."

In the first poem in *Myricae*, "All Souls' Day," Pascoli envisions the dead members of his family speaking from their graves one cold rainy night. The storm rages, the water streams down the crosses, and his father moans his ever-yearning words amid the rhythms of the pelting rain. Ruggero Pascoli forgives his unknown killer, adding that if the murderer has no children, he can never know what sorrow he has caused. He asks a blessing for his own surviving children, that they be granted the capacity to forget, because for him there is no forgetting, and no rest.

"Romagna" ("The Romagna"), dedicated to Pascoli's friend Severino Ferrari, who is addressed in the second line of the poem, is generally taken as one of the poems which most clearly reveals the influence of Carducci, but it already shows in tone and detail the individual route that Pascoli would take. Sunny Romagna, the scene of his happy childhood, is recalled: the farmhands eating lunch, the child taking refuge from the dazzling sun in the shade of a mimosa tree to read tales of chivalry. Then, one black day, all the Pascolis scatter like swallows, and "homeland" for the poet is now merely "where one lives."

In the epigrammatic "Morte e sole" ("Death and the Sun"), Pascoli plays with the irony that the sun, supposedly the source of light and life, while symbolic of enlightenment, is also a symbol and revelation of death. When the eye looks upon the sun, it does not see light but instead blackness, a void. Nicholas Perella observes that Pascoli has here taken François de La Rochefoucauld's maxim ("One cannot look fixedly upon either the sun or death") and, by emphasizing the blackness, has refashioned La Rochefoucauld's original intention into an existential joke.

POEMETTI

Pascoli's next work, *Poemetti* (minor poems), later incorporated in *Primi poemetti* (first minor poems) and *Nuovi poemetti* (new minor poems), shifts from the lyrical emphasis of *Myricae* to the short narrative. Modeled upon Homer and Vergil and championing the outdated position that an emphasis on agricultural interests produces a healthy society, the poems chronicle the seasonal activities of a peasant family. Pascoli is also concerned here for the plight of Italians forced to emigrate for economic reasons, and in a longer poem titled "Italy" (the original title is in English), he writes of a family returning to Italy from Cincinnati, Ohio; they speak a kind of pidgin Italian that incorporates many English words.

CANTI DI CASTELVECCHIO

Pascoli's next book of poetry, *Canti di Castelvecchio*, contains more autobiographical poems and is often viewed as the peak of his poetic achievement. It includes the classic "La cavalla storna" ("The Dapple-grey Mare"), written in *laisses* of rhymed hendecasyllabic couplets that many Italian schoolchildren have been required to memorize. Pascoli felt great affection for the mare that loyally drew her master's body to his home and who alone knew the identity of his murderer, and the poem recalls Pascoli's mother's attempt to extract an identification from the little mare by means of a sign or a sound. The poem "La voce" ("The Voice") was a product of Pascoli's dark and lean years after his expulsion from the university. One night, while crossing the river Reno, weeping bitterly because he feels he must commit suicide, he hears his mother address him by his childhood nickname, "Zvanì," and the mysterious message blocks his resolution to die, imbuing him instead with the courage to live. The sentimentality inherent in the poem is counteracted somewhat by Pascoli's grotesquely effective assertion that his mother cannot be speaking to him, for in reality "her mouth is full of earth."

CONVIVIAL POEMS

In *Convivial Poems*, named for the impressive but short-lived review *Convito* (1895-1907) of Adolfo De Bosis in which Pascoli first published some of the poems included in the collection, the poet directs his attention to those readers capable of appreciating the values of the classical world. He refers to the demise of the review in the opening line of the first selection, "Solon" ("Sad is a banquet without song, sad as/ a temple without the gold of votive gifts"), and proceeds to discuss the enduring nature of poetry. In "Anticlus," the poet attempts to convey the incomparable beauty of the Greek Helen, and in the "Poemi di Psiche" ("Poems of Psyche"), the pantheism of the first segment, "Psiche" ("Psyche"), stands in contrast to the immortality of the soul put forth in the second, "Il gufo" ("The Owl"), a retelling of the story of the death of Socrates. In "Alèxandros" ("Alexander the Great"), the great conqueror appears at the end of his career to lament that there is nothing more on earth for him to win ("Oh! happier was I when a longer road/ lay before me"). He concludes that it is better to be able to hope and dream ("the dream is the infinite shade of the Truth") than to possess material things.

The atmospheric effects of Pascoli's introspective poems invite comparison with the work of such poets as Thomas Hardy, Paul Verlaine, Stéphane Mallarmé, and Maurice Maeterlinck. Indeed, Pascoli is a difficult poet to translate precisely because much of his work depends more on atmosphere and vocabulary than on form and idea. Pascoli did Italian literature an inestimable service by extending the vocabulary of poetry beyond the bounds of tradition and by offering it the benefit of countless new and daring images and analogies. His influence on later writers has been so great that the large body of distinguished Italian poetry written during the twentieth century would probably have been far less impressive without his example and leadership.

OTHER MAJOR WORKS

NONFICTION: *Minerva oscura*, 1898; *Sotto il velame*, 1900; *La mirabile visione*, 1902; *Pensieri e discorsi*, 1907; *Scritti danteschi*, 1952; *Lettere a Maria Novaro e ad altri amici*, 1971.

EDITED TEXTS: *Epos*, 1897; *Lyra*, 1899; *Sul limitare*, 1900; *Fior da fiore*, 1902.

BIBLIOGRAPHY

Brand, Peter, and Lino Pertile, eds. *The Cambridge History of Italian Literature*. Rev. ed. New York: Cambridge University Press, 1999. Includes introductory information on Pascoli's life and work and pertinent historical background.

Donadoni, Eugenio. *A History of Italian Literature*. Translated by Richard Monges. New York: New York University Press, 1969. Contains introductory biographical and critical information on Pascoli's life and work.

LaValva, RosaMaria. *The Eternal Child: The Poetry and Poetics of Giovanni Pascoli*. Chapel Hill, N.C.: Annals of Italian Studies, 1999. A critical interpretation of Pascoli's "Il fanciullino" with the text of the poem in English and Italian. Includes bibliographical references and index.

Perugi, Maurizio. "The Pascoli-Anderton Correspondence." *Modern Language Review* 85, no. 3 (July, 1990): 595. An analysis of the correspondence between Isabella Anderton and Pascoli, including the text of some of their letters.

_____. "Pascoli, Shelley, and Isabella Anderton, 'Gentle Rotskettow.'" *Modern Language Review* 84, no. 1 (January, 1989): 50. A discussion of the English attributes of Pascoli's work and the influence Percy Bysshe Shelley had on Pascoli's poetry.

Phelps, Ruth Shepard. *Italian Silhouettes*. Freeport, N.Y.: Books for Libraries Press, 1968. Provides brief historical background to the works of Pascoli and other Italian literature.

Truglio, Maria. *Beyond the Family Romance: The Legend of Pascoli*. Toronto, Ont.: University of Toronto Press, 2007. Truglio takes a Freudian approach to Pascoli, placing him in the context of the fin de siècle and Scapigliatura movement. Works discussed include *Convivial Poems* and poems from *Myricae*.

Jack Shreve

PIER PAOLO PASOLINI

Born: Bologna, Italy; March 5, 1922
Died: Ostia, Italy; November 2, 1975

PRINCIPAL POETRY

Poesie a Casarsa, 1942
La meglio gioventù, 1954
Le ceneri de Gramsci, 1957 (*The Ashes of Gramsci*, 1982)
L'usignolo della chiesa cattolica, 1958
La religione del mio tempo, 1961
Poesia in forma di rosa, 1964
Poesie, 1970
Trasumanar e organizzar, 1971
La nuova gioventù, 1975
Poems, 1982
Roman Poems, 1986
Poetry, 1991

OTHER LITERARY FORMS

Pier Paolo Pasolini (pos-oh-LEE-nee) was a critic, philologist, film director, playwright, translator, and novelist as well as a poet. His first novel, *Ragazzi di vita* (1955; *The Ragazzi*, 1968), based on rigorous sociological, ethnographic, and linguistic observation, chronicles the street life of shantytown adolescents through dialogue, flashbacks, and direct intrusions by the author; Pasolini makes original and abundant use of slang and street language. Within three months after the book appeared, the prime minister's office reported it to the public prosecutor in Milan for its "pornographic content," and Pasolini was brought to trial. Similar controversies recurred throughout Pasolini's career as a writer and film director.

ACHIEVEMENTS

Outside Italy, Pier Paolo Pasolini is better known as a director of films than as a poet, and even within Italy, it was not until nearly a decade after his death that his poetic talent was fully appreciated. His poetry is considered the most important in Italy after Giuseppe Ungaretti's generation and ranks with the work of Bertolt Brecht and Pablo Neruda as among the most powerful political poetry of the twentieth century. At the time of Pasolini's early education, a triad of nineteenth century poets (Giosuè Carducci, Giovanni Pascoli, and Gabriele D'Annunzio), fond of artificial language and classical literary convention, ruled Italian letters; they were followed by the Hermetic school of poetry (Umberto Saba, Ungaretti, Eugenio Montale), which emphasized personal expression and symbolic density.

Both schools were disdainful of social commentary in poetry. After the fiasco of Italian fascism, however, the politically responsive neorealist was born in Italy, and it was within the framework of neorealism that Pasolini worked. When *The Ashes of Gramsci* appeared in 1957, it broke a long line of pure lyric and Hermetic poetry in Italy: The poet described his own inner conflict between reason and instinct, between nostalgia for the past and the need for a new order, using a straightforward Italian diction free of the Latinate loftiness to which his poetic predecessors had necessarily been bound.

BIOGRAPHY

Pier Paolo Pasolini was the first of two sons born to Carlo Alberto Pasolini and Susanna Colussi Pasolini. Pasolini's father, though from an aristocratic Bolo-

gnese family, was reduced to poverty and became a soldier. Until his death in 1958, his life was a dream of military and fascist ideals, and after his discharge from the military, he became an alcoholic. It was with the petite bourgeoisie background of his mother's family of the Friuli area (in the northeastern corner of Italy, bordered by Austria and Yugoslavia) that the poet identified. Pasolini's mother, who had inherited her Hebrew name from a great-grandmother who was a Polish Jew, was a schoolteacher and already thirty when she was married.

Pasolini's family followed his father to wherever he was stationed in Northern Italy. His parents' marriage was turbulent and marked by frequent temporary separations, and his mother channeled all her love into her relationship with her sons, especially her older son. Indeed, the relationship between Pasolini and his mother, whom he would one day cast as the Virgin Mary in his film *Il vangelo secondo Matteo* (1964; *The Gospel According to St. Matthew*, 1964), was animated by an un-

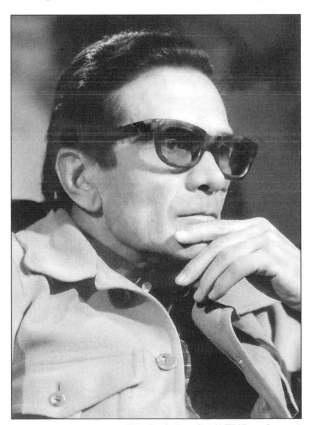

Pier Paolo Pasolini (AFP/Getty Images)

equivocally incestuous tension. When Pasolini and his mother moved to Rome without his father in 1945, his mother took a position as a maid to support her son's literary aspirations. The image of his "artless, eternally youthful mother" pervades all the poet's work.

In high school in Bologna, after Pasolini's inevitable exposure to the poetry of Carducci, Pascoli, and D'Annunzio, one of his teachers read to him a poem by Arthur Rimbaud. Later, Pasolini claimed that his conversion away from fascism dated from that day; he also wrote that after Rimbaud, poetry was dead. William Shakespeare was another early discovery, and Pasolini's reading of Niccolò Tommaseo's compilation, *I canti del popolo greco* (1943; songs of the Greek people), did much to awaken Pasolini's appreciation of the folk culture of his mother's Friuli. Shakespeare, Tommaseo, and Carducci constituted Pasolini's personal triad, recognized as such in "La religione del mio tempo" (the religion of my time). He came early under the spell of the Provençal *trobar clus* as well, and he considered himself a disciple of the Spanish poet Antonio Machado.

In the winter of 1942-1943, Pasolini's mother moved back to Friuli to avoid the bombings in the larger cities. Most of the following year, which Pasolini called the most beautiful of his life, was spent there with his mother and brother. That September, he was drafted, but a week later, on the day of Italy's truce with the Allies, he escaped into a canal as his column of recruits was marched to a train en route to Germany. In April, 1944, his brother Guido went to the mountains to join the Osoppo-Friuli partisan division. He and some comrades were captured by the Communist Garibaldi Brigade, politically tied to Marshal Tito's fighters and favoring the incorporation of Friuli into the emerging nation of Yugoslavia; the comrades were later slain. The death of Guido was deeply traumatic to Pasolini and embarrassing to him as the Communist he would soon become.

Pasolini taught briefly in a private school, became involved in the local politics of Friuli, wrote for the local newspapers, and at length established himself as a Communist. With his maturity in the 1940's, he began to feel increasing guilt for his homosexuality, guilt he dwelt on in his unpublished diaries (written from 1945 to 1949), from which he later extracted the completed whole of *L'usignolo della chiesa cattolica* (the nightingale of the Catholic Church). Repeatedly, he writes of "being lost," of being dominated by the "slave penis." By 1949, Pasolini's sexual acts with other men were such that attempts were made to blackmail him, and he was formally charged by the magistrate of San Vito al Tagliamento with corrupting minors and committing lewd acts in public. Before the *carabinieri* of Casarsa, by whom he was also summoned, he defended himself by invoking the name of André Gide, who had won the Nobel Prize in Literature in 1947, and by describing his activities as an "erotic and literary experiment." Although Pasolini was acquitted in 1952, the fact that he did not deny the charge led the executive committee of the Communist Federation of Pordenone to expel him from the Italian Communist Party for moral and political unworthiness. It was a triple blow: Friuli had turned its back on him, his party had rejected him, and he had lost his teaching position. In a letter to a member of the Udine Federation, he declared his intention to remain a Communist and to persist in living for the sake of his mother, although another person might consider suicide. In the winter of 1949, he fled with her to Rome.

Pasolini's first few years in Rome were difficult, but the eternity and modernity of Rome captivated him, and he thrived on the sexual freedom that the metropolis afforded him. A teaching position was secured for him in 1951, and soon he was writing for *Il popolo di Roma, Il giornale* of Naples, and *Il lavoro* of Genoa. He cemented friendships with writers such as Giorgio Bassani, Alberto Moravia, Elsa Morante, Attilio Bertolucci, and Federico Fellini, whom he helped with the Roman dialect of Fellini's 1956 film *Le notti di Cabiria* (*The Nights of Cabiria*, 1957). In 1952, Pasolini tied for second place and won 50,000 lire in the Quattro Arti contest in Naples for his article on Ungaretti.

The years from 1953 to 1961 were the most productive of Pasolini's career. He published two novels, four books of poetry, and the critical essays collected in *Passione e ideologia* (1960; passion and ideology), and from 1955 to 1959, he directed the literary magazine *Officina*. He wrote thirteen film scripts, translated the *Oresteia* of Aeschylus, and directed and scripted his first film, *Accattone* (1961). Rome was alive in those years with intellectual creativity and political ferment, but as exciting as it was for Pasolini, it also took its toll on him. For the first time, he found himself getting involved with literary projects merely because he needed a public; he was plagued by litigation and by vicious journalistic attacks.

After his debut in the world of filmmaking, Pasolini's life changed course. His fertile mind seethed with new ideas, and the names of far-flung places began to appear in his work. In 1966, he made his first visit to New York, where he sought out young revolutionary blacks in Harlem and was mightily impressed by the potential he discovered in the United States. Two years later, he was deeply disillusioned by the "tragedy-revolt" of the student riots of 1968; in his view, the youth, who had been cradled by the class struggle, had sold out to the bourgeoisie. Between 1970 and 1975, he made a successful and controversial trilogy of films—*Il decamerone* (1971; *The Decameron*, 1975), *I racconti di Canterbury* (1972; *The Canterbury Tales*, 1975), and *Il fiore belle mille e una notte* (1974; *The Arabian Nights*, 1975)—based on his belief that the "last bastion of reality seemed to be the 'innocent' bodies, with the archaic, dark, vital violence of their sexual organs." In the *Corriere della Sera* of June 5, 1975, however, he repudiated this notion, claiming that "even the 'reality' of innocent bodies has been violated, manipulated, tampered with by the power of consumerism." Pasolini's polemics against the consumer society had become harangues, and the poet did not seem to have any cures to offer for the ills he so vehemently identified. His output in his last years was increasingly complex and contradictory.

The exact circumstances of Pasolini's death may never be clearly established. Late on the evening of November 1, 1975, Pasolini set off in his Alfa Romeo GT and picked up a street hustler named Giuseppe Pelosi. On the beach at Ostia, the two of them struggled, Pasolini was struck on the head with a board, and Pelosi subsequently ran over Pasolini with his own car. Because the boy was unmarked, however, and because he gave a confused testimony, there is some reason to believe that Pelosi was merely an agent for others who had more reason than he to eliminate Pasolini.

ANALYSIS

As a writer and as a man, Pier Paolo Pasolini was one of the most complex figures of twentieth century literature, and his life and work are replete with paradoxes. Despite his belief that his leftist poetry was different from all other poetry being written, he employed the hendecasyllable, the most widely used meter in all Italian verse in all periods, and the terza rima of Dante. He rebelled against Italy's long-entrenched cultural traditionalism yet declared himself a lover of tradition whom it pained to witness the disappearance of Italian peasant culture. He was a Marxist and at the same time did not abandon the Roman Catholic Church; he condemned abortion and called on the Church to lead the fight away from the materialism that was gaining such a stranglehold on capitalistic societies everywhere. With his romantic spirit of identifying with the outcasts of the earth, Marxism came easily to him, but as a gay man, his Marxism demanded a morality that allowed for the individual. His religion was the liberation of the masses, yet he chose to focus not on their struggle but rather on their vindicated joy. Although he professed to love the common people, such people as individuals figure little in his poetry. His style in both his poetry and his films was stark and unsentimental, yet he could wax fulsome and self-indulgent when writing on the subject of his mother.

POESIE A CASARSA

To some extent, these contradictions were apparent in Pasolini's earliest, dialect poems. As a result of the breakup of the Roman Empire and the late emergence of Italy as a political entity, Italy inherited a multiplicity of dialects, substantially more varied than the dialects of most other Western European nations. Pasolini by nature felt attracted by the sound of his mother's dialect, Friulian, and, impressed by Paul Valéry's "hésitation prolongée entre le sens et le son," he opted for the sound element. He wrote his first volume of poetry, *Poesie a Casarsa* (poetry to Casarsa), in Friulian, publishing it privately in Bologna in 1942 and dedicating it to his father. When the slim volume of forty-six pages was reviewed, the review had to be printed in Switzerland, for dialect literature was very much anathema to the fascist regime. In addition to the scandal implicit in using an Italian dialect for a literary endeavor, Pasolini's medium was a special, less-recognized dialect within Friulian, distinct from the standardized jargon used by Friulian poets Ermes de Colloredo in the seventeenth century and Pietro Zorutti in the nineteenth century.

Pasolini consolidated *Poesie a Casarsa* with a group of Resistance poems known as Il testamento Coran (the Qurʾān testament) and with several others written in Friulian, and published *La meglio gioventù* (the finest youth) in 1954. In all these poems, the poet yearns for a recovery of moral health to be achieved through a reacquaintance with the peasant's world, and he treats the themes of nature, a boy's happiness with his mother, and the exhilaration of the company of beautiful young men. In "Il dí la me muàrt" ("The Day of My Death"), for example, the poet tells of one who loved boys and "wrote/ poems of holiness/ believing that in this way/ his heart would become larger." In 1975, Pasolini made another consolidation and published *La nuova gioventù* (the new youth), in which he combined the poetry of *La meglio gioventù* with a reworked version of two parts of that book and with some new Italo-Friulian pieces composed in 1973-1974.

THE ASHES OF GRAMSCI

The Ashes of Gramsci contains poems, dated carefully but not arranged in chronological order, that probe the poet's difficulties with a Marxism that in actual practice seeks to limit the expression of the individual spirit. The title poem, "The Ashes of Gramsci," takes its name from the words on Antonio Gramsci's grave in the English cemetery in Rome, not far from Percy Bysshe Shelley's. Gramsci, the Italian Marxist political philosopher whose works were written while he was imprisoned by the fascists, had made loud charges that Italian literature was run by elitists more interested in eloquence and style than in people.

The first poems in *The Ashes of Gramsci*, "L'Appennino" (Apennine) and "Il canto popolare" (the popular song), written during the poet's early days of residence in Rome, compare the grand Italy of the past with present conditions, in which major cities are besieged by hordes of impoverished immigrants from the poorer southern regions. It is in these poor people, however, living in pigsty encampments "between the shining modern churches and skyscrapers," that the poet's

hope resides. In "Picasso," the poet focuses on the committed and socially responsive artist amid a decaying society, decreeing that "The way out/ . . . is by remaining/ inside the inferno with the cold/ determination to understand it," and not in Picasso's "idyll of white orangutans." "The Ashes of Gramsci," the central poem in the collection, probes the contrast between bourgeois society and Marxist commitment, between the ideal of freedom and the imperfect and irrational life as it is. Before Gramsci's grave and addressing him on a cloudy May day in a "scandal of self-contradiction," the poet declares himself to be "with you and against you." The poem is replete with oxymorons which create a mood of excruciating tension.

"Récit" stems from the poet's outrage at the obscenity charges brought against him for *The Ragazzi*, while the last three poems in the volume, all written in 1956, in some way reflect the trauma of Nikita Khrushchev's anti-Stalin campaign, the revelation of Joseph Stalin's crimes, and the subsequent Soviet invasion of Hungary. In "Il pianto della scavatrice" ("The Tears of the Excavator"), the symbolic machine transforms the earth and wails for change. This longest poem in the collection contains bright glimmers of hope, as the poet speaks glowingly of a Rome that taught him the grandeur of little things and taught him how to address another man without trembling—a Rome where the world became for him the subject "no longer of mystery but of history."

"Una polemica in versi" (a polemic in verse), clearly the result of the news of the Soviet invasion of Hungary, accuses the party of usurping the glory that rightfully belongs to the people and urges a hypothetical militant Communist to declare his error and his guilt. The poem ends with a panorama of the hopeful young characterized by "shameless generosity" against a backdrop of older people, aware of defeat and in various states of drunkenness, uncertainty, and disappointment.

The last poem in the volume, "Land of Work," stands in contrast to the first poem, "L'Appennino," in its less sanguine view of the potential of the poor. The Southern Italian peasants that the poet observes here belong more to the realm of the dead than to the living, and their prehistorical condition is underscored by a series of subhuman similes involving dogs, sheep, and other animals. Where there had been a hunger "taking the name of hope," now "every inner light, every act/ of conscience" seems to be a thing of yesterday. For once, the poet has no compassion to give: "You lose yourself in an inner paradise/ and even your pity is their enemy."

LA RELIGIONE DEL MIO TEMPO

La religione del mio tempo appeared the same year (1961) as Pasolini's first film, *Accattone*. The poet seems deliberately to abstain from direct political involvement here, but he is humiliated by the corruption of all attempts to renew society. For the first time, Pasolini experiments with epigrams, but often they do not rise above expressing a mere self-pity. Africa, unsullied by the bourgeois taint, comes into view for the first time as the poet's "only alternative." There are poems of memory, poems of love for boys, and poems wherein little hope abides. In "To an Unborn Child," Pasolini grieves not at all for his "first and only child" who can never exist. In "To a Boy," a poem of praise for the inquisitiveness of young Bernardo Bertolucci, later to become a prominent film director in his own right, Pasolini concludes in the style of Giacomo Leopardi: "Ah, what you wish to know, young man/ will end up unasked, it will be lost unspoken." In "Sex, Consolation for Misery," he characterizes sex as "filthy and ferocious as an ancient mother" but concedes that "in the easiness of love/ one who is wretched can feel like a man." The title poem, "La religione del mio tempo" ("The Religion of My Time"), is the longest in the collection; in it, the poet isolates cowardice and its product, materialism ("All possessions are alike: whether/ industry or pasture, ship or pushcart"), as the disease and symptom plaguing modern society, and points an accusing finger at the "Vile disciples of a corrupted Jesus/ in the Vatican salons . . ./ strong over a people of serfs."

If there is any light in all this gloom, it shines forth from Pasolini's mother alone, and in an unusually self-indulgent "Appendice alla 'Religione': Uno luce" ("Appendix to the 'Religion': A Light"), Pasolini celebrates her "poor sweet little bones" and longs for the day when they will be together in the Casarsa cemetery, where "passion/ keeps the bones of the other son/ still alive in frozen peace."

POESIA IN FORMA DI ROSA

Poesia in forma di rosa (poetry in the form of a rose), which appeared in 1964, is a poetic diary that includes Pasolini's description of the trial provoked by the episode titled "La Ricotta" in the film *Rogopag* (1962); Pasolini was charged with insulting the Roman Catholic Church. Another section, "Worldly Poems," represents the diary he kept during the filming of *Mamma Roma* (1962); there is also a "Progetto di opere future" ("Plan of Future Works") and an account of his tours of Israel and Southern Italy while filming *The Gospel According to St. Matthew*. In the first part of the book, he employs the tercet, but in the rest, he employs the loose hendecasyllable, rhythmic prose, and a geometric arrangement of words on the page. The poetry is imbued with Pasolini's sense of his own unidentifiable, obsessive error: "I who by the excess of my presence/ have never crossed the border between love/ for life and life." Ideology is a drug, and the moralists have made socialism as boring as Catholicism. When the poet cries that "only a bloodbath can save the world/ from its bourgeois dreams," the effect is immediately undone by "This is what a prophet would shout/ who doesn't have/ the strength to kill a fly." His insistent pursuit of the consolation of sex with strangers is defended: "Better death/ than to renounce it"; the search, he claims, is for the "enchantment of the species" rather than for the perfect individual. His mother is here as well, the object of his prayer in "Supplica a mia madre" ("Prayer to My Mother") requesting that she please not die and proclaiming that she is, as his readers well know, irreplaceable to him.

TRASUMANAR E ORGANIZZAR

In 1971, Pasolini published *Trasumanar e organizzar* (to transfigure and to organize). The volume consists of three parts: a private diary; a collection of lyrics written to Maria Callas, with whom Pasolini worked while filming *Medea* (1969; *Medea*, 1970), and a section of wholly political poems. The collection also contains Pasolini's first elaboration in poetry of his frustrated relationship with his father, and his single serene love poem, written in 1969 to Nino Davoli, whom Pasolini had discovered in the Roman slums while preparing for *The Gospel According to St. Matthew*. Not all the poems are dated, but most of them were written after 1968. The title refers to the polarity between the spiritual ascent and the institutionalization or organization of humankind, the thematic points between which Pasolini moves with alternating sarcasm and heartbreak. The title piece is a polemic against the Italian Communist Party; youth protest, in which he had placed so much hope, is now represented as the irrational behavior of unknowingly bourgeois children. The keynote of the collection is the contradictory, bewildering nature of contemporary reality and the poet's pathetic awareness that he can neither enter into that reality nor even claim a precise role in it: a fitting note for the conclusion of Pasolini's turbulent poetic career.

OTHER MAJOR WORKS

LONG FICTION: *Ragazzi di vita*, 1955 (*The Ragazzi*, 1968); *Una vita violenta*, 1959 (*A Violent Life*, 1978).

SCREENPLAYS: *Accattone*, 1961; *Mamma Roma*, 1962; "La Ricotta," 1962; *Comizi d'amore*, 1964; *Il vangelo secondo Matteo*, 1964 (*The Gospel According to St. Matthew*, 1964); *Uccellacci e uccellini*, 1966; *Edipo re*, 1967 (*Oedipus Rex*, 1967); *Teorema*, 1968 (*Theorem*, 1969); *Medea*, 1969 (*Medea*, 1970); *Il decamerone*, 1971 (*The Decameron*, 1975); *I racconti di Canterbury*, 1972 (*The Canterbury Tales*, 1975); *Il fiore belle mille e una notte*, 1974 (*The Arabian Nights*, 1975); *Il padre selvaggio*, 1975 (*The Savage Father*, 1999); *Salò o le 120 giornate de Sodoma*, 1975 (*Salò: Or, 120 Days of Sodom*, 1975).

NONFICTION: *Passione e ideologia*, 1960; *La poesia populare italiana*, 1960; *Scritti corsari*, 1975; *Lettere luterane*, 1976 (*Lutheran Letters*, 1983); *The Letters of Pier Paolo Pasolini*, 1992.

EDITED TEXTS: *Poesia dialettale del novecento*, 1952; *Canzoniere italiano: Antologia della poesia popolare*, 1955.

MISCELLANEOUS: *Alì dagli occhi azzurri*, 1965; *La divina mimesis*, 1975 (*The Divine Mimesis*, 1980); *San Paolo*, 1977 (*Saint Paul*, 1980).

BIBLIOGRAPHY

Baranski, Zygmunt G., ed. *Pasolini Old and New: Surveys and Studies*. Dublin: Four Courts Press, 1999. A collection of biographical and critical essays on Pasolini. Includes bibliographical references and indexes.

Chiesi, Roberto, and Andrea Mancini, eds. *Pier Paolo Pasolini: Poet of Ashes*. San Francisco: City Lights Books, 2007. This work is a mixture of poetry in Italian with English translations, essays, and interviews. Provides information on his life and critical analysis of his works.

Gordon, Robert S. C. *Pasolini: Forms of Subjectivity*. New York: Oxford University Press, 1996. Gordon analyzes Pasolini's intensely charged, experimental essays, poetry, cinema, and narrative, and their shifting perspectives of subjectivity.

Lawton, Ben, and Maura Bergonzoni, eds. *Pier Paolo Pasolini: In Living Memory*. Washington, D.C.: New Academia, 2009. This work examines the legacy of Pasolini and his influence on art in Italy and abroad.

Pasolini, Pier Paolo. *The Letters of Pier Paolo Pasolini*. Edited by Nico Naldini. London: Quartet Books, 1992. A collection of Pasolini's correspondence translated into English that provides invaluable insight into his life and work.

Rohdie, Sam. *The Passion of Pier Paolo Pasolini*. Bloomington: Indiana University Press, 1995. A critical study that is primarily concerned with Pasolini's work in film but also provides valuable biographical information.

Rumble, Patrick, and Bart Testa, eds. *Pier Paolo Pasolini: Contemporary Perspectives*. Buffalo, N.Y.: University of Toronto Press, 1994. A collection of essays that explore the work of Pasolini and his time with the Communist Party. From the 1990 conference "Pier Paolo Pasolini: Heretical Imperatives" held in Toronto.

Jack Shreve

CESARE PAVESE

Born: Santo Stefano Belbo, Italy; September 9, 1908

Died: Turin, Italy; August 27, 1950

PRINCIPAL POETRY

Lavorare stanca, 1936, expanded 1943 (*Hard Labor*, 1976)

La terra e la morte, 1947

Verrà la morte e avrà i tuoi occhi, 1951

Poesie edite e inedite, 1962

A Mania for Solitude: Selected Poems, 1930-1950, 1969

Disaffections: Complete Poems, 1930-1950, 2002

OTHER LITERARY FORMS

Cesare Pavese (pah-VAY-zay) was primarily a novelist. He wrote nine novels, beginning with *Paesi tuoi* in 1941 (*The Harvesters*, 1961). His nonfiction *Dialoghi con Leucò* (1947; *Dialogues with Leucò*, 1966) and the novel *La luna e i falò* (1950; *The Moon and the Bonfire*, 1952) are considered his masterpieces. Pavese is noted for dealing with classical myths and writing about characters from the countryside. R. W. Flint translated a selection of his fiction, and many of his works of fiction continue to be available in English.

Pavese was also a respected essayist. In his expanded edition of *Hard Labor*, published in 1943, he included two highly valued essays: "The Poet's Craft" and "Concerning Certain Poems Not Yet Written." His other essays were published posthumously as *La letteratura americana e altri saggi*, edited by Italo Calvino, in 1951. In 1970, they were translated in English by Edwin Fussell as *American Literature: Essays and Opinions*.

Pavese was also an accomplished translator of English works into Italian. He began with Sinclair Lewis's *Our Mr. Wrenn* in 1931. He went on to translate such authors as Herman Melville, James Joyce, Sherwood Anderson, and William Faulkner. His diaries and letters were also published.

ACHIEVEMENTS

Cesare Pavese was one of a group of writers to come to maturity during the mid-1930's. He is noted for his antifascist efforts and his commitment to other left-wing causes, and he was even imprisoned for his activities. His first volume of poetry, *Hard Labor*, published in 1936 and expanded in 1943, considered one of his major achievements, has been translated into English by such writers as Margaret Crosland and William Arrowsmith. Several poems were censored by the authorities, a testimony to Pavese's subversive political thinking. Pavese concentrated on prose in the years following World War II, but he returned to verse a few years before his death, first publishing a group of poems called *La terra e la morte* in a magazine. These poems have a stark, lyrical quality to them. In 1950, Cesare Pavese received the Strega Prize, Italy's greatest literary award.

BIOGRAPHY

Cesare Pavese was born to parents Eugenio Pavese and Consolina Pavese in 1908, at their family vacation spot in the Piedmont region of Italy. The family, which included an older daughter, lived in Turin. His father worked as a bailiff in the court system. When Pavese was six years old, his father died. He started writing poetry while still in secondary school. In 1923, Pavese entered the Liceo Massimo d'Azeglio to complete his high school studies. Agusto Monti became his teacher and mentor. In 1926, Pavese entered the University of Turin. It was here that he began his lifelong interest in American literature. He did his thesis work on Walt Whitman, getting a degree from the university in 1930. His mother died the same year. He also started work on a cycle on poems that would become part of *Hard Labor*.

To help support himself during his postgraduate years, Pavese translated Melville's *Moby Dick: Or, The Whale* (1851), as well as works by Joyce, John Dos Passos, and Anderson. Pavese also joined antifascist groups; in 1935, he was arrested for holding letters of a jailed antifascist that he received from his girlfriend Tina Pizzardo, who was a member of the Communist Party. Pavese served seven months of a three-year sentence under house arrest and in exile.

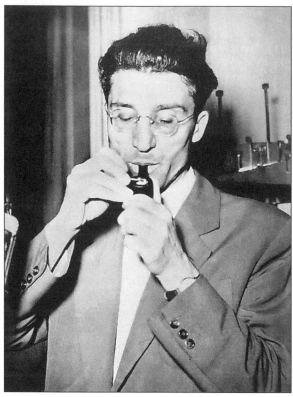

Cesare Pavese (The Granger Collection, New York)

His first book, *Hard Labor*, was published in 1936, but censors reduced the number of poems by four. Pavese would later publish this volume in a much larger edition. After his arrest, Pavese continued to write but stopped publishing for some time. His friend Guilio Einaudi restored a publishing company, and Pavese worked for and published most of his works with this publishing house. In 1941 and 1942, Pavese published two novels, as well as a translation of Faulkner's *The Hamlet* (1940). He left Turin in 1943, when the city fell under Nazi control. After the war, he returned to Turin and joined the Communist Party. After the war, Pavese published three books, *Feria d'agosto* (1946; *Summer Storm, and Other Stories*, 1966), *La terra e la morte*, and *Dialogues with Leucò*. In 1949, Pavese met and fell in love with the American actress Constance Dowling. Their affair lasted a year. Pavese was known as a troubled person. He seemed to embody the modern existentialist despair of his day. In August of 1950, despondent over a broken love affair, Pavese killed himself with an overdose of sleeping pills.

ANALYSIS

Though influenced by American writers such as Whitman, Cesare Pavese is not particularly well known in the United States. However, he has a worldwide reputation and is a very important figure in twentieth century modern Italian literature. Pavese's work has influenced many modern poets, including Denise Levertov. Her volume *Life in the Forest* (1978) contains a section of poems inspired by Pavese's work.

HARD LABOR

Pavese once said of *Hard Labor* that it "might have saved a generation." For a volume in which he wished to speak to and for a generation, it is striking to note that one of its major themes is silence—and another solitude. It is a silence at times wished for, and freeing: "Here, in the dark, alone,/ my body rests and feels it is the one master of itself" (in "Mania di solitudine," "Passion for Solitude"); at other times it seems to crush the person who cannot escape it: "every day the silence of the lonely room/ closes on the rustle of movement, of every gesture, like air" (in "La voce," "The Voice"). In his early poem "Antenati" ("Ancestors"), Pavese strongly suggests that the inability to speak is passed down through generations of rough men: "I found out I had lived, before I was born,/ in tough, sturdy, independent men, masters of themselves./ None of them knew what to say, so they just kept quiet." The women in the family also endure a hard silence: "In our family women don't matter./ What I mean is, our women stay home/ and make children like me, and keep their mouths shut." They suffer their own hard labor.

In "Gente spaesata" ("Displaced People"), the natural landscape can induce a hypnotic silence between men: "We've seen too much of the sea./ Late afternoon—the colorless water stretches dully away, disappearing into air. My friend's staring at the sea,/ and I'm staring at him, and neither says a word." The antidote to the sea is the hills, which supplant the earlier barren landscape. In Pavese's words, almost like a drinking song or boast, the hills become fleshy and fertile, ripe for dreams—dreams of women. In such a dream landscape, imagined conversation is possible: "We could stroll through the vineyards and, maybe,/ meet with a couple of girls, dark brown, ripened by the sun,/ we could strike up a conversation, we could sample their grapes." A harsh landscape swirls with levels of talk: simple talk, drunken talk, imaginary talk—all transformed by the poet's language.

Though the individual suffers in silence, a kind of collective is available that unites these lonely, working people: "All he feels is the pavement, which other men have made—/ men with calloused hands, hands like his" (in "Lavorare stanca," "Hard Labor"). The old pastoral ode of a shepherd following his flock, has fallen away to reveal a flintier modern man—worn down but bearing up—in silence: if not a part of, at least within, his or her community. In these kinds of poems, the solitary wanderer is not the only person to hold dreams or to suffer dreams being crushed. Poems such as "Pensieri di Deola" ("Deola Thinking"), "La moglie del barcaiolo" ("The Boatman's Wife"), and "Atlantic Oil" show people beaten down, exhausted, by the world of work, by the necessity of getting by, which is the hard soil to which all men must cling: "The long days work has left them dead" (in "Crepuscolo di sabbiatori," "Sand-Diggers' Twilight").

In "Atlantic Oil," a working mechanic is invited by the landscape to fall away into dreams: "And the story ends with the mechanic marrying the vineyard of his choice,/ and the girl that goes with it. He'll work outdoors in the sun." His heady dreams are contrasted with the knowledge of a drunken mechanic who sleeps in a ditch by the road. All these worlds will spiral down, "plunging in the valley below, down in the darkness."

Sometimes, memories of the past are all that are available, or fantasies of an imagined future with someone, a future that will never happen. The poems, despite their hard realities, contain romantic and lyric qualities that seem to hold out some hope of rescue. Usually it is an imagined woman who holds out the most hope for a man, as in "Paternità" ("Fatherhood"): "Every man,/ alone with a drink, will see her again. She'll always be there." Her permanent absence, her fleshly invisibility, ultimately creates longing and confusion and a return to silence in "Incontro" ("Encounter"): "I created her from the ground of everything/ I love the most, and I cannot understand her."

The poems in *Hard Labor* are often crafted with a long, proselike line. The people in the city and countryside seem fresh from a young poet's developing vision and seem to take their inspiration from another solitary wanderer: Whitman.

VERRÀ LA MORTE E AVRÀ I TUOI OCCHI

After a period of time when Pavese wrote only novels, he returned to verse. In the later poems, he uses a more spare line length. The poems are stark lyrics, often addressed directly to a "you." In 1945, he published in a magazine a group of nine poems called *La terra e la morte*. These poems were later collected in Pavese's posthumous volume *Verrà la morte e avrà i tuoi occhi* (death will come and it will have your eyes).

The later poems resonate with several of Pavese's familiar themes. The land and sea are ever-present, as is the quixotic search for a love that cannot be possessed. As always, silence pervades, and it assumes even darker forms, as in "La terre et la morte" ("Earth and Death"): "You are earth and death./ Your season is darkness/ and silence." In the series of love lyrics connected to the title poem, love becomes an open wound, a fatality, subsumed by silence:

Death will come, and it will have your eyes.
It will be like ending a vice, like seeing a dead face
emerge from the mirror,
like hearing closed lips speak.
We'll go down in silence.

A few months after these last poems were written, Pavese took his own life. He was only forty-one.

OTHER MAJOR WORKS

LONG FICTION: *Paesi tuoi*, 1941 (*The Harvesters*, 1961); *La spiaggia*, 1942 (*The Beach*, 1963); *Il compagno*, 1947 (*The Comrade*, 1959); *La bella estate*, 1949 (includes *Il diavolo sulle colline* and *Tra donne sole*; *The Beautiful Summer*, 1959); *Il carcere*, 1949 (*The Political Prisoner*, 1959); *La casa in collina*, 1949 (*The House on the Hill*, 1956); *Il diavolo sulle colline*, 1949 (*The Devil in the Hills*, 1954); *Prima che il gallo canti*, 1949 (includes *Il carcere* and *La casa in collina*); *Tra donne sole*, 1949 (*Among Women Only*, 1953); *La luna e i falò*, 1950 (*The Moon and the Bonfire*, 1952; also known as *The Moon and the Bonfires*); *Fuoco grande*, 1959 (with Bianca Garufi; *A Great Fire*, 1963); *The Selected Works of Cesare Pavese*, 1968.

SHORT FICTION: *Feria d'agosto*, 1946 (*Summer Storm, and Other Stories*, 1966); *Notte di festa*, 1953 (*Festival Night, and Other Stories*, 1964); *Racconti*, 1960 (*Told in Confidence, and Other Stories*, 1971); *The Leather Jacket: Stories*, 1980; *Stories*, 1987.

NONFICTION: *Dialoghi con Leucò*, 1947 (*Dialogues with Leucò*, 1966); *La letteratura americana e altri saggi*, 1951 (*American Literature: Essays and Opinions*, 1970); *Il mestiere di vivere: Diario, 1935-1950*, 1952 (*The Burning Brand: Diaries, 1935-1950*, 1961; also known as *The Business of Living*); *Lettere*, 1966 (partially translated as *Selected Letters, 1924-1950*, 1969).

TRANSLATIONS: *Il nostro signor Wrenn*, 1931 (of Sinclair Lewis's *Our Mr. Wrenn*); *Moby-Dick*, 1932 (of Herman Melville); *Riso nero*, 1932 (of Sherwood Anderson's *Dark Laughter*); *Il 42 parallelo*, 1935 (of John Dos Passos's *Forty-second Parallel*); *U omini e topi*, 1938 (of John Steinbeck's *Of Mice and Men*); *Tre esistenze*, 1940 (of Gertrude Stein's *Three Lives*); *Il borgo*, 1942 (of William Faulkner's *The Hamlet*).

BIBLIOGRAPHY

Hacht, Anne Marie, and David Kelly, eds. *Poetry for Students*. Vol. 20. Detroit: Thomson/Gale, 2004. Analyzes Pavese's "Two Poems for T." Contains the poem, a summary, and discussions of the poem's themes, style, historical context, critical overview, and criticism. Includes bibliography and index.

Lajolo, Davide. *An Absurd Vice: A Biography of Cesare Pavese*. New York: New Directions, 1983. Lajolo was a friend of Pavese and his first biographer. His friendship with Pavese gave him special insights, but later scholars distrusted some of his psychological and political speculations about Pavese.

O'Healy, Áine. *Cesare Pavese*. Boston: Twayne, 1988. This short, excellent biography clears away many of the myths about Pavese. It is an excellent place to begin a study of Pavese and his work.

Pavese, Cesare, and Anthony Chiuminatto. *Cesare Pavese and Anthony Chiuminatto: Their Correspondence*. Edited by Mark Pietralunga. Toronto, Ont.: University of Toronto Press, 2007. This collection of letters between Pavese and Italian American musician and educator Chiuminatto between 1929 and 1933 sheds light on the Italian poet.

Simborowski, Nicoletta. *Secrets and Puzzles: Silence and the Unsaid in Contemporary Italian Writing*. Oxford, England: Legenda, European Humanities Research Center, 2003. Traces self-censorship in postwar Italy in the writings of Pavese, Primo Levi, Natalia Ginzburg, and Francesca Sanvitale. Chapter 3 focuses on Pavese's political commitment.

Smith, Laurence G. *Cesare Pavese and America: Life, Love, and Literature*. Amherst: University of Massachusetts Press, 2008. This biography of Pavese examines his relationship with the United States, which turned from admiration into criticism. Discusses his brief affair with American actress Constance Dowling.

Robert W. Scott

MIODRAG PAVLOVIĆ

Born: Novi Sad, Voyvodina, Serbia; November 28, 1928

PRINCIPAL POETRY

87 pesama, 1952
Stub sećanja, 1953
Oktave, 1957
Mleko iskoni, 1963
Velika Skitija, 1969
Nova Skitija, 1970
Hododarje, 1971
Svetli i tamni praznici, 1971
The Conqueror in Constantinopole: Poetry, 1976
Zavetine, 1976
Karike, 1977 (*Links*, 1989)
Pevanja na viru, 1977 (*Singing at the Whirlpool*, 1983)
Bekstva po Srbiji, 1979
Vidovnica, 1979
Izabrana dela Miodraga Pavlovića, 1981 (4 volumes)
Divno čudo, 1982

Nova pevanja na viru, 1983

Glas pod kamenom = A Voice Locked in Stone,
   1985

The Slavs Beneath Parnassus: Selected Poems,
   1985

Sledstvo, 1985

Bezazlenstva, 1989

Knjiga staroslovna, 1989

Ulazak u Kremonu, 1989

Cosmologia profanata, 1990

Esej o coveku, 1992

Pesme o detinjstvu i ratovima, 1992

Knjiga horizonta, 1993

Medustepenik: Pesme, 1994

Izabrane i nove pesme, 1946-1996, 1996

Nebo u pecini: Sa crtezima autora, 1996

Posvecenje pesme: Izbor iz poezije, 1996

Izvor: Poezija II, 2000

Život u jaruzi: Ktitorov san, 2007

OTHER LITERARY FORMS

Miodrag Pavlović (PAHV-lo-vihch) has published
two books of short stories, *Most bez obala* (1956;
a bridge without shores) and *Bitni ljudi: Price sa
Uskrsnjeg ostrva* (1995; fundamental folk), and two
books of short plays, *Igre bezimenih* (1963; the plays
of the nameless) and *Koraci u podzemlju: Scensko
prikazanje u dva dela* (1991; steps in the underworld).
Although his stories and plays are not nearly as successful as his poetry, they illuminate his approach to
other genres. More important are his essays on various
aspects of literature in general and of Serbian and
Yugoslav literature in particular; these are contained
in *Rokovi poezije* (1958; the realm of poetry), *Osam
pesnika* (1964; eight poets), and *Poetika modernog*
(1978; modern poetry). Equally important is Pavlović's work on several anthologies, one of which,
Antologija srpskog pesništva, XIII-XX vek (1964; an
anthology of Serbian poetry, eighteenth to twentieth
centuries), has continued to provoke animated discussion. He has also edited anthologies of Serbian lyric
folk poetry, modern English poetry, and the poetry of
European Romanticism. Finally, he has translated extensively from classical and modern literatures, especially German, English, French, and Italian.

ACHIEVEMENTS

Miodrag Pavlović is a powerful and significant poetic figure. Together with Vasko Popa and other poets,
he was instrumental in bringing about the revolution in
Serbian poetry in the early 1950's, when a more mod-
ernistic approach won over the more traditional and realistic one. He has written a great number of enduring
poems; with his protest against the senselessness and
injustice of existence, with his untiring quest for truth
and for roots, and with his elevation of Serbian poetry
to a high level of technical excellence and spiritual richness, he has ploughed a deep furrow in Serbian, Yugoslav, and world poetry. Pavlović already has a large
group of followers among younger poets, and he has
been translated into many languages. In 1978, he was
elected to the Serbian Academy of Sciences and Arts.
When he has written his last verse, there is no doubt that
critics will rank him as one of the most significant Serbian poets of the twentieth century.

BIOGRAPHY

Miodrag Pavlović was born in 1928 in Novi Sad,
Voyvodina (later, Yugoslavia; now Serbia). He attended medical school at the University of Belgrade
and, after he graduated, practiced medicine for a short
while. Soon, however, he abandoned medicine to devote all his time to writing. He was briefly a director of
the Theater of Belgrade and then was an editor in a leading Belgrade publishing house, Prosveta, from 1961 to
1984.

ANALYSIS

Miodrag Pavlović's first volume of poetry, *87
pesama* (87 poems), was one of those exceptional
books that usher in a new era in literature. Together
with Vasko Popa, Pavlović entered the scene at a crucial time in the history of contemporary Yugoslav literature—a time when World War II literature was
decreasing in popularity and Yugoslav writers were
once again becoming aware of the outside world. Of
great significance is Pavlović's emphasis on a distinctly Anglo-Saxon way of conceiving, writing, and
appreciating poetry. He was one of the first to heed
the call for regeneration and to lead Serbian poetry
away from Romanticism or pragmatic utilitarianism

and toward a more disciplined, analytical, and intellectual approach.

In his essays on literature, especially on poetry, Pavlović reveals his thoughts, tastes, and preferences. Explaining the principles of selection that underlie his anthology of Serbian poetry, Pavlović has said that he chose poems that "speak about the fundamental questions of individual and collective existence, poems that either convey a thought or lead through their content directly to cognition." In the same book, he acknowledged that he had selected poems, not poets. This de-emphasis of personality is a reflection of T. S. Eliot's view that literature should be as depersonalized and unemotional as possible. A longtime student of Eliot and other English and American poets, Pavlović found it natural to implement their views and ideas in his poetry, adding, to be sure, his own approach.

87 PESAMA

Pavlović's significance as a poet is not, however, limited to the historical role that he has played. The purely artistic quality of his poetry, his many innovations, the influence he has exerted on younger poets— all these add to his stature. The first poem in *87 pesama*, "Whirlwind," is almost a programmatic poem, fully indicative of Pavlović's early stage:

> I wake up
> over the bed a storm
> Ripe sour cherries fall
> into the mud
> In the boat
> disheveled women
> wail
> The whirlwind
> of wicked fingernails
> chokes the dead
> Soon
> nothing will be known
> about that

Many recurring elements of Pavlović's poetry— elements that startled and even provoked some of his early readers—are present in "Whirlwind." This poem reveals the poet's anxiety and a certain revulsion against existence, undoubtedly caused in part by the horrors of the war. Similar images of anxiety, horror, and despair can be found in other poems in this collec-

tion. Man is compared to an ant standing at the bottom of the cellar stairs, whose cry simply "does not reach." When someone nearby dies, "the world becomes lighter by a human brain" ("Requiem"). Corpses swim under the ground, and "lost days and dissipated suns drown in a river like dead clouds" ("The Damned Forest"). The collection is dominated by images of darkness, night, death, destruction, chaos, and apocalypse: a skull, a funeral, a headless hen hanging by the leg from a cloud. The overwhelmingly bleak atmosphere is relieved only by the last poem, "Hope Should Be Found Again."

STUB SEĆANJA

This despairing mood of *87 pesama* is carried over to Pavlović's second collection, *Stub sećanja* (a pillar of memory). Skulls and heads without faces or hair reappear; cries are heard again. Yet, one feels that Pavlović is trying to escape the hopeless setting of his first book, embarking on a long quest for a meaning. It is not coincidental that the title of this collection refers to the power of memory, for it is in one's memory that the answers to life's riddles should be sought. Death is no longer the end of everything; rather, it is a key ("Variations on the Skull"). In the central poem of this book, "The Defense of Our City," the poet reiterates: "I have hopes for this city" ("this city" is a symbol of human existence).

OKTAVE

In Pavlović's third collection, *Oktave* (octaves), the poet continues his quest. He moves out of the city into nature's wide-open spaces; at the same time, he turns inward to the unconscious. The figure of a sleeping tiger whose head rests on the poet's shoulder symbolizes the potent forces of the unconscious, which reside in humans like an animal. There are formal changes in this volume as well: Instead of brief poems consisting almost entirely of metaphors, images, and terse statements, there are long descriptive poems of eight stanzas, some of which rhyme—a rare occurrence in Pavlović's verse. Nevertheless, the central theme of these poems remains the merciless search for origin and identity: "On the ridge of the desert the chorus of stars is asking me:/ who are you?" ("Ulcinj").

MLEKO ISKONI

To answer such questions, Pavlović entered a new phase of development, a change that resulted in an entirely different kind of poetry. In *Mleko iskoni* (primeval milk), the poet turns to prehistoric times and Greek antiquity. Framed by poems about the creation and the end of the world, this cycle of fourteen poems depicts the downfall of the once-proud Greek civilization. Various witnesses of this downfall express their despair. Thus, Orestes laments: "On the bald earth/ another man stands/ and not a single god" ("Orestes on the Acropolis"). Odysseus complains: "Not even gods want to be born any more" ("Odysseus Speaks"). Pindar expresses doubt concerning the need for poetry: "I don't want to be a poet any more,/ heroes are buried" ("Pindar on a Stroll"). The decay has reached such proportions that "No one will join our secret society any more . . . ,/ Eternity no longer has a form nor a substance./ No one will be accepted any more" ("Eleusinian Shadows").

Nevertheless, this cycle marks a significant departure from the pervasive despair of Pavlović's previous volumes. Here, he depicts the downfall of a mighty civilization in mythical terms. The dying Greek civilization is replaced in the poet's scheme with the advent of the Slavic tribes who had begun to settle in the north.

VELIKA SKITIJA AND NOVA SKITIJA

Pavlović devoted his next two books to these primitive but virile warriors and peasants who swooped down from the north and spread destruction in their wake, at the same time signaling a new beginning. *Velika Skitija* (great Scythia) and *Nova Skitija* (new Scythia) represent the high point in Pavlović's return to the past in his quest for the roots of his nation. Some of his best poems, such as "The Slavs Before Parnassus," "Epitaph of the Old Slavic Bard," "The Foundling," "The Song of the Bogomils," and "Dušan Before Constantinople," are to be found in these books. Touching on the important events in the history of his people, the poet is at the same time searching for universal values and for the meaning of collective experience.

HODODARJE

The next stage in Pavlović's poetic wanderings took him to Western European civilization. In *Hododarje* (sacrificial procession), he visits important places of this civilization, including Amiens, Chartres, Rouen, and Mainz. He also muses on the achievements of native figures such as Njegoš and Dis, visits some modern churches in the Balkans, and ends with a pilgrimage to Mount Athos. In all these poems, he strives to find a connecting link among the Hellenic world, the Southern Slavs, and Western European civilization.

SVETLI I TAMNI PRAZNICI

With *Hododarje*, Pavlović completed a full circle: Starting from the modern city and moving back to primeval times, Greek antiquity, and the ancient Slavs, he returned to Western Europe, of which the modern big city of his youth is an integral part. A kind of synthesis of this circular quest and its findings can be found in *Svetli i tamni praznici* (bright and dark holidays), a book of poems with pronounced religious overtones. The emphasis on the Mother of God and the Savior, seen not in a conventional, church-oriented way but on the poet's own terms, seems to indicate that he has found unifying figures that give the road traveled by humanity an ultimate meaning. It may also indicate that the quest is over and that the tortuous wandering of Pavlović as a poet has found a fruitful end. That this may be so is indicated by his later books of poetry. Lacking a unifying feature, these poems resemble in theme and form those of the various stages of his development. To be sure, new books take him to new places (Lepenski vir, for example, a newly discovered prehistoric site by the Danube in Serbia), but the discoveries seem to confirm the earlier findings; the difference is in degree, not in kind. Moreover, some of the latest poems reflect the poet's further development, so that when familiar motifs are repeated, they are offered in much more luxurious garb.

THE 1960'S

Pavlović's poetry of the 1960's established his international reputation and allowed him to travel widely. Visits to India and China allowed him to research the mythologies and oral traditions of Eastern cultures, which began to appear in his poems alongside his native South Slavic traditions in books such as *Bekstva po Srbiji* (flights through Serbia) and *Divno čudo* (a divine miracle). The discovery in the 1970's of a Mesolithic archaeological site, Lepenski vir, inspired him to further explore the origins of human creativity in *Zavetine* (spells), *Links*, and *Nova pevanja na viru* (new singing at the whirlpool).

THE 1970'S AND 1980'S

His poetry throughout the 1970's and 1980's drew links between myth and poetry, tracing the unbroken connections from archaic life to the modern world. Beginning with *Pesme o detinjstvu i ratovima* (1992; poems about childhood and wars), Pavlović's poems began to become more intimate and biographical. The childhood of the title is his own; the war is World War II, although it foreshadows the events in Serbia at the end of the twentieth century.

This marks a distinct change in approach for Pavlović, whose previous poetry had been marked by a strong intellectualism. As mentioned, Pavlović has sought from the beginning to rid Serbian poetry of excessive Romanticism. He agrees with T. S. Eliot's view that poetry is not a turning loose of emotion but an escape from personality—provided one has a personality and emotions from which to escape. Though an intellectual and reflective poet, Pavlović is not devoid of emotion; he is an aloof but not an impassive observer, so that a certain cool passion emanates from his poems. If he were impassive, why would he raise his voice against the horrors of existence? Why would he search for explanations of life's riddles? Because he is against Romantic emotionalism and in favor of an intellectual approach to poetry, he offers a rational solution: "The spark of reason,/ the most human of all humanities" ("A Cry Should Be Repeated"). Thus, in his efforts to depersonalize poetry, Pavlović keeps the individual in the background while interceding passionately on his behalf.

UNIVERSAL CONCERNS

Another feature of Pavlović's poetry is the universal scope that governs his entire outlook. Even when he speaks of geographically limited areas, such as ancient Greece, the old Slavic territories, the West, or his city, he always speaks for all humankind. All people have a common origin, and they still strive "toward the home of brotherly unity where our cradles are swaying/ . . . we seek the melody of our common lament in the moonlight" ("Idyll"). Such universality has given Pavlović's poetry a dimension that has greatly enhanced his appeal among poets and critics abroad.

FORM AND STYLE

Pavlović's poetry also demonstrates his technical mastery. The significance of his appearance in the early 1950's derived not only from new themes but also from formal innovations. Above all, his oeuvre is characterized by a great variety of form, ranging from the sketchy, concise, almost laconic early poems to longer forms, and from the inner monologue and confessional style of the early poems to the narrative, descriptive, and dramatic verse of his later period.

Pavlović's language is rich, economical, precise, and lapidary. He has a gift for striking metaphors, such as "A skull/ the sword of nature/ the only raft on the black river" ("Variations on the Skull") and "Pieces of meat lie on the window/ from which the sinews hang down to the ground" ("Funeral"). Many of his images defy conventional logic: "two knives play on the piano" ("On the Death of a Hen"); "a rain of blood falls from the earth to the sky" ("Lament of Hector's Wife"). These predilections may reflect the influence of the prewar Surrealist poets, whom Pavlović knows well, although he is a strongly original poet who has assimilated all influences to his own purposes. Finally, Pavlović has enriched the language of Serbian poetry with many felicitous neologisms. It is his combination of thematic novelty, artistic boldness, and formal excellence that has made Pavlović one of the most important and accomplished of contemporary Serbian poets.

OTHER MAJOR WORKS

SHORT FICTION: *Most bez obala*, 1956; *Bitni ljudi: Price sa Uskrsnjeg ostrva*, 1995.

PLAYS: *Igre bezimenih*, pb. 1963; *Koraci u podzemlju: Scensko prikazanje u dva dela*, pr. 1967.

NONFICTION: *Rokovi poezije*, 1958; *Osam pesnika*, 1964; *Poezija i kultura*, 1974; *Poetika modernog*, 1978; *Kina: Oko na putu*, 1983; *Prirodni oblik i lik: Likovni ogledi*, 1984; *Govor o nicem*, 1987; *Poetika zrtvenog obreda*, 1987; *Hram i preobrazenje: Jedna knjiga*, 1989; *Eseji o srpskim pesnicima*, 1992; *Ogledi o narodnoj i staroj srpskoj poeziji*, 1993; *Obredi poetickog zivota*, 1998; *Uzurpatori neba: Preludijum I fuga*, 2000.

EDITED TEXTS: *Antologija savremene engleske poezije*, 1956 (with Svetozar Brkić); *Antologija srpskog pesništva, XIII-XX vek*, 1964; *Pesništva evropskog romantizma*, 1969; *Antologija lirske narodne poezije*, 1982.

BIBLIOGRAPHY

Johnson, Bernard. Introduction and notes to *The Slavs Beneath Parnassus: Selected Poems*, by Miodrag Pavlović. St. Paul, Minn.: New Rivers Press, 1985. Johnson's introduction and notes on his translations of Pavlović's works offer rare biographical and critical information on the poet.

McAllister, Lesley. "Serbian History: A Tale of Optimism Under Suppression and Exile." Review of *A Voice Locked in Stone. Toronto Star*, May 17, 1986, p. M4. This short, favorable review of the work finds Pavlović expressing hope for his nation's future.

Mihailovich, Vasa D. "The Poetry of Miodrag Pavlović." *Canadian Slavonic Papers* 20 (1978): 358-368. A critical analysis of selected poems by Pavlović.

Vasa D. Mihailovich (including original translations)

CHARLES-PIERRE PÉGUY

Born: Orléans, France; January 7, 1873
Died: Near Villeroy, France; September 5, 1914
Also known as: Marcel and Pierre Baudouin

PRINCIPAL POETRY

Jeanne d'Arc, 1897 (as Marcel and Pierre Baudouin)

La Chanson du roi Dagobert, 1903

Le Mystère de la charité de Jeanne d'Arc, 1910 (*The Mystery of the Charity of Joan of Arc*, 1950)

Le Porche du mystère de la deuxième vertu, 1911 (*The Portico of the Mystery of the Second Virtue*, 1970)

"Châteaux de Loire," 1912 ("Chateaux of the Loire")

Le Mystère des saints innocents, 1912 (*The Mystery of the Holy Innocents, and Other Poems*, 1956)

"Les Sept contre Thèbes," 1912 ("Seven Against Thebes")

La Tapisserie de sainte Geneviève et de Jeanne d'Arc, 1912

Ève, 1913

La Tapisserie de Notre-Dame, 1913

Sainte Geneviève, patronne de Paris, 1913

"Les Sept contre Paris," 1913 ("Seven Against Paris")

Quatrains, 1939

Œuvres poétiques complètes, 1941

God Speaks: Religious Poetry, 1945

OTHER LITERARY FORMS

Most of the prose of Charles-Pierre Péguy (pay-GEE) falls into the category of journalism. His articles, which first appeared in *La Revue socialiste* (1897) and *La Revue blanche* (1899), are available in *Notes politiques et sociales* (1957). Other prose works by Péguy have been collected in *Œuvres en prose, 1898-1908* (1959) and *Œuvres en prose II, 1909-1914* (1961), both edited by Marcel Péguy. Gallimard has also published the *Œuvres complètes* (1917-1955) in twenty volumes, including *Deuxième Élégie XXX, L'Esprit de système, Un Poète m'a dit, Par ce demi-clair matin, Situations*, and *La Thèse*, all posthumous publications or fragments. *Les Œuvres posthumes de Charles Péguy* (1969) was edited by Jacques Viard.

Very few of these works have been translated into English in their entirety. Selections from Péguy's prose are available in *Basic Verities: Prose and Poetry* (1943), *Men and Saints: Prose and Poetry* (1944), and *God Speaks*. In *Temporal and Eternal* (1958), translated by Alexander Dru, there are selections from *Notre Jeunesse* (1910; our youth), *Clio* (1917), and *Deuxième Élégie XXX*. Péguy's correspondence is published in *Lettres à André Bourgeois* (1950). Marcel Péguy has edited a volume of selected correspondence titled *Lettres et entretiens* (1927).

ACHIEVEMENTS

Charles-Pierre Péguy, the militant journalist, the unswerving socialist, the ardent defender of Alfred Dreyfus, was a writer who might be unknown to the world at large and even to France today if it were not for his poetry. In the last four years of his life, having "found the faith anew," he turned to poetry as a medium of expression. This intensely personal verse, in colloquial but correct French, in which God speaks with people as if he were one of them, touches the reader with its simplicity.

Péguy is able to personify hope as a little child in *The Portico of the Mystery of the Second Virtue*; God himself is taken off guard by the unassuming courage of this girl who can change the world. Péguy sees hope in the possibility of beginning anew: "Le premier jour est le plus beau jour" (the first day is the most beautiful day). His Joan of Arc is also a defenseless child who nevertheless believes in action: One must not save, but spend, oneself. Thus, Péguy offers a message of simple heroism, much needed in prewar France and still appealing two wars later.

Péguy extols France, perhaps a bit too much when the God of the Holy Innocents says that the French are his favorite people. Péguy weaves a rich tapestry of French heroes and saints, most of whom are drawn from the Middle Ages: King Dagobert, Saint Genevieve, Joan of Arc, Saint Louis, and Jean de Joinville. Perhaps the only nonmedieval heroes admitted are Pierre Corneille, Jules Michelet, and Victor Hugo. The cathedrals of France, Notre-Dame de Paris and Chartres, are woven into the tapestry, itself a cathedral with its images of porches, mysteries, and saints. With a profound sense of history, a theme that always fascinated Péguy, the ship of the ages approaches Paris, bearing France's sins and virtues, victories and failures, from the day when the Île-de-France was first inhabited by the Romans.

All of Péguy's poetry is deeply religious, in contrast to his socialist prose. A nonpracticing Catholic convert who claimed that he had never left the Church, Péguy puzzled his many friends and has continued to fascinate critics—among them Pie Duployé, who has dedicated a sizable volume to the question of Péguy's religion. The faith which informs Péguy's poetry is universal; it touches believer and nonbeliever alike, for it is moral without being dogmatic, uncompromising but gentle. Deeply rooted in the soil of France yet revealing a profound understanding of universal human concerns, Péguy's poetry has found a small but devoted audience.

BIOGRAPHY

Charles-Pierre Péguy was born at Orléans in the Faubourg Bourgogne on January 7, 1873, the only son of a poor working woman who was to lose her husband within a few months. Péguy was always proud to be a member of a hardworking family, and he regarded France's peasants and workmen as its greatest strength. He grew up under the care of his mother and grandmother, attending local schools. He was able to attend the *lycée* at Orléans in 1885 because of a scholarship and because of the new system of public education which he was later to extol. Higher education even became possible; thus, he attended both the Lycée Lakanal at Sceaux in 1891 and the École Normale Supérieure in 1894, which was eventually to deny him the *agrégation*. For this, as well as for its adherence to the values of the modern world, Péguy was to immortalize the school as "l'école dite normale, autrefois supérieure" (called normal, formerly superior). Around 1895, he became attracted to socialism, not in the Marxist sense but rather in the idealistic tradition of the early nineteenth century—the tradition of Pierre Proudhon and Pierre Leroux, as Jacques Viard has demonstrated. Péguy founded a socialist group and at the turn of the century actively supported Dreyfus for idealistic reasons, "so that France will not be in the state of mortal sin." When, in Péguy's view, other socialist leaders began to use Dreyfus for their own ends, when what he originally envisioned as "mystique" degenerated into "politique," Péguy went his own way. In 1900, he founded his *Cahiers de la quinzaine*, "pour dire bêtement la vérité bête" ("to tell the stark truth starkly").

Several years earlier, in 1896, Péguy's best friend, Marcel Baudouin, had died, yet Péguy kept his memory alive. Indeed, Péguy's first poetic work, *Jeanne d'Arc* (Joan of Arc), a long drama in blank verse, was published by "Georges Bellais" (a pseudonym for Péguy) under the names "Marcel and Pierre Baudouin" (also pseudonyms for Péguy) in 1897. All his subsequent works (with the exception of two posthumously published works) were first published by Péguy himself in the *Cahiers de la quinzaine* (1900-1914). He married Marcel's sister, Charlotte-Françoise, in 1897. They had four children and were to remain faithful to each other, though not always happy. Péguy's main work was his *Cahiers de la quinzaine*, by no means lucrative, for he had a talent for antagonizing his subscribers through the uncompromising honesty of many of the articles he printed, which were nevertheless of the highest literary quality.

In 1908, Péguy surprised his friend Joseph Lotte by declaring, "J'ai retrouvé la foi" (I have returned to the faith). Perhaps, however, because of Péguy's civil marriage and his wife's anti-Catholic convictions, he did not practice his religion or have his children baptized. The whole tenor of his work, however, changed at this time, becoming more reflective, often mystical. His best prose works, such as *Clio*, *Notre Jeunesse*, and *L'Argent* (1913; money), and most of his poetry date from his conversion. In 1912-1913, he made several pilgrimages to Chartres for the cure of his sick child Marcel, immortalizing the experience in his poem "Présentation de la Beauce à Notre-Dame de Chartres." Indeed, the Chartres pilgrimage has been reestablished in France as a result of Péguy's inspiration.

Péguy's last years were troubled by spiritual and emotional uncertainties. He derived particular help and consolation from his friendship with Henri Bergson, whose lectures at the Collège de France Péguy attended faithfully. At the outbreak of World War I in August, 1914, Péguy—then forty-one years old—immediately enlisted as a lieutenant in the infantry. Killed near Villeroy on September 5, 1914, by a bullet in the forehead, Péguy became the model of those heroic soldiers who died for their country. Ironically, during World War II, a bullet was to strike the forehead of the bust erected in front of his birthplace, 48 rue Bourgogne.

ANALYSIS

Like that of his contemporary, Paul Claudel, the style adopted by Charles-Pierre Péguy recalls the Psalms, yet Péguy has none of Claudel's triumphant exuberance. Péguy's verse has been called a "piétinement": It is plodding, a step-by-step advancement, like a pilgrimage to Chartres or a Corpus Christi procession. Péguy says that it is not important to arrive but simply to go. His verse is repetitive, yet the reiterations serve to emphasize, to clarify, and to articulate his thought.

Péguy's three *tapisseries* (tapestries) are written in four-line rhymed stanzas in the traditional Alexandrine, while the *Quatrains* and *La Chanson du roi Dagobert* are ballads with a very folkloristic air. All the rest of Péguy's major poems are written in free verse.

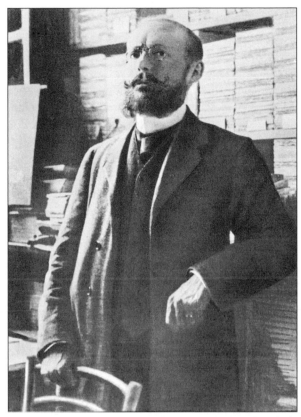

Charles-Pierre Péguy (The Granger Collection, New York)

Péguy's free verse is idiosyncratic, ranging from brief lines consisting of only a word or two to proselike paragraphs; some stanzas are only a line long, while others continue for pages. In his first work, the dramatic poem *Jeanne d'Arc*, Péguy baffled the printers by leaving entire pages blank, without any explanation.

Péguy is known for his use of contrasts and paradoxes. The most important of these in his poetry are the polarities spiritual and physical, aging and newness, and temporal and eternal. The theme of aging and newness, which is not peculiar to his poetry, is also basic to his later prose, especially *Clio*. Clio, the Greek Muse of history, is a symbol of aging, as are Ève, deadwood, and paper. Péguy sees newness in the Virgin Mary, the medieval world, Joan of Arc, and hope, the second theological virtue. These elements are characterized by powerlessness and abandonment and are symbolized also by the dawn, the first bud of April, the first day of creation, or fresh springs of water, all suggesting originality, spontaneity, and a freshness of vision. Péguy infinitely prefers this attitude to one of conformity and habit, symbolically connected with aging and decay.

In contrasting the spiritual and the physical, Péguy does not use the word *charnel* (physical) in its usual sexual connotation, but simply to insist that a human being is composed of both body and soul. He imagines the soul and the body as a horse hitched to a plow, with the soul pulling the body but the two closely united. The temporal and the eternal are also contrasted throughout Péguy's work. Among his favorite symbols for the temporal is Ève, while the Virgin Mary represents the eternal, yet here again he prefers to integrate them into a single concept, the human condition. He also refuses to dichotomize the secular and the sacred. These ideas echo the Bergsonian philosophy of time and duration that was very popular in Péguy's day—a philosophy which Péguy learned from Bergson himself.

Péguy's first poetic works were dramatic, and much of his verse maintains a dramatic orientation. The *mystères* are essentially dialogues; in them, God speaks in a very human tone. Throughout his verse, Péguy assumes an intimacy with God, Christ, and the saints. Péguy recounts biblical events with a sense of immediacy and personal involvement, and he frequently addresses the Virgin Mary in a tone that recalls medieval courtly love poems or the confidence of a small child in his mother.

Péguy's poetic universe is peopled largely by women, a point which has attracted the attention of many critics. Only in the *Quatrains* is there any indication of romantic love. These women do not represent the typical feminine image in literature, nor are they the Eternal Feminine of wisdom and beauty; they are, rather, symbols of Péguy's ideals.

Open to all nations and races, and particularly sympathetic to the oppressed, Péguy nevertheless insisted on the importance of the "race" (his conception of race was essentially nationalistic) embodied in France. Its fundamental unit, Péguy believed, was the parish, and his choice of images suggests the rural France of a bygone—indeed, a mythical—era in which the Church and the French nation were mystically united. In Péguy's imagery, France is a garden and the French people are God's gardeners. "La Beauce" is the "océan des blés" ("ocean of wheat") over which shines the Star of the Sea, the Virgin of Chartres. Nothing is as great as plowing the fields, says Péguy, as he mentions each tool by name. The rhythm of the seasons and the centuries suggests the presence of the eternal in the temporal and the temporal in the eternal. Thus, Péguy's poetry, disconcerting and sometimes tedious, moves into a cosmic dimension, making him truly a poet of the twentieth century.

JEANNE D'ARC AND THE MYSTERY OF THE CHARITY OF JOAN OF ARC

Of all Péguy's poetic subjects, Joan of Arc seems to have fascinated him the most. Two works are completely devoted to her—*Jeanne d'Arc*, a "drama in three plays," and *The Mystery of the Charity of Joan of Arc*—and she plays a considerable role in seven others. For Péguy, the ardent socialist, she was in 1897 the heroine of the new socialist city, but his bulky *Jeanne d'Arc* was unbelievable, unsalable, and unstageable. This first verse play has three parts: "Domrémy," "Les Batailles" (the battles), and "Rouen." The first part, "Domrémy," was the source for *The Mystery of the Charity of Joan of Arc* in 1910.

The Mystery of the Charity of Joan of Arc is dedicated to all who wish to remedy evil in the world, a major preoccupation of Péguy, especially after 1908, when he transferred socialist problems to a spiritual level. The work contains three characters: Madame Gervaise, Hauviette, and Jeannette. Madame Gervaise is a twenty-five-year-old Franciscan nun who has evolved from the stereotyped religious figure of the *Jeanne d'Arc* of 1897, in which she had retired to a convent for her individual salvation. Here, she is a mature woman who recognizes the involvement of everyone in the problem of evil and who frequently represents the traditional Catholic viewpoint. Her dialogues with Jeannette are almost monologues, for Jeannette prefers to pray rather than to engage in dialogue.

In her dialogue with Hauviette, Jeannette's extraordinary vocation comes to light. Jeannette is unhappy because people suffer. She wants to relieve their misery, as she expresses in her Our Father, a prayer that might be Péguy's own. She is especially concerned about the problem of eternal damnation, an enigma which haunted Péguy throughout his life. Jeannette articulates the need of a saint who will succeed and faintly sees her own vocation in these words.

Jeannette is called not only to liberate France but also to participate with Christ in saving the world, for Péguy places great emphasis on human and divine cooperation. This is perhaps the reason for the lengthy account of the Passion of Christ which occupies almost half of the play. At the end of the Passion, Jeannette asks whom one must save and how. She learns that she must save everyone, in imitation of Christ, by prayer and suffering. Jeannette also asks for a sign—namely, the safety of Mont Saint-Michel. She receives it and welcomes it in a glorious hymn of praise. In one of several unpublished conclusions, Jeannette receives her vocation to save France in words that echo the call of the prophets in the Old Testament. Why Péguy never published these conclusions is not clear. Perhaps he wished to emphasize Jeannette's agony; perhaps, too, he meant the next two *mystères* as a response to her dilemma.

THE PORTICO OF THE MYSTERY OF THE SECOND VIRTUE

Written between June, 1910, and 1911, *The Portico of the Mystery of the Second Virtue*, the second of the *mystères*, was published in the *Cahiers de la quinzaine* on September 24, 1911. A lengthy work, it occupies 140 pages in the Pléiade edition and contains Péguy's most important poetic themes. Romain Rolland called it Péguy's best work, and with the *The Mystery of the Holy Innocents, and Other Poems*, Pie Duployé considers it Péguy's most authentically religious poem. Surprisingly, neither poem attracted great attention at the time of its publication.

The Portico of the Mystery of the Second Virtue is Péguy's poem of abandonment, in the spirit of the "little way" of Saint Thérèse of Lisieux, as Marjorie Villiers observes (*Charles Péguy: A Study in Integrity*, 1965). It is his most overtly autobiographical work, containing references to Péguy's (then) three children; to their ages, names, and patron saints; to the illness of his son, Marcel; and to his own reconciliation with God. It is very biblical and rests more on the parables of the lost sheep and the prodigal son, and on the Book of Wisdom, than on the catechism which Péguy recalled from his boyhood days at St. Aignan. The prayers to the

Virgin Mary echo the Hail Mary and the famous litanies.

As in all of Péguy's works, the digressions here are many and mysterious, yet he never loses sight of the central theme, hope, personified as a powerless little child who is powerful in her nothingness. Here, and in *The Mystery of the Holy Innocents, and Other Poems*, Hope returns like a refrain, continuing to amaze God, who narrates the poem through the person of Madame Gervaise. Péguy contrasts Hope with her grown sisters, Faith and Charity, who do not astound God. Christ came to Earth, however, to make hope possible, to give the lost sheep a second chance, to allow humans to transmit his message to one another and to share in his creative work. The poem ends with a beautiful celebration of night and sleep, the virtue of a confident child and the sign of the triumph of hope.

THE MYSTERY OF THE HOLY INNOCENTS, AND OTHER POEMS

The Mystery of the Holy Innocents, and Other Poems, written in 1912 and published on March 24 of the same year, returns to many themes already treated in the preceding work: the three theological virtues (faith, hope, and charity) and a beautiful hymn to night that again evokes the burial of Christ, freedom, and abandonment. Péguy announced its theme as paradise, a thread which runs through the poem and serves as its conclusion. The title *The Mystery of the Holy Innocents, and Other Poems*, referring to the unbaptized Jewish victims of Herod's jealousy, may suggest Péguy's own unbaptized children. He mentions the Holy Innocents only at the end of the poem, along with a beautiful eulogy of childhood and children.

Again in this poem God speaks, commenting on his love of night and his astonishment at hope. He prefers the person who does not calculate for tomorrow. He loves especially the French people, builders of cathedrals and leaders of Crusades, worthy descendants of Saint Louis and champions of freedom. Madame Gervaise gives an instruction on prayer, especially the Our Father, as an example of trust and hope. Péguy also develops his favorite parable, that of the prodigal son, a subject which he had intended for a fourth *mystère* but which never grew beyond a few pages. His portrayal of Hope as the youngest of the family suggests the story of

Benjamin, the youngest of Jacob's sons. Thus, Madame Gervaise and Jeannette relate the biblical narrative of Joseph and his brothers, with a sympathy for the Jewish people habitual in Péguy. In Péguy's narrative, the Old Testament story of Joseph and his brothers represents the temporal, while the New Testament, from which the story of the prodigal son is taken, represents the eternal. Here, as elsewhere in his poetry, Péguy attempts to integrate the two concepts.

LA TAPISSERIE DE SAINTE GENEVIÈVE ET DE JEANNE D'ARC

In addition to the *mystères*, Péguy wrote several *tapisseries*. He defined a *tapisserie* as a lengthy succession of stanzas on the same theme, frequently following the same rhyme scheme as well; many of the stanzas begin with the same line. The first of Péguy's three *tapisseries*, *La Tapisserie de sainte Geneviève et de Jeanne d'Arc*, published December 1, 1912, was planned as a novena beginning on the feast of Saint Genevieve, January 3, 1913. It is dedicated to the patrons of Paris and France, Saint Genevieve and Saint Jeanne d'Arc, respectively, and it contains nine poems of varying length, with several sonnets among them.

Péguy calls upon Saint Genevieve, the shepherdess, to guard the flock of Paris in the twentieth century as she defended the city against the Huns in her own day. In poems 4 and 5, Péguy compares Saint Genevieve and Jeanne d'Arc. In poem 8, the longest of the series, he compares the weapons of Christ with those of Satan, which are sometimes identical. In poems 8 and 9, Jeanne is not named, but it is evident that the poems refer to her. She takes part in a battle and like Christ is led to death at the end of the last poem. Jeanne here is not the anguished Jeannette of *The Mystery of the Charity of Joan of Arc*, but rather the victorious leader of the French forces and the courageous martyr of the fifteenth century.

LA TAPISSERIE DE NOTRE-DAME

The second tapestry, *La Tapisserie de Notre-Dame*, consists of five poems, four short ones dedicated to Notre-Dame de Paris and one longer one, "Présentation de la Beauce à Notre-Dame de Chartres." Perhaps the richest in images among all the *tapisseries*, these poems depend on the symbol of a ship, and of the Virgin Mary as the star of the sea. Mary becomes the refuge of sinners, for she will obtain forgiveness from her Son for the sins that weigh down the boat. "Présentation de la Beauce," rhythmic and melodic, eventually loses its effect. Despite its excessive length, however, it is a sensitive portrayal of pilgrims wending their way through the fertile wheat fields to pay homage to the heavenly Queen.

ÈVE

In its conception, *Ève*, the last of Péguy's *tapisseries*, was his most ambitious work. Unfinished at his death, it already ran to some nine thousand lines, including a "suite" discovered after his death. It is a dense and difficult work, brilliantly studied by Joseph Barbier, Albert Béguin, Jean Onimus, and other scholars.

Péguy defined its subject as salvation. He begins with Ève's expulsion from the earthly paradise, a place he describes with great poetic beauty. It echoes the harmonious city that he had created in his early socialist works, a utopia modeled on Plato's *Politeia* (fourth century B.C.E.; *Republic*, 1701). Péguy sees Ève as the mother of humanity, as the representative of all women, responsible for their change in status. He muses on the human condition, the intransigence of the sinner, and the solitude of humanity without God. He evokes the ancient world, which Christ was to inherit, and Judgment Day. Perhaps the most popular lines of Péguy's entire oeuvre appear in the middle of the poem, in the otherwise tedious monologue addressed to Ève. These lines refer to soldiers who have died for country in a just war: "Heureux ceux qui sont morts pour la terre charnelle...." ("happy are they who have died for this land of flesh"). This was soon to become Péguy's epitaph, for he was to die for his country in September, 1914.

OTHER MAJOR WORKS

NONFICTION: *Notre Jeunesse*, 1910; *L'Argent*, 1913; *Clio*, 1917; *Lettres et entretiens*, 1927; *Lettres à André Bourgeois*, 1950; *Notes politiques et sociales*, 1957; *Œuvres en prose, 1898-1908*, 1959 (Marcel Péguy, editor); *Œuvres en prose II, 1909-1914*, 1961 (Marcel Péguy, editor); *Temporal and Eternal*, 1958.

MISCELLANEOUS: *Œuvres complètes*, 1917-1955 (20 volumes); *Basic Verities: Prose and Poetry*, 1943; *Men and Saints: Prose and Poetry*, 1944; *Les Œuvres posthumes de Charles Péguy*, 1969.

BIBLIOGRAPHY

Aronowicz, Annette. *Jews and Christians on Time and Eternity: Charles Péguy's "Portrait of Bernard-Lazare."* Stanford, Calif.: Stanford University Press, 1998. An insightful book that explains clearly Péguy's deep sympathy for Jews and his strong opposition to anti-Semitism.

Hill, Geoffrey. *The Mystery of the Charity of Charles Péguy.* 1985. Reprint. New York: Oxford University Press, 1997. This poem by a notoriously difficult modern poet is an elegy for and rumination of Péguy's life and his political thought.

Humes, Joy. *Two Against Time: A Study of the Very Present Worlds of Paul Claudel and Charles Péguy.* Chapel Hill: University of North Carolina Press, 1978. A clearly written book which describes the profound differences between Paul Claudel and Péguy, who were the most important Catholic poets in France during the early twentieth century.

Kimball, Roger. "Charles Péguy." *New Criterion* 20, no. 3 (2001): 15-21. A profile of Péguy emphasizing the interrelationship of events in his life with his work, especially *Notre Jeunesse.*

St. Aubyn, F. C. *Charles Péguy.* Boston: Twayne, 1977. This book remains the best introduction to the rich diversity of Péguy's life and works. It contains an annotated bibliography of his works and important critical studies on his writings.

Savard, John. "The Pedagogy of Péguy." *Chesterton Review* 19, no. 3 (August, 1993): 357-379. This essay compares masterful uses of paradox by Péguy and the English Catholic writer G. K. Chesterton. Savard argues that through paradoxical arguments, both writers lead their readers to deal with complex moral issues.

Schmitt, Hans A. *Charles Péguy: The Decline of an Idealist.* Baton Rouge: Louisiana State University Press, 1967. A biography of Péguy by an accomplished historian of modern Europe. Includes bibliographic references.

Villiers, Marjorie. *Charles Péguy: A Study in Integrity.* 1965. Reprint. Westport, Conn.: Greenwood Press, 1975. A classic, well-researched biography of Péguy.

Wessling, H. L. *Certain Ideas of France: Essays on French History and Civilization.* Contributions to the Study of World History 98. Westport, Conn.: Greenwood Press, 2002. Contains a chapter looking at the relationship between Charles de Galle and Péguy.

Wilson, A. N. "World of Books: Péguy, Leader of a Life Less Ordinary." *Daily Telegraph,* July 11, 2007, p. 25. Wilson discusses his interest in the poem on Péguy by Geoffrey Hill and his fascination with the life of the French poet, which was marked by contradictions. He remarks on the quality of Villiers's 1965 biography and its lasting value.

Irma M. Kashuba

NIKOS PENTZIKIS

Born: Thessaloníki, Greece; October 30, 1908
Died: Thessaloníki, Greece; January 13, 1993

PRINCIPAL POETRY

Ikones, 1944
Anakomidhi, 1961
Paleotera piimata ke neotera, 1980 (includes *Ikones* and prose pieces)
Psile e perispomene, 1995

OTHER LITERARY FORMS

Nikos Pentzikis (pehnt-ZEE-kees) might be called the odd case of modern Greek literature, for he combines in his poetry as well as in the much larger body of his prose a restless and inquisitive spirit typical of the modern era with a kind of pre-Renaissance, more particularly Byzantine, religious mysticism. The young hero of his first novel, *Andréas Dhimakoudhis*, published in 1935, suffers from unrequited love and commits suicide. This death is symbolic of Pentzikis's own early disappointments in love, the "death" of his sentimental self. His second book, *O pethamenos ke i anastasi* (wr. 1938, pb. 1944; the dead man and the resurrection), a stream-of-consciousness narrative, deals again with a young man (unnamed this time, but an obvious persona of his creator), who, though he regains his trust in life, regains it at the level of myth. He upholds the religious traditions of his country and accepts a metaphysical explanation of the world while returning and developing his sense of the concrete, his love for the world of shapes and colors. From that time on, Pentzikis cultivated his metaphysical and physical certainties in the parallel activities of writing and painting.

Pentzikis's love of the concrete is particularly evident in his book *Pragmatognosia* (1950; knowledge of things), which deals mostly with the realities of Thessaloníki, his native town, and in two works in diary form, *Simiosis ekato imeron* (1973; notes of one hundred days) and *Arhion* (1974; filing cabinet). These idiosyncratic works catalog dry data of all kinds, from skin diseases to bus fares and theater tickets (the writer sorts out and reorders cartons of souvenirs); they also rework religious information from old Greek Orthodox texts. The methodology behind these as well as other, stylistically more traditional works, such as *Arhitektoniki tis skorpias zois* (1963; architecture of the scattered life), *Mitera Thessaloniki* (1970; *Mother Salonika*, 1998), *Sinodhia* (1970; retinue), and *Omilimata* (1972; homilies), is based upon the so-called copying memory. Pentzikis spurns self-consciously aesthetic writing, which he finds hubristic. Instead, he favors an itemized record of reality as a fitting homage to God for the world which is his handicraft. The beautiful and the ugly, the banal and the exalted—all must find a place in Pentzikis's work, under the unifying veil of Christian myth, especially its Greek Orthodox version.

Pentzikis's later narrative method also incorporates a system of numerology. He writes or paints in clustered units of words, both religious and secular, that are ordered by their numerical values as defined by ancient Pythagorean and Neoplatonic tenets. The method is mechanical but true to his belief that a writer cannot rely entirely on his own mind but must have some external reference hallowed by time and practice.

ACHIEVEMENTS

Nikos Pentzikis's principal achievement was to have survived at all as a writer, to have persisted in his own idiosyncratic ways of seeing the world and so registering it in his poetry and prose. In his unswerving commitment to an utterly individual metaphysical vision only tangentially shaped by the currents of his time, Pentzikis shared affinities with Elias Canetti and Jorge Luis Borges.

In the context of modern Greek letters, Pentzikis successfully integrated national and personal memory with the stuff of his everyday experience, producing prose narratives and poems which explore both the human condition and the nature of writing. In the words of the distinguished translator Kimon Friar, Pentzikis's texts are

> a dizzying depository of words that are demotic, purist, formal, colloquial, archaic, modern, medieval, ecclesiastical, obsolete, scientific—all strung together in an eccentric syntax of his own devising. By flying beyond convention and good taste, by concentrating on things and not on rhythms or cadences or composition, he has evolved an inner style of his own, a "nonstyle" that is the man.

BIOGRAPHY

Nikos Gabriel Pentzikis was born in Thessaloníki, Greece, on October 30, 1908. Pentzikis's father operated a successful pharmaceutical business; his sister, Zoe Karelli (née Hrisoule Pentzikis), became a poet and translator, an active figure on the Greek literary scene. Pentzikis completed his elementary schooling at home and, beginning in 1919, attended a regular high school. Two years later, he was writing his first poems. Between 1926 and 1929, while studying pharmacology in Paris and Strasbourg, he read extensively in literature, particularly the Symbolists. Returning to his native city to take charge of the family business (his father had died in 1927), Pentzikis published some of his writings, but dissatisfied with the reaction they provoked, he burned them.

Pentzikis's first book, *Andréas Dhimakoudhis*, reflected his student days in France and his emotional, restless nature. His second publication in book form, *O pethamenos ke i anastasi*, marked his return to, and conscious acceptance of, the traditions of his native land, particularly the traditions of the Greek Orthodox Church. This reconciliation was also evident in his collection of poems *Ikones* (icons). The war years, although difficult for Pentzikis, were also formative for his subsequent literary production and rich in contacts with other Greek writers. Between 1945 and 1947, he issued—with the help of others—the literary journal *Kohlias*, an avant-garde publication that welcomed both original material and translations.

By 1950, Pentzikis had achieved a measure of stability in his life. Married in 1948, he was professionally secure as the representative in northern Greece of Geigy, the Swiss pharmaceutical company. Both his prose work *Pragmatognosia* and the poems which he wrote and published in the late 1940's and throughout the 1950's exuded a new self-confidence, celebrating the concrete realities of his land, his native city, and the religious and folk traditions of his people. During this period, Pentzikis was also active as a painter. He began to concentrate on his own work and rarely translated or reviewed the work of others. An exception, in 1960, was his brief but incisive article on the poet George Seferis, a man and a writer very dissimilar to himself.

In the 1960's, Pentzikis continued to write and paint and began lecturing and giving interviews about his work. In 1970, he published no fewer than three books, to which he added three more between 1972 and 1974. After 1976, he concentrated on producing revised and expanded editions of his earlier works and also began painting steadily. Having retired with a pension from Geigy, he devoted all his time to his literary and artistic work, which continues to be controversial and is still rejected by many readers and critics for its apparent shapelessness. For Pentzikis, however, this was his *askissi*, his own way of practicing the solitary, virtually monastic life of the visionary artist. It must be noted that, over the years, Pentzikis managed to enlarge, albeit slightly, the circle of his readers and admirers. A small but growing readership has discovered the wisdom and the flashes of genius sometimes obscured by the forbidding surface of his work.

ANALYSIS

Poetry is often a substitute or corrective for life. Nikos Pentzikis rounded out his first collection of poems, *Ikones*, during the difficult years of World War II. His family's diminished status and his own disappointments had already induced him to find solace in Christianity, particularly in the Greek Orthodox faith, and

not, like so many other men of his generation, in political engagement. If life seemed absurd, he would espouse the Christian myth, whose special kind of absurdity harked back to Tertullian's early declaration of faith: "Credo quia absurdum" ("I believe because it is absurd").

Pentzikis's poems, however, proved that being a Greek Orthodox writer did not necessarily mean the conventional repetition of religious formulas and articles of faith. He shunned such abstractions and aimed, instead, for the concrete. In long, flowing verses which one could compare to deep breaths, he named all objects that had set his senses in motion, even the most humble, in order to place in relief the universal sympathy that governs them. He copied or reaffirmed objective reality in a way that helped him dissolve or forget his ego. The "I" became "we" or remained "I" in relation to others, not in isolation from them.

IKONES

Ikones comprises responses to old letters, photos, and other souvenirs stored in a carton. (Much of Pentzikis's work has taken its inspiration from the miscellaneous contents of such cartons.) The Greek title, *Ikones*, is ambiguous; it might mean "images," "pictures," or "icons" proper (that is, Byzantine religious paintings). In his introduction to the collection, Pentzikis stated that all but the last poem had been written while he was looking at a number of photos of sculptures from the Louvre. He then took great care to list all those items, filling nearly a page, but not before he expressed some thoughts that made the list more meaningful. He believed that he should get down to basics, that his reactions to the world should be unclouded by emotions and thoughts, which tend to compartmentalize and distort reality. The *Ikones* are not self-contained poems, based more or less on mood or offering a particular message; they are rather stages in a process, tentative attempts at developing an objective relationship with the world:

> By dying I myself become an object, a statue of life,
> a replica like the face which I now hold before me
> admiring it, as the artist of the Renaissance admired
> a vertebra of the human body. The truth of the human
> body's life with all its possible variations excels
> over any idea.

Working with a pile of mementos in front of him, Pentzikis both challenged and surrendered to his memory. He was deliberate when he extracted from memory its secrets, but he also found in memory an escape from actuality—in the case of *Ikones*, the actuality of war and personal failure. The dual mechanism of memory is clear in "Dhidhahi" (instruction), the first poem of the volume. The impatient and heavily charged lines of this poem suggest the struggle waged by the observing mind with its memories. These, like roses pressed between the pages of an old book, preserve enough of their fragrance to interfere with the mind's resolution to break out into a state of pure essence, an indivisible objective reality.

The poetry of *Ikones* is much more angular than mere summaries or descriptions of it can show. In its convolutions, one discerns Pentzikis's constant and insistent search for a rhythm. He looked for a pattern, a method of living that would honor both the complexity and the simplicity of life. This search is more explicit in the sixth poem (which, like all the poems in the volume except the first and the last, is untitled):

> I must not fail anything
> more of the components of being
> in the matrix that is being put
> together
> the beautiful in simple forms
> simplicity and complicated structure
> progressing all the time

This is the flow, the vital flow—often undercut or reversed by its own rashness but also persistent—of the subject to the object. As Pentzikis writes in the fourth poem, "the object has its own value/ if I love life I should not subdue it/ its not coming to see me does not matter."

The last poem in *Ikones*, "Rapsodhia skeseon" (rhapsody of relationships), comprises more than five hundred lines. In a brief note appended to the poem, Pentzikis informed his readers that its composition had been bracketed by two deaths, that of a cousin of his mother and that of an old lady who used to clean his drugstore. One death heralded the poem and another underscored it. The poem itself also contains visions of death, among which is a recollection of the funeral of

Pentzikis's own father. Dryly descriptive scenes alternate with meditative passages in which the experience of death is reevaluated in the light of religion.

THE MIDDLE POEMS

Between 1949 and 1953, Pentzikis published in successive issues of the journal *Morfes* a series of poems which one might call his "middle poems," because they fall between *Ikones* and the later series of poems, *Anakomidhi* (transferal of relics) and were given no general name. The "middle poems" are more lyric and topical than the poems of *Ikones*; they tell stories and evoke legends associated mostly with Greek Macedonia, describing various geographical areas and combining reality with myth in an effort to enlarge upon the central theme by means of concrete detail.

The poem "Topoghrafia" (topography) is in free verse, but the lines are grouped in quatrains. As its title promises, the poem provides an exact topographical and historical description of a particular spot in Thessaloníki, but the description ends on a sentimental note which is the secret core of the poem. Here, Pentzikis confounds the reader's expectations. He might have started with the image of the sitting girl, the poet's beloved, and then located or described the surrounding landscape outward. Instead, he progresses from the borders to the center of the scene, through allusions to the life and martyrdom of Saint Demetrius, Thessaloníki's patron saint. Thus, the image of the sitting girl at the end of the poem comes as a revelation. It is a lyric image, but the sentiments it evokes have been colored and deepened by the girl's precise placement in a space hallowed by time.

In the much longer poem "Symvan" (event), a group of soldiers on leave visit a country chapel. One of the soldiers narrates an old story of the miraculous rescue of Thessaloníki by Saint Demetrius from a hostile invasion from the north. The soldiers gain a vision of the city not as a group of buildings but as a living person. The past comes alive, and the present becomes meaningful. Pentzikis uses the same method in the poem "Messa ston paleo nao" (in the old church), in which he describes the interior of a church while musing on the faith which motivated the church's builders.

Not all these "middle poems," however, structure and control the poet's feelings around some historical or topographical reality. In the poem "Strophil" ("Turn," or "Turning Point"), exclamation seems to be the dominant note:

> I want to sing of you, flowers of the earth
> as I plunge my hand in the past of the race
> through heaps of fallen dead leaves
> to the stem that raises its head high.
> The head that will be reaped at some moment
> to the most heartfelt satisfaction of God
> reading it we are able to die
> serene in our intimacy with another life.

The message is similar to that of a number of the "middle poems"—indeed, of Pentzikis's entire oeuvre: The "other" life, the truer life, can be gained via death. The manner of this particular poem, however, is unusually lyric, like a dance. It expresses no doubts; Pentzikis lets himself go on simple faith.

ANAKOMIDHI

In the later series of poems, *Anakomidhi*, Pentzikis reverted to a looser and more abstract form. He no longer grouped lines in stanzas of four lines each but ran them consecutively. The poems collected in *Anakomidhi* are very much like pieces of prose, but they are also dense and allusive. They reminded Pentzikis's readers of *Ikones*, with which they are linked by the introductory poem, "Horos kimitiriou" (space of cemetery). This poem was written in the late 1940's, while the other thirteen poems in the collection—twelve of them numbered with Greek numerals and the thirteenth entitled "Sinanastrofi sinchis" (constant association)— were written in 1960 and 1961 in response to the transferal of the remains of Pentzikis's mother.

The spade which unearths the bones of the dead mixes deeply buried memories and feelings with the soil. The poems are like bones, so to speak, suddenly exposed to light together with the contents of the grave. Images, thoughts, impressions, and sentiments jostle against one another and at the same time struggle to cohere. All the poems in *Anakomidhi* are transpositions of things into poetry, avenues of traffic between the present and the past, between life and what is wrongly thought to be dead and gone.

A similar rhythm can be felt throughout Pentzikis's verse as he moves up into the realm of myth and down into the world of doubt and despair, the world of perishable things, which he rediscovers and embraces only in the light of myth. Thus, for Pentzikis, a human being is insignificant, a particle of dust or a "garbage can," but also a vehicle of memory and a reflection of the Godhead.

OTHER MAJOR WORKS

LONG FICTION: *Andréas Dhimakoudhis*, 1935; *O pethamenos ke i anastasi*, pb. 1944 (wr. 1938).

NONFICTION: *Pragmatognosia*, 1950; *Arhitektoniki tis skorpias zois*, 1963; *Mitera Thessaloniki*, 1970 (*Mother Salonika*, 1998); *Sinodhia*, 1970; *Omilimata*, 1972; *Simiosis ekato imeron*, 1973; *Arhion*, 1974; *Pros ekklesiasmo*, 1986.

BIBLIOGRAPHY

Friar, Kimon. *Modern Greek Poetry*. New York: Simon & Schuster, 1973. Translations of Greek poetry in English with some commentary on the biographical and historical backgrounds of the poets.

Thaniel, George. *Homage to Byzantium: The Life and Work of Nikos Gabriel Pentzikis*. St. Paul, Minn.: North Central, 1983. A critical study of Pentzikis's work. Includes bibliographic references and an index.

Voyiatzaki, Evi. *The Body in the Text: James Joyce's "Ulysses" and the Modern Greek Novel*. Lanham, Md.: Lexington Books, 2002. While this text concentrates on the modern novel, it features a chapter on Pentzikis, which sheds light on his poetry.

George Thaniel

SAINT-JOHN PERSE
Alexis Saint-Léger Léger

Born: Guadeloupe, French Antilles; May 31, 1887
Died: Giens, France; September 20, 1975

PRINCIPAL POETRY

Éloges, 1911 (English translation, 1944)
Amitié du prince, 1924 (*Friendship of the Prince*, 1944)

Anabase, 1924 (*Anabasis*, 1930)
Exil, 1942 (*Exile*, 1949)
Pluies, 1943 (*Rains*, 1949)
Éloges, and Other Poems, 1944 (includes *Éloges*
    and *Friendship of the Prince*)
Neiges, 1944 (*Snows*, 1949)
Vents, 1946 (*Winds*, 1953)
Exile, and Other Poems, 1949 (includes *Exile*,
    Rains, and *Snows*)
Amers, 1957 (*Seamarks*, 1958)
Chronique, 1960 (English translation, 1961)
Oiseaux, 1962 (*Birds*, 1966)
St.-John Perse: Collected Poems, 1971, 1982

OTHER LITERARY FORMS

Some 440 pages of the Pléiade edition of the *Œuvres complètes* (1972) of Saint-John Perse (pehrs), which was supervised by the poet himself, are given to letters. Perse's letters provide the reader not only with a wealth of details about his life but also with comments about his poems and political and cultural events during more than half a century. In Perse's letters to his family and to literary figures such as André Gide, Paul Claudel, Jacques Rivière, Archibald MacLeish, Allen Tate, and T. S. Eliot, one can find clues to the duality of Saint-John Perse the poet and Alexis Saint-Léger Léger the diplomat. An English translation of these letters by Arthur Knodel, *St.-John Perse: Letters* (1979), gives them the same emphasis as Gide's or Claudel's journals.

Perse's Nobel Prize acceptance speech, "Poésie" ("On Poetry"), delivered in Stockholm on December 10, 1960, and his address "Pour Dante" ("Dante"), delivered in Florence on April 20, 1965, to mark the seventh centenary of Dante's birth, are available in *St.-John Perse: Collected Poems*, a bilingual edition. Perse's manuscripts, his annotated personal library, his notebooks on ornithology, several scrapbooks with clippings, and other documents have all been gathered by the Saint-John Perse Foundation in Aix-en-Provence, France.

ACHIEVEMENTS

Saint-John Perse is a "poet's poet." Although he won international recognition with the Nobel Prize in Literature in 1960, preceded by the Grand Prix National des Lettres and the Grand Prix International de Poésie in 1959, his readership has remained small. Poets as diverse as Eliot and Czesław Miłosz have paid him tribute; it is in the tributes of Perse's fellow poets that one finds the measure of his work, rather than in the standard literary histories of his age, for he remained aloof from fashionable movements of the century.

Indeed, Perse is characterized above all by a self-conscious detachment. During his diplomatic career, from 1914 to 1940, he maintained a sharp division between his public and his poetic persona. In these years, he published only two works, *Anabasis* and *Friendship of the Prince*. His choice of a partly English pseudonym emphasized his aloof stance.

Perse's exile to the United States in 1941 marked the end of his political career but the revival of his poetic creation. *Exile*, his first poem written in the United States, was first published in French in *Poetry* magazine in 1941. Although Perse never wrote in English, his poems were always published in the United States in bilingual editions and followed by numerous articles and reviews by American critics. Perse disdained literary factions and did not give public readings of his works. He twice refused the Norton Chair of Poetry at Harvard, in 1946 and 1952, but he was officially recognized by the American Academy of Arts and Letters in 1950, when he received the Award of Merit Medal for poetry.

In his poetry, Perse maintained distance by seldom including place-names or markers of any kind that would locate his work in a specific place or time. In Perse's conception, the poet's task, like the scientist's, is to explore the universe, the elements, and human consciousness. The distinguishing quality of Perse's poetry is its universality, its endeavor to celebrate the cosmos and humankind beyond the limits of the personal, beyond the literary currents of the time. In this conception, poetry is not a re-creation or a transcription of reality; rather, poetry is reality, continually in flux, with all its tensions and its complexity. Perse's long poems, free from a specific form or traditional meter, and his symphonic compositions, with echoes and variations of the same phrase, achieve a musical quality seldom surpassed by his contemporaries.

BIOGRAPHY

Alexis Saint-Léger Léger (who wrote using the pseudonym Saint-John Perse) was born on May 31, 1887, on a small island near Pointe-à-Pitre in Guadeloupe. His parents were both of French descent and came from families of plantation owners and naval officers established in the islands since the seventeenth and eighteenth centuries. Perse spent his childhood in Guadeloupe, where his father was a lawyer. The young poet and his sisters were brought up on family plantations among servants, private tutors, and plantation workers. It was not until the age of nine that Perse started school. In 1899, a few years later, earthquakes, the Spanish-American War, and an economic crisis compelled the family to leave for France, where they settled in Pau. In 1904, Perse began studying law, science, literature, and medicine at the University of Bordeaux. He wrote his first poems there, and between 1904 and 1914, he met a number of writers, among them Francis Jammes, Claudel, Paul Valéry, Gide, and Rivière. After his military service in 1905 and 1906, Perse divided his time between traveling and studying political science, music, and philosophy; he soon extended his circle of friends to include Erik Satie and Igor Stravinsky.

Perse spent the years from 1916 to 1921 in Peking, where he wrote *Anabasis*. After serving in the Ministry of Foreign Affairs, he was promoted in 1933 to secretary general, a position that he held until 1940, when the war and the Vichy government forced him to leave for England and, shortly after, for the United States. It was MacLeish who encouraged him to accept an appointment at the Library of Congress. In 1942, Perse published *Exile* and became known officially as Saint-John Perse. He spent the following seventeen years in the United States, where his voluntary exile provided him with an endless array of new scenery, including rare species of birds and plants that he painstakingly detailed in his notebooks. In 1946, he published *Winds*, followed by *Seamarks* in 1957; in the latter year, he returned to France, where he continued to spend most of his summers. In 1958, he married Dorothy Milburn Russell in Washington, D.C. Limited editions of his last two major works, *Chronique* and *Birds*, were illustrated with color etchings by Georges Braque. Al-

though the years that followed his Nobel Prize in 1960 were rich in translations, new editions, and tributes, Perse's publications after *Birds* were limited to a few short poems. He spent his last years in France at the Presqu'île de Giens, where he died in 1975 at the age of eighty-eight.

ANALYSIS

When asked why he wrote, Saint-John Perse always had the same answer: "to live better." For him, poetry was a way of life, not self-centered but open to the world. In his work, the universe predominates over the self, and very little space is left in the texts for the poet's own life and feelings. Perse recorded details of travels and carefully described the flora and fauna that he encountered; these details constitute the only "autobiographical" elements in his *Œuvres complètes*. Perse was a close observer of nature, often compared to the Swedish botanist Carolus Linnaeus, Henry David

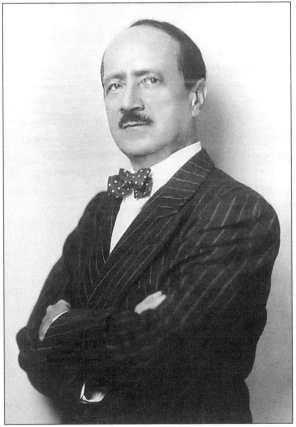

Saint-John Perse (©The Nobel Foundation)

Thoreau, and Walt Whitman. He was not only a scientist who named things but also a thinker and wanderer. The constant tension between the microcosm and the macrocosm, the precise words for small details, provided Perse with a means to stop, to reverse, or to capture what the Romantics cried for: the passage of time. Few poets have been so at ease with the concept of time and space; for Perse, these concepts are not limited by nihilism or religion. Perse rejected the alternatives represented by Jean-Paul Sartre and Claudel: Neither humanity nor God is the center of his vision. There is only the universe and the beyond, the symbiosis of humanity and the elements. Perse goes beyond traditional spatiotemporal limits. He is everywhere and nowhere in particular; in his sweeping vision, time and space merge in one eternal movement.

This universality was recognized by the Swedish Academy, which awarded Perse the Nobel Prize for "the soaring flight and the evocative imagery of his poetry, which in a visionary fashion reflects the conditions of our time." Perse's oeuvre leaves an impression of wholeness. He saw his poems as "one long uninterrupted phrase," as if they belonged to the same mold or flow.

ÉLOGES

In Perse's first collection, *Éloges*, one can find the roots of his later, more solemn, longer poems: the mysterious forces of the elements, the insistent presence of the sea, the celebration of life as well as the yearning for other shores, for a place *outre-mer* (beyond the sea) and *outre-songe* (beyond the dream). The figure dominating Perse's works has no proper name; "Navigator" and "Poet" together provide enigmatic suggestions of anonymity and leadership.

Perse's manuscripts, with their lists of variations and echoes of other poems or lines, sometimes more than half a century apart, show that the final version of a given poem was often highly condensed, frequently a synthesis of passages written at different times. His oeuvre is characterized by an unusual consistency of style and vision; a complex network of recurring motifs provides an inner structure that belies the prosaic "formlessness" of his verse.

ANABASIS

Anabasis, Perse's first major poem, recounts an expedition through the desert, the symbol of humankind's march through time and space and through consciousness. Although it was written in China in a Daoist temple in the Gobi Desert, it echoes the *Kyrou anabasis* (n.d.; *Anabasis*, 1623; also known as *Expedition of Cyrus*, and *The March Up Country*) of the Greek historian Xenophon, describing the retreat of a mercenary force of ten thousand Greeks after the failure of an expedition organized by Cyrus the Younger against his older brother Artaxerxes. Emphasizing the literal meaning of "anabasis," an expedition beyond geographical boundaries (in this case, both inland and inward, toward the essence of Being), Perse sets his poem outside a particular time and place. In addition to the narrative and epic aspects of the poem, it is perhaps this very movement of the expedition and march that has inspired composers such as Alan Hovhaness and Paul Bowles in their musical transcriptions of passages from *Anabasis*. They were preceded by the Swedish composer Karl-Birger Blomdahl, a disciple of Paul Hindemith and Béla Bartók, who composed an oratorio using the original French version of the poem. Blomdahl saw *Anabasis* as an "uninterrupted dialogue" and compared the work to a Byzantine mosaic. This fragmented aspect of some of the more elliptical and condensed passages in *Anabasis* perhaps results from the fact that the published poem was the condensed version of an original poem four times as long.

This epic poem has ten cantos framed by two songs in which the birth of a colt, the passage of a stranger, and the "feminine" soul are related parts of Perse's main network of motifs. In the first group of cantos, the stranger reappears, contemplating his land. Through the figure of the stranger, Perse explores the conflict between the restless urge to conquer new lands and the civilizing impulse to build a city. Tracing a cycle of exploration, achievement, and renewed restlessness, the poem conveys the movement of human history.

SEAMARKS

Seamarks, Perse's longest poem, recalls classical Greek drama with its imagery, its chorus and altar, and the sea being the theatrical arena where man and woman celebrate life. In French, the title *Amers* also suggests a fusion of "sea" (*mer*) and "love" (*amour*). The poem's four parts are divided in turn into cantos of uneven length. In the first part, "Invocation," ritual preparation for the celebration of the sea is accompanied by ritual preparation for the poem, unifying reality and poetry. The second part, "Strophe," or "movement of the chorus around the altar," introduces the different groups and individuals confronting the sea for "questioning, entreaty, imprecation, initiation, appeal, or celebration." The second part ends with a very long canto, "Étroits sont les vaisseaux . . ." ("Narrow Are the Vessels . . ."), the high point of the poem, which celebrates the physical and psychological union of man and woman. They are navigating on a ship as narrow as a couch, and the woman's body has the shape of a vessel; thus, the sea, which seems to protect and "bear" the lovers, becomes feminine and a synonym for love.

In the third part, "Choeur" ("Chorus"), one collective voice exalts the sea on behalf of humankind, and the procession from the city to the shore led by the poet is, according to Perse, the "image of humanity marching towards its highest destiny." In the concluding fourth part, "Dédicace" ("Dedication"), it is noon; the drama is over, and the poet removes his mask, after having brought his people to the highest point in time and space, where humanity is immortal. One finds the same ascension and defiance of death in Perse's next poem, *Chronique*, which is the "chronicle" of the earth, of humanity, and of the poet himself in pursuit of nomadism toward higher elevations and a "higher sea," beyond death.

BIRDS

Perse's last major poem, *Birds*, is more a meditation on art and on poetry than a continuation of the cosmic cycle of *Anabasis*, *Seamarks*, and *Chronique*. The limited first edition of the poem was illustrated with twelve lithographs by Braque; the references to Braque's birds were added after Perse had already written most of the poem. They add a new dimension to the bird in flight, now caught on the canvas, where it continues to live, not as a visual image but as a living part of reality. The descriptive, the technical, and the metaphysical passages of the poem, although very different from one another, all convey the movement of the bird in flight— on the canvas, in the air, and in poetry.

The poem is divided into thirteen parts, the first part introducing the migratory bird, which searches for "an uninterrupted summer," as do the painter and the poet. The asceticism and the "combustion" of his flight have a symbolic import, reinforced in the last part, in which the bird's wings are like a cross. Part 2 presents a very technical description of the anatomy of the bird compared to the structure of a ship, as was the woman in *Seamarks*. It is followed in parts 3 through 7 by the description of the bird perceived by Braque's eye, like the eye of a bird of prey, and painted on the canvas, where it continues to live and fly in its metamorphoses throughout the successive stages of the painting. The finished painting is like the launching of a ship, and the needle of the nautical compass, shaped as a bird, now becomes the symbol for direction and equilibrium. In parts 8 through 10, the bird, defying the seasons, night, and gravity, continues its migration, searching for eternity and "the expanse of Being." In parts 11 and 12, Perse returns to Braque, but only to give a long list of legendary or historical birds that are different from Braque's anonymous birds on the canvas. Thus, the bird becomes the poet's sacred messenger and a symbol for the nomadism of his poetic creation.

Perse's epic vision of the universe informs his entire oeuvre—a timeless vision that will endure when many celebrated poems, tied too closely to their time and place, have faded into oblivion.

OTHER MAJOR WORKS

NONFICTION: *St.-John Perse: Letters*, 1979; *The Poet and the Diplomat: The Correspondence of Dag Hammarskjöld and Alexis Leger*, 2001 (Marie-Noëlle Little, editor).

MISCELLANEOUS: *Œuvres complètes*, 1972 (includes poetry and letters).

BIBLIOGRAPHY

Baker, Peter. *Obdurate Brilliance: Exteriority and the Modern Long Poem*. Gainesville: University Press of Florida, 1991. Critical interpretation of some of Perse's works with an introduction to the history of American poetry in the twentieth century. Includes bibliographical references and index.

Galand, René. *Saint-John Léger*. Boston: Twayne, 1972. A standard critical biography of Perse.

Knodel, Arthur. *Saint-John Perse*. Edinburgh: Edinburgh University Press, 1966. Critical analysis of selected works by Perse. Includes bibliographic references.

Kopenhagen-Urian, Judith. "Delicious Abyss: The Biblical Darkness in the Poetry of Saint-John Perse." *Comparative Literature Studies* 36, no. 3 (1999): 195-208. Kopenhagen-Urian examines Saint-John Perse's oxymoron "delicious abyss" in relation to four functions observed in Perse's use of the Bible: the contrasting perspective, the structured allusion, the repeated motif, and the "collage."

Loichot, Valérie. *Orphan Narratives: The Postplantation Literature of Faulkner, Glissant, Morrison, and Saint-John Perse.* Charlottesville: University of Virginia Press, 2007. Loichot compares and contrasts Perse's *Éloges* with works by William Faulkner, Édouard Glissant, and Toni Morrison.

Ostrovsky, Erika. *Under the Sign of Ambiguity: Saint-John Perse/Alexis Léger.* New York: New York University Press, 1984. A thorough biography, with aesthetic and psychological insights into Perse's life and accomplishments.

Poiana, Peter. "The Order of *Mimesis* in Saint-John Perse's *Vents.*" *Neophilologus* 91 (2007): 33-49. This extensive examination of how mimesis functions in Perse's *Winds* sheds light on many aspects of his poetic vision.

Rigolot, Carol. *Forged Genealogies: Saint-John Perse's Conversations with Culture.* Chapel Hill: University of North Carolina Press, 2002. Analyzes Perse's multiple strategies of dialogue within his poems.

Sterling, Richard L. *The Prose Works of Saint-John Perse: Towards an Understanding of His Poetry.* New York: Peter Lang, 1994. A critical study of the prose works of Perse that is intended to give a fuller understanding of his poetry. Includes bibliographical references and index.

Marie-Noëlle D. Little

PERSIUS

Born: Volaterrae, Etruria (now Volterra, Italy); December 4, 34 C.E.
Died: Campania (now in Italy); November 24, 62 C.E.

PRINCIPAL POETRY

Saturae, first century C.E. (*Satires*, 1616)

OTHER LITERARY FORMS

Persius (PUR-shee-uhs) is remembered only for his satires.

ACHIEVEMENTS

Modern critics slight Persius for lacking the *felicitas* of Horace and the *indignatio* of Juvenal; ancients were apparently satisfied to allow him to occupy his own space. The *Life of Persius* reports that Lucan, upon hearing a reading of the satires, cried that these works were true poetry while he himself was composing trifles. Persius clearly influenced Juvenal, although Juvenal chooses not to mention him by name. Martial and Quintilian, however, single him out for praise, emphasizing that Persius wrote only one book. Quintilian also cites him often for lexical or grammatical illustrations.

That the satires are preserved in several manuscripts is evidence of their continuing popularity in the Middle Ages. Persius's luster began to tarnish when modern critics decided that the difficulties of his language did not repay their efforts, but interest in his work has been renewed by later studies and commentaries. He is, indeed, not Horace or Juvenal. Persius has his own distinct style and persona. He is worth reading not only for his place in the tradition of Roman satire but also for the use to which he put the genre: an exhortation to moral goodness.

BIOGRAPHY

Most of the information about Aulus Persius Flaccus comes from the anonymous *Life of Persius* attached to various manuscripts. Persius belonged to the equestrian order; he was of distinguished Etruscan lineage and prosperous circumstances. His father died when he was six, and a stepfather died within a few years of marriage to his mother. At the age of twelve, Persius went to Rome to study with the grammarian Remmius Palaemon and the rhetorician Verginius Flavus. When he was sixteen, he attached himself to Lucius Annaeus Cornutus, author, teacher, and freedman from the house of the Annaei, to which the Senecas and Lucan belonged. In satire 5, Persius describes Cornutus's acceptance of him in terms which properly refer to a father's acknowledging a child; Cornutus, however, was more mentor than parent. Persius credits Cornutus with "sowing his ears with Cleanthean fruit"—that is, with inculcating in him the Stoic way of life. He was a relative of the famed Arriae, the elder of whom showed her condemned husband how to die by stabbing herself. The younger Arria was the wife of the Stoic Thrasea Paetus, himself condemned by Nero in 66 C.E. Persius was cherished by Thrasea, sharing with him an earnest adherence to Stoicism.

Very little biographical material can be gleaned from Persius's satires apart from the relationship with Cornutus and his friendship with a certain Macrinus and the poet Caesius Bassus, addressed in satires 2 and 6, respectively. In satire 3, someone tells an anecdote of his school days when he put oil on his eyes to appear ill and so to avoid a recitation to be attended by his father and his father's friends. Persius is sometimes assumed to be the speaker. If so, the anecdote is a fiction, because Persius's father, and probably also his stepfather, would have been dead. The passage more naturally belongs to the primary voice of the satire, one of Persius's companions who is urging him to virtue. The *Life of Persius* calls him temperate and chaste, a man of the gentlest character, of maidenly modesty, fine reputation, and exemplary devotion to his mother, sister, and aunt. This description has prejudiced many against him and has influenced the interpretation of the satires, especially of the obscenity present in satires 1 and 4. Persius makes few references to women and no specific ones to his female relatives. Unbiased reading of the satires themselves provides no justification for the labels "priggish" and "cloistered" that are often associated with him.

Persius died from some kind of stomach ailment before he turned twenty-eight. His very early poetic attempts and some verses about the elder Arria were suppressed by Cornutus, who also shortened the last poem to make it appear finished. The *Life of Persius* says he wrote "both rarely and slowly." Some 650 lines in six satires and 14 lines of prologue are left. These were published by Bassus and were popular immediately and for several hundred years after Persius's death.

ANALYSIS

Any evaluation of Persius's poetry must begin with satire 5 of the *Satires*, which presents Cornutus's supposed judgment of Persius's proper manner and goals of composition:

> You follow the words of the toga, skillful at striking juxtaposition . . . expert at scraping pale morals and at pinning down fault with the humor worthy of a gentleman.

Like the rest of Persius's language, these words involve controversy and present problems of interpretation; nevertheless, they clearly assert the place of Persius within the satiric tradition. His role is to criticize moral failings with humor. Again, at the end of the programmatic first satire, when he associates himself with Lucilius, inventor of satire, and with Horace, his great predecessor in the genre, the terms of the association are criticism and humor.

WIT, HUMOR, AND VISUAL IMAGES

While Stoicism and the Stoic sage provide the standard against which others are criticized, Persius's claim to humor is usually denied. His humor is most apparent when seen against a Ciceronian background. The *ingenuo ludo* (humor worthy of a free man) can be traced back to Cicero. In the *Orator* (46 B.C.E.; also known as *Orator ad M. Brutum* and *De optimo genere dicendi*; *The Orator*, 1776) and *De Oratore* (55 B.C.E.; *On Oratory*, 1742), Cicero treats sources of laughter for the orator, divided into wit and humor. Wit is based on words and is suitable for attacking or responding to attack; humor is based on substance of thought or facts and is displayed in sustained narration and caricature. Although examples from all the Ciceronian categories can be found in Persius's satires, various kinds of verbal ambiguities and vivid scene painting in narration are the most important for appreciating his wit and humor. When Persius describes a scene, it requires visualization, because the picture is more humorous than the words themselves.

The visual aspect of Persius's art is pertinent also to his use of other poets, especially Horace. In *Lines of Enquiry: Studies in Latin Poetry* (1976), Niall Rudd shows that Persius knew Horace by heart and that association of visual images accounts for the pattern of his imitation of Horace. This imitation—or rather, the extensive use of Horatian vocabulary—has obfuscated modern interpretation and commentary. The language of Persius is Horatian but the thought is not, and a case can be made that Persius considered that he was, if not outstripping, at least challenging Horace with his own words.

Apart from his Horatian language, Persius presented other difficulties caused to a large degree by frequent neologisms, use of metaphor, and "striking juxtapositions." Horace had named his satires *Sermones* (conversations) and had affected an easy conversational manner, frequently expressed in dialogue. Persius's conversational style and dialogues are of another sort. The conversation follows its own flow, almost in a stream of consciousness; respondents or adversaries appear and disappear with disconcerting abruptness; nevertheless, the satires are coherent and their meanings are clear.

SATIRE 1

All except satire 1 are primarily explications of Stoic doctrine. Satire 1 is an extended joke, based on the Ovidian story of King Midas, whose ears Apollo changed into those of an ass because he could not distinguish good music from bad. In satire 1, Persius separates himself from his literary milieu and sets himself within the satiric tradition, content with only a few discriminating readers. The joke is established in the eighth line. Persius does not care if he has no readers; one should not seek standards outside himself, for "who at Rome does not—." The conclusion comes in line 121: "Who does not have ass's ears?" Between lines 8 and 121, the diminutive *auriculae*, the word for "ears," is put to curious uses. The goal of contemporary poetry, and even forensic oratory, is to offer sexual titillation to the audience. Persius first says this straightforwardly by having the poems enter the loin and scratch the internal organs. Then by repetition of *auriculis*, he equates the parts of the word; that is, *auri-* (ear) equals *-culis* (buttocks). Simultaneously, he establishes the ears as

hungry and poetry as food. Through these two perversions of poetry, as sexual stimulus and as food, Persius disparages other poets and their audiences. By contrast, the ear of his reader will be whole (*aure*) and clean (*vaporata*).

SATIRE 2

In most of the other satires, the humor is more spice than substance, used to relieve the seriousness of the message. Nominally, satire 2 is a birthday poem to Persius's friend Macrinus, otherwise unknown. In fact, the poem is about prayer: the wicked or foolish things people pray for, habits of life counterproductive to their prayers, imputation to the gods of their own venal character. Persius acknowledges that there is a proper use of externals while denying the efficacy of gold in supplication. From petitioners, the gods desire a soul disposed to what is just and right, pure recesses of the mind, and a heart steeped in noble virtue. With such a nature, one can offer a sacrifice of grain.

SATIRE 3

The whole of satire 3 is ironic. Persius is making fun of himself. He sets the scene, speaks near the beginning and end, and falls asleep in the middle. The premise is that he was carousing the previous night and so has overslept. He is awakened by a friend who sees the drinking as a clear sign that Persius has taken the first step on the path to moral degradation. A lecture is, therefore, in order. The lecture most resembles that given by the worried parent of a college student in a similar condition. The friend appeals to his sense of guilt and shame; he points out all the advantages Persius had that were not available to himself; he provides negative examples of similar behavior; he wonders what will become of him. The premise allows for a presentation of Stoic teaching, and most of what there is, is couched in medical metaphor. The passage, however, is straightforward Stocisim:

Wretches, learn and understand the causes of things: what we are and what life we are born to live; what ranking has been given or where and from where the bend around the goal is easy; what the limit is for silver; what it is right to pray for; what use harsh money has; how much it is fitting to bestow on country and dear kin; whom god has bidden you to be; and in what part of the human sphere you have been placed.

What some centurion would say to all this abruptly ends the sermonizing. For Persius, the centurion is the prototype of the nonphilosophical man; his speech, an example of illiberal humor, is a caricature of philosophers which is apt, occasions laughter, and is funny.

The satire ends with the proposal that Persius is afflicted by the disturbing passions of avarice, lust, fear, and anger, such that even mad Orestes would judge him mad. Single references to madness at the beginning and in the middle of the poem, together with this one to Orestes, suggest that the whole satire illustrates the Stoic paradox that all fools are impious.

SATIRE 4

In satire 4, the level of irony and ambiguity is such that the politician as male prostitute has been named the dominant metaphor. In fact, the whole satire contains seemingly innocent words which also have sexual or, at least, genital connotations. The problem in concentrating on the double meanings is that on the sexual level, the poem is not coherent. Persius seems to be simply teasing.

Although there is no attempt to make the scene Athenian, the reader is asked to pretend that Socrates is talking to Alcibiades. The message of the satire is serious: Know yourself, have internal standards before applying external ones, and see your own faults before criticizing others. The satire is, however, structured in terms of sucking and spitting. Socrates sucked hemlock, Alcibiades should suck hellebore, and the miser sucks flat vinegar. The stranger spits out abuse against Alcibiades, and Alcibiades should spit back what he is not. A carefully constructed image of Alcibiades the precocious politician is destroyed by a reference to his "vaunting his tail to the flattering rabble."

Two caricatures illustrate the observation that no one tries to descend into himself but each looks at the pack on the back in front. Alcibiades prompts the ridicule of Vettidius, but if he should sun himself, some stranger would make fun of him. Exaggeration makes both characterizations humorous, but unrelenting obscenity combines with the exaggeration in the tirade against Alcibiades.

At the end, Socrates alludes to the passions of avarice, lust, and ambition. If Alcibiades is influenced by these, "for nothing would he give his thirsty ears to the people." The final verse is haunting: "Live with yourself; know how damaged your furniture is."

SATIRE 5

Satire 5 is a discussion of the nature of freedom. For this, Persius needs a serious style and so begins by identifying with bards of epic and tragedy who require a hundred voices for their subjects. Persius cannot sustain the level, and the conceit of the hundred voices deteriorates, becoming in turn a hundred mouths, tongues, and, finally, throats into which are heaped globs of hearty song. Cornutus corrects Persius: for him the words of the toga and the moderate style, plebeian meals and not the heads and feet of Mycenaean banquets.

Persius first defines freedom by implication. He, as a legally free Roman citizen, subjected himself to Cornutus. This subjection to Cornutus represents subjection to reason; his "mind is constrained by reason and labors to be conquered." Paradoxically, such a subjection to reason is almost a definition of Stoic freedom, as a comparison with a later section of the satire shows. Only the wise man is free. As Persius "labors to be conquered" by reason, others are conquered by such passions as avarice, gluttony, athletics, gambling, and lust. They realize too late that they have wasted their lives.

Such a sequence of thought leads to the dramatic, open introduction of the discussion: "There is need for freedom." The freedom desired is not the legal freedom possessed by Persius, granted to slaves by masters and praetors. The real masters are those within, the passions mentioned briefly before. Now Persius offers longer illustrations of these masters. One slave to passion is torn between Avarice and Luxury, both of whom address him. Avarice's appeal is urgent; that of Luxury, sensuous. A scene from comedy shows a slave to love. Ambition makes an aedile sponsor an extravagant Floralia. Superstition provokes adherence to foreign cults whose most conspicuous features are held up for ridicule. The litany and the satire are abruptly ended by the laughter of another centurion.

SATIRE 6

The sixth satire is the least humorous and perhaps the least successful of the collection. It is addressed to Bassus, the poet and friend who published Persius's work after his untimely death. Bassus and Persius are spending the winter at their respective country estates. As in satire 2, the address to the friend is only the preface to another subject, here the proper use of wealth. Persius's treatment can be seen as an answer to questions posed indirectly in satire 3: What use does money have? How much should one bestow on country and kin? For his part, Persius claims a middle course. He does not envy others who are richer, he will be neither miserly nor lavish, he will live within his means, and when necessary, he will share his resources with less fortunate friends. Such a way of life calls forth a voice suggesting that Persius's heir will resent the diminution of his inheritance and that importation of Greek philosophy is responsible for such heretical attitudes. The heir himself is summoned. If he is displeased, Persius will leave his money to a beggar, since, ultimately, all are related. He refuses to deprive himself now for the pleasures of some future prodigal. The avarice of the heir must be satisfied by his own efforts, but such avarice knows no limits.

In all the satires on Stoic themes, Persius seeks an unobtrusive pretext for his message. Although based on Stoic doctrine, the calls to virtue have almost universal applicability and are not weighed down by specific references to time or circumstances. Such a universality makes Persius profitable reading in any age.

BIBLIOGRAPHY

Anderson, William, ed. *Essays on Roman Satire.* Princeton, N.J.: Princeton University Press, 1982. The essays "Part vs. Whole in Persius' Fifth Satire" and "Persius and the Rejection of Society" are useful to students of Persius.

Bramble, J. C. *Persius and the Programmatic Satire: A Study in Form and Imagery.* New York: Cambridge University Press, 1974. After a brief study of satire 5, Bramble focuses on satire 1 with a close analysis of how the satire form best suits the thematic material.

Conte, Gian Biagio. *Latin Literature: A History.* Translated by Joseph B. Solodow, revised by Don Fowler and Glenn W. Most. Baltimore: The Johns Hopkins University Press, 1994. Briefly but completely places the poet and his achievements within the overall framework of Roman art and society.

Harvey, R. A. *Commentary on Persius.* Leiden, the Netherlands: E. J. Brill, 1981. Provides an overview of each satire, then close commentary on the texts line by line, clarifying words and phrases and explaining the cultural context of references and allusions. Includes a history of editions.

Hooley, Daniel M. *The Knotted Thong: Structures of Mimesis in Persius.* Ann Arbor: University of Michigan Press, 1997. A monographic treatment of "allusive artistry" in Persius's satires, especially his use of Horace. Hooley treats this use of mimesis in a thematic rather than systematic and comprehensive way, producing an admittedly exploratory rather than definitive work.

_____. *Roman Satire.* Malden, Mass.: Blackwell, 2007. Examines the development of the genre of satire in Rome, placing Persius in his historical time and place.

Hutchinson, G. O. *Latin Literature from Seneca to Juvenal: A Critical Study.* New York: Oxford University Press, 1993. An illuminating review of Persius in terms of his contemporary counterparts.

Morford, Mark. *Persius.* Boston: Twayne, 1984. A brief biography and critical overview of Persius and his six satires, in Twayne's World Authors series. The biography is quite concise, but the treatment of Persius's works is detailed as both criticism and commentary.

Plaza, Maria, ed. *Persius and Juvenal.* New York: Oxford University Press, 2009. This collection of essays looks at both Persius and Juvenal and their works.

Reckford, Kenneth J. *Recognizing Persius.* Princeton, N.J.: Princeton University Press, 2009. Reckford examines the *Satires,* looking at topics such as freedom and integrity.

Carrie Cowherd

FERNANDO PESSOA

Born: Lisbon, Portugal; June 13, 1888
Died: Lisbon, Portugal; November 30, 1935
Also known as: Alberto Caeiro; Álvaro de Campos;
    Ricardo Reis; Alexander Search; Bernardo Soares

PRINCIPAL POETRY

Thirty-five Sonnets, 1918 (as Alexander Search)
English Poems I-III, 1921 (3 volumes, as Search)
Mensagem, 1934 (*Message*, 1992)
Obras completas, 1942-1956
Selected Poems, 1971
Sixty Portuguese Poems, 1971
The Poems of Fernando Pessoa, 1986
*A Little Larger than the Entire Universe: Selected
    Poems*, 2006 (Richard Zenith, editor)
The Collected Poems of Alberto Caeiro, 2007
Selected English Poems, 2007 (Tony Frazer, editor)

OTHER LITERARY FORMS

In addition to his verse, Fernando Pessoa (PEHS-wah) published many critical essays and polemical tracts during the course of his career. Most of these were published in the many Portuguese journals with which he was associated, or as short-run pamphlets for particular occasions. He also accumulated a large body of nonliterary writing of a speculative, philosophical nature that was never intended to be published during his lifetime. Moreover, Pessoa was a prolific letter writer, and he left a large body of uncollected correspondence containing some of his clearest and most detailed commentary on his own work. The vast bulk of this material is now available in the following posthumous collections: *Páginas de doutrina estética*, 1946; *Páginas de estética e de teoria e crítica literárias*, 1966; *Páginas íntimas e de auto-interpretação*, 1966; *Textos filosóficos*, 1968; *Cartas a Armando Côrtes-Rodrigues*, 1945; and *Cartas a João Gaspar Simões*, 1957.

ACHIEVEMENTS

Although very little of Fernando Pessoa's work was collected and published in book form during his lifetime, his poetry—appearing mainly in small literary journals that he founded, supported, or helped to edit—has come to be considered an important expression of the modern sensibility. Pessoa is considered to be a major poet of the twentieth century—and, in the opinion of many of his countrymen, the greatest of all Portuguese poets since Luís de Camões.

This is evident in the increasing influence that his posthumously published work has had on the modern Portuguese tradition in poetry—in which he has come to be considered the seminal figure—and in his effect on the work of such prominent later poets as José Régio and João Gaspar Simões, and, finally, in the works of his many admirers among poets writing in Spanish, English, and many other languages.

Pessoa's preoccupations—the introspective, philosophical nature of his poetry, the epistemological doubts that it expresses, and the anxiety-ridden existential atmosphere that pervades his work—are not provincial but universal in character, and they convey the central concerns found in the work of countless modern writers. Among the recurring themes of Pessoa's work is a persistent concern with understanding the essential nature of the self and its difficulties when subjected to the contingencies of life. Like many other modern writers, Pessoa sought to discover through his writing the psychological truth about the artist's identity: Who is the artist, and what is his or her role among all the fictional selves that inhabit the work? These two concerns are clearly expressed in the reflexive nature of Pessoa's work, where the "I" is constantly turning back upon itself, asking: Who is speaking? and Who is speaking now?

Until 1942, when Pessoa's work began to be published in collected form, his reputation was based mainly on his early poems in English. These were published under the pseudonym Alexander Search and were written mostly between 1903 and 1905, although not published in collected form until a decade later. Otherwise, there was the collection *Message*, the only volume of Pessoa's Portuguese verse published before his death, assembled and submitted to a poetry contest sponsored by the Portuguese Secretariat of National Propaganda in 1934. Neither of these two volumes, however, is representative of the poet's best work, for the verse written in English is imitative, while the poetry of *Message* is fervently nationalistic and hence deliberately provincial. The remainder of his work was known only to the small readerships of short-lived Portuguese literary journals such as *A Águia*, *A Renascença*, *Orpheu*, *Centauro*, *Exílio*, *Portugal futurista*, *Contemporânea*, *Athena*, and *Presença*, in which the majority of his published work—both poetry and prose—appeared between 1912 and 1928.

BIOGRAPHY

Fernando António Nogueira Pessoa was born in Lisbon, Portugal, on June 13, 1888. After the early death of his father, Joãoquim de Seabra Pessoa, in 1893, and the subsequent remarriage of his mother, Maria Madalena Pinheiro Nogueira, to Commandante João Miguel Rosa, the newly appointed Portuguese consul to Durban, South Africa, Pessoa and his mother left Portugal for South Africa in December of 1894. Here, Pessoa received his education in English. From 1894 until August of 1905, when he returned to Lisbon to attend the university there, Pessoa was developing the skills which were later to have such an important effect upon his career: his bilingual abilities in Portu-

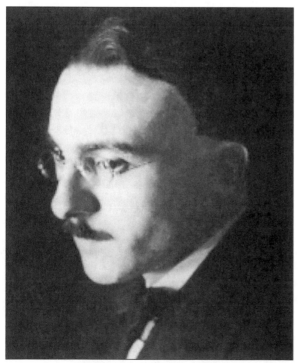

Fernando Pessoa (Centro de Turismo de Portugal)

guese and English and his interest in business and international commerce, which led to a lifelong career as a commercial translator in Lisbon. This position gave Pessoa the flexibility of movement and the leisure necessary to participate in his literary activities, which consisted of the founding and editing of numerous literary journals whose purpose, it became increasingly clear, was to further the development of an indigenous, innovative, modern Portuguese literature.

This developing literary nationalism is evident in the change from Pessoa's early poetry, written in English between 1905 and 1909, to the appearance in that year of his first verse in Portuguese. That early work in Portuguese is clearly reflected in *Message*, much of which was written long before its publication in 1934. It was, however, with the development of his "heteronyms" (three distinct pseudonymous personalities, each with a different style), which first appeared in 1914 and were later widely employed in the many poems he published in small magazines, that the mature work that contributed to his growing international reputation came into being.

This fame, however, was late in coming. Pessoa rarely left Lisbon after his return from South Africa in 1905, and he never left Portugal again. When he died on November 30, 1935, in Lisbon—a victim of alcoholism at the age of forty-seven—he was virtually unknown outside his own country, and to those Portuguese readers who did know him, his greatest accomplishment was thought to be his allegorical collection of nationalistic poems, *Message*. Pessoa's real fame, however, was to come later—through the work of his surrogate selves, of heteronyms (as later critics described them), when the posthumous publication of his complete works, beginning in 1942, revealed the large body of Pessoa's work that had been published under the names Álvaro de Campos, Alberto Caeiro, and Ricardo Reis.

ANALYSIS

During several decades of intense and sustained critical interest, initiated by Simões's *Vida e obra de Fernando Pessoa* (1950; life and works of Fernando Pessoa), Fernando Pessoa's status as a poet has been transformed from that of a literary oddity—combining an intense nationalistic provincialism with an affinity for the faddish avant-garde literary movements of the early twentieth century—into that of a major figure in modern European literature. His poetry is now seen by many critics to express—in both content and form— the deepest concerns of the modern age. Ronald W. Sousa, his "rediscoverer," expresses this new perception of Pessoa's work in *The Rediscoverers*:

Pessoa's writing . . . while not "philosophical" in a strict sense, nonetheless not only treats in practical application the systematic intellectual problems of the day but also does so at a level of abstraction and in a mode of presentation that approach many of the formal properties of traditional philosophy.

This modernist sensibility is characterized by two strong emphases in Pessoa's work: the assertion of the relative or subjective nature of the interior psychological world of the self, and the epistemological reduction of the external world of objects and persons to the status of concrete phenomenological data that exist in a wholly different order of reality from that of the reflecting mind. For this reason, Pessoa's work has come, in recent years, to be associated with the work of two better-known writers: Jorge Luis Borges and Alain Robbe-Grillet.

In the stories and parables of Borges, such as "Borges y yo" ("Borges and I"), "Las ruinas circulares" ("The Circular Ruins"), and "De alguien a nadie" ("From Someone to No One"), one finds an intense questioning of the reality of the self which explores in a more self-conscious, didactic way the identical questions of existence that Pessoa considers in his "Passos da cruz" ("Stations of the Cross"). There, the narrator is the incarnate Christ, Jesus, who reveals his bewilderment in the course of a confusing series of events.

"STATIONS OF THE CROSS"

"Stations of the Cross," written under Pessoa's own name, consists of a series of fourteen sonnets that retell the story of Christ's Passion from the perspective of the suffering victim. In this work, Pessoa's literary kinship with Robbe-Grillet is made evident, for, like the central characters of Robbe-Grillet's New Novels (*nouveaux romans*)—*Les Gommes* (1953; *The Erasers*, 1964) and *Le Voyeur* (1955; *The Voyeur*, 1958)—the speaker of the "Stations of the Cross" sequence is plagued by a split in consciousness that finds him acting out a role in a drama of whose ultimate purpose he is not consciously aware. This epistemological dilemma is well illustrated in sonnet 6, where Jesus speculates on his role in history: "I come from afar and bear in my profile,/ If only in remote and misty form,/ The profile of another being." The puzzled speaker, reflecting on the role into which he has been cast unaware (unlike the biblical account of Christ's Passion, in which he is granted foreknowledge), concludes: "I am myself the loss I suffered." Like Borges's narrators, this speaker seems intended to be a figure representing modern humanity's existential bewilderment.

MESSAGE

Also included in Pessoa's orthonymic poetry (that part of his work published under his own name) are the fervently nationalistic poems of *Message*. These poems constitute the only collection of his poems in Portuguese published during his lifetime. Fortunately, the collection was put together shortly before his death, so that the volume contains work spanning nearly the entire period during which he wrote verse in Portuguese. It would be a mistake, however, to see this collection as representative of his work. For one thing, the collection is dominated by a tone of intense longing for the restoration of Portugal's once-illustrious past. Furthermore, as Sousa has shown in his work on Pessoa, the volume has an elaborate, systematic, symbolic structure (not characteristic of Pessoa's other work) which gives it the thematic unity of a sustained political allegory. Sometimes the nostalgia of *Message* is expressed as a generalized attitude, as in his reminiscence of an unidentified sea explorer in "Mar Português" ("Portuguese Sea"). At other times, Pessoa speaks through the personage of a historical figure such as the sixteenth century king of Portugal Dom Sebastian, who is elevated to the status of a legendary hero in the poem bearing his name: "Mad, yes, mad, because I sought a greatness/ Not in the gift of Fate./ I could not contain the certainty I felt."

This concern with the relativity of the self goes beyond being merely a theme of much of Pessoa's best poetry; it is also expressed in the very manner of its presentation. The writer now known as Pessoa wrote much of his mature work under the assumed identity of a series of three "heteronyms," for each of which Pessoa created not only a biographical background but also a distinctive style.

ÁLVARO DE CAMPOS

The first of the three heteronyms that Pessoa adopted was Álvaro de Campos, whose writing was characterized by the use of long verse lines of uneven length, informal, colloquial diction, and the organic forms of free verse. This style is illustrated in the long, overlapping lines of a poem such as "Na noite terrível" ("In the Terror of the Night"), a poetic meditation on a common existential theme—the creation of oneself by one's own actions. As in much of Pessoa's work, the poem is pervaded by a tone of elegiac regret: "In the terror of the night—the stuff all nights are made of,/ . . . I remember what I did and could have done with life,/ . . . I'd be different now, and perhaps the universe itself/ Would be subtly induced to be different too." This poem exhibits Campos's tendency to mold entire lines—and at times entire poems—around subtle variations of key words. In the example above, this is done with the noun "night," the verb "to do," and the adjective "different," where Pessoa carefully retains their grammatical functions consistently throughout the passage. Another characteristic of Campos's style illustrated in the poem is the use of the paradoxes, oxymorons, and non sequiturs that has frequently led critics to compare his style to that of the French Surrealists.

"TOBACCO-SHOP"

The surreal quality of Campos's work is best seen in "Tabacaria" ("Tobacco-Shop"), in which verbal irrationality is used to create a subtly ironic form of black humor reminiscent of the best poetry of Benjamin Péret, the master comedian of the French Surrealist movement. The speaker of this poem, self-characterized as a metaphysical "genius," sits dreaming in a garret, out of which he observes a little tobacco shop far below in the street. He finally concludes that dreams and fantasies are humankind's only certainty, though they can never have more than an accidental correspondence with the external world.

ALBERTO CAEIRO

Pessoa's second major Portuguese heteronym, Alberto Caeiro, which he employed from time to time between 1914 and 1920 (when he "killed him off" at the tragically young age of twenty-six), is predominantly a nature poet. As Caeiro himself says in a poem titled "If, After I Die":

I am easy to describe.
I lived like mad.
I loved things without sentimentality.
I never had a desire I could not fulfil, because I
   never went blind.
. . . And by the way, I was the only Nature poet.

This epitaph illustrates well Caeiro's simple, colloquial style, which has been described by many critics as essentially prosaic. In creating an informal style for Caeiro which imitates the structure and content of ordinary speech, Pessoa eschews traditional poetic devices such as elevated diction, figures of speech, meter, rhyme, and predictable stanzaic patterns, and employs rhetorical locutions that call attention to the poems as conversation.

"I'M A SHEPHERD" AND "THE KEEPER OF FLOCKS"

These qualities of Caeiro's style are best illustrated in his most famous work, a series of forty-nine brief poems collectively titled "O guardador de rebanhos" ("The Keeper of Flocks"). There are also, however, other characteristic elements of Caeiro's work. One of the most important of these is what critics have called the "antimetaphysical" nature of his thought. As Peter Rickard, one of Pessoa's translators, puts it:

Fundamental to his worldview is the idea that in the world around us, all is surface: things are precisely what they seem, there is no hidden meaning anywhere.

This attitude of calm, naturalistic objectivity toward the world is prominent in poems such as "Sou um guardador de rebanhos" ("I'm a Shepherd"):

I'm a shepherd.
My sheep are my thoughts.
And my thoughts are all sensations.
I think with my eyes and ears
And with my hands and feet
And with my nose and mouth.
And so on a warm day,
. . . I feel my whole body lying full-length in reality,
I know the truth and I'm happy.

Some critics see in Caeiro's thought a foreshadowing of existentialism's assertion of the primacy of existence over essence—where humanity's immediate physical experience in the world is valued above the rational productions of its reflecting consciousness.

RICARDO REIS

It was Pessoa's third major Portuguese heteronym, Ricardo Reis, that served him longest. Works by Reis appeared from 1914, the first year of Pessoa's adoption of the heteronyms, until 1935, the year of his death. Under this guise, Pessoa produced some skillful imitations of Latin poetry, writing a series of Horatian odes the style of which is characterized by archaic, formal diction and the use of free verse. Reis's odes, like those of Horace, are governed by classical conventions that constrain not only the language of the poem but its theme as well. As Pessoa later said of Reis's classicism in a letter to one of his friends: "He writes better than I do, but with a purism which I consider excessive."

Equally important, however, is Reis's attitude toward the world, for in many ways his resigned attitude of detachment from life is the psychological converse of Caeiro's engagement with it. This important contrast in attitude is succinctly characterized by F. E. G. Quintanilha, one of Pessoa's translators:

In opposition to Caeiro's constant discovery of things . . . Reis assumes a stoic and epicurean attitude towards Existence. As he assumes that he can learn nothing more, he shuts himself up in his world and accepts life and destiny with resignation.

"THE ROSES OF THE GARDENS OF ADONIS"

These attitudes and techniques are well illustrated in one of Reis's best odes, "As rosas amo dos jardins do Adónis" ("The Roses of the Gardens of Adonis"), which illustrates a number of characteristic elements: The elevated poetic diction, the Latinate syntax, the perfect strophic form, the use of conventional symbolism drawn from mythology—even the name by which the beloved is addressed is a poetic convention. However, the imitative nature of this ode is not limited to its style, form, or content. The didactic conclusion that the speaker reaches at the end of the poem expresses the carpe diem (seize the day) theme common in classical poetry:

Like them, let us make of our lives *one day*—
Voluntarily, Lydia, unknowing
That there is night before and after
The little that we last.

As Pessoa himself suggested, this degree of imitative purity cannot help but strike the modern reader as "excessive," however skillfully it might be accomplished.

CREATING SELVES

Pessoa's attempt to resolve the epistemological doubts that have plagued the artist in the modern age led him to consider the essential nature of the self, which constituted for him the core of the problem. He concluded that the self is multiple, that it contains many conflicting potentialities. To prove the truth of this proposition, he created the heteronyms, giving each of them a distinctive personality which was reflected in the work they wrote. To Campos, he gave a painful awareness of the reflexive nature of thought and language; he granted Caeiro an absolute, almost inhuman, objectivity; and he provided Reis with a stoic detachment. Each of these selves is thoroughly consistent within itself yet is challenged by the equal though quite different reality of the other two.

Perhaps Pessoa's greatest challenge, however, is not to the reader but to the modern artist himself. To the question of the relation of the author to the fiction that he creates, Pessoa's work provides a clear answer. The mere existence of the heteronyms suggests that the author himself is as much a fiction as the work he creates. To assume that a poem signed Fernando Pessoa is somehow more honest or authentic than one signed by a heteronym—who, after all, is just a name, not someone who really lived—would be to ignore the radical critique of thinking about literature and reality that his accomplishment clearly represents.

OTHER MAJOR WORKS

NONFICTION: *Cartas a Armando Côrtes-Rodrigues*, 1945; *Páginas de doutrina estética*, 1946; *Cartas a João Gaspar Simões*, 1957; *Livro do desassossego*, 1961 (*The Book of Disquiet*, 1991); *Páginas de estética e de teoria e crítica literárias*, 1966; *Páginas íntimas e de auto-interpretação*, 1966; *Textos filosóficos*, 1968; *Always Astonished: Selected Prose*, 1988; *A educação do estóico*, 1999 (*The Education of the Stoic: The Only Manuscript of the Baron of Teive*, 2005; Richard Zenith, editor); *The Selected Prose of Fernando Pessoa*, 2001; *Lisbon: What the Tourist Should See*, 2008.

BIBLIOGRAPHY

Klobucka, Anna M., and Mark Sabine, eds. *Embodying Pessoa: Corporeality, Gender, Sexuality*. Toronto, Ont.: University of Toronto Press, 2007. This collection of essays examines Pessoa's heteronyms and the question of sexual identity in his works.

Monteiro, George. *Fernando Pessoa and Nineteenth-Century Anglo-American Literature*. Lexington: University Press of Kentucky, 2000. The critic searches for the poet's literary influences rooted in the English language. His European models and precursors included John Keats, Elizabeth Barrett Browning, and Lord Byron. Edgar Allan Poe was the most influential of his American models, along with Nathaniel Hawthorne and Walt Whitman. The critic traces elements of influence in Pessoa's work as he identifies the poet's own legacy of influence.

Pessoa, Fernando. *A Little Larger than the Entire Universe: Selected Poems*. Edited and translated by Richard Zenith. New York: Penguin Books, 2006. This excellent translation of Pessoa's work provides an idea of the scope of the works he wrote under his own and other names. The introduction contains background information and some analysis.

Sadlier, Darlene J. *An Introduction to Fernando Pessoa: Modernism and the Paradoxes of Authorship*. Gainesville: University Press of Florida, 1998. This study focuses on the diminished value of authorship in twentieth century literature and the modernist pursuit of source. This vision is consistent with Pessoa's personas, as his heteronyms relate their literary creation to source. This study also explores links between Pessoa's heteronomous writings and his literary predecessors. The critic seeks to broaden an understanding of European modernism by demonstrating that Pessoa's authorship was a mimetic textual performance.

Santos, Irene Ramalho. *Atlantic Poets: Fernando Pessoa's Turn in Anglo-American Modernism*. Hanover, N.H.: University Press of New England, 2003. Examines Pessoa as a modernist, comparing him with Walt Whitman, Emily Dickinson, and other American poets.

Sousa, Ronald W. *The Rediscoverers: Major Writers in the Portuguese Literature of National Regeneration*. University Park: Pennsylvania State University Press, 1981. Addresses Pessoa in the context of Portuguese literature and the modern age. Bibliography.

Steven E. Colburn

SÁNDOR PETŐFI

Born: Kiskörös, Hungary; January 1, 1823
Died: Segesvár, Hungary; July 31, 1849

PRINCIPAL POETRY

A helység-kalapácsa, 1844 (*The Hammer of the Village*, 1873)
Versek, 1842-1844, 1844 (*Poems, 1842-1844*)
Cipruslombok Etelke sírjáról, 1845 (*Cypress Leaves from the Tomb of Etelke*, 1972)
János Vitéz, 1845 (*Janos the Hero*, 1920; revised as *John the Hero*, 2004)
Szerelem gyöngyei, 1845 (*Pearls of Love*, 1972)
Versek II, 1845 (*Poems II*, 1972)
Felhok, 1846 (*Clouds*, 1972)
Összes költeményei, 1847, 1848 (*Collected Poems*, 1972)
"Széchy Mária," 1847
Az apostol, 1848 (*The Apostle: A Narrative Poem*, 1961)
Sixty Poems, 1948
Sándor Petőfi: His Entire Poetic Works, 1972

OTHER LITERARY FORMS

Sándor Petőfi (PEHT-uh-fee) wrote several short narrative pieces for the fashion magazines and periodicals of his day. "A szökevények" (the runaways) was published in the *Pesti Divatlap* in 1845. The following year, his melodramatic novella *A hóhér kötele* (*The Hangman's Rope*, 1973) was published in the same magazine. In 1847, he published two tales in *Életképek*: "A nagyapa" (the grandfather) and "A fakó leány s a pej legény" (the pale girl and the ruddy boy). "Zöld Marci," a drama written in 1845, was destroyed by the author when it was not picked up for theatrical production; the bombastic *Tigris és hiéna* (tiger and hyena) was withdrawn from production but published in 1847. The most valuable prose Petőfi wrote was the personal essay and brief diary entries relating to the events of March, 1848. "Úti jegyzetek" ("journal notes") was serialized in *Életképek* in 1845; in 1847, *Hazánk* published his "Úti levelek Kerényi Frigyeshez" (travel notes to Frigyes Kerényi). *Lapok Petőfi Sándor naplójából* (pages from the diary of Sándor Petőfi) appeared in 1848. In addition, his letters, published in the 1960 *Petőfi Sándor összes prózai muvei és levelezése* (complete prose works and correspondence of Sándor Petőfi), provide good examples of his easy prose style. Early in his career, Petőfi earned some money doing translations of works by such authors as Charles de Bernard, George James, and William Shakespeare. In 1848, Petőfi's translation of Shakespeare's *Coriolanus* (pr. c. 1607-1608) appeared. He also began a translation of *Romeo and Juliet* (pr. c. 1595-1596) but died before finishing it.

ACHIEVEMENTS

Sándor Petőfi has been called Hungary's greatest lyric poet. He made the folk song a medium for the expression of much of the national feeling of the nineteenth century, establishing a new voice and introducing new themes into Hungarian poetry. Building on past traditions, he revitalized Hungarian poetry. Though a revolutionary, he did not break with all tradition, but rather sought a return to native values. Choosing folk poetry as his model, he endorsed its values of realism, immediacy, and simplicity. He also exploited to the fullest its ability to present psychological states through natural and concrete images, with an immediacy that had an impact beyond the poetic sphere.

Petőfi's poetry is the "poetry of Hungarian life, of the Hungarian people," according to Zsolt Beöty. However, although Petőfi drew on popular traditions, he did so with the conscious art of a cultivated poet. This combination of Romantic style and realistic roots gives his poetry a freshness and sincerity that has made him popular both in Hungary and abroad. More important, it has assured him a place in the development of Hungarian lyricism.

Petőfi's impact, however, goes beyond Hungary. He appeals to the emotions yet maintains a distance: His themes seldom lose their universality. For Petőfi, the revolutionary ideal of the nineteenth century applied equally to politics and poetics. Folk orientation and nationalism were equally an organic part of his poetry, and his revolutionary ideals were unthinkable without a popular-national input. Thus, he both mirrors and creates a new world, a new type of person, and a new society. He is an iconoclast and revolutionary only when he perceives existing values and systems as denying the basic value of human life. His endorsement of conventional values of family, home, and a just social order can be understood only in this context.

Style and form, matter and manner were never separate for Petőfi. A consummate craftsperson and a conscious developer of the style and vocabulary of mid-nineteenth century Hungarian poetry, he knew that in helping to create and enrich the new poetic language, he was bringing poetry to the masses. In exploring the language, he made poetic what had been commonplace.

Following in the footsteps of the great Hungarian language reformers and poets of the late eighteenth and early nineteenth centuries, Petőfi expanded the scope of poetry in both theme and language. Like William Wordsworth and Robert Burns in English literature, he placed emphasis on everyday themes and the common person. It would be unfair to the earlier molders of Hungarian poetry, from Mihály Csokonai Vitéz through Károly Kisfaludi, Dániel Berzsenyi, and Mihály Vörösmarty, to minimize their influence on Petőfi. To a great extent, they created a modern Hungarian poetic medium no longer restricted by the limitations of language. Simultaneously, they created a poetic language and encouraged the taste of the public for native themes and native styles. Classical and modern European influences had been absorbed and naturalized by these men. The German influence, strong for both political and demographic reasons, had also been greatly reduced. The intellectual and cultural milieu, in fact, changed so dramatically in these years that German-language theaters and publications were becoming Hungarian in language as well as sentiment. For example, *Hazánk* (homeland), a periodical to which Petőfi contributed regularly, was called, until 1846, *Vaterland*.

As a poet of a many-faceted national consciousness, Petőfi was always committed to the simple folk, to the common person. He did not categorically support the unlettered peasant in favor of the clerk, nor did he condemn the class hierarchy of earlier times without cause. He did condemn, however, inequity and petrified institutions that did not allow for the free play of talent. He endorsed human values above all.

BIOGRAPHY

Sándor Petőfi was born on January 1, 1823, in Kiskörös—a town located on the Hungarian plain—to István Petrovics, innkeeper and butcher, and his wife, Mária Hruz. Petőfi's father's family, in spite of the Serbian name (which Petőfi was to change when he chose poetry as his vocation), had lived in Hungary for generations. His mother, Slovak by birth, came from the Hungarian highlands in the north. Such an ethnic mix was not unusual, and the young man grew up in what he himself considered the "most Magyar" area of all Hungary, the region called Kis Kúnság (Little Cumania) on the Great Plains. Much of his poetry celebrates the people and the landscape of this region: Though not the first to do so, he was more successful than earlier poets in capturing the moods of the region known as the Alföld (lowlands).

Petőfi's father was wealthy, and desiring his sons to be successful, he determined to educate them. The young Petőfi was sent to a succession of schools that were designed to give him a good liberal education in both Hungarian and German, among them the lower gymnasium (high school) at Aszód, from which he graduated valedictorian. He was active in various literary clubs and, through the zeal of several nationalistic teachers, became acquainted with the prominent authors of the eighteenth century: Berzsenyi, József Gvadányi, and Vitéz, as well as the popular poets of the day, Vörösmarty and József Bajza.

The year spent at Selmec, in the upper division of the gymnasium, was marred by his father's financial troubles and by Petőfi's personal clashes with one of his teachers. As a result of these pressures, he yielded to his penchant for the theater and on February 15, 1839, when he was barely sixteen, ran away with a group of touring players.

Petőfi's decision to become an actor was not made lightly, for he knew the value of an education, and he made every effort to complete his studies later. The years that followed were particularly hard ones. Petőfi roamed much of the country, traveling mostly on foot. He took advantage of the hospitality offered at the farms and manor houses, and thus he came to know a wide spectrum of society. On these travels, he also developed his appreciation for nature, uniting his love for it with the objectivity of one who lives close to it. Since acting could not provide him a living, Petőfi decided to join the army, but he was soon discharged for reasons of ill health. In the months following, he became friends with Mór Jókai, later a prominent novelist but at that point a student at Pápa. Petőfi, determined to complete his studies, attended classes there. He joined the literary society and gained recognition as a poet: "A borozo" (the wine drinker), his first published poem, appeared in the prestigious *Athenaeum* in May, 1842, and he also won the society's annual festival.

Petőfi, then nineteen, considered himself a poet; he was determined that this would be his vocation. He planned to finish his studies, to become a professional man able to support himself and to help his parents and also to pursue his chief love, poetry. When a promised position as tutor fell through, however, he was once more forced to leave school and to make his living as an actor, or doing whatever odd jobs (translating, copying) he found. In the winter of 1843-1844, ill and stranded in Debrecen, he copied 108 of his poems, determined to take them to Vörösmarty for an opinion. If the verdict was favorable, Petőfi would remain a poet and somehow earn his living by his pen; if not, he would give up poetry forever. The venture succeeded, and this volume, *Poems, 1842-1844*, firmly established his reputation.

A subscription by the nationalistic literary society Nemzeti Kör provided Petőfi with some funds, and on July 1, 1844, he accepted a position as assistant editor of the *Pesti Divatlap*. From this time on, he earned his living chiefly with his pen. Besides submitting shorter pieces to a variety of journals, he published two heroic poems and a cycle of love lyrics. In March of 1845, he left the *Pesti Divatlap* to tour northern Hungary. A rival journal, *Életképek*, published the series of prose letters, "Journal Notes," in which Petőfi reported his impressions of the people and scenes he encountered. Two more volumes of poetry, *Pearls of Love* and *Poems II*, appeared. Although he became increasingly dedicated to *Életképek*, Petőfi continued to publish in a variety of journals.

In 1846, while campaigning for better remuneration for literary contributors to journals—founding the Society of Ten and even leading a brief strike—Petőfi published another volume of poetry, *Clouds*, and a novella, *The Hangman's Rope*. In the fall, he took a trip to eastern Hungary, intending to publish a second series of travel reports. Early in the trip, however, he met Júlia Szendrey, and the travelogue, as well as his life, changed dramatically. He fell in love with her almost at their first meeting. They were engaged and, despite parental opposition, gained a grudging approval and were married a year later. Júlia was to provide the inspiration for Petőfi's best love lyrics. Sharing his political and national convictions, she encouraged his involvement in politics, even in the campaigns of 1848 and 1849. Petőfi's "Úti levelek Kerényi Frigyeshez" (travel notes to Frigyes Kerényi) thus became more than an account of the customs and sights of Transylvania and the eastern part of the country; they show the development of the relationship between Petőfi and Júlia, their courtship and marriage.

The year 1846 also marked the beginning of Petőfi's friendship with János Arany. Petőfi had been drawn to Arany when the latter won a literary prize with his epic *Toldi* (1847; English translation, 1914). Feeling that they were kindred spirits, Petőfi wrote immediately—and also composed a poem in praise of the then-unknown man from Nagyszalonta. Later, after they met, their friendship deepened and, with it, Arany's influence on the younger man. Arany helped form the objective vein in Petőfi's poetry. Thus, the influence of a worthy mentor who could rein the excesses of his emotions helped Petőfi attain the perfection of the poems he wrote between 1846 and 1849.

Finally, Petőfi also achieved a measure of financial independence through a contract signed in August of 1846 with the publisher Gustáv Emich for the publication of his *Collected Poems*. This relationship assured Petőfi a regular, if modest, income and gave him a friend and adviser who would stand him in good stead in his last, troubled years.

After his marriage and brief honeymoon at Koltó, the hunting castle lent to him by Count Teleki, Petőfi and his wife returned to Pest in November of 1847. Several poems commemorate the weeks at Koltó, including "Szeptember végen" (at the end of September), regarded by many critics as one of the masterpieces of world literature. In Pest, too, Petőfi continued to write, contributing to various journals. His poetry of this period included political themes, and he became increasingly involved in the liberal movements that were sweeping the city. While the seat neither of the Diet nor of the king, Buda and Pest were still regarded by many Hungarians as the rightful center of the country. There was agitation to have the capital returned from Pozsony, now that the reason for its move, the presence of the Turks, no longer existed. Social, legal, and economic reforms were sought, and the cessation of certain military measures, such as the special occupation status of Transylvania and parts of the southeastern region of the country; simply, the Hungarian people desired the reunion of their artificially divided country.

As one of the leaders of the young radicals, Petőfi took part in these political activities, which were to culminate in the demonstrations of March 15, 1848. He had written his "Nemzeti dal" (national ode) the previous day for a national demonstration against Austria. During the day, when his poem, along with the formal demands expressed in the Twelve Points, was printed and distributed without the censor's approval as an affirmation of freedom of the press, Petőfi was in the forefront, reciting the ode several times for the gathering crowds. Through a series of negotiations, acceptance in principle of the program of reform was won. The revolution—as yet a peaceful internal reform—had begun.

When both public safety and national security seemed threatened by the invitations of the Croatian army of Count Josef Jellačić and similar guerrilla bands, Petőfi became a member of the Nemzetor (national guard), which he was to commemorate in one of his poems. He joined the staff of the *Életképek*, which had been edited by his friend Jókai since April, 1848. He published his diary on the events of March and April, 1848, a lively if fragmented account of his activities and thoughts in those days, and also a translation of Shakespeare's *Coriolanus*. In September, he undertook a recruiting tour, and in October, he joined the regular army. The War of Independence was in full force by this time, relations between the Hungarians and the Habsburgs having deteriorated completely. Even the fact that Júlia was expecting the couple's first child in December did not allow Petőfi to draw back from the struggle he had so often advocated in his poems.

Commissioned as a captain in the army on October 15, 1848, Petőfi was assigned to Debrecen. He had difficulties with the discipline and procedures of army life, however, until transferred to the command of General Józef Bem, a Polish patriot and skillful general who was winning the Transylvanian campaign. Through the first half of 1849, Petőfi participated in the Transylvanian campaigns, visiting his wife and son whenever a lull in the fighting or his adjutants' duties allowed. On July 31, 1849, he took part in the Battle of Segesvár and was killed by Cossack forces of the Russian army, which had come to aid the Austrians according to the agreements of the Holy Alliance. Petőfi's body was never found, because he was buried, according to eyewitnesses, in a mass grave. This fact, however, was not known until much later, and many rumors of his living in exile, in hiding, or in a Siberian labor camp were circulated in the 1850's, proof of the people's reluctance to accept his death. His widow's remarriage was severely criticized, though eventually the poet's death had to be accepted. His poetry, however, continues to live.

ANALYSIS

Antal Szerb remarked in his 1934 work, *Magyar irodalomtörténet* (history of Hungarian literature), "Petőfi is a biographical poet. There is no break between the experience and its poetic expression." Sándor Petőfi's poetry, although best analyzed from a biographical perspective, is not autobiographical; its

themes and topics span a surprisingly broad range for a career compressed into such a few years.

THE HUNGARIAN TRADITION

In the early poems, written from 1842 to 1844, Petőfi had already established his distinctive style and some of his favorite themes. Although he was influenced both by classical poets (especially Horace) and by foreign poets of his own era—Friedrich Schiller, Heinrich Heine, the Hungarian-born Austrian poet Nikolaus Lenau, and probably the English poets Lord Byron and Percy Bysshe Shelley—Petőfi believed that Hungarian poetry must free itself of its dependence on foreign rules of prosody in order to reflect native meters and patterns.

In this, he was not the first: The tradition of medieval verse and song had survived and had been revived by previous generations of poets; the seventeenth century epic of Miklós Zrinyi had continued to inspire poets; the folk song, too, had been cultivated by earlier poets, notably Csokonai in the late eighteenth century and Kisfaludi in the early nineteenth century. What was new in Petőfi's approach was his conscious effort to establish a poetic style that put native meters and current speech at the center of his art. Proof of his success is found not only in the immense and ongoing popularity of his poetry among all classes of the population, but also in the recognition accorded him by Arany, who was later to define the "Hungarian national meter" chiefly on the basis of a study of Petőfi's use of native rhythms.

Petőfi's early poems were written primarily in the folk-song style. In subject, they ranged from Anacreontics to love lyrics to personal and meditative poems. The love poems are light and playful exercises without great emotional commitment, but they present the people and locale Petőfi was later to make his own: the *puszta*, its people, plants, and animals. In "Egri hangok" (sounds of Eger), however, the Anacreontic is used for a serious and patriotic purpose, anticipating Petőfi's later use of this genre.

The poem grew out of a personal experience: Walking from Debrecen to Pest in February of 1844, in his gamble to be recognized as a poet or to abandon this vocation, he was welcomed by the students of the college. The poem opens with a quiet winter scene: On the ground, there is snow; in the skies, clouds; but for the poet everything is fine, because he is among friends in a warm room, drinking the fine wines of Eger. The mood is not rowdy but serene and content. Juxtaposing natural imagery and emotion in a manner reminiscent of folk song, he states: "If my good spirits would have seeds:/ I'd sow them above the snow,/ And when they sprout, a forest of roses/ Would crown winter." The mood here, however, only sets the stage for the patriotic sentiment that is the poem's real purpose. Petőfi moves on to consider the historical associations of the city of Eger, the scene of one of the more memorable sieges of the Turkish wars; thus, he examines the decline of Hungary as a nation. He does not dwell long on nostalgia, however, but turns back to the good mood of the opening scenes to predict a bright future for the country.

THE FAMILY

Petőfi's early poems about his family reveal the emotional depth of his best work. They are full of intense yet controlled feeling, but the setting, the style, and the diction remain simple; a realistic note is never lacking. Contemplating a reunion with the mother he has not seen for some time, he rehearses various greetings, only to find that in the moment of reunion he "hangs on her lips—wordlessly,/ Like the fruit on the tree."

The felicitous choice of image and metaphor is one of the greatest attractions of Petőfi's poetry. "Egy estém otthon" (one evening at home) and "István öcsémhez" (to my younger brother, István) reflect the same love and tender concern for his parents. The emotions are deep, yet their expression is restrained: He sees his father's love manifest in the grudging approval bestowed on his "profession" and his mother's love manifest in her incessant questions. Objective in his assessment of his father's inability to understand him, he knows that the bond between them is no less strong. His own emotions are described in a minor key, coming as a comment in the last line of the quatrain, a line that has the effect of a "tag," because it has fewer stresses than the other three.

THE HAMMER OF THE VILLAGE

Petőfi's two heroic poems use the same devices to comment on society—albeit in a light and entertaining manner. *The Hammer of the Village*, written in mock-

heroic style, satirizes both society and the Romantic epic tradition, which by this time had become degraded and commonplace. Using a mixture of colloquialism and slang, the parody is peopled with simple villagers who are presented in epic terms. The characters themselves behave unaffectedly and naturally; it is the narrator who assumes the epic pose and invests their jealousies and Sunday-afternoon amusements with a mock grandeur. Thus, Petőfi shows his ability to use the heroic style, though he debunks certain excesses in the heroic mode then fashionable, presenting the life he knows best; he does this not by ridiculing simple folk but by debunking pretentiousness. Though popular, the poem understandably failed to gain the critical approval of the journal editors, whose main offerings were often in the very vein satirized by Petőfi.

JANOS THE HERO

In contrast, *Janos the Hero* received both critical and popular support. It has served as the basis of an operetta and has often been printed as a children's book especially in foreign translations. Much more than a fairy tale cast in folk-epic style, the work has several levels of meaning and explores many topics of deep concern for the poet and his society.

The hero and his lover, his adventures, his values, and his way of thinking are all part of the folktale tradition. The epic is augmented by more recent historical material: the Turkish wars and Austrian campaigns, events that mingle in the imagination of the villagers who have fought Austria's wars for generations and who fought the Turks for generations before that. The characterization, however, remains realistically rooted in the village. The French king, the Turkish pasha, even the giant are recognizable types. The hero, Janos, remains unaffected and unspoiled, but he is never unsophisticated. His naïveté is not stupidity; he is one to whom worldly glory has less appeal than do his love for Iluska and his desire to be reunited with her.

The style of the poem reinforces this "obvious" level: It is written in the Hungarian Alexandrine, a ten- to eleven-syllable line divided by a caesura into two and two, or two and three, measures. The language is simple and natural, but, as in the folk song, the actual scene is merged with the psychological world of the tale. The similes and metaphors of the poem reflect the method of the folk song and thus extend the richness of meaning found in each statement. The use of the devices goes beyond their traditional application in folk song. Through the pairing of natural phenomena and the protagonist's state of mind, a higher level of meaning is suggested: The adventures of Janos become symbolic of the struggle between good and evil. Iluska becomes the ideal for which he strives as well as the force that keeps him from straying from the moral path; he does not take the robbers' wealth to enrich himself, nor does he accept the French throne and the hand of the princess. Helping the weak and unfortunate, he continues to battle oppression, whether in the form of an unjust master or the Turks or giants and witches who rule over the forces of darkness.

The images used by the lovers on their parting illustrate these principles quite well: Janos asks Iluska to remember him in these words: "If you see a dry stalk driven by the wind/ Let your exiled lover come to your mind." His words are echoed by Iluska's answer: "If you see a broken flower flung on the highway/ Let your fading lover come to your mind." The cosmic connections are suggested, yet nothing inappropriate on the literal level is said. Furthermore, the dry stalk is an appropriate symbol for the grief-stricken and aimlessly wandering Janos. The faded flower as a symbol of the grieving girl becomes a mystical metaphor for her; in the concluding scenes, Janos regains Iluska when he throws the rose he had plucked from her grave into the Waters of Life.

The realism of the folk song and the quality of Hungarian village life are not restricted to the description of character or to the imagery. The setting, particularly when Janos is within the boundaries of Hungary, is that of the Hungarian plain. He walks across the level, almost barren land, stops by a sweep well, and encounters shepherds, bandits, and peddlers, as might any wanderer crossing these regions. These touches and Janos's realistic actions—such as eating the last of the bacon that he had carried with him for the journey, using the brim of his felt hat for a cup and a mole's mound for a pillow, and turning his sheepskin cloak inside out to ward off the rain—reaffirm the hero's basic humanity. He is not the passive Romantic traveler in the mold of Heine or of Byron. He never becomes a mere ob-

server; instead, he naturally assumes an active role and instinctively takes charge of his own life and of events around him. Even in the more mythical setting of the second half of the poem, his sense of purpose does not waver.

The years 1845 and 1846 were intensely emotional ones for Petőfi, and many of his works of this period suffer from a lack of objectivity and of emotional distancing. Love, revenge, and patriotism, a struggle between national priorities, the gulf between the rich and the poor—all sought a voice. The simple lyric of the traditional folk song was not yet strong enough to carry the message, and Petőfi sought a suitable medium of expression. In this time of experimentation, he found in the drama of the Hungarian people an objective correlative for his own emotions.

CLOUDS

The collection *Clouds* contains occasional poems in the world-weary mood of the previous year, but new forms and a new language show that to a great extent Petőfi had mastered the conflicting impulses of the earlier works. The best poems lash out against injustice, or they are patriotic poems that become increasingly militant in tone. In "A Csárda romjai" (the ruins of the Csárda), Petőfi takes a familiar landmark of the arid, deserted lowlands and makes it a metaphor for the decline of the country. The poem opens as a paean to these plains, the poet's favorite landscape because it reminds him of freedom; in succeeding stanzas, he seems to digress from the objective scene into sentimentality. He stops himself, however, before this train of thought goes too far; inasmuch as it is the ruin before him that has inspired these thoughts, the poem is also returned to the concrete scene. The ruin is of stone—a rarity here— so he seeks an explanation, which is soon given: A village or city once stood here, but the Turks destroyed it and left only a half-ruined church. A parenthetical expression brings the poem back to the idea of lost liberty ("Poor Hungary, my poor homeland,/ How many different chains you have already worn"), and the narrative is then resumed.

In time, an inn was built from the church, but those who once lodged there are now long dead. The inn has lost its roof, and its door and window are indistinguishable; all that remains is the sweep of the well, on top of which a lone eagle sits, meditating on mutability. In the final four lines, the scene is expanded to encompass the entire horizon, which serves to give it an optimistic and magical tone. The melancholy scene is bathed in sunshine and surrounded by natural beauty. The parallelism between the decline of the nation and the slow ruin of the church-inn has been established, and a note of optimism for the nation's future has been introduced, but precise development of this idea is only suggested. The point is not belabored.

"A NÉGY-ÖKRÖS SZEKÉR"

The poems of these years showed great variety; not all are in the meditative-patriotic vein. In "A négyökrös szekér" (the ox cart), for example, Petőfi returned to a more personal theme: a nighttime ride in an oxcart. The poem is set in the country; the speaker is on a visit home. With a group of young friends, he returns to the next village in an oxcart to prolong the party. The magic of the evening is suggested in the second stanza—"The merchant breeze moved over the nearby leas/ And brought sweet scents from the grasses"—but the refrain anchors the scene in reality: "Down the highway, pulling the cart,/ The four oxen plodded slowly." The poem remains a retelling of the evening, although a pensive note is introduced when the poet turns to his companion, urging that they choose a star "which will lead us back/ To the happy memories of former times." The poem then closes with the calm notes of the refrain.

"TÜNDÉRÁLOM"

The culmination of this process of revaluation and poetic development comes in "Tündérálom" (fairy dream). This lyric-psychological confession is written in iambic pentameter and eight-line stanzas with a rhyme scheme of *abcbbdbd* so that the *b* rhyme subtly connects the two halves. Its real theme, despite the poet's explicit statement that he has here conjured up "first love," is the search for happiness. As such, the poem fits Petőfi's preoccupations in 1845 and 1846. Although many of the trappings of Romanticism are found in the poem, the longing for an unattainable ideal is given its own expression. It is almost impossible to trace specific influences, yet the poem expresses some of the quintessential notions of the Romantic movement without ever quite losing touch with reality.

The poem owes its success partly to its images, through which the everyday world is constantly brought into contact with the ethereal without disturbing it in the slightest:

> I'm a boatman on a wild, storm-tossed river;
> The waves toss, the light boat shakes,
> It shakes like the cradle that is rocked
> By the violent hands of an angry nurse.
> Fate, the angry nurse of my life.
> You toss and turn my boat,
> You, who like a storm drove on me
> Peace-disturbing passions.

Throughout, the ambiguity between realistic phenomena and magical manifestations is maintained: The dreamer seems to imagine the latter, but the former are asserted. Thus, the mysterious sounds he hears are identified as a swan's song, and, as he leaps from a mountain peak into the sky to gain his ideal, he falls back to awake to a lovely yet earthly maiden. Thus, the idyll is again returned to reality.

The ambiguity can be sustained so successfully because it is the imagery that creates the mood, and Petőfi's sure handling of imagery never allows it to get out of control. The description of the progress of the idyll illustrates this well:

> Dusk approached. On golden clouds
> The sun settled behind the violet mountains;
> A pale fog covered this dry sea,
> The endlessly stretching plain.
> The cliff on which we stood glowed red
> From the last rays, like a purple pillow
> On a throne. But truly, this was a throne
> And we on it the youthful royal couple of happiness.

In a sense, this poem was for Petőfi the swan song of the purely internal lyric. Appropriately, it exhibits the best qualities of his subjective, Romantic early verse. It is melodious, and it unfolds the story in a series of rich and sensuous images. The objective world is completely subordinated to the imaginative one, but it is not ignored. Symbols abound, but they are suggestive, not didactic. The girl in the poem is Imagination and Inspiration; she is the ideal goal of those starting their careers. When she is lost, the ideal is lost, but Petőfi suggests in the closing lines that such an ideal can be held for only a moment. It must give way to reality; thus, it is not lost, only changed. The impractical dreams of youth are supplanted by the practical programs of adulthood which will implement these goals.

"LEVÉL VÁRADY ANTALHOZ"

Two more poems of this fertile period deserve mention: "Levél Várady Antalhoz" (letter to Antal Várady) and "Dalaim" (my songs). Each of these poems serves as an *ars poetica*. In the former, Petőfi states that the beauty of nature has revived him and cured him of his world-weariness, and he affirms his commitment to social and political causes. The six stanzas of "Dalaim" are a masterful expression of the variety of themes and moods found in Petőfi's poetry, from the landscape poetry of his homeland to joy, love, Anacreontics, patriotism, and the desire to free his homeland of foreign rule, as well as to the fiery rage that makes his songs "Lightning flashes of/ his angry soul."

"DALAIM"

"Dalaim," like "Tündérálom," serves as a transition to the final, mature phase of Petőfi's poetry, characterized by a harmonious fusion of the often divergent trends identified so far in his poetry. Personal experiences and national events play as important a part in the formation of this style as do the experimentations of his earlier years. Structure and mood, internal and external scenes merge as his themes become more complex and his subjects more serious. "Naïve realism" is supplanted by a deeper realism, and the personal point of view is gradually replaced by a conscious spokesman for the Hungarian people. The intense emotions of Petőfi's mature poems continue to be expressed in a restrained style, and even the deep love poetry addressed to his wife finds expression in a controlled style that continues to reflect the Hungarian folk song and the European traditions that influenced him at the beginning of his career.

"RESZKET A BOKOR, MERT"

The objective lyric style that marks the best of Petőfi's poetry had two inspirations. One was his wife, Júlia; the other was his friend and fellow poet Arany. Though Petőfi's love for Júlia was deep and passionate, the poetry in which he celebrates that love is both objective and universal.

The poems of his courtship and marriage show a progression from an emphasis on physical beauty to a desire for spiritual identification. The style remains that of the folk song and the direct personal lyric, but the imagery brings a wealth of associations to bear on the relationship. Most prominent are images of blessedness and fulfillment. In "Reszket a bokor, mert" (the bush trembles, because), the intensity of feeling is almost too much for the classic folk-song pattern, yet the poet retains the delicate balance between form and content. Written shortly after their meeting, before Petőfi had a firm commitment from Júlia, the poem is essentially a question posed through a range of associations: "The bush trembles, for/ A little bird alighted there./ My soul trembles, for/ You came to mind." In the following lines, the balance between the exterior, natural scene and the interior, psychological one is maintained. The beloved is likened to a diamond—pure, clear, and precious—and to a rose. This latter image receives emphasis and gains freshness as Petőfi uses the word *rozsaszálam*—that is, a single, long-stemmed rose. To the usual associations, grace and slenderness are added, along with the suggestion of something individual, unique.

The last stanza poses a question: Does Júlia still love him in the cold of winter, as she had loved him in the warmth of summer? Through the reference to the seasons, Petőfi not only retains the parallelism on which the poem is built but also refers to the actual moment from which the poem springs. All this, even the gentle note of resignation in these lines, leads to the statement: "If you no longer love me/ May God bless you,/ But if you do still love me,/ May He bless you a thousandfold." Júlia's answer was, "A thousand times," and from that time on, Petőfi seems to have had no doubt that her commitment to him was as complete as his to her.

"SZEPTEMBER VÉGEN"

The poems continue to chronicle the events and emotions of the courtship, marriage, and honeymoon. "Szeptember végen" (at the end of September) records a day of meditative peace touched by melancholy. The images raise it to extraordinary heights, and the skillful use of meter and mood, image and meaning makes it a masterpiece. It unites the virtues of folk poetry and the gentle philosophy of Petőfi's peaceful moments in an eternal tribute to his wife. Its three stanzas of eight lines each, written in dactylic tetrameter, a relatively slow and descending cadence, are meditative yet grand, suggesting that the poet's soliloquy is not merely a personal matter. The images reflect the scene at Koltó in the foothills of the eastern Carpathians and the autumn setting with its associations of death. The atmosphere created again depends on the union of the natural and the psychological. The poet addresses his wife, calling her attention to the contrast between summer in the garden and the snow already on the mountaintops. He, too, feels this contrast:

> The rays of summer are still flaming in my young heart,
> And in it still lives spring in its glory,
> But see, gray mingles with my dark hair;
> The hoarfrost of winter has smitten my head.

A line that rivals François Villon's "Où sont les neiges d'antan?" (Where are the snows of yesteryear?) introduces the next stanza: "The flower fades, life fleets away." This line gently leads the poem to the next topic, the brevity of life and the poet's premonition that he will precede his wife to the grave. Will she mourn him, or will she soon forget their love?

The gradual movement of the poem, revealing the manner in which one emotion fades into another, enables the poet to escape excesses of sentimentality and melancholy in spite of the topic. As always, realistic touches help bring the reader to accept the closing lines. On one level, the poem is a metaphysical statement concerning the enduring reality of love. On another, it is a deeply felt personal declaration of love set in a specific time and place. The poet's control of his material enables him to assert, without a trace of the maudlin, that life has no more durability than a flower, that permanence is to be found only in the love that endures beyond the grave. The themes of love, nature, and death are united in such a way that not one of them is slighted, not one of them is vague and impersonal.

"RÓZSABOKOR A DOMBOLDALON"

Though his married years were also years of increasingly greater involvement in public affairs and politics, Petőfi continued to write beautiful love poems to his wife. In "Rózsabokor a domboldalon" (rosebush on the hillside), he returns to the happy, carefree tones of the folk song as he compares his wife's leaning on him to the wild rosebush hugging the hillsides. "Minek nevezzelek?" (what shall I name you?) also uses a lighter style, as the poet seeks to explain just what his wife means to him. A catalog of her ethereal charms and spiritual qualities tumbles forth, for he cannot summarize her essence in a word. The directness of his approach, as well as the seeming paradoxes in which the description is couched, again invites the reader to go beyond the surface to think about the thesis of the poem.

"SZERETLEK, KEDVESEM"

Shortly before his death, Petőfi wrote "Szeretlek, kedvesem" (I love you, my dear). Again, there is what seems to be a breathless profession of love as Petőfi lists the ways in which he loves Júlia. The eighty lines of the poem constitute essentially one sentence. Its form, free verse in lines ranging from two to four measures, reflects this quality. The message is not frivolous, however, for he succeeds in conveying a depth of love that excludes all other feelings yet encompasses all. Theirs is a fully mutual relationship, as he states in the last line, for he has learned all he knows of love from her.

"BOLOND ISTÓK"

In Petőfi's objective poetry of the time, also, the mood of these years of married happiness is seen. The verse narrative "Bolond Istók" (crazy Steve) reflects this mood in its story of a wandering hero who finds a haven and a loving wife through his dedication and service. The objectivity and restrained style of the poem balance the hardships of the student with the sentimental overtones of the grandfather, who is disillusioned with his son. Even the romantic flight of the granddaughter to escape a marriage her father wishes to force on her is spared sentimentality. Tongue-in-cheek hyperbole is often the key: The deserted farm "seems to be still in the throes of the Tatar raids," and the old housekeeper and host seem about as civil as Tamburlaine's forces when Istók first comes upon them. The young man's optimism serves to offset this mood and also to introduce the new theme: the arrival of the granddaughter, whose plea for help is to bring hope and new life to the old farmstead. In time, he marries the girl, and in due course a cradle is rocked by the hearth. The cycle of life reasserts itself over the disruption caused by evil.

Other poems, such as "A vńdor" (the wanderer), "A kisbéres" (the hired man), and "A téli esték" (winter evenings), return to the theme of domestic bliss, as do two prose works written during this period: "A nagyapa" (the grandfather) and "A fakó leány s a pej legény" (the pale girl and the ruddy boy).

FRIENDSHIP WITH ARANY

Petőfi's friendship with Arany also reinforced the objective orientation of his poetry. The two men shared many of the same goals, though they did not always agree on the methods to be followed in achieving them. Poetically, too, they differed, yet the friendship was fruitful for both. In the years following their first exchange of letters, their correspondence ranged from their common concern with creating a national poetry, to their families, to a general exchange of information and ideas. The naturally more reserved as well as more pessimistic Arany was often shaken out of his soberness by the playful letters of Petőfi.

The two friends, occasionally joined by others, undertook several projects together. As a result of their collaborative efforts, Petőfi wrote "Széchy Mária" (1847) and began his translation of Shakespeare. It was in Petőfi's genre and landscape poems, however, that the influence of Arany's calmer, more objective style seems to have borne the richest fruit.

PATRIOTIC POEMS

Nationalism, a sense of commitment to and concern for the Hungarian people, and patriotism, a commitment to the political institutions of a free and independent Hungarian nation, are themes found throughout Petőfi's poetry. Often, these concerns appear in an oblique way. Increasingly, after March 15, 1848, however, they became open topics of his poetry while continuing to influence the other genres in the same indirect fashion as earlier. As early as 1846, in "Egy gondolat bánt engement" (one thought troubles me), Petőfi had expressed a desire to die on the battlefield in defense of liberty. The next year, he stated the obligation of the poet to sacrifice personal feelings in the interests of patriotic and human duty in "A XIX: Század költői" (the poets of the nineteenth century). After the events of March, 1848, Petőfi plunged into these responsibilities fully; it is perhaps this which gives his poetry the masculine quality not captured by Western European poets of his time: He calls for action with the conviction of one who is ready to be the first to die in battle. These sentiments are skillfully stated in "Ha férfi vagy, légy férfi" (if you are a man, then be one)—a poetic declaration of principles in which didacticism does not detract from poetic value.

A sense of responsibility to his wife and family did not interfere with Petőfi's commitment to his people; if anything, it contributed to the commitment. Júlia shared his sentiments and supported her husband, and he considered her his partner in his work. "Feleségem és kardom" (my wife and my sword) must be read in conjunction with "Ha férfi vagy, légy férfi," for it balances the picture. His wife, an equal partner, will tie the sword on her husband's waist and send them off together, if necessary. Her heroism is to be admired no less than bravery on the battlefield.

In the early years, Petőfi's patriotic poetry had some nostalgic moments. By 1846, however, he had moved beyond the glorification of the past to the criticism of the present and suggestions for reforms. He called on poets to be active in bringing about reforms, and he urged his readers to take pride in Hungarian traditions. In "Magyar vagyok" (I am a Hungarian), he stated his unequivocal loyalty; "Erdélyben" (in Transylvania) shows the dedication to this eastern region of Hungary that had preserved Hungarian traditions and language in the trying years of the Turkish wars and the Austrian Partition—a dedication echoed by Hungarian poets today.

"NEMZETI DAL"

The events of March 15, which were to transform not only Petőfi's life but also the history of his country, seemed to crown with success the efforts of the reformers. Petőfi's "Nemzeti dal" (national ode) inspired the demonstrators, and the Twelve Points made clear to everyone the goals they were espousing. The spirited call to arms in the refrain—"By the God of the Magyars,/ We swear/ We swear that captives/ We'll no longer be!"—became the rallying cry of the nation. In the poem, nostalgia for the past is united with faith in the future, and the urgency and immediacy of the situation are emphasized in the words that virtually leap at the listener: "Up Magyar, the country calls!/ Here's the time, now or never!/ Shall we be free or captives ever?/ This the question you must answer!" In contrast to the direct address here, the refrain is in a collective mode. A dialogue is thus established, with the poet calling on his audience to respond and prompting their response through the oath phrased in the refrain.

In the six stanzas of this poem, Petőfi chides his countrymen for enduring servitude. It is time for the sword to replace the chain, he urges, so that the Hungarian name will again be great and future generations will bless them. The language and the images are as direct as the tone, and throughout, the poet emphasizes the need for heroic action regardless of the consequences. Understandably, the poem had great impact. If Petőfi had made only this contribution to the independence movement, he would have been remembered, but he did much more.

The Revolution that had begun peacefully, and seemed, at first, to accomplish its goals through legal reform, escalated into war when Hungarian territory was invaded, first by the Croatian armies of Jellačić, who had Imperial support, and later by Austrian forces, as the Chancery consolidated around the new king, Franz Joseph. National minorities within the country were urged by the Austrian government to attack the Hungarians, and some did. Others, notably the German towns, remained neutral or espoused the Hungarian cause. As the war became an open struggle between the Hungarian Ministry and the Habsburgs, Hungarian leader Lajos Kossuth was able to force a final break with Austria, and the Habsburgs were formally deprived of their position as monarchs of Hungary. Petőfi became increasingly involved in both the political and the military events, seeing a break with Austria and the establishment of a republic as the only means of achieving social reform. Of the nearly 150 short lyrics he wrote in 1848 and 1849, almost all deal with the political and military turmoil in Hungary. Some are antimonarchist or anti-Habsburg, some chide the nationalities for turning on the land that gave them shelter earlier, and an increasing number glorify national virtues and ancient constitutional rights that had long been ignored by the monarchs.

WAR POEMS

Petőfi was not sanguine, however, and hopeful poems such as "1848" alternate with ones that express bitter disappointment, such as "Európa csendes, ujra

csendes" ("Europe is quiet, is quiet again"). He saw that Europe had given up its democratic ideals, and no hope of support was left. However, he did not speak of Hungary's cause as a hopeless if glorious one. Even the combined forces of Austria and Russia were no match for his poetic belief in victory, expressed in "Bizony mondom, hogy gyoz most a magyar" ("truly I say, now the Hungarians will win").

Though they constitute a relatively small percentage of his poetic work, Petőfi's war poems deserve attention. For the most part, they are spirited, upbeat marches or a lively mixture of narrative and lyric moods, emphasizing the dedication and heroism of the soldiers. They do not glorify war for its own sake, but rather emphasize the patriotic reason for the combat. "Bordal" (wine song) returns to a traditional genre to urge all men to defend their homeland, "draining blood and life" from anyone who seeks to destroy it just as they "empty the glass of wine."

Petőfi's confidence in the ultimate triumph of his cause, if not on the battlefield or in the treaty rooms then at least in the judgment of history, can be sensed in one of the last battle songs he wrote, "Csatában" (in battle). This poem is also notable for the personal involvement of the poet. He begins the poem by recreating a battle in vivid natural images and giving it a cosmic frame:

> Wrath on the earth,
> Wrath in the sky!
> The red of spilt blood and
> The red rays of the sun!
> The setting sun glows
> In such a wild purple!
> Forward, soldiers,
> Forward, Magyars!

Through such images and a wonderfully effective onomatopoeia, the whole universe seems to become involved in the strife. The poet's own involvement, symbolic of the involvement of the nation, is signaled in the change in the refrain from "Forward" to "Follow me."

Shortly after composing this poem, Petőfi died on the battlefield of Segesvár. Within weeks, the Hungarian Resistance was also over, but Petőfi lives on in legend and in his poetry.

LEGACY

Petőfi's short poetic career established him as a poet of the first rank. The variety of themes and styles he handled with success is amazing; even the less powerful lyrics of his early years have enriched Hungarian literature and music, many of them having been set to music and passing into the modern "folk-song" repertory. His early fame and his fame abroad rested on both his republican sentiments and his romantic early death. Early translations into German were followed by English versions based on the German. His popularity grew with the worldwide interest in the Hungarian Revolution of 1848 and its brutal suppression; it also waned as political realities changed. The Petőfi behind the legend was neglected even in Hungary for a long time; abroad, he is still mostly known as a revolutionary hero, not as a poet. Translations, prepared with enthusiasm but lack of knowledge or skill, seldom do him justice. In Hungary, the most talented of his contemporaries recognized his talents independent of his political views. Today, there is general agreement about his position as a central figure in Hungarian literature and in the development of the Hungarian lyric. His republican, nationalistic, and patriotic ideas are also recognized; they are an essential part of the poet who spoke from the heart of his generation, who spoke for his people, and who spoke for the masses and indeed to give all classes of society a voice. He was truly a poet of national consciousness.

OTHER MAJOR WORKS

LONG FICTION: *A hóhér kötele*, 1846 (novella; *The Hangman's Rope*, 1973).

SHORT FICTION: "A szökevények," 1845; "A fakó leány s a pej legény," 1847; "A nagyapa," 1847.

PLAYS: *Tigris és hiéna*, pb. 1847; *Coriolanus*, pb. 1848 (translation of William Shakespeare's play).

NONFICTION: "Úti jegyzetek," 1845; "Úti levelek Kerényi Frigyeshez," 1847; *Lapok Petőfi Sándor naplójából*, 1848; *Petőfi Sándor összes prózai muvei és levelezése*, 1960; *Petőfi Sándor by Himself*, 1973; *Rebel or Revolutionary? Sándor Petőfi as Revealed by His Diary, Letters, Notes, Pamphlets, and Poems*, 1974.

MISCELLANEOUS: *Works of Sándor Petőfi*, 1973.

BIBLIOGRAPHY

Basa, Enikő Molnár, ed. *Hungarian Literature*. New York: Griffon House, 1993. This overview of Hungarian literature helps place Petőfi in context.

_____. *Sándor Petőfi*. Boston: Twayne, 1980. An introductory biography and critical study of selected works by Petőfi. Includes bibliographic references.

Ewen, Frederick. *A Half-Century of Greatness: The Creative Imagination of Europe, 1848-1884*. New York: New York University Press, 2007. Contains a chapter on Petőfi, examining his role as a soldier and discussing his work.

Illyés, Gyula. *Petőfi*. Translated by G. F. Cushing. 1973. Reprint. Budapest: Kortárs Kiadó, 2002. An exhaustive biography and critical examination of the life and works of Petőfi.

Szirtes, George. Foreword to *John the Valiant*, by Sándor Petőfi. Translated by John Ridland. London: Hesperus Press, 2004. Noted translator Szirtes provides background and some literary analysis for this bilingual translation of *János Vitéz*.

Enikő Molnár Basa (including original translations)

PETRARCH

Born: Arezzo, Tuscany; July 20, 1304
Died: Arquà, Carrara (now in Italy); July 18, 1374

PRINCIPAL POETRY

Epistolae metricae, 1363 (*Metrical Letters*, 1958)
Bucolicum carmen, 1364 (*Eclogues*, 1974)
Africa, 1396 (English translation, 1977)
Rerum vulgarium fragmenta, 1470 (also known as *Canzoniere*; *Rhymes*, 1976)
Trionfi, 1470 (*Tryumphs*, 1565; also known as *Triumphs*, 1962)
Rime disperse, 1826 (also known as *Estravaganti*; *Excluded Rhymes*, 1976)

OTHER LITERARY FORMS

The other writings of Petrarch (PEH-trahrk), except for some prayers in Latin hexameters, are all in Latin prose and consist of epistles, biographies, a collection of exempla, autobiographical works, psalms, orations, invectives, assorted treatises, and even a guidebook to the Holy Land, which he never visited and knew only through the eyes and books of others. Ironically, although the author believed that he would achieve lasting fame because of his Latin compositions, he is remembered today largely for his vernacular poetry. Contemporary scholars do study his Latin works, but primarily to gain insight into his Italian poems. A knowledge of his classically inspired writings, however, is essential to anyone who would understand the cultural milieu that led to the birth of the Renaissance in Italy.

ACHIEVEMENTS

Two words sum up Petrarch's profound historical legacy: Petrarchianism and Humanism. The first stands for the widespread influence of the author's vernacular poetry, especially his love sonnets but also *Triumphs*, on Western European culture from the late fourteenth century to the mid-seventeenth century. It refers to the imitation in literature and the representation in art of the themes and images so carefully crafted in Petrarch's Italian verse: in literature, for example, the expression of the lover's torment through the use of antithesis, oxymoron, hyperbole, and other appropriate rhetorical figures, or the description of the beloved as an ideal yet real lady with golden hair, ivory skin, and pearl teeth; in art, the reproduction of *Triumphs* on canvas and wedding chests and in other media, such as woodcuts, enamels, tapestries, and stained glass, as well as in pageants, ballets, and theatricals. The second term, Humanism, refers to the intellectual and cultural movement that derived from the study of classical literature and civilization during the late Middle Ages and that was one of the main factors contributing to the rise of the Renaissance. Petrarch is commonly called the founder of Humanism because his intense interest in antiquity led him to be the first in modern times to collect ancient manuscripts, compose letters to great Roman and Greek figures of the past, imitate Cicero in his prose and Vergil in his epic poetry, and examine classical writings in their own context, with waning regard for accrued medieval traditions and superstitions. Early

fifteenth century Italian Humanists, such as Coluccio Salutati and Leonardo Bruni, were followers of Petrarch and saw him as the enlightened initiator of a new age, the epoch now known as the Renaissance. In reality, although Petrarch does embody many of the qualities of a Renaissance man because of his well-rounded nature and varied accomplishments, he is neither wholly in the Renaissance nor entirely in the Middle Ages. Rather, he is a transitional or pivotal figure. His vernacular amorous poetry, with its emphasis on the unreciprocated love for an idealized woman, is in many ways only a culmination of the Provençal troubadour tradition; his *Triumphs*, written in Dante's terza rima, could hardly be more medieval; and his psalms and autobiographical dialogues mirror the Middle Ages' confessional literature. Yet the genres and classical style of most of his Latin compositions, his anti-Scholastic attitudes, and his love of secular learning for its moral and civic teachings clearly place him in what would become the mainstream of the Renaissance cultural tradition.

BIOGRAPHY

Petrarch was born Francesco Petrarca in Arezzo, Tuscany (now in Italy), on July 20, 1304, the oldest child of Pietro di Parenzo, an exiled Florentine notary. Di Parenzo, more commonly called Ser Petracco ("Ser" indicates a notary), was a White Guelph and, like Dante, had been exiled from Florence and its territory in 1302. (Petrarch later formed his own surname by ingeniously reworking Petracco into an elegant Latinate form.) Early in 1305, Petrarch's mother, Eletta Canigiani, took her son to her father-in-law's home in Incisa, north of Arezzo and in Florentine territory. There, she and Petrarch lived until 1311, when her husband moved them to the independent state of Pisa. In 1312, the family moved to Carpentras, in Provence, to be near the papal seat, which Clement V had moved to Avignon in 1309. In Carpentras, Petrarch began his study of the *trivium* with Convenevole da Prato and continued his studies there until 1316, when, at the tender age of twelve, he was sent to the University of Montpellier to study law. In 1320, he and his younger brother Gherardo, of whom he was very fond, moved to Bologna to continue their legal studies. Petrarch, how-

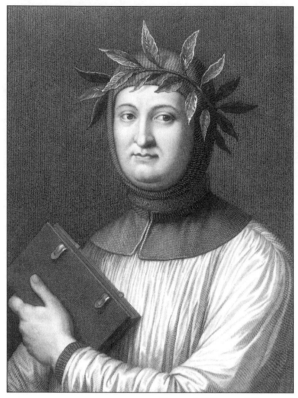

Petrarch (Library of Congress)

ever, never completed the work for his degree because of his many varied interests. Upon the death of his father in 1326, he abandoned forever his pursuit of law and returned with his brother to Avignon. There, the two of them began ecclesiastical careers to improve their financial situations. Petrarch received the tonsure, but he never went further than the minor orders. Gherardo, on the other hand, later became a Carthusian monk.

On Good Friday, 1327, Petrarch saw a woman in the Church of Santa Chiara in Avignon and fell in love with her. The poet identifies her only as Laura, except once when he calls her "Laureta"; her exact identity has never been definitively established. While many critics believe her to be Laura de Noves, who married Hugues de Sade in 1325, others question her very existence. Whatever the case, the figure of Laura, ever reluctant to return the poet's love, is the inspiration or motivation for most of Petrarch's Italian poetry. He even records her death from the plague on April 6, 1348, in his precious copy of Vergil, an indication of the reality and depth of his devotion to her.

In 1330, Petrarch entered the service of Cardinal Giovanni Colonna and remained under that family's patronage for almost two decades. Petrarch soon became, as he characterized himself, a *peregrinus ubique* ("pilgrim everywhere"). In 1333, he traveled through northern France, Flanders, and Germany. He visited Paris, where Dionigi da Borgo San Sepolcro gave him a copy of Saint Augustine's *Confessiones* (397-401; *Confessions*, 1620); Liège, where he discovered two new orations by Cicero; and Aachen, where he visited the tomb of Charlemagne. In 1336, he climbed Mount Ventoux with his brother. At the top, he read from his copy of the *Confessions* a passage on the vanity of man. He meditated at length on what he had read, and the experience marked the beginning of the serious introspection that characterized the rest of his life. From the top of the mountain, he also looked down on Italy and felt a strong desire to return to his native country. This he accomplished in a trip to Rome, where he visited Giacomo Colonna toward the end of that year.

Petrarch returned to Avignon in 1337, desirous of solitude, which he found fifteen miles away, in Vaucluse, a valley that afforded him a quiet place to study and write. In that same year, his first illegitimate child, Giovanni, was born. The mother is unknown, and the son died from the plague in 1361. By Petrarch's midthirties, he was well known in Italy and France for his Latin verse, and in 1340, he received letters from the Senate in Rome and the University of Paris offering him the poet laureate's crown. He chose to receive the honor in Rome and left the next year for Naples, where King Robert examined him on various questions and proclaimed him worthy of the prize. On Easter Sunday, 1341, he accepted the laurel crown in Rome and delivered a coronation speech on the nature of poetry. It was the first time that such a ceremony had been held since classical times, and it dramatized the significance that the literary models of antiquity were assuming. From Rome, he traveled to Pisa, then to Parma, where he spent about a year working on his epic *Africa*.

In 1342, Petrarch was back in Avignon, where the following year, his illegitimate daughter Francesca was born. In October, 1343, he traveled again in Italy, this time as ambassador of the new pope, Clement VI, to the new queen, Joan I. In December, he left Naples, disgusted with the corruption of the court, and went to Parma, where his stay was cut short by the outbreak of war. He escaped through enemy lines and visited Modena, Bologna, and Verona before returning to Avignon by the end of 1345. Soon after arriving in Avignon, he retired to Vaucluse, where he spent all of 1346. In the summer of 1347, he learned that Cola di Rienzo had been elected tribune of Rome. Delighted with the election, Petrarch wrote him a congratulatory Latin eclogue in which he rebuffed all the Roman nobles, including members of the Colonna family, who were hostile to the tribune. At this time, he became entirely independent of Colonna patronage. In November, he headed toward Rome, but in Genoa, he learned of the despotic actions of the tribune and decided to interrupt his trip. He selected Parma as his main residence but traveled around Italy at will for three years. In the autumn of 1350, on his way to Rome for the Jubilee, he stopped in Florence, where he visited Giovanni Boccaccio. They met again in Padua in April of the following year. In June, 1351, Petrarch was back in Vaucluse, whence he traveled back and forth to Avignon in hope of papal assistance. The death of Clement VI and the election of Innocent VI to the papacy in December, 1352, caused Petrarch to lose all hope of support from the papacy, as Pope Innocent suspected him of necromancy. Petrarch bid his brother farewell for the last time in April of the next year and left in May for Italy.

Back in his native land, Petrarch accepted an offer from the Visconti family to live in Milan, where he remained for eight years (1353-1361). In June, 1361, he left Milan because of the spread of the plague and traveled to Padua, where he was a guest of Francesco da Carrara. In early 1362, he returned to Milan, but because of renewed danger from the plague, he was back in Padua in the spring. In September, he went to Venice, where he remained until 1368, alternating his sojourn there with repeated trips to Padua, Milan, and Pavia. In 1363, Boccaccio paid him a visit in Venice that lasted for a few months. In 1368, Petrarch moved to Padua and from there, in 1370, to nearby Arquà with his daughter Francesca and her family. He spent his final years in Padua and in Arquà, where he died during the night on July 18, 1374.

ANALYSIS

Petrarch was both an Italian and a Latin poet, and any analysis of his poetry must take into consideration both aspects of his career. He continually and extensively revised most of his compositions; the exact chronology of his works, therefore, whether poetry or prose, is difficult to establish. His first book in Italian is *Rhymes*, poems written and revised between 1336 and 1374 but not printed until 1470, almost a full century after his death. Any "publication" prior to that date refers, more precisely, to the circulation of a manuscript. The earliest edition of Petrarch's collected Latin works dates from 1496; his complete works, including Italian verse, titled *Opera quae extant omnia*, were first published in Basel in 1554 and later reprinted there in 1581. No modern edition of the complete works exists, although a national edition has been in progress since 1926.

Although he longed to be remembered, as has been indicated, for his prodigious production in Latin, the smaller body of his Italian verse has been much more widely appreciated since the end of the fifteenth century. In both cases, however, his compositions have been widely influential because of the basic principle of imitation that he endorsed and that the Renaissance accepted as canon. Petrarch believed in the necessity of imitating the great Latin authors to produce works of lasting significance. His adherence to this doctrine in the bulk of his poetry and prose established the precedent for *imitatio* that later Humanists refined. Curiously, the subsequent refinement of the principle led to compositions that were much more Ciceronian, in terms of correct grammar and pure style, than Petrarch ever achieved in his own prose. This fact may account for the declining interest in his Latin prose after the fifteenth century. In his Italian poetry, Petrarch himself was not concerned with the imitation per se of preceding traditions as much as with the application of the best of those traditions, such as certain images found in the troubadour lyrics, to a real model: Laura. In the early sixteenth century, however, Pietro Bembo cited Petrarch's Italian lyrics as the best model for those who would write vernacular poetry. With the flourishing of the printing press at the same time as the cardinal's endorsement, Petrarch's Italian poems, already outstanding for their lyric quality and psychological insights, became destined to serve as models and to achieve prominence in the literature of the Western world.

RHYMES

Drawing on a literary-historical examination of the past, Petrarch's Latin writings, as critic Aldo Bernardo has emphasized, "contain a virile and noble view of mankind [and] exalt the achievements of ancient heroes and thinkers as indications of the heights that man can attain." Petrarch discovered in the classical era examples of moral and civic virtue capable of instructing modern humans, who, with the additional light of Christianity, could then surpass the accomplishments of pagan antiquity. Petrarch also shows the boundaries or limitations of paganism, with its bent for the things of this world, such as earthly fame and glory. The tension caused by attempting to balance the appeal of this world's attractions with the Christian's hope of a better life hereafter finds its ultimate expression in the poet's Italian lyrics.

In the collected *Rhymes*, Laura is both a *figura Christi* and a *figura Daphnae*, a symbol of Christ's purity and Daphne's sensuality. More than a study of Laura, however, the poems constitute a keen analysis of the poet's struggle to keep the attractions of this world in proper perspective. For the Christian, the eternal happiness of the next life should outshine the fleeting pleasure of this world; for Petrarch, this knowledge simply compounded his internal conflicts, as he struggled to bring his passions and desire for worldly renown under control and to submit to God. As in Saint Augustine's *Confessions*, the final word of the *Rhymes* is "peace," something that Petrarch's revered saint achieved but of which the poet claims only to have caught glimpses.

The Latin inscription at the head of the Vatican holograph of Petrarch's collected Italian poems is *Rerum vulgarium fragmenta* ("fragments of vernacular rhymes"). This title emphasizes the nonunitary nature of the collection of 366 lyrics. First, the poems, although mostly sonnets, include a variety of types and may be divided into the following categories: sonnets, canzones, sestinas, ballads, and madrigals. The total number corresponds to the maximum number of days in a year and makes the collection a sort of breviary.

Second, the poems treat many topics in addition to the poet's love for Laura, including the themes of friendship, papal corruption, and patriotism. Petrarch continually reordered the poems from 1336 until his death, but the criteria for their final ordering are unclear. Except for the universally accepted grouping of a few sonnets either according to shared themes (such as poems 41 through 43, dealing with Laura's departure for an unknown place, and poems 136 through 138, treating the corruption of the Church in Avignon) or to juxtapose one idea to another (such as poems 61 and 62, expressing respectively the exaltation of love and reason), no single organizational principle, such as a meaningful chronology, has been established. Because of the blank pages that separate poems 263 and 264 in Vatican manuscript 3195, a two-part division of the overall framework traditionally has been made. The first 263 poems, which depict Laura as a real woman who moves, talks, laughs, cries, and travels, are usually designated "In vita di madonna Laura" (in the lifetime of Laura). The last 103 poems, which present Laura as a more ethereal being whose carnal presence is not felt, then receive the label "In morte di madonna Laura" (after the death of Laura). Although the headings are not original to Petrarch, they seem generally appropriate.

The true subject of the poems in which Laura appears, either in person or more often in the form of a conceit, such as the laurel tree or the dawn (*l'aurora*, in Italian), is not really Laura. Rather, it is the love of Petrarch for Laura. The *Rhymes* is the intimate story of the poet's emotions, perceptions, feelings, and changing moods produced by the sight or memory of his beloved. The actual descriptions of Laura, whose hair is always blond like gold and whose skin is white like snow or ivory, are not nearly as significant as the depictions of the poet's melancholic or exalted states as he contemplates her beauty or ruminates over his unreciprocated love. Closely connected with the repeated motif of one-sided love are the themes of the transitoriness of time, the brevity of life, and the vanity of earthly objects and honors.

Two famous canzones, "Spirito gentil" ("Noble Spirit") and "Italia mia" ("My Italy"), best exemplify the category of patriotic or political poems in the *Rhymes*. The first poem was probably written either to

Cola di Rienzo in 1347, when he attempted to reinstate the Roman Republic, or to Bosone de' Raffaelli da Gubbio, a Roman senator. It pleads with the "noble spirit" to call Rome's erring citizens back to its ancient path of virtue and glory. Rivalries should be put away and a sense of national pride engendered to wake Italy from its lethargy. "My Italy" constitutes an eloquent plea for peace and is addressed to Italy's warring lords; the most famous section, "Ancient Valor Is Not Yet Dead in Italic Hearts," was chosen by Niccolò Machiavelli to conclude *Il principe* (1532; *The Prince*, 1640). The sonnet sequence previously referred to, poems 136 through 138, represents possibly the most colorful and violent depiction of the corruption of the Church, but references to the papal court at Avignon as "Babylon" occur throughout the *Rhymes*. The best-known poems of friendship treat members of the Colonna family: "Gloriosa columna" ("Glorious Column") and "Rottalè l'alta colonna" ("Broken Is the High Column"). Whatever the theme, all Petrarch's vernacular rhymes are characterized by a sensitivity to beautiful images and sounds that is almost without parallel in the history of Italian versification. In addition, the poet perfected the sonnet form.

TRIUMPHS

Begun in 1351 or 1352 and revised between 1356 and 1374, *Triumphs* was never completed by Petrarch. Like Dante's *La divina commedia* (c. 1320, 3 volumes; *The Divine Comedy*, 1802), Petrarch's *Triumphs* is an allegorical poem written in interlocking rhymed tercets. Its main divisions are six in number and relate the following story: "Triumphus amoris" ("Triumph of Love"), in four chapters, has Love—in a chariot and surrounded by classical figures—appear to the poet in a dream; as the poet observes the spectacle, Laura appears and he falls in love with her; thus enslaved, he follows the chariot to Cyprus, where Love's triumph is celebrated. "Triumphus pudicitiae" ("Triumph of Chastity"), in one chapter, shows Love vainly attempting to imprison Laura, who—armed with her virtues—succeeds in taking Love prisoner; then, surrounded by a court of ladies famous for their virtue, Laura ultimately celebrates her triumph in the temple of Chastity in Rome, where Love is left a prisoner. "Triumphus mortis" ("Triumph of Death"), in two chapters, has

Laura die without suffering and then visit Petrarch in a dream, at which time she reveals that she always loved him. "Triumphus famae" ("Triumph of Fame"), in three chapters, has Fame arrive as Death leads Laura away; surrounded by famous literati, Fame explains that she has the power to take a man from the grave and give him life again. "Triumphus temporis" ("Triumph of Time"), in one chapter, shows the Sun, envious of Fame, accelerating time so that the poet will realize that Fame is like snow on the mountain and that Time triumphs over her. Finally, "Triumphus aeternitatis" ("Triumph of Eternity"), in one chapter, depicts the poet's realization that everything in the world passes away; as the poet turns his thoughts to God, he sees a new world, more beautiful and outside time and space; there the righteous triumph, and there the poet hopes to see Laura.

The individual triumphs are successive until the sixth and final one, which provides a vision of the future. The allegorical meaning of the poem points to the need for humans to look to God for the ultimate fulfillment of their aspirations. The tone of the work, therefore, is undoubtedly medieval and reminiscent of Dante. Although Petrarch claimed in a letter to Boccaccio that he had never read *The Divine Comedy*, his allegorical poem, with its many Dantean echoes and allusions, including borrowed phrasing, stands as proof that he knew Dante's work very well. Unfortunately, the lyric quality of the unfinished poem fails to match that of the *Rhymes*. This is true for at least two reasons: First, the catalogs of characters are almost interminable and serve to break up the poetic rhythm almost before it is established; second, the allegorical frame, too obvious even from the brief summary provided, is so heavy as to be oppressive. Nevertheless, this composition, although vastly inferior to the collected lyrics, exerted a dramatic influence on Renaissance art because of the esteem in which its author was held. The representation of its processionals in all the major and most of the minor artistic media was an essential part of the phenomenon of Petrarchianism.

AFRICA

Petrarch believed that *Africa*, his epic poem composed in Latin hexameters and divided into nine books, was his most promising work. He began writing the poem in 1338 or 1339, reworking and revising it during the next thirty-five years but never finishing it. Because it was never completed, it was never more than promising. Part of it was presented to King Robert in Naples before Petrarch received the crown of poet laureate, but the poem never circulated during the author's lifetime. After his death, friends circulated it, and it was poorly received. In truth, the poem has never enjoyed critical acclaim or approval, except for rare passages such as the tragic love story of Masinissa and Sophonisba. The epic hero is Scipio Africanus; the sources on which the poem is based include Cicero's "Somnium Scipionis" ("Dream of Scipio") at the end of *De republica* (51 B.C.E.; *On the State*, 1817) and Livy's history.

The story begins with an account of Scipio's dream of his deceased father, who died gloriously in the Roman defeat of the Carthaginians in Spain. The father carries Scipio to Heaven, where the son sees a vision of the rise and fall of their beloved Rome and learns that to follow virtue is the duty of man on Earth. His father assures him of victory over Hannibal in the upcoming African campaign and promises him lasting fame because of a poet to be born in the distant future—a not-too-subtle reference to Petrarch himself. The poem, regrettably, is almost completely lacking in both subtlety and dramatic tension. Scipio, brimming with virtue, foils his ally Masinissa's illicit love affair and proves himself an unbelievable character. The outcome of the battle is known before it begins: Hannibal will be defeated, and Scipio will return to Rome victorious. On the voyage home, the conquering general and his friend Ennius discuss the nature of poetry. The latter relates a dream he had of Homer, in which a young poet of great genius figures prominently; the future poet of renown sits in an enclosed valley (read Petrarch seated in Vaucluse). The epic, with its initial and final dream sequences in which Petrarch enjoys a conspicuous place, strikes most critics as too self-congratulatory and ill conceived from beginning to end. As Thomas Bergin has stated, the poem lacks a reading public, "for a reader of Latin epics will want to read true Latin epics and not late medieval imitations."

ECLOGUES

Petrarch's Latin eclogues number twelve, one for each month of the year. As was common in the tradition of Roman and medieval pastoral poems, the bucolic setting disguises quite contemporary events. The pastors or shepherds in a faraway idyllic landscape parallel people close at hand; rustic dialogues find their analogue in contemporary issues. In brief, Petrarch's compositions are a series of allegories placed in rural settings. The themes have all been encountered before: the Roman revolution of Cola di Rienzo, the poet's love for Laura, his coronation in Rome, the corruption of the Church, the conflict in Petrarch between worldliness and spirituality, the death of King Robert, the usefulness of sacred and secular poetry, the destructiveness of the Black Death, and the poet's decision to leave the service of the Colonna family. The eclogues, although neither notably influential nor necessarily inferior, testify to Petrarch's ability to compose countless variations on any number of themes, many of which are notably personal. His life provided almost as much source material for his work as his scholarly studies did. Most of the eclogues were composed between 1346 and 1348, with the definitive version completed in 1364.

METRICAL LETTERS

The *Metrical Letters* make up a collection of sixty-six epistles in Latin hexameters, subdivided into three books. Petrarch dedicated the collection to his friend Marco Barbato di Sulmona, who was chancellor to King Robert. Beginning in 1350, the poet reorganized the letters during a period of more than a decade, completing his task in 1363. The subjects treated range from personal confessions and descriptions of autobiographical happenings to political exhortations and stirring praises for Italy. In purpose, these varied and unequal epistles are not unlike the prose letters found in four other Petrarchan collections. Their intent is to present the poet as he wished to be remembered by posterity. Consequently, they are not filled with spontaneous comments and casual observations, no matter how they may appear at first glance. Every comment and every observation is calculated; this is especially true in those letters that have been carefully rewritten in hexameters. Petrarch's desire, from the first letter to the last, is to interpret for future readers the events of his life, to analyze the results of his studies, and to speculate on the significance of his work. What may have started as another exercise in introspection quickly evolved into a new form of autobiography: an epistolary account revised through time with the reader constantly in mind.

OTHER MAJOR WORKS

NONFICTION: *Rerum familiarium libri*, wr. 1325-1366 (English translation, 1975-1985, also known as *Books on Personal Matters*); *Collatio laureationes*, 1341 (*Coronation Oath*, 1955); *Psalmi penitentiales*, 1342-1347; *Rerum memorandum libri*, 1343-1345; *De vita solitaria*, 1346 (*The Life of Solitude*, 1924); *De viris illustribus*, 1351-1353 (later reorganized as *Quorundam virorum illustrium epithoma*, with a preface by Petrarch, completed by Lombardo della Seta); *Secretum meum*, 1353-1358 (also known as *De secreto conflictu curarum mearum*; *My Secret*, 1911); *Invectiva contra quendam magni status hominem sed nullius scientiae aut virtutis*, 1355; *Itinerarium Syriacum*, 1358 (also known as *Itinerarium breve de Ianua*); *Sine nomine*, 1359-1360 (*Book Without a Name*, 1973); *Senilium rerum libri*, wr. 1361-1374 (*Letters of Old Age*, 1966); *Rerum familiarium libri xxiv*, 1364-1366 (*Books on Personal Matters*, 1975); *De remediis utriusque fortunae*, 1366 (*Physicke Against Fortune*, 1597; also as *On Remedies for Good and Bad Fortunes*, 1966); *De sui ipsius et multorum ignorantia*, 1367 (*On His Own Ignorance and That of Many*, 1948); *Posteritati*, 1370-1372 (*Epistle to Posterity*, 1966); *Invectiva contra eum qui maledixit Italiae*, 1373; *De otio religioso*, 1376; *Miscellaneous Letters*, 1966.

MISCELLANEOUS: *Opera quae extant omnia*, 1554, 1581.

BIBLIOGRAPHY

Bloom, Harold, ed. *Petrarch*. New York: Chelsea House, 1989. Well-chosen collection of eight previously published essays by major Petrarch scholars.

Braden, Gordon. *Petrarchan Love and the Continental Renaissance*. New Haven, Conn.: Yale University Press, 1999. Sticking close to the works themselves, Braden studies Petrarch's poems and their effects on the likes of Giovanni Boccaccio, Pietro Bembo, Pierre de Ronsard, and Garcilaso de la Vega. He emphasizes the continuity of subject matter and the poets' "creative narcissism."

Fubini, Riccardo. *Humanism and Secularization: From Petrarch to Valla*. Durham, N.C.: Duke University Press, 2003. An examination of Humanism and its relationship with Petrarch, Bracciolini, and Poggio. Bibliography and index.

Jones, Frederic J. *The Structure of Petrarch's "Canzionere": A Chronological, Psychological, and Stylistic Analysis*. Rochester, N.Y.: Boydell and Brewer, 1995. An analysis of Petrarch's poetry, particularly his *Rhymes*. Bibliography and indexes.

Kennedy, William J. *The Site of Petrarchism: Early Modern National Sentiment in Italy, France, and England*. Baltimore: The Johns Hopkins University Press, 2003. An examination of Petrarch's nationalism as it manifested itself in literature and its effect. Bibliography and index.

Kirkham, Victoria, and Armando Maggi, eds. *Petrarch: A Critical Guide to the Complete Works*. Chicago: University of Chicago Press, 2009. A collection of essays that cover Petrarch's works, including poetic works such as *Triumph* and *Rhymes*.

McLaughlin, Martin, and Letizia Panizza with Peter Hainsworth, eds. *Petrarch in Britain: Interpreters, Imitators, and Translators over Seven Hundred Years*. New York: Oxford University Press, 2007. This collection of twenty essays by prominent Petrarch scholars in Italy and Britain discusses the legacy of Petrarch in Britain, including his effect on love poetry, his decline during Romanticism, and his subsequent revival.

Mazzotta, Giuseppe. *The Worlds of Petrarch*. Durham, N.C.: Duke University Press, 1993. A critical look at the poetry and other works of Petrarch, including the *Rhymes*. Also examines his Humanism. Bibliography and index.

Quillen, Carol E. *Rereading the Renaissance: Petrarch, Augustine, and the Language of Humanism*. Ann Arbor: University of Michigan Press, 1998. Examines Petrarch as a reader and writer as well as his correspondence in relation to Humanism. Also looks at Saint Augustine. Bibliography and index.

Sturm-Maddox, Sara. *Petrarch's Laurels*. University Park: Pennsylvania State University Press, 1999. The relationship between Petrarch's concerns for love and for glory is encased in that of "Laura" and "the laurel." This study of their relationship in his poetry examines the conflicts, metamorphoses, and parallels that entwine the two.

Madison U. Sowell

PINDAR

Born: Cynoscephalae, near Thebes, Boeotia, Greece; c. 518 B.C.E.
Died: Argos, Greece; c. 438 B.C.E.
Also known as: Pindaros; Pindarus

PRINCIPAL POETRY
Epinikia, 498-446 B.C.E. (*Odes*, 1656)

OTHER LITERARY FORMS
Pindar (PIHN-dur) is remembered only for his poetic achievement.

ACHIEVEMENTS
Pindar's victory odes are among the greatest achievements of ancient Greek poetry, but they are also probably the most consistently misunderstood. Composing in a genre (*epinikion*) and mode (choral lyric poetry) foreign even to later Greek audiences, Pindar stands alone as the chief Archaic Greek poet whose works survive in any bulk. The Archaic Age itself—that period from the time of Homer in the eighth century B.C.E. to the rise of classical literature in fifth century B.C.E. Athens—is relatively obscure. The events, manners, and traditions of the period were not those of later times, so that it is hard to extrapolate from literary activity at Athens when analyzing the work of Pindar. The additional difficulty of having little to compare with Pindar's work in his own genre (only some poems by his contemporaries Bacchylides and Simonides) means that any assessment of his achievement is necessarily limited. What comparison one can make shows Pindar to have a distinctive style, complex and exciting. So highly compressed is the style, in fact, that the general opinion of Pindaric odes, from antiquity on, can be summed up in the remark of the English poet

Abraham Cowley: "If a man should undertake to translate Pindar word for word, it would be thought that one madman had translated another." However, Cowley is only one among a number of poets who have been fascinated by Pindar, in whom they have found a model for "inspired" verse (Pierre de Ronsard and Friedrich Hölderlin are among the great poets deeply influenced by Pindar). Even Horace, the astute transposer of old Greek lyric verse into Roman poetry, failed to get beyond the fixation on Pindaric style, which later led to Pindar's image as that of a rather wild, raving, "natural" bard:

Rushing down like a mountain stream
Which rains have swollen over its known banks,
Unmeasurable Pindar boils and flows, deep mouth. . . .

Pindar's legacy, then, has little to do with his real achievement. His imitators dwelt on style; divorced from the context and conventions of the poetry, this style is bound to seem odd at best and at worst, incomprehensible. In his own terms, however, Pindar might best be judged by determining whether he has achieved what he set out to do. In that case, he has been a successful composer of *epinikia*, because he has fulfilled the promise that lies behind this genre: He preserves the names and victories (often otherwise unknown) of fifth century aristocrats who desired the prestige of Pindar's poetry to commemorate their participation in the Panhellenic games. Pindar, like the epic poet Homer before him, conferred immortality on heroic deeds, this being the ideology behind his poetry as expressed in *Nemean Ode* 7:

if a man succeeds in an exploit, he casts
a delightful theme upon the streams of the Muses
for great deeds of strength, if they lack songs,
are sunk in deep obscurity.

BIOGRAPHY
Little is known about Pindar beyond what has been recorded by ancient scholars in elucidating the circumstances of composition for various poems. This produces a sort of lifelong itinerary around the Greek world rather than a clear biography of the poet. Clearly, his life was spent in aristocratic circles. He was born into a socially superior family having connections with

the Aegid clan, a far-flung kinship group that included members of the Spartan ruling elite. Ancient tradition records that Pindar went to Athens for schooling in the art of choral poetry; the district of Boeotia was apparently backward in such matters (as Pindar implies, referring to the old insult "Boeotian sow," that his poetry has cast aside). Pindar's first recorded poem, *Pythian Ode* 10, was written when he was about twenty and performed in Thessaly for an aristocratic patron.

Pindar's later life was ruled by this pattern. He traveled throughout the Greek world at the invitation of local tyrants, self-made absolute rulers (not despots, as implied by the modern sense of the word), who were at that time in the process of replacing hereditary kings as the supreme authority in the Greek city-states. They needed the prestige that an internationally known poet such as Pindar could bring to their accomplishments—not only athletic, but military and political as well. Pindar was not the first poet to be patronized by tyrants: The sixth century poet Ibycus and, later, Simonides and Bacchylides also celebrated the deeds of these wealthy and powerful men. All, including Pindar, were certainly paid for their efforts, in money and lavish hospitality.

Pindar would either write a choral ode for his patrons, then oversee its performance, or send a poem with instructions for the accompanying song and dance, while he himself remained in Thebes. Pindar seems, at times, to have accompanied the victor from the games to his hometown, where the ode would then be performed at festival occasions. It is even possible that a few odes were actually composed extempore at the games. These compositions survive, it appears, because the aristocratic patron families handed down manuscripts as treasured heirlooms. The Alexandrian scholars Zenodotus and Aristophanes helped to collect Pindar's poetry in the third century B.C.E.

Further, acquaintance with one aristocratic family often led to commissions from others. Thus, after celebrating the victory of Xenocrates at Delphi in 490 B.C.E., Pindar became known to the family and, in 476 B.C.E., was invited to compose *epinikia* for Xenocrates' brother Theron and for Hieron, another tyrant, in Sicily. In such a fashion, Pindar's patrons came to include aristocrats in Sparta, Rhodes, Corinth, Cyrene, and

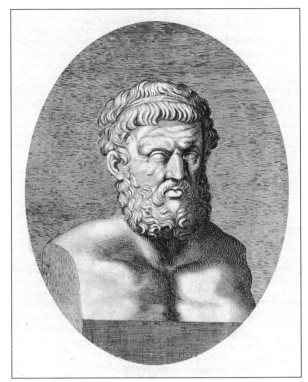

Pindar (Time & Life Pictures/Getty Images)

Athens. His international reputation is reflected in the geographical distribution of the *epinikia*: Only five of the surviving forty-five poems are addressed to victors from Pindar's home state of Thebes; fifteen are for Sicilians and eleven for victors from the island of Aegina, for which Pindar had a special affection.

The patron-poet bond, however, based as it was on traditional Panhellenic codes of behavior, led to conflicts for Pindar when the political situation during the years of the Persian invasions of 490 B.C.E. and 480 B.C.E. polarized the Greek city-states. Pindar tended to identify his patrons' families with their homelands. In praising Athens, then, as he did in *Nemean Ode 2*, the poet risked offending the citizens of Aegina, with whom Athens was at war during the decade after Marathon in 490 B.C.E. Similarly, his continuing affirmations of support for the Theban oligarchy, even when it joined with the Persians against most of the other Greek states, posed problems of loyalty. Nevertheless Pindar, in most instances, was able to reconcile his conflicting affiliations by an appeal to the common Greek ideals and myths; references to both occur frequently in the *epinikia*. Once, however, shortly after the Persians were repulsed, the jealous rivalry between Thebes and Athens did affect Pindar, resulting in the levy of a heavy fine on the poet by the Thebans after he praised Athens in a dithyramb, calling it "defense of Greece, Athens renowned, divine citadel," and recalling the Athenian naval victory over the Persians at Salamis in 480 B.C.E.

Although Pindar fascinates historians because of the unusual perspectives he offers on the turbulent events of the fifth century B.C.E., to look to his poetry for reasoned historical judgments would be as much in vain as it would be to seek therein a coherent picture of his life. His poetry was not meant to be either biography or chronicle, but rather a celebration of a series of victorious moments, which, by their semisacred nature, move personal and political history into the background.

ANALYSIS

Of the seventeen books representing Pindar's vast production in a variety of poetic genres, only four books of one genre, the victory odes (*epinikia*), survived antiquity intact. These odes are named for the periodic Panhellenic festival games held at Olympia (the Olympian odes), Delphi (the Pythian odes), Nemea (Nemeans), and Corinth (Isthmians).

The remaining books of Pindar survive as several hundred fragments, some of them only a line long. As was usual in Greek Archaic poetry, his compositions were most often meant for public performance, and the now lost books were arranged by third century B.C.E. editors according to the social occasions for which the poems were written: *encomia* (praise poems), *threnoi* (dirges), hymns, *paians* (hymns to Apollo), dithyrambs (to Dionysus), *hyporchemata* (dance songs), *parthenia* (maiden songs), and *prosodia* (processionals). While the modern reader might regret the loss of the huge mass of verse Pindar wrote, the fragments of these other genres make it clear that the Pindaric style known from the *epinikia* is representative of his works as a whole.

VICTORY ODES

To understand the *epinikia* requires an appreciation of both their occasional nature and the nature of those occasions for which they were written. The most prestigious games—Olympian, Pythian, Nemean, and Isthmian—occurred at regular intervals and united the independent Greek city-states as few other traditions, with the exception of Homeric poetry, could. So important were these Panhellenic athletic and musical contests that a sacred truce prevailed whenever they were held. To their local communities, victors became heroes; although their immediate reward at the games consisted only of a wreath of laurel leaves, their later perquisites very often included free meals at public expense, statues, coins with their imprint, and inscriptions. In this context, poetry was yet another reward for victory.

In many ways, Pindar's odes mimic the rituals they celebrate. For example, just as a sacred herald would proclaim the victor, the event won, and the city and father of the winner in footraces, wrestling, boxing, pancratium, pentathlon, or chariot, horse, or mule races, so Pindar was obliged to include these details in the program of his poem for the victor. The *epinikia* are thus amplified announcements of the event. Pindar, on the other hand, also associates himself with the athletic victor and the poem with a feat of skill (in Pindar, *sophia*, "skill," is used with respect to both poetry and other forms of wisdom, including the knowledge which trainers impart to athletes): "Let someone dig me a wide jumping pit . . . there's a spring in my knees," exclaims the poet as he embarks on one song of praise. This extended metaphor implies that the victory provides an opportunity for Pindar to compete in performance with the victor, as he attempts to produce a poem as perfect as the feat that it commemorates.

ODES AS PERFORMANCE ART

Performance was central to the *epinikia*, so that the text of each poem in fact represents only a third of Pindar's work. That each poem was sung and danced by a trained chorus explains much about the form of the compositions: usually a repeated series of strophe, antistrophe, and epode, representing dance instructions (literally, "turn," "counterturn," and "added song"—all performed while standing in place). Gestures probably highlighted the often tersely narrated myths which Pindar employs. Perhaps most important, the poet could use the chorus, as in Greek tragedy, to reflect upon the greater implications of the hero's victory for the city-state, which the chorus personifies. Since Archaic Greek ethical thought constantly reminds one that wealth, good fortune, and all types of victory are threatened by jealous gods (as one author writes, "The tallest trees are struck by lightning"), the danger of the victor's newly acquired status must be kept before his eyes by his lesser fellow citizens, the chorus: Again, as in Greek tragedy, the chorus warns. Finally, the presence of the chorus means that the "I" which appears commonly in the *epinikia* should not be taken as equivalent to the poetic self. It is more often a sort of shorthand for the opinion of the chorus; it can also simply be a device for making transitions within the poem, from praise to narrative myth to gnomic utterances.

RITUAL FUNCTION OF THE ODES

Thus, the ode both incorporates the heroic athlete into the community (by warning of excess in good fortune) and distances him from it (by praise). In Pindar's hands, the poetry of victory also integrates the past with the present, as the poet draws on local mythological examples in comparing the celebrated athlete with the city-state's earlier heroic figures. Again, both praise and warning are served by the myth: The victor is like Achilles or Heracles or Pelops, Pindar says; he should avoid being like Ixion or the ungrateful Tantalus. In this, Pindar's use of myths, though idiosyncratic and innovative in details that he considers sacrilegious, fairly represents the outlook of much Archaic Greek poetry from Homer on; it is conventional and traditional. As Frank Nisetich explains in *Pindar's Victory Songs* (1980), "to see the general behind the particular, to grasp one thing by contrast with its opposite, to trace human vicissitudes to the will of the gods and explain, appreciate, or find the right response to a present situation through reference to myth or proverb"—these purposes represent the dominant forms of style in Archaic poetry; they are certainly Pindar's.

PYTHIAN ODE 10

In his earliest surviving *epinikion*, Pindar constructs the poem in the manner in which he will become adept: Praise of a victor precedes and follows a mythical narrative, which is in some way related to his topic. In *Pythian Ode* 10 (498 B.C.E.), the victor Hippokleas has won a race for boys: Both his name and the event are mentioned in the first series of strophe-antistrophe epode. The poem begins, however, with a bit of complex mythological genealogy, in the fashion Pindar sometimes follows: "Lacedaemon is happy, Thessaly is blest; both have their kings descended from one father, Heracles. . . ." This reference to the kinship bonds of Spartan and Thessalian royal houses ends suddenly, with a transition question in the first person, another Pindaric device: "Why am I declaiming in this way?" Pindar answers that he was commissioned to write; yet he includes Pytho (that is, Delphi, home of Apollo's sacred shrine and site of the Pythian games) as his inspiration. The appearance of spontaneity is important to Pindar, and he often downplays, as here, the more mercantile aspects of his craft in favor of the almost mystical lure of the games and their ideals and the effect victory has on him, compelling his praises.

In the first counterturn of this ode, Pindar typically uses a gnomic statement to direct attention to a new topic—in this case, from the victor to the victor's father. The statement here acknowledges the role of the gods in bringing human deeds to fulfillment; with them, the victor's father "has found all the happiness our mortal race can come to." A contrast immediately follows: the happy race which mortals cannot reach, the mythical Hyperboreans, who live (as their name denotes) beyond the North Wind, feasting and singing continually, freed from the fear of death. Pindar works his way into describing them by reference to the Gorgon slayer, Perseus, who is said to have dined with this race. Is this relevant? Contemporary notions of a poem's unity would probably reject the detail; here, the aesthetics of Archaic Greek poetry differ. In social context, Perseus's myth is exactly right for the occasion, since he was the great-grandfather of Heracles, the mythical progenitor of the very family Pindar is praising (and of the rulers of Sparta, mentioned earlier). Poetically, Perseus fills the role of the praiseworthy athlete, corresponding to his descendant in real life. As the victor has returned from Delphi northward to his Thessalian home, so Perseus, in the myth, once moved north to the celebrations of the immortal race; Pindar makes the comparison implicit and complimentary. The poem's conclusion contains more praise, this time of Hippokleas's beauty; a warning ("there is no telling what will be a year from now"); and an affirmation of the social bond between patron and poet, expressed in athletic imagery (the patron Thorax has "yoked the chariot of the Muses").

Already in *Pythian Ode* 10, the imagery is Pindaric by being animated—that is, a static image (counterturn two: one cannot reach the Hyperboreans on a ship) becomes part of the "piloting" of the poem by Pindar: "Stay the oar now," says the poet as he steers clear of a digression in the third epode. The poem, after being a ship, immediately becomes a bee, digressively flitting; his song is honey, the poet says; then the poem is a chariot; finally, the ship image returns at the end of the poem, when Pindar praises Thorax's brothers: "In their hands belongs the piloting of cities. . . ."

OLYMPIAN ODE 1

A highly developed, rapidly shifting scheme of imagery is characteristic of Pindar. *Olympian Ode* 1 (476 B.C.E.), one of his finest and most difficult compositions, shows the technique in abundance, illustrating how Pindar can redouble the messages of gnomic utterance and myth by the way in which he chooses and structures images. Consider, for example, the constellation of images which opens the poem in symphonic fashion:

> Water is preeminent and gold, like a fire
> burning in the night, outshines all possessions
> that magnify men's pride. But if, my soul,
> you yearn to celebrate great games,
> look no further for another star shining
> through the deserted ether brighter than the sun,
> or for a contest mightier than Olympia. . . .

Water and fire will recur in the myth that Pindar proceeds to tell (how Pelops was allegedly cut and boiled in a pot); gold and the sun echo each other within this passage, as primary elements, one by day, one by night. Beyond this, however, the arrangement of images is itself a contest: Pindar names the "victor" substances in each sphere, and the contest of Olympia wins. There are few more exciting collocations of imagery that enacts its subject.

Mention of the Olympian victor (Hieron), his horse, and his kingly status brings Pindar shortly to tell of "Pelops's land"—Olympia itself—and thus of the myth of Pelops. Here one notes a characteristically Pindaric

way of retelling the old story: He claims that the received version is wrong, that the gods could never have chopped up the boy and consumed him; this, says Pindar, is a myth concocted by jealous neighbors upon the boy's disappearance to become cup-bearer of Zeus, a great favor to the boy's family. Pindar typically does not tell the story in straightforward manner, even when not revising the myth; here he also backtracks to tell of the misfortunes of Tantalus, Pelops's father, which caused Pelops to be cast out of Olympus, the home of Zeus, back into the world of men. Then Pindar leaps ahead to Pelops's marriage to Hippodameia; as in *Pythian Ode* 10, the young hero of myth, striving against obscurity, becomes an ideal image of the young athlete-king for whom the poem is performed. As Pelops won a chariot race to win his bride, so Hieron wins fame by victory in a horse race.

Finally, Pindar ends *Olympian Ode* 1 with another redoubling of imagery within the poem: Pelops had prayed to Poseidon to win the strength for a victory; thus, in conclusion, Pindar prays for a double boon (again, victor and poet are united): that Hieron win another victory with the gods' favor, and that he himself "consort with victors, conspicuous for my skill among Greeks everywhere." This is indicative of growing confidence in his art.

PYTHIAN ODE 8

Pindar's last datable poem, *Pythian Ode* 8 (446 B.C.E.), shows the effects of controlled compression of myth, in a format reminiscent of the ending of *Olympian Ode* 1; this time, the entire poem is a prayer. It opens with an address to Hesychia (Peace); at turn four, Pindar prays to Apollo to help in the singing of the song; next, the gods in general are invoked to "look with unjealous eyes" upon the fortunes of the victor's father (again, the warning motif occurs); finally, the poem ends with invocations of Aegina, the nymph who gave her name to the island home of the victor, and to Zeus and several heroes of the city-state, that they guide the island's fate. Evident here is a significant aspect of Pindar's mature art. The myth itself is expressed in direct quotation of a mythical figure: Amphiarus, a prophet and soldier, is given oracular words of wise counsel, ostensibly to the second wave of invaders against Thebes (his son among them), but clearly intended to remind the athletic victor of aristocratic ideals. The prophet is quoted as saying that "the spirit of the fathers lives in their sons"; Pindar himself has often said the same thing, but here he makes it more dramatic by placing the sentiment in a hero's mouth.

Pythian Ode 8 represents the most concise statement of Pindar's ideas on his own art, while at the same time showing him distancing himself from the moralizing maxims inherent in the genre. Thus, he claims, after narrating the Amphiarus myth, to have actually met the hero's son, Alcman, and to have received a true prophecy from him. Pindar says elsewhere, in a poetic fragment, that he is "prophet of the Muses"; here he dramatizes that status. Because he can foretell the future, he can make the victor fly ahead into that time on the "wings of devising." In the end, he foresees that his poetic/athletic ideal—for it is one notion—will survive. The expression of his confidence can serve as the capstone to Pindar's lifework: "What is someone? What is no one? Man: A shadow's dream. But when god-given glory comes, a bright light shines upon us and our life is sweet. . . ."

BIBLIOGRAPHY

Boeke, Hanna. *The Value of Victory in Pindar's Odes: Gnomai, Cosmology, and the Role of the Poet.* Boston: Brill, 2007. Examines gnomai and cosmology in the odes of Pindar.

Bowra, C. M. *Pindar.* 1964. Reprint. New York: Oxford University Press, 2000. This classic work on Pindar remains the standard introduction to the poet and his works.

Currie, Bruno. *Pindar and the Cult of Heroes.* New York: Oxford University Press, 2005. Combines a study of Greek culture and religion, in particular the hero cults, with a literary study of Pindar's odes.

Hamilton, John T. *Soliciting Darkness: Pindar, Obscurity, and the Classical Tradition.* Cambridge, Mass.: Department of Comparative Literature, Harvard University, 2003. An examination of Pindar's works as they fit into the larger tradition of Greek poetry.

Hornblower, Simon. *Thucydides and Pindar: Historical Narrative and the World of Epinikian Poetry.* New York: Oxford University Press, 2006. Hornblower argues that there is a relationship between the writings of Thucydides and Pindar, finding stylistic similarities and shared values.

Hornblower, Simon, and Catherine Morgan, eds. *Pindar's Poetry, Patrons, and Festivals: From Archaic Greece to the Roman Empire.* New York: Oxford University Press, 2007. This collection of essays examines the festivals, the games, and the patronage system, as well as Pindar's odes.

Itsumi, Kiichiro. *Pindaric Metre: "The Other Half."* New York: Oxford University Press, 2009. A close examination of the meters used by Pindar in the original Greek.

Mackie, Hilary. *Graceful Errors: Pindar and the Performance of Praise.* Ann Arbor: University of Michigan Press, 2003. Mackie looks at Pindar's odes as public performances and argues that Pindar had to take into account the various groups in his audience as well as balance an athlete's accomplishments against those of a mythical figure.

Rutherford, Ian. *Pindar's Paeans: A Reading of the Fragments with a Survey of the Genre.* New York: Oxford University Press, 2001. The paean, or sacred hymn to Apollo, had a central place in the song-dance culture of classical Greece. The most celebrated examples of the genre in antiquity were Pindar's paeans. Rutherford offers a comprehensive reevaluation of the poems.

Richard Peter Martin

POLIZIANO
Angelo Ambrogini

Born: Montepulciano, Tuscany (now in Italy); July 14, 1454

Died: Florence (now in Italy); September 28, 1494

Also known as: Politian

PRINCIPAL POETRY

Manta, 1482 (*Manto,* 2004)

Rusticus, 1483 (*The Countryman,* 2004)

Ambra, 1485 (English translation, 2004)

Nutricia, 1491 (English translation, 2004; the 4 previous works collectively known as *Sylvae*; English translation, 2004; Charles Fantazzi, translator)

Stanze cominciate per la giostra del magnifico Giuliano de' Medici, 1518 (commonly known as *Stanze*; *The Stanze of Angelo Poliziano*, 1979)

Rime, 1814

OTHER LITERARY FORMS

Poliziano (poh-leets-YAHN-oh) was a great scholar, a professor, critic, and translator of Greek into Latin, as well as a great poet. At age sixteen, he won the title of *Homericus juvenis* (Homeric youth) by translating books 2 through 5 of Homer's *Iliad* (c. 750 B.C.E.; English translation, 1611) into Latin hexameters. His translations of works by Epictetus, Herodian, Plutarch, Plato, Alexander Aprodisias, Galen, and Hippocrates delighted his contemporaries with their stylistic grace. His love of philology, as seen in his *Miscellaneorum centuria prima* (1489; commonly known as *Miscellanea*), which treats the origins of classic institutions and ceremonies, the significance of fables, words and their uses, and even spelling, made him one of the founders of modern textual criticism. He was also interested in jurisprudence and composed a recension of Justinian's *Digesta* (533 C.E., also known as *Pandectae*; *The Digest of Justinian*, 1920), which, though not a milestone in juristic erudition, gave impetus to further criticism of the scholarly code. He wrote many letters to Lorenzo de' Medici, Marsilio Ficino, and a wide range of other friends and contemporaries, which were translated into English in 2006 as *Letters*. Near the end of his life, Poliziano wrote to King John II of Portugal, tendering him the thanks of the civilized world for dragging from secular darkness into the light of new worlds and offering his services to record these great voyages.

ACHIEVEMENTS

Poliziano is important in Italian letters both as an interpreter of Italian humanism and as the most significant writer in the language between Giovanni Boccaccio and Ludovico Ariosto. Poliziano mastered the art of Italian versification and gave to the octave a new capacity for expression that would be utilized in the following centuries by Ariosto, Torquato Tasso, and Giambattista Marino. In Poliziano, to quote John Addington Symonds, "Faustus, the genius of the Middle Ages, had wedded Helen, the vision of the ancient world."

BIOGRAPHY

Poliziano was born Angelo Ambrogini in the Tuscan town of Montepulciano, the Latin name of which, Mons Politianus, was the source of the appellation by which the poet is known. His father, Benedetto Ambrogini, a capable bourgeois jurist, was murdered for championing the cause of Piero de' Medici in Montepulciano, whereupon the ten-year-old Poliziano was sent to Florence to seek consolation in his studies. He studied Latin under Cristoforo Landino, who was remarkable for instilling in his pupil the notion that the Tuscan vernacular was in no way inferior to Latin and that, like Latin, it ought to be subject to rules of grammar and rhetoric. Poliziano studied Greek under Giovanni Argyropulos, Andronicus Callistos, Demetrius Chalcondyles, and Marsilio Ficino; and he also studied Hebrew. At sixteen, he began writing epigrams in Greek; at seventeen, he was writing essays on Greek versification; and at eighteen, he published an edition of Catullus. By 1473, Poliziano was in the service of Lorenzo de' Medici, the ruler of Florence and the chief patron of the arts in Italy. To provide Poliziano with an income, Lorenzo appointed him secular prior of the College of San Giovanni. Poliziano obtained the degree of doctor of civil law, took clerical orders, and was appointed to the canonry of the Cathedral of Florence. In 1475, Lorenzo made him tutor to his sons Piero (who succeeded his father for a brief time) and Giovanni (later Pope Leo X), but his wife, Clarice Orsini, who was pious and conventional, preferred a religious education for her sons rather than the secular one Poliziano offered, and she lobbied for his removal as tutor.

Following the tradition set by Luigi Pulci, who wrote a tribute in octaves to Lorenzo's tournament held in 1469, Poliziano wrote a celebration of the tournament of Lorenzo's brother Giuliano, held on January 28, 1475, in honor of the latter's beloved, Simonetta Cattaneo, the wife of Marco Vespucci. The undertaking, however, was ill-starred. First, Simonetta died

(April 26, 1476), and she had to be changed from the heroine of book 1 of the *Stanze* to her role as resurrected Fortune in book 2. Exactly two years later, on April 26, 1478, Giuliano was murdered at Mass by members of the Pazzi family, who hoped to murder both Medici brothers and thus wrest Florence from Medici control. This second calamity robbed the poem of its hero, and Poliziano never progressed beyond the first stanzas of the second canto. Instead, he wrote a prose memorial in Latin against the Pazzi conspiracy, titled *Conjurationis pactianae commentarium* (1498).

In 1479, Poliziano was dismissed from the Medici household; after six months of wandering in northern Italy, he was finally readmitted to Lorenzo's favor, but he was never to regain his position as sole tutor to the Medici children. At the Court of Mantua in 1480, in only two days according to his own boast, he wrote his *Orfeo* (pr. 1480; English translation, 1879; also known as *Orpheus*), the first secular play in Italian. There is, however, a great deal of uncertainty as to the date of the play's composition, and other sources date the work as early as 1471. In 1480, Poliziano was made professor of Greek and Latin literature at the University of Florence, and he continued to hold that position until his death.

Poliziano was not involved in public affairs, and his private life seems to have been uneventful. He did not marry; judging from his Greek epigrams on the youth Chrysocomus, it is possible that the homosexual sentiments he placed in the mouth of Orfeo were really his own. In one of Poliziano's *canzoni a ballo*, he pokes light fun at a priest who has a pig stolen from him and then hears the confession of the thief but cannot press charges. Poliziano's comparison of his own situation to that of the priest, "Woe, by what a grief I'm hit;/ I can never speak of it!/ I too suffer like the priest," may be a reference to his homosexuality.

Poliziano's letters reveal how much he enjoyed the rustic pleasures of his villa at Fiesole in the neighborhood of his friends Count Giovanni Pico della Mirandola at Querceto and Marsilio Ficino at Montevecchio. Away from Florence but still close enough to enjoy its panorama, the solitude which he could savor at Fiesole was "beyond all price." He expatiates on this pleasure in the *Rusticus*: "Give unto me the life of a tranquil

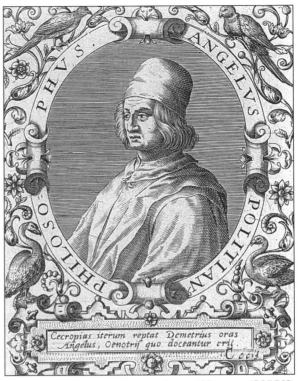

Poliziano (©Bettmann/CORBIS)

scholar, amongst the pleasures of the open fields; for serious thought in hours of study, give me my books; I ask but for moderate wealth, well-earned without weary toil, but I desire no Bishop's mitre nor triple tiara to rest as a burden upon my brow."

Poliziano's devotion to Lorenzo was steadfast, and he was at his patron's bedside when Lorenzo died on April 8, 1492; in a Latin monody written after Lorenzo's death, Poliziano cried, "Oh that my head were waters and mine eyes a fountain of tears, that I might weep day and night!" He survived his friend and patron by only two years; influenced by the spiritual revival of Girolamo Savonarola, Poliziano was buried as a penitent in the cowl of a Dominican friar.

ANALYSIS

Although the subject matter of Poliziano's poetry has not traveled well into modern times, he has never lost his place in literary history; both his name and his rather unattractive face, with its prominent aquiline nose, are familiar to those who have studied the Italian Renaissance. He was considered the foremost scholar of his day; Erasmus called him a "miracle of nature," and Pietro Bembo, who succeeded him as arbiter of Italian letters, called him the "master of the Ausonian lyre." The enthusiasm with which he applied himself to his teaching of Homer and Vergil drew students from all over Europe, who took his humanistic learning back to their homelands. Among his non-Italian students were the German Johann Reuchlin, the Englishmen William Grocyn and Thomas Linacre, and the Portuguese Arias Barbosa. Linacre, a physician under whom Erasmus studied, introduced the first secular study of Greek at Oxford, and Barbosa introduced the study of Greek at Salamanca. Pulci, an older poet whose *Giostra* (c. 1470) had set a precedent for the *Stanze* of Poliziano, was in turn aided by Poliziano in the composition of Pulci's parody of the French epic, the *Morgante maggiore* (1483; *Morgante: The Epic Adventures of Orlando and His Giant Friend Morgante*, 1998), which work is concluded with a good word for Pulci's "Angel" from Montepulciano. Outside Italy, Poliziano's Italian verse directly influenced the poetry of Juan Boscán in Spain half a century later.

It seems likely that passages in Poliziano's *Stanze* inspired as many as three of Sandro Botticelli's paintings: *The Birth of Venus* (1484), *Primavera* (1478), and *Venus and Mars* (1477). According to Giorgio Vasari and Condivi, Poliziano advised the young Michelangelo on classical subjects. It has also been suggested that Poliziano's version of the myth of Polyphemus and Galatea in the *Stanze* provided the model for Raphael's frescoes in the Villa Farnesina in Rome.

The best of Poliziano's Latin odes on the death of Lorenzo were set to music by Heinrich Isaac, who had succeeded Antonio Squarcialupi as organist at the Medici Court in 1475. George Chapman used a passage from the *Ambra* in the dedication of his translation of the *Odyssey* in 1615, and he reworked the ode on the death of Albiera degli Albizzi into his "Epicede or Funerall Song" on the death of Henry, Prince of Wales (1612).

ORFEO

Poliziano's idyllic *Orfeo* is the earliest secular play in Italian literature and marks the beginning of that characteristic Renaissance genre of the dramatic mythological pastoral that would culminate in Tasso's *Aminta*

(pr. 1573; English translation, 1591). Because the playlet was also accompanied by music, now unfortunately lost, it is seen as a forerunner of modern opera, and because of the author's attempts to individualize the psychology of his characters, it is deemed important in the evolution of the tragicomedy as well.

Although Poliziano's *Orfeo* is technically more a dramatic work than it is a poem, it is actually better poetry than it is drama. As drama, it is flawed and illogical; as poetry, according to Symonds, "the very words evaporate and lose themselves in floods of sound." Its hero, Orpheus, who represents Renaissance Italy, is a lover of art and beauty who dares to invade the dark depths of Hades in search of his lost lover, Eurydice. *Orfeo* is a short work of only 454 lines, written mostly in octaves, but also containing one passage in terza rima, two *ballate*, two *canzonette*, and two bits of Latin verse. The first third of the play is pastoral; the middle third, in which Orpheus pleads passionately before Pluto in Hades for the release of his lady, is the most lyrical:

> Therefore the nymph I love is left for you
> When Nature leads her deathward in due time:
> But now you've cropped the tendrils as they grew,
> The grapes unripe, while yet the sap did climb:
> Who reaps the young blades wet with April dew,
> Nor waits till summer hath o'erpassed her prime?
> Give back, give back my hope one little day!
> Nor for a gift, but for a loan I pray.

The last third culminates in the brutal murder of the hero. When Orpheus turns to look at Eurydice before the stipulated time, she disappears, and the embittered lover launches into a wild lament: "And since my fate hath wrought me wrong so sore,/ I swear I'll never love a woman more." He proceeds to decry the man who mopes and moans for a woman's love, and then declares that, after all, it is the love of males that is "sweetest, softest, best." He invokes the names of gods who have loved boys, and then is silenced by an indignant maenad who invites her followers to slay the slanderous Orpheus for his insult to their sex. They tear him limb from limb and soak the forest in his blood; after boasting of their deed, the maenads join in the drunken *ballata* that concludes the playlet. This final song, which resembles the *trionfo* in form and its spirit of recklessness, appears to be Poliziano's own contribution to the Orphic legend. It was indeed a remarkable innovation; neither the Greek nor the Roman maenads were characterized to this extent by drunkenness or lust for drink.

STANZE

If Poliziano adapted classical material to contemporary form in *Orfeo*, in the *Stanze*, he dressed contemporary material in classical style. Despite its complete title, *Stanze cominciate per la giostra del magnifico Giuliano de' Medici* (stanzas begun for the tournament of the magnificent Giuliano de' Medici), the poem offers no details of the joust itself: The subject disappears beneath the strata of decoration. While there is little that is original in the poem, which might accurately be called a collage of snippets taken from such authors as Statius, Claudian, Theocritus, Euripides, Ovid, Vergil, and Petrarch, its sheer ornamentation is lush and impressive.

The poem addresses three of the most fervent interests of the fifteenth century Italian public: the love of classical literature, the search for artistic beauty, and the enjoyment and appreciation of nature. As the narrative begins, Giuliano is indifferent to love while amorous nymphs sigh over him. He prefers instead to ride his Sicilian steed, and as a simple hunter untroubled by other passions, he often makes his home in the forest, protecting "his face from the rays of the sun with a garland/ of pine or green beech." He has no sympathy for frenzied lovers; love, he reasons, is but the result of lust and sloth. Cupid decides to challenge the young man's indifference and sends a white doe to lure him to a flowery glade under the shadow of gnarled beech trees, where he is smitten by the nymph identified as Simonetta. The fair-skinned, white-garmented Simonetta is ornamented with roses, flowers, and grass, and there are ringlets of her golden hair upon her "humbly proud" forehead. When Giuliano asks what friendly star makes him worthy of a sight so beautiful, Simonetta demurs, answering that she is not what he is searching for, that she is not worthy of an altar, and that furthermore she is already married.

Cupid reports the success of his mission to his mother, Venus, and there ensues a lengthy description of the realm of Venus on the island of Cyprus, a "realm where every Grace delights, where Beauty/ weaves a garland of flowers about her hair,/ where lascivious Zephyr flies behind Flora and/ decks the green grass with flowers." It was this passage (octave 68) that inspired Botticelli's painting *Primavera*, which itself may have served as a kind of frontispiece to Poliziano's *Stanze*. Here, in the realm of Venus, on the doors of her palace, "splendid with gems and with such/ carvings that all other works would be crude and lifeless in comparison," there is one carving of "a young woman not with human countenance/ carried on a conch shell, wafted to shore by playful zephyrs." These lines (octave 99) were probably the source of Botticelli's masterpiece *The Birth of Venus*.

Venus decides to provoke Giuliano to hold a tournament in honor of his new lady, and the second canto of the *Stanze* begins triumphantly with wonderful dreams and prophecies of the glory to be achieved by Giuliano in the tournament, for which the entire first canto had been an introduction. The death of the actual Simonetta, however, required the conversion of the nymph bearing her name to a personified Fortune, who governs Giuliano's life in a different capacity. After discussing the futility of tears in the face of this disaster, the poet proffers this bit of realistic advice: "Blessed is/ he who frees his thoughts from her [Fortune] and encloses/ himself completely within his own virtue." The work breaks off abruptly at the end of octave 46; the political murder of the actual Giuliano robbed the poet of his hero.

RISPETTI AND STRAMBOTTO RHYMES

From 1470 to 1480, Poliziano used Italian for many of his lyrics. He wrote as many as two hundred *rispetti*, eight-line or occasionally six-line love poems rhyming alternately and followed by a concluding couplet with a new rhyme, that are called *strambotti* elsewhere in Italian literature. The *strambotto* may in its origin reflect an original link with folk dance. The poems of Poliziano are not quite folk songs, and although unhampered by erudite language, their accomplished phraseology and carefully selected metaphors are obviously the work of a master. Their expression aspires to a collective rather than a personal essence. Here, instead of the *contadino* willing to mortgage heaven for his *dama*, there is the scholar-courtier dabbling at love as a pastime and imitating "the gold of the heart with the baser material of fine rhetoric," according to Symonds. Less generous than Symonds's judgment is the appraisal of Francesco De Sanctis. He finds even less originality in the *rispetti* of Poliziano than is found in the *Stanze*, and De Sanctis further charges the poet with haste and inattentiveness, lamenting the lack of the personal and subjective touch achieved in similar works by Petrarch. In Poliziano, the same ideas are repeated with only slight variation: The catalog of folk themes was small, and Poliziano did little to make it larger. These few popular ideas move in a circle around the most uncomplicated of situations, such as the beauty of the lover, jealousy, leave-taking, waiting, hope, provocation, despair and thoughts of death, avowals of love and crushing rejections.

CANZONETTE

The best of Poliziano's Italian lyrics are his thirty or so dance songs in the *ballata* form, sometimes classed variously as *canzoni a ballo* or *canzonette*, written in ottava rima but longer and more sophisticated than the *rispetti*. They certainly fail as poetry if judged by Matthew Arnold's definition of poetry as a "criticism of life," but Symonds has made a valiant attempt to coax modern readers to a sympathetic appreciation of these curiously time-bound lyrics. If, proposes Symonds, one transports oneself back to Florence on a summer night, as Prince Lorenzo wanders in the streets with Poliziano, his singing-boys joining hands with beautiful workshop girls and apprentice lads and marble carvers, one can appreciate such lines as these:

> For when the full rose quits her tender sheath,
> When she is sweetest and most fair to see,
> This is the time to place her in thy wreath,
> Before her beauty and her freshness flee.
> Gather ye therefore roses with great glee,
> Sweet girls, or ere their perfume pass away.

These lines are from Poliziano's dance song "I' mi trovai fanciulle un bel mattino" ("I Went A-Roaming, Maidens, One Bright Day"). The title recurs five times as the refrain between four stanzas that describe the violets and the lilies of the landscape, relate the poet's discovery of the incomparable roses and the rapture

that their perfume induces in him, and culminate with the poet's instinct to pluck the blooming flowers before they fade and are lost, ending with the carpe diem lesson of the stanza quoted above.

"MY BRUNETTE" AND "OH, WELCOME MAY"

Another May song is "Ben venga maggio" ("Oh, Welcome May"), which, in addition to its now clichéd topos, suffers a further indignity in its transference to modern English: the loss of sonority and cadence when its refrain word, *maggio*, becomes the lackluster monosyllable *May*. The mirth and exuberance of the original do, however, survive in translation: "With rose and lily crowned,/ and your lips a thirst,/ Love, laughing, comes a ground./ Welcome him to your feast./ Who will, of you, be first/ to give him buds of May?" The birds and flowers of this poem are not merely a backdrop but rather an integral part of the whole exhilarating ritual. Every word contributes to the enthralling gaiety.

The Tuscan peasants' songs of Maying and wooing were those most often reworked by Poliziano when he wrote in Italian. Of his wooing songs, the best is "La brunettina mia" ("My Brunette"), a poem which Symonds judged untranslatable. The brunette of the title is a village beauty who bathes her face in the fountain and wears upon her hair a wreath of wild flowers. She is a blossoming branch of thorn in spring; her breasts are May roses, her lips are strawberries. It should be noted, however, that one of Poliziano's editors, Giosuè Carducci, concluded that this poem was in fact not written by Poliziano.

Departing from the aristocratic tradition of poetry that dictates restraint and decorum, Poliziano, like Lorenzo, wrote *canti carnascialeschi*, street songs that could be satirical, gibing, or even ribald and to which Savonarola accordingly took exception. It was precisely the disrespectful tone of such poems that typified to the patriot-priest Savonarola the decadence of his age.

GREEK EPIGRAMS AND LATIN POEMS

Poliziano's output in Greek was limited to fifty-seven epigrams that appeared in his *Opera omnia* (1498). Poliziano's Greek vocabulary is "unexceptionable" and "simple"; he writes in the ordinary dialect of the epigrammatic poets as well as in Doric. Thematically, Poliziano follows the ancient practice of reworking familiar ideas; his epigram on Chalcondyles, for example, was modeled on Plato's epigram in praise of Aristophanes. Six of the epigrams, written about 1492, praise the scholarly Alessandra Scala, "whose immortal beauty could not be the effect of art but only of simple nature." There are also the Doric couplets on two beautiful boys and the love sonnet to the youth Chrysocomus.

Poliziano's poems in Latin were among the most accomplished written since antiquity. His use of Latin was more original than his use of Greek; rather than merely culling phrases from classical works, he trusted his own ear, which did, however, cause him to mix dictions from different periods. In addition to composing Latin poems in established forms such as elegy, epigram, satire, and idyll, he struck out in a new direction and poured forth torrents of hexameters that testified to his remarkable intellectual energy. About one hundred epigrams in Latin by Poliziano have survived, many of which are addressed to Lorenzo and other heads of state and to his friends; some are epitaphs, such as the one for Fra Lippo Lippi and Squarcialupi; and some are inscriptions, such as the one for the bust of Giotto by Benedetto da Maiano. Others are harangues against humanist rivals, and still others are love poems. Among Poliziano's longer Latin poems are odes and elegies on, for example, the death of Lorenzo and the death of Albiera degli Albizzi, a young and lovely lady soon to have been married.

Written from 1480 to 1490 and based on Poliziano's lectures at the University of Florence were four pieces collectively titled *Sylvae*. Poliziano borrowed the title from Statius; the poems combine classical scholarship with great poetic skill. The *Manta* is a panegyric of Vergil. The *Rusticus* celebrates the joys of country life and prefaces the study of the bucolic poets, primarily Hesiod and Vergil. The *Ambra*, from the name of Lorenzo's favorite villa, contains an idyllic description of the Tuscan landscape and a eulogy of Homer. The *Nutricia* is a general introduction to the study of ancient and modern poetry, from the legendary and real poets of Greece and Rome to Dante, Petrarch, Giovanni Boccaccio, and Guido Cavalcanti, closing with a characterization of some of Lorenzo's poems. Poliziano's brief dismissal in this work of the great triad of Greek trage-

dians is quaintly revealing of how little fifteenth century Italians valued the drama of ancient Greece.

Poliziano, the most brilliant classical scholar of his age, was a true philologist in the etymological sense of the word; he loved learning, and his scholarly writings are remarkably free of the pedantry that had marred and unnecessarily complicated such writing before his example. Poliziano was charged with the fire of his classical studies, and he saw no contradiction in rendering the poetic offshoots of his glorious lore in the lowly vernacular. Despite his vast learning, the diction of his vernacular poetry is down-to-earth and uncomplicated, and if he was accused of composing his Latin verses "with more heat than art," it was because he actually responded to his craft as an ancient rather than as an imitator.

OTHER MAJOR WORKS

PLAY: *Orfeo*, pr. 1480 (English translation, 1879; also known as *Orpheus*).

NONFICTION: *Miscellaneorum centuria prima*, 1489 (commonly known as *Miscellanea*); *Conjurationis pactianae commentarium*, 1498; *Letters*, 2006.

MISCELLANEOUS: *Opera omnia*, 1498.

BIBLIOGRAPHY

Brand, Peter, and Lino Pertile, eds. *The Cambridge History of Italian Literature*. Rev. ed. New York: Cambridge University Press, 1999. Includes introductory information on Poliziano and pertinent historical background.

D'Amico, John F. *Theory and Practice in Renaissance Textual Criticism: Beatus Rhenanus Between Conjecture and History*. Berkeley: University of California Press, 1988. Gives a short account of Poliziano's achievements.

Donadoni, Eugenio. *A History of Italian Literature*. Translated by Richard Monges. New York: New York University Press, 1969. Contains biographical and critical information on Poliziano's life and work.

Godman, Peter. *From Poliziano to Machiavelli: Florentine Humanism in the High Renaissance*. Princeton, N.J.: Princeton University Press, 1998. Godman presents an intellectual history of Florentine humanism from the lifetime of Poliziano in the late fifteenth century to the death of Niccolò Machiavelli in 1527. Making use of unpublished and rare sources, Godman traces the development of philological and official humanism.

Grafton, Anthony. *Defenders of the Text: The Traditions of Scholarship in an Age of Science, 1450-1800.* Cambridge, Mass.: Harvard University Press, 1991. Grafton summarizes Poliziano's innovations as a classical scholar.

Poliziano, Angelo. *Letters.* Edited and translated by Shane Butler. Cambridge, Mass.: Harvard University Press, 2006. The correspondence of Poliziano reveals a great deal about his life and writings, including his relationship with the philosopher Pico della Mirandola.

_____. *Silvae.* Edited and translated by Charles Fantazzi. Cambridge, Mass.: Harvard University Press, 2004. Fantazzi's introduction to his translation of Poliziano's poetry provides background and some analysis of the poetry.

Jack Shreve

FRANCIS PONGE

Born: Montpellier, France; March 27, 1899
Died: Le Bar-Sur-Loup, France; August 6, 1988

PRINCIPAL POETRY

Douze Petits Écrits, 1926
Le Parti pris des choses, 1942 (*Taking the Side of Things*, 1972; also known as *The Nature of Things*, 1995)
Le Carnet du bois de pins, 1947
Proêmes, 1948
La Seine, 1950
La Rage de l'expression, 1952 (*Mute Objects of Expression*, 2008)
Le Grand Recueil, 1961 (3 volumes: *Lyres, Méthodes,* and *Pièces*)
Tome premier, 1965
Nouveau Recueil, 1967
Le Savon, 1967 (*Soap*, 1969)

La Fabrique du Pré, 1971 (*The Making of the Pré*, 1979)
Things, 1971
The Voice of Things, 1972 (includes *Taking the Side of Things* and selected other poems and essays)
Comment une figue de paroles et pourquoi, 1977
L'Écrit Beaubourg, 1977
The Sun Placed in the Abyss, 1977
Selected Poems, 1994

OTHER LITERARY FORMS

Although Francis Ponge (PON-zhuh) did admit to writing poetry, he was reluctant to call his works poems, inventing instead other names for them, such as "prétextes," "définitions-descriptions," and "proêmes." Most of his works are generally classified as prose poems, ranging from a few sentences in length to those which are book length, such as *Soap*. Certain of his texts, however, are not readily classifiable. Commentary on the act of writing poetry is a feature of many of Ponge's works; the transcripts of his conversations with Philippe Sollers, for example, are prose texts about poetry, while a work such as "Le carnet du bois de pins" ("The Notebook of the Pine Woods") is clearly a poetic piece which also features a level of metacommentary about the act of writing. There are, however, other works, many of them contained in a volume titled *Méthodes* (1961), that are basically theoretical works expounding Ponge's aesthetic, but whose structural and poetic qualities effectively blur the distinction between theoretical work and literary text. Ponge's interest in the creation of the literary text as process is evidenced by two of his other works, *The Making of the Pré* and *Comment une figue de paroles et pourquoi* (how a fig of words and why). In each of these two works, a comparatively short poem is preceded by the notes, doodles, dictionary definitions, preliminary drafts, and the like that chronicle the various stages of evolution toward the finished poem. Also worthy of mention, as constituting a separate literary form, are Ponge's works of art criticism, which have been collected in the volume *L'Atelier contemporain* (the contemporary workshop), published in 1977.

ACHIEVEMENTS

During the first thirty-five years of Francis Ponge's career, he was known only within limited artistic circles. His reputation grew slowly, and in 1956, *La Nouvelle Revue française* devoted an entire issue to his work. In 1959, Ponge received a prize for his poem "La Figue (séche)" ("The [Dried] Fig"). In that year, he also received the medal of the French Legion of Honor. Between 1965 and 1971, he lectured extensively in the United States, Canada, and Great Britain, and in 1966-1967 he was a visiting professor at Columbia University. He received the Ingram Merrill Foundation Award for 1972 and the Books Abroad/Neustadt International Prize for Literature in 1974. In 1975, at the prestigious international colloquium at Cerisy-la-Salle, his oeuvre was the subject of study by a distinguished group of his literary colleagues (the proceedings of this conference were published in 1977).

BIOGRAPHY

Francis Jean Gaston Alfred Ponge was born on March 27, 1899, in the city of Montpellier, in the south of France. His father was a bank manager, and his Protestant parents provided him with a secure and loving middle-class upbringing. His childhood in this Mediterranean environment often brought him in contact with the remains of Roman architecture and monuments with their Latin inscriptions; his early awareness of France's cultural and linguistic links with classical civilization is everywhere evident in his poetry.

In 1909, the Ponge family moved to Normandy, where Ponge attended secondary school. He studied Greek and Latin and grew to love their precision; this classical training taught him to appreciate the historical depth of the French language. His study of the natural sciences familiarized him with the scientific method and developed in him the habit of careful observation and the minute recording of details which char-

acterize his poetry. He also excelled in philosophy, taking top honors for his *baccalauréate* essay, titled "L'Art de penser par soi-même" (the art of thinking for oneself).

In 1916, Ponge entered a *lycée* in Paris to prepare himself for university study. In 1917, he began reading philosophy at the Sorbonne and law at the École de Droit. His tastes in philosophy led him to study Arthur Schopenhauer, John Locke, and Benedict de Spinoza, rather than currently popular figures, such as the vitalist Henri Bergson. In 1918, and again in the following year, his hopes for admission to the École Normale Supérieure were blocked by a traumatic inability to speak during crucial oral examinations. This unhappy failure may have been symptomatic of some greater emotional disturbance during that period of his life, or, as some critics have suggested, it may have been caused by a fear of being unable to express himself orally in a precise manner. In any case, there appears to be a connection between these events and the development of Ponge's restrained, meticulous poetic style.

Ponge's awareness of social and political problems was heightened by the chaotic events of World War I and the Russian Revolution. Ponge was becoming thoroughly disgusted with what he perceived to be the weakness and corruption of a society lacking strong moral

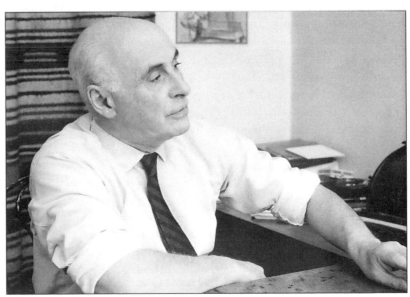

Francis Ponge (AFP/Getty Images)

principles. In April, 1918, he joined the army. The indignities he suffered as a common soldier serving in an army that rewarded mediocre performance and crushed the individual's spirit only compounded his negative feelings about the deficiencies of French society.

Demobilized in 1919, Ponge spent the next three or four years on the edges of Left Bank literary circles. During this time, he published some poems and made a few important contacts with critics and editors. He judged the Parisian literary world to be generally snobbish and affected, however, and refused to play the role of attentive young disciple which might have gained for him greater exposure. Preferring to work alone, he began to search for his own aesthetic voice that would express the spirit of revolt he felt against social and literary decadence.

Whether because of his Protestant upbringing, his parental influence, his education, or certain other factors, even at a young age Ponge had exhibited a marked strength of character and independence, high ideals, and a belief in the individual's responsibility for his or her own actions. These traits influenced his literary and political development. Throughout his adult life, he was attracted to various political, literary, and philosophical movements because of affinities with certain of their beliefs; his refusal to adopt completely any system of beliefs but his own, however, made most of these alliances rather brief. He associated himself with the Surrealists because of their spirit of literary and linguistic revolt, but he was uncomfortable with their undisciplined approach to composition and the excessive Hermeticism of some Surrealist writings. Ponge joined the French Communist Party in 1937 because he saw it as the only viable means of improving living and working conditions for French workers, but his inability to accept the dogmatism of the party and its doctrinaire attitudes toward art eventually led him to resign. His beliefs about the limitations and moral imperatives governing humankind's actions in the world have much in common with those of Albert Camus and other Existentialist writers, although Ponge's ultimate view of the human condition is more optimistic than that of Camus. Aspects of Ponge's philosophy and aesthetics can be labeled materialist, mechanist, phenomenological, Stoic,

and Epicurean, but Ponge's individualism resists categorization.

After the death of his father in 1923, Ponge's mother came to live with him in Paris. With the exception of an interlude in 1927 when a small inheritance allowed him to live comfortably and write full time, Ponge was almost constantly plagued by financial difficulties for the next twenty years of his life. A succession of minor jobs with publishing houses and insurance companies, punctuated by periods of unemployment, often left him with no more than twenty minutes a day to devote to his writing.

Ponge's association with the Surrealist movement came in the late 1920's. He met André Breton and other prominent Surrealists, participated in some of their less extravagant activities, and followed their literary experiments with interest. His involvement with them was brief, however. He discovered that he wished to marry, and not wanting to offend his fiancé's middle-class family by continuing to affiliate with an artistic movement so thoroughly disliked by the French bourgeoisie, he abandoned his lukewarm connections with the Surrealists. He accepted an appropriately respectable job with the publishing firm Messageries Hachette in 1931. He and Odette Chabanel were married in that same year, and their daughter Armande was born in 1935.

The drudgery and demeaning nature of his "respectable" job inspired great sympathy in Ponge for his fellow workers. A desire to see the quality of life improved for all workers, as well as a growing concern about fascism, led him to become a labor union official in 1936 and a member of the Communist Party in 1937. His role as a union activist resulted in his losing his position in 1937.

Unemployed for a time, Ponge subsequently worked for an insurance firm until he joined the army in 1939. Demobilized in 1940 after the fall of France, he was active in the Resistance movement in the south of France, both as a journalist and in the underground. He continued to write poetry, and his first major collection of poems, *Taking the Side of Things*, was published in 1942.

Returning to Paris after the Liberation in 1944, Ponge became the literary and art editor for *Action*, a communist weekly newspaper. This brought him into stimulating contact with the work of such literary and artistic figures as Louis Aragon, Paul Éluard, Camus, René Char, Pablo Picasso, Georges Braque, and Jean Dubuffet. In 1944, Jean-Paul Sartre drew attention to Ponge; his essay on *Taking the Side of Things* was influential in introducing Ponge to the French literary public.

Ponge became increasingly irritated with the dogmatic attitudes of both *Action* and the Communist Party, and by 1947, he had resigned his editorship and allowed his membership in the Communist Party to lapse. For the next few years, Ponge found little employment, and he and his family were reduced to extreme poverty. His literary work was becoming better known, but in spite of occasional publications and speaking engagements, he was from time to time forced to sell personal possessions to pay his debts. Not until 1952, when he was fifty-three years of age, was Ponge to know a fair degree of financial security; in that year, he was offered a teaching position at the Alliance Française in Paris, which he held until he reached retirement age. Subsequently, he lived and wrote in Provence, with occasional visits abroad as a visiting professor or guest lecturer, until his death in 1988.

Most of Ponge's literary recognition came late in his career, although essays by Sartre and Camus helped to generate some early interest in his work. In the 1960's, the Tel Quel group, headed by Philippe Sollers, and exponents of the French New Novel such as Alain Robbe-Grillet, discovered their kinship with Ponge's aesthetic and linguistic explorations.

ANALYSIS

The title of Francis Ponge's first major book of poems epitomizes his aesthetic philosophy and poetic style. Usually translated as *Taking the Side of Things*, it announces both Ponge's preference for things over ideas and his desire to correct what he saw as a human anthropocentric conception of the universe. Ponge disapproved of the human tendency to regard abstract ideas as absolutes rather than as linguistic constructs whose truth is only relative. He was also unhappy with commonplace cultural notions which deem certain subjects unworthy of poetic consideration. Rejecting such assumptions, Ponge adopted an ironic anti-intellectualism by devoting his literary endeavors to the defense of the concrete things of the world. As subjects for his poems, he chose ordinary objects encountered in daily life that are often taken for granted. He perceived them as relegated to a kind of second-class citizenship by their inability to express themselves, and he sympathetically imagined them as pleading with him to speak for them.

Ponge thus designated himself as the advocate of things. In his poems, he declined to describe the object as though it were a human being, and he resisted the lure of lyric excess that might tempt him to forget his self-appointed task. Choosing an object such as a door, a pebble, a loaf of bread, or a bar of soap, he observed it with the concentration of a scientist. He avoided preconceived ideas and linguistic formulas unless he could transform them to offer the reader fresh insights into the nature of the object or the functioning of language. He sought not to render the object from a human point of view, but rather to find a literary form whose structure, density, and character would be the verbal equivalent of the object.

Ponge labeled his works *définitions-descriptions*, a term he invented to describe a literary form that would combine the functions of encyclopedias, etymological dictionaries, and dictionaries of synonyms, rhymes, and analogous words. Whereas the traditional dictionary definition uses words devoid of connotation to describe each object, Ponge chose words with greater affective content for his descriptions; he repeatedly evoked the object by words whose sound, spelling, etymology, or secondary meanings reflected and echoed the object.

For Ponge, the ideal result of this faithful attention to the object was a literary text that had as much material solidity as the object it represented. Although manifestly not the same as the object itself, this kind of poetic formulation has characteristics similar to those of the object. The words which make up the poetic text are thus to be reckoned with as material presences, not as transparent signs which are to be transcended in search of the "real" object to which they refer. In addition, each object poem has its own unique structure; Ponge avoided established literary forms because they required the poet to make compromises. In Ponge's view, for example, the requirements of the sonnet's structure might cause a poet to reject that word that best reveals the object's essence because it does not satisfy the requirements of meter or rhyme.

An insistence upon the irreducible materiality of language is central to Ponge's approach to poetry. He spoke of words as objects which are "strangely concrete, with two dimensions, for the eye and the ear, and the third is perhaps something like their meaning." Language has an often startling ability to reveal the essential characteristics of the things it describes, but careless use of language devalues it, allowing historically acquired meanings to be lost. With a rigor which is classical in its insistence on proportion and in its rejection of subjective emotionalism, Ponge sought forms so apt that they would resist the ravages of time, much, as he has suggested, as the Roman inscriptions of his beloved Provence have weathered the centuries.

"ESCARGOTS"

For Ponge, the ability to use language was not a reason to elevate humanity to a position of superiority in the world. He did not often refer to human beings in his poetry of objects, fearing that he could not be objective; Ponge's object lessons, however, reveal that he held human beings to be neither more nor less important than any other part in the mechanistic workings of the universe. In a poem titled "Escargots" (snails), Ponge contrasted the snail's evanescent secretion, its "silvery wake" of slime, to its enduring shell. He then drew the analogy to human beings' own "secretions"—their mundane, everyday language, which will disappear as quickly as does the snail's trail—and humans' literary creations, which, fashioned with care, can be as lasting as the snail's shell. Ponge admired the snail, whose art is an inherent product of its life and whose modest shell will endure as a monument even after the snail is gone. Its shell is perfectly proportioned to the snail and is eminently suited to its nature. The analogous conclusion, for Ponge, was that language is the essential property of human beings and that it is their ethical duty to use it as deliberately as possible, so that what they produce is as perfectly suited to humans as the shell is to the snail.

"LE CYCLE DES SAISONS"

Ponge viewed the entire world as expressive, although most of its objects have severely limited vocabularies. In "Le Cycle des saisons" (the cycle of the sea-

sons), for example, trees manifest their exuberance in an eloquent profusion of "words"—that is, their leaves. Because each tree "utters" the same leaf again and again, however, the trees can only repeat their single-word vocabulary. Since humans represent the sole creatures whose language enables them to speak about, and on behalf of, other things, they can, like Ponge, use their talent so that the poetic "monuments" they leave behind dignify not only humanity but also the objects that so faithfully serve it.

EQUIVALENCE

Ponge's belief that the poem should perfectly suit its object-subject led him to formulate a compositional ideal which he called *adéquation*, best translated from its Latin components—*ad* (to) and *aequus* (equal)—as "equivalence." A perfect realization of this ideal results in a poem with almost magical qualities; its words, while remaining true to language's own laws of syntax, so perfectly conjure up the object they describe that the poem becomes the verbal equivalent of the object. Ponge attempted to achieve *adéquation* through the use of various compositional techniques: the creation of forms that are tailor-made for their subjects, the frequent use of word associations, the exploration of etymologies, the innovative and often humorous use of figurative language, the coining of puns and portmanteau words, and the enlistment of typography in support of a poetic idea.

FITTING FORM TO OBJECT

Ponge attempted to fit the form of the poem to the object it describes, both on the level of overall structure and on the level of syntax. "L'Huître" (the oyster), for example, has three sections. The first describes the outward appearance of the oyster, stressing its obstinate refusal to reveal its inner self. The second section uses a metaphor that describes the shell's contents as a separate world whose sky is a hard mother-of-pearl *firmament*. Finally, a single sentence refers to that rarity, the pearl, as a *formule* ("tiny form," but also "formula"). This mimetic approach to form is not without its humorous side; the "Ode inachevée à la boue" (unfinished ode to mud) is as formless as the substance it describes, covering several pages and finally trailing off in midsentence. In *Soap*, words froth and bubble and proliferate in imitation of the effervescence of soap and in-

clude such airy coinages as *ebullescence* (ebullience).
In "Le Papillon" (the butterfly), soft fricative and plo-
sive sounds abound, and the poem's breathless manner
cleverly mimics the whimsical and erratic flight of the
butterfly: "Dès lors, le papillon erratique ne se pose
plus qu'au hasard de sa course, ou tout comme" ("From
then on, the erratic butterfly no longer alights except
by chance in its flight, or just about").

"PLUIE" AND "LE MIMOSA"

Sometimes Ponge's poems present an intentional
air of formlessness. Composed of numerous short sections with labels such as "Variant" and "Other," these
alternative versions approach the same subject from
slightly different points of view in a manner reminiscent of the multiple perspectives of cubist art. For example, in "Le Mimosa" (the mimosa), Ponge subtly
demonstrated the process of poetic creation by catching
the reader off guard with a mélange of false starts and
complaints about how difficult it is to capture the essence of the mimosa in words. The effect of all this
"beating around the bush" is a poem that simultaneously communicates a great deal both about the elusive fragility of flowers and about the mysterious nature of the creative process.

However winding the linguistic route through a typical Ponge poem may be, the end is reached when, after
having led the reader on a thorough search of all the levels and relations of meaning, the object of the poem is
present in the reader's consciousness with an unprecedented, harmonious clarity. For example, "Pluie" (rain)
ends its detailed description of a shower with the brief
phrase "il a plu" (it has rained). Here, the rain, which
first appeared in the poem as an object (noun), is finally
seen as a process (verb), and as one that is not finished.
Ponge avoided the simple past tense, more common in
literary texts but clearly connoting finality. Instead he
used the present-perfect tense, which in French indicates the strong link between this past action and the
present time; in this line resonates the memory of all
that has transpired in the poem. Furthermore, since *plu*
is the past participle of the verb *plaire* (to please) as
well as of the verb *pleuvoir* (to rain), an additional interpretation of this last line is, "It has been pleasing"—a
modest judgment on the part of the poet with which
most readers would concur.

ETYMOLOGIES, PUNS, AND PORTMANTEAU WORDS

Ponge maintained that language contains truths
about the essential nature of the objects it is capable of
describing, if only writers are willing to work hard
enough to find these truths. Once the inherent harmony
between language and the objects of the world is struck,
the poet will find that the words intertwine to form a
network of secondary meanings and serendipitous etymologies.

In an essay on his creative method, Ponge gave an illustration of the inherent ability of language to form
metonymical links that illuminate the world with sudden insights: Once, when writing in Algeria, the word
sacripant (roguish) continually occurred to him as an
adjective descriptive of the harsh red color of the Sahel
at the foot of the Atlas mountains. Curious about the
etymology of the word, he traced it to the name of
Ludovico Ariosto's characters. He then discovered to
his delight that this name, Sacripant, was linked to that
of Rodomont—a king of Algeria, whose name (red
mountain) furnished Ponge with the sort of felicitous
coincidence in which his poems abound.

Sometimes Ponge puns on words in such a way that
their literal meaning is revealed in a fresh and unexpected manner. In "L'Orange" (the orange), Ponge describes a squeezed orange; in a play on the French
pression (pressing or squeezing), he portrays the orange as having undergone an ordeal of "expression"
and of having submitted to a forced "oppression." In
yet another punning excursion, Ponge compares the
"aspirations" of the squeezed orange to regain its
"countenance" (an allusion not only to its shape or disposition, but also to its contents) to those of a sponge;
he remarks that, whereas the sponge will soak up any
liquid, even dirty water, "l'orange a meilleur goût"—
"the orange has better taste." These and other clever
plays on words seem particularly apt as they are applied
to the orange. The reader comes away glad that Ponge
has tried to render it "aussi rondement que possible"—
as loyally, as ardently as possible (which *rondement*
ordinarily means in French)—but in the case of the
orange, also adding a further layer of meaning, in that
rondement is a word originally derived from that round-
ness so descriptive of an orange.

Such puns are typical of Ponge's playful approach to words. He is also very sensitive to the ability of word associations to trigger poetic observations and to create stylistic unity. In "La Huître" (the oyster), the circumflex and *-tre* ending of the poem's title inspire Ponge's use of the French suffix *-âtre*, as in *blanchâtre* (whitish), *verdâtre* (greenish), *noirâtre* (blackish), and *opiniâtrement* (obstinately). In "Le Pain" (the loaf of bread), Ponge compares the crusty surface of the loaf to the raised surface of a relief map or a globe. This novel view of the loaf's surface suddenly yields a panoramic impression of the geography of Earth, thus trading on an imaginative link between the words *pain* (bread) and *panoramique* (panoramic), which appear in the first lines of the poem.

Ponge is not above inventing etymologies for words when it suits his purpose. His discussion of "L'Ustensile" (the utensil) is a product of his imaginative conjecture that *ustensile* is derived from a combination of the words *utile* (useful) and *ostensible* (ostensible); this latter word refers to the fact that a utensil is usually hung in plain sight on the kitchen wall, ready to be of service.

Ponge also delights in creating portmanteau words in the manner of Lewis Carroll. Describing the change of seasons in "La Fin de l'automne" (the end of autumn), Ponge pictures a marshy, rain-drenched bit of earth as a *grenouillerie*, a "frog-preserve," characterized by an *amphibiguïté salubre*—a "salubrious amphibiguity." This latter phrase suggests an ambiguous region—neither lake nor dry land—that is inhabited by amphibians, and a rainy season of autumn becoming winter that affords its creatures a healthy period for cleansing reflection before the onset of spring.

VISUAL POETRY

Ponge was fascinated by the graphic possibilities of the written word. Although he created at least one visual poem, "L'Araignée mise au mur" (the spider placed on the wall), that is reminiscent of Guillaume Apollinaire's *Calligrammes* (1918; English translation, 1980), Ponge does not ordinarily write purely concrete poetry; the dominant role of language in his poems is always that of a verbal rather than a graphic medium. Nevertheless, he is intrigued by the ability of the shapes of the letters of the alphabet to participate

in the process of symbolization. In an essay from *Méthodes* titled "Proclamation et petit four" (proclamation and petit four), Ponge points out that the modern reader's acquaintance with poetry is almost exclusively an acquaintance with the printed page; only infrequently does one hear poetry spoken aloud. He thus finds it appropriate to explore the link between the subject of the poem and the poem's typography. In this same essay, he expresses the hope that readers of his poem "L'Abricot" (the apricot) will be aware of the resemblance between the *a* in "apricot" and the fruit itself. Other links between typography and meaning are made explicit in the poems themselves. In "La Chèvre" (the goat), Ponge sees the goat's little beard in the accent mark in its name; his poem "La Cruche" (the pitcher) begins with the observation that its *u* is as hollow as the container it describes; and in "Notes prises pour un oiseau" (notes taken for a bird), Ponge sees the silhouette of the resting bird in the *s* of *oiseau*. The role of typography as an active participant in Ponge's poems ranges from a minor one in which the letters in the object's name are shown to illustrate certain of its qualities, to poems inspired almost entirely by typographical observations. "Le 14 juillet" (July 14, or Bastille Day) is generated from the characters of its title, whose letters and numbers are transformed into French citizens carrying flags and wielding weapons in a miniature reenactment of the drama of the French Revolution.

Although Ponge's various compositional techniques have seemed contrived to some readers, at their most apt, woven together into a tightly composed prose poem, these techniques approach Ponge's ideal of "equivalence." This sense of focus and unity is perhaps strongest in Ponge's shorter poems, in which virtually every word is linked to every other word through etymology, assonance, visual links, or word associations. The Ponge poem at its best delights the reader, bringing to light unnoticed qualities of the object it describes; it inspires, as well, a deep understanding of the expressive potential of language. In a Ponge poem, language becomes another kind of object, whose profoundly established connections to the things of the world reveal much about that world.

Ponge has conceded that human involvement can

never be eliminated from the process of writing about things, yet he firmly relegates humans to the role of simple participants in a functioning system. This view is very much in keeping with modern trends in French scholarship, which increasingly portray humans as products of the cultural structures into which they are born rather than as their master.

LEGACY

Although predicated on the notion of "equivalence"—an aesthetic ideal difficult if not impossible to achieve—Ponge's approach to poetry was yet a pragmatic one, based both upon careful observation of his object-subjects and upon diligent mining of the language for the insights it provides. Ponge asserted that the resistance posed by a centuries-old system of structures such as language actually helped him write better poetry. The poet's commitment to a meticulous use of language prevented the annexation or the taking for granted of objects by human beings and, at the same time, furnished insights into human behavior.

Like Camus, Ponge acknowledged the impossibility of attaining philosophical absolutes and recognized the absurdity of the human condition. Like Stéphane Mallarmé, he endeavored to develop a poetic language capable of a perfect rather than an approximate rendering of the world. Unlike these two writers, however, Ponge was not greatly distressed by the realization that such efforts are doomed to fall short of perfection. Refusing to be conquered by a daunting quest for absolutes, he adopted a pragmatic and ultimately optimistic attitude toward human potential. For Ponge, human dignity was to be found in the faithful performance of a person's duty to strive for proportion and perfection in the use of that most uniquely human of all human attributes—language. There is a kind of heroism or sainthood in accepting time and again the challenge to find in language a perfect equivalent for the things of the world; in striving to meet this challenge to the best of his ability, humans perfect themselves morally. Ponge invited humans to learn a lesson from the snail, whose patient work of construction is necessary to its existence and is perfectly suited to—and is a perfect expression of—its nature. In a like manner, human nobility or sainthood is attained by perfecting one's self, by knowing and accepting one's limitations and by obeying one's own nature. "Perfect yourself morally," Ponge advised, "and you will produce beautiful poetry."

OTHER MAJOR WORKS

NONFICTION: *Méthodes*, 1961; *Pour un Malherbe*, 1965; *Entretiens de Francis Ponge avec Philippe Sollers*, 1970; *L'Atelier contemporain*, 1977.

BIBLIOGRAPHY

Andrews, Chris. *Poetry and Cosmogony*. Atlanta: Rodopi, 1999. Andrews analyzes references to science and to the creation of the universe in the works of Raymond Queneau and Ponge. Includes bibliographical references and index.

Higgins, Ian. *Francis Ponge*. London: Athlone Press, 1979. Critical assessment of Ponge's oeuvre. Includes bibliographic references.

Meadows, Patrick Alan. *Francis Ponge and the Nature of Things: From Ancient Atomism to a Modern Poetics*. Lewisburg, Pa.: Bucknell University Press, 1997. Critical interpretation of Ponge's works. Includes bibliographical references and index.

Minahen, Charles D. *Figuring Things: Char, Ponge, and Poetry in the Twentieth Century*. Lexington, Ky.: French Forum, 1994. A collection of critical essays on the poetic works of René Char and Ponge. Includes bibliographical references.

Puchek, Peter. *Rewriting Creation: Myth, Gender, and History*. New York: Peter Lang, 2001. Critical interpretation of the works of selected twentieth century poets including Ponge. Includes bibliographical references and index.

Rowlands, Esther. *Redefining Resistance: The Poetic Wartime Discources of Francis Ponge, Benjamin Peret, Henri Michaux, and Antonin Artaud*. New York: Rodopi, 2004. Presents a critique of linguistic resistance in the poetic texts compiled between 1936 and 1946 of Ponge, Peret, Michaux, and Artaud.

Sorrell, Martin. *Francis Ponge*. Boston: Twayne, 1981. An introductory biography and critical analysis of selected works. Includes bibliographic references.

Janet L. Solberg

VASKO POPA

Born: Grebenac, Serbia, Kingdom of Serbs, Croats, and Slovenes (now in Serbia and Montenegro); July 29, 1922

Died: Belgrade, Yugoslavia (now in Serbia and Montenegro); January 5, 1991

PRINCIPAL POETRY

Kora, 1953 (*Bark*, 1978)

Nepočin-polje, 1956 (*Unrest-Field*, 1978)

Sporedno nebo, 1968 (*Secondary Heaven*, 1978)

Selected Poems, 1969

The Little Box, 1970

Uspravna zemlja, 1972 (*Earth Erect*, 1973)

Kuća nasred druma, 1975

Vučja so, 1975 (*Wolf Salt*, 1978)

Živo meso, 1975 (*Raw Flesh*, 1978)

Collected Poems, 1943-1976, 1978 (includes *Bark*, *Unrest-Field*, *Secondary Heaven*, *Earth Erect*, *Wolf Salt*, *Raw Flesh*, and selections from *Kuća nasred druma*)

The Blackbird's Field, 1979

Homage to the Lame Wolf: Selected Poems, 1956-1975, 1979

Ponoćno sunce: Zbornik pesnićkih snovidenja, 1979

Rez, 1981 (*The Cut*, 1986)

Collected Poems, 1997

OTHER LITERARY FORMS

In addition to poetry, Vasko Popa (POH-pah) published *Urnebesnik: Zbornik pesničkog humora* (1960), a selection of Serbian wit and humor, and *Od zlata jabuka* (1966; *The Golden Apple*, 1980), a collection of folk poems, tales, proverbs, riddles, and curses, which Popa selected from the vast body of Yugoslav folk literature.

ACHIEVEMENTS

When Vasko Popa's first book of verse appeared in 1953, it was rejected by many readers and critics who did not believe that Yugoslav poetry was in need of modernization. In the struggle against traditional forms

and themes, Popa's poetry, like that of Miodrag Pavlović, played a prominent role and contributed decisively to the victory of the modernists. Since then, he gained steadily in stature and popularity so that many critics have come to regard him as a major Yugoslav poet of the twentieth century.

Popa's contributions were manifold. He not only helped rejuvenate Serbian and Yugoslav poetry but also brought it to the level of world poetry—one of the few Yugoslav poets to do so. His profound interest in finding the primeval roots of his nation's culture; his creation of myths for modern times; his probings into the deepest recesses of the subconscious; his gift for striking visions, images, and metaphors; and his highly accomplished, seemingly effortless poetic skill—he brought all these elements to twentieth century Yugoslav poetry. Popa's wrestling with fundamental human problems—death, fate, the meaning of life, love—makes his poetry universal and enduring. Uncompromising when his poetic freedom is questioned, determined to reconfirm the superiority of poetry, and captivated by his craft almost to the exclusion of all other concerns, he is a poet's poet, whose place at the top of all Serbian and Yugoslav literature seems assured.

BIOGRAPHY

Vasko Popa was born on July 29, 1922, in Grebenac, a village near Bela Crkva in the Banat region of the Kingdom of Serbs, Croats, and Slovenes (now in Serbia and Montenegro). He studied literature at the universities of Belgrade, Bucharest, and Vienna and graduated from Belgrade in 1949. He settled in Belgrade, working as an editor in various publishing houses, chiefly Nolit, one of the largest publishers in Yugoslavia, from which he retired in 1982. Popa began to publish poetry in 1951, and his first book appeared in 1953. He traveled widely and was highly respected outside his native land. He received numerous literary awards, and his poems were translated into many languages.

ANALYSIS

Vasko Popa's poetry displays many unique features. From the very first, he showed a predilection for objects, for specifics rather than generalities, for the concrete rather than the abstract. As if to restore the equilibrium disturbed in his early manhood during the war, he felt a need to call everything by its proper name, to relegate each object to its appointed place.

BARK

Among Popa's first poems, which appear in *Bark*, are those titled simply "Chair," "Plate," and "Paper." In such poems, Popa attempted to penetrate the outer shell of objects, arriving at their core. One gets the impression that he stared persistently at an inanimate object until it appeared to breathe and to move. In one of his finest poems, "The Quartz Pebble," he extolled the magnificent beauty of a stone in its seeming immobility and indifference to its surroundings ("headless limbless"). Soon, however, the smooth white stone began to move "with the shameless march of time," holding everything "in its passionate/ Internal embrace." Thus, the essential traits of the quartz pebble are illuminated in a very few lines. Although not a living being, it moves, breathes, smiles, and shows passion. (This poem first appeared in *Bark* and was repeated and expanded into a cycle in Popa's second collection, *Unrest-Field*.) The secret of Popa's propensity for things lies in the fact that they were not merely things for him but beings, which only the sixth sense, or the inner eye, of a poet could discern.

Popa's dead world pulsates with a weird life that is more intense than that of living beings in the familiar world. Speaking of a cigarette in "In the Ashtray," he calls it "a tiny sun/ With a yellow tobacco hair" being extinguished in an ashtray while "the blood of a cheap lipstick suckles/ The dead stumps of stubs." In "On the Hat Stand," "collars have bitten through the necks of hanging emptiness." "In a Smile" describes a scene where "Blue-eyed distances/ Have coiled up into a ball." The culmination of this anthropomorphism is found in the cycle "Spisak" ("List"). In addition to the quartz stone mentioned above, this cycle comprises a duck that "will never learn/ How to walk/ As she knows/ How to plough mirrors"; a horse that has eight legs and drags the whole earth behind him; a pig that runs joyfully toward "the yellow gate," only to feel the "savage wild knife in her throat"; a dandelion that is "A yellow eye of loneliness/ On the sidewalk edge/ At the end of the world"; and a chestnut tree that "lives on the adventures/ Of his unreachable roots." A dinner plate is "A yawn of free lips/ Above the horizon of hunger." Popa's obsession with things reveals not only his uncanny ability to see the world from their perspective but also his intention to speak through natural symbols, to present graphically the mysterious nature of human destiny.

UNREST-FIELD

Popa's closeness to things was undoubtedly accentuated by the war experience of his impressionable years, when the language spoken around him was blunt, terse, bloody, and final. From this experience stem two haunting cycles of poems in *Unrest-Field*, "Igre" ("Games") and "Kost kosti" ("One Bone to Another"). "Games" is Popa's response to the frightening games of war. The poems of this cycle resemble an eerie pantomime of creatures beyond the natural and comprehensible, for Popa's "games" defy logical explanation, symbolically reflecting the cruelty, grotesqueness, and fatuity of human existence. In "The Seducer," one person fondles a chair leg until it gives him

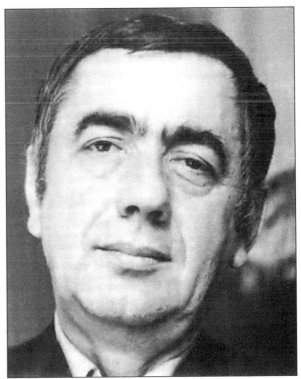

Vasko Popa (©Lufti Özkök)

"the glad"; another kisses a keyhole while a third person gapes at them, turning his head until it falls off. In "The Chase," people bite arms and legs off one another and bury them like dogs, while others sniff around, searching for buried limbs; whoever finds his own is entitled to the next bite.

Even more drastic is the cycle "One Bone to Another." By stripping human beings to their bones and allowing the bones to express the feelings of their former bodies, Popa speaks the subterranean language of life beyond the grave. This *danse macabre* suggests the life that was or might have been. When, in the first section (the poem "At the Beginning"), one bone says to another, "We've got away from the flesh," the stage is set for a new existence entirely different from the human, yet the bones proceed to emulate their former "owners": "It's marvelous sunbathing naked," "Let's love each other just the two of us"; "Then we'll . . ./ Go on growing as we please." Soon, flesh commences to grow back on them, "As if everything were beginning again/ With a more horrible beginning" ("In the Moonlight"). They have no place to go: "What shall we do there/ There long awaiting us/ There eagerly expecting us/ No one and his wife nothing" ("Before the End"). Finally, they devour each other: "Why have you swallowed me/ I can't see myself any more . . ./ All is an ugly dream of dust" ("At the End"). Again, the application to human conditions is all too obvious.

In these bleak conditions, Popa assails his nemesis—his fate or death—head-on, demanding the return of his "little rags": the minimum requirements for existence. He calls his nemesis a "monster"; he threatens it ("Flee monster . . ./ We're not meant for each other") and challenges it to a showdown, trying all the while to build an immunity against adversity, albeit unsuccessfully. It is a valiant protest just the same, capable of restoring one's dignity ("I've wiped your face off my face/ Ripped your shadow off my shadow"). Thus, Popa can even be called an optimist, despite the macabre atmosphere of his world.

In such an atmosphere, the love experience, too, undergoes a Popa-esque metamorphosis. In the cycle "Daleko u nama" ("Far Within Us"), from *Bark*, Popa tries to save his love from a nightmarish dream:

> Horror on the ocean of tea in the cup
> Rust taking a hold
> On the edges of our laughter
> A snake coiled in the depths of the mirror . . .
> Murky passages flow
> From our eyelashes down our faces—
> With a fierce red-hot wire
> Anger hems up our thoughts . . .
> The venomous rain of eternity
> Bites us greedily

In such moments of acute danger, the poet expresses unabashed tenderness: "The streets of your glances/ Have no ending/ The swallows from your eyes/ Do not migrate south"; "I would steal you from silence/ I would clothe you in songs." Even the hours of fear ("The pillars supporting heaven crumble/ The bench with us slowly/ Falls into the void"), of parting ("Only in sleep/ we walk the same paths"), of threatening loss ("I go/ From one side of my head to the other/ Where are you?") are only temporary. In Popa's world, love seems to be the only power capable of overcoming the adversities of fate and death.

SECONDARY HEAVEN

From the small, seemingly insignificant objects of his early verse, Popa moved to the larger arena of his native land and from there to the universe itself, in the collection *Secondary Heaven*. In Popa's cosmology, the sun rules in his empire, but his rule is marred by the struggle between the forces of darkness and light. Popa uses this allegory to suggest his worldview and to treat complex human problems in an oblique fashion.

Secondary Heaven begins with a symbol of emptiness in the form of zero: "Once upon a time there was a number/ Pure and round like a sun/ But alone very much alone." No matter how much the zero adds or multiplies itself, the result remains zero. The forces of light, represented by King Sun, are engaged in a battle against the world of nothingness (zero). Tragically, the heir to King Sun, Prince Sun, is a blind bastard led by two crippled rays. Hope seems betrayed, and the chances of the forces of light are slim, yet the struggle goes on. This is the bare outline of *Secondary Heaven*. Popa's allegory should be seen not as a metaphysical or mythological interpretation of reality but rather as a reflection of humanity's fate in a celestial mirror.

The force of the poet's idiom, the familiar simplicity, the use of old legends and folklore, and the original humor and charming irony make his collection a great achievement. Above all, it shows that Popa's poetic thought has come full circle. By way of the universe, he has reached his final destination—his own self.

WOLF SALT, RAW FLESH, AND KUĆA NASRED DRUMA

Of Popa's later collections, *Wolf Salt* is centered on the myth of a wolf as an old Slavic symbol of vitality, not of evil and destruction. The wolf is depicted as a benign creature, lame yet possessing indestructible tenacity, symbolizing the vitality of the Serbian people. He is connected with the Serbian historical and legendary figure Saint Sava, who is his shepherd. Popa's characteristic terseness and directness of expression add to the exceptional quality of this book, making it one of the best in his entire opus. *Raw Flesh* represents a slight departure from Popa's customary manner in that it is more personal and realistic. The poet returned to his native region, evoked memories of his childhood, and even named names. Although the poems have a realistic surface, they resonate with ancient myths, popular beliefs, and superstitions, all indicating the depth of Popa's immersion in the soul of his people. These poems seem somewhat lighter than his usual poetry, as if to show another, less somber side of the poet. *Kuća nasred druma* (the house on the high road) is a heterogeneous collection lacking a tight cyclical unity, but even here one can perceive a potentially unifying subject matter that could eventually lead to the further development of this cycle and possibly give birth to other cycles.

Stylistically, Popa's poetry is marked by several distinct characteristics. Rather than composing individual, self-contained poems, he generally worked in cycles of poems dealing with the same subject matter and written in the same vein. In turn, these cycles are related to one another; for this reason, Popa frequently changed the order of cycles in new editions, where they acquire new pertinence.

TERSE VERSE, HUMOR, IRONY

Perhaps the most conspicuous feature of Popa's verse is its terseness. His poetry is often aphoristic, and his language is reduced to a bare minimum. When he wanted to underscore the maddening intensity and chaos of a battle, he described a river turning and twisting, unable to find its shores again. The agility of a horse is illustrated by its eight legs—the impression one gets when observing a galloping horse. Popa always used fewer rather than more words, to the point of being cryptic and difficult to fathom at times.

There is also a certain playfulness in Popa's poetry, connected with his predilection for games and pantomime amid the horrors of war. It can be good-natured fun (a picture of a donkey that cannot be seen for its large ears), often turning, however, into the nervous, biting humor of a sensitive man dissatisfied with his world. Not infrequently, Popa's humor takes a mordant, even macabre twist, but more often he laughs at the absurdity, the tragicomedy, of human life. In his most exalted poetry, in *Secondary Heaven*, the old sun stopped "Three paces from the top of heaven . . ./ And went back to his rising/ (So as not to die in our sight)"; similarly, two lame rays lead a blind sun, and "morning is out somewhere seeking his fortune." Such humor is hard to separate from the irony with which Popa's worldview was suffused.

Popa's irony, too, assumed various forms. The most noticeable is his almost chatty approach to problems facing his creatures or things. At a crucial moment, when a solution is expected, the poet half jestingly quips, "What shall I tell you?," meaning, "Oh, what's the use!" His ironic attitude arose for the most part from his awareness that he was locked in a losing battle with his old nemesis, although he stubbornly refused to admit defeat.

LANGUAGE AND IDIOM

Popa's language requires a study in itself. No other Yugoslav poet (save perhaps Laza Kostić or Momčilo Nastasijević) has shown such originality and resourcefulness—indeed, virtuosity—of language. Particularly notable is Popa's ability to distill the existing lexicon, to select the mot juste, and even to coin words. Striking also is the deceptive simplicity of Popa's idiom—deceptive because his "simple" expressions often harbor a variety of meanings, depending on the context. That is why he is both easy and difficult to translate. His language also reveals elements of folk speech, evident also in other aspects of his poetry, especially in *Secondary Heaven*:

A transparent dove in the head
In the dove a clay coffer
In the coffer a dead sea
In the sea a blessed moon

A stanza such as this ("A Dove in the Head") resembles a folk poem or riddle in both content and form. Popa's poetry abounds in similar examples.

Popa's prosody is idiosyncratic: He eschews rhyme and strict meter, but he also avoids free verse. His lines are roughly metric, by no means following a regular pattern yet possessing a strong underlying rhythm.

INFLUENCES

There is no critical consensus concerning the extent to which Popa was influenced by other poets, in part because the uniqueness and elemental power of his poetry belie any simple notion of imitation. Early in his career, Popa was attracted by the Surrealists, whose Yugoslav offshoot was very strong between the two wars, but he refused to follow their prescriptions blindly, believing that each period brings its own problems and solutions. Another source of influence was Nastasijević, one of the most unusual and enigmatic of modern Yugoslav poets. This dark genius, creating his art outside, and often against, the mainstream of Yugoslav poetry between the two wars, had always attracted Popa, even when Nastasijević was almost a forgotten poet. (Popa edited Nastasijević's collected works.) How much direct influence Nastasijević exercised on Popa is indeed difficult to ascertain, because both poets followed the dictates of their own strong personalities; that there has been some influence, however, is beyond doubt. Other poets mentioned as influences on Popa are Léon-Gontran Damas, Francis Ponge, and even Rainer Maria Rilke.

Popa's own influence on Yugoslav poetry is just as difficult to establish. At the beginning of his career, he was shunned by the established poets; poets who followed him do not show clearly what they have learned from him, their reverence for him notwithstanding; his forceful originality and unconventional style are difficult to imitate without the appearance of mere copying. Although he has been emulated and has doubtless influenced his fellow poets, like many great poets, he remained a poetic world unto himself and without legitimate offspring.

OTHER MAJOR WORKS

SHORT FICTION: *Urnebesnik: Zbornik pesničkog humora*, 1960 (selection of Serbian wit and humor); *Od zlata jabuka*, 1966 (*The Golden Apple*, 1980).

BIBLIOGRAPHY

Alexander, Ronelle. *The Structure of Vasko Popa's Poetry*. Columbus, Ohio: Slavica, 1985. A critical analysis of Popa's linguistic technique in selected works. Includes bibliographic references.

Katz, Joy, and Kevin Prufer, eds. *Dark Horses: Poets on Overlooked Poems—An Anthology*. Urbana: University of Illinois Press, 2007. Susan Wheeler provides commentary on Popa's "Blandulla, Tenella, Vagula."

Lekić, Anita. *The Quest for Roots: The Poetry of Vasko Popa*. New York: Peter Lang, 1993. Lekić's study of Popa and his work provides the complex background where Popa's imagination and metaphysics have their beginnings. Includes bibliographical references and index.

Mihailovich, Vasa D. "Vasko Popa: The Poetry of Things in a Void." *Books Abroad* 53 (1969): 24-29. A basic introduction to the themes in Popa's poetry.

Vasa D. Mihailovich